Bone Tumors

Jayasree Kattoor • Sindhu Nair P
Jayasree Geothe

Bone Tumors

Evidence-based Approach in Diagnosis and Management

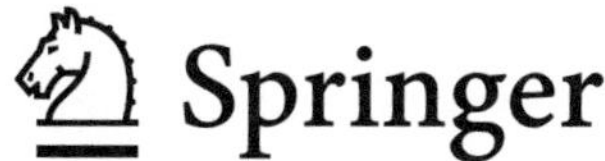

Jayasree Kattoor
Department of Pathology
Regional Cancer Center
Thiruvananthapuram, Kerala, India

Sindhu Nair P
Department of Pathology
Regional Cancer Center
Thiruvananthapuram, Kerala, India

Jayasree Geothe
Department of Pathology
Sree Mookambika Institute of Medical Sciences
Kulasekharam, Tamil Nadu, India

ISBN 978-981-99-4740-9 ISBN 978-981-99-4738-6 (eBook)
https://doi.org/10.1007/978-981-99-4738-6

This Springer imprint is published by the registered company Springer Nature Singapore Pte Ltd.
The registered company address is: 152 Beach Road, #21-01/04 Gateway East, Singapore 189721, Singapore

To
Our teachers
Our patients
Our students
and
Our family

Foreword

I am honoured to write a foreword for this excellent work, "Bone Tumors: Evidence-based Approach in Diagnosis and Management."

I congratulate Dr. Jayasree and co-authors for concisely capturing the essence of bone pathology. They have coherently systematized relevant histopathology details, clinical manifestations and radiological findings, ruling out differentials, breaking down complex topics with utmost efficiency, clarity and excellent illustrations and including immunological profile, molecular studies, therapy and management. Also, there are inclusions of revisions and illuminating case studies.

This publication is unequivocally superior to the other books available in the same subject.

I would definitely recommend this amazing work not just for PG students, but also for practicing pathologists and academicians.

Professor. A.Vijayalakshmi
Former Head of Pathology
Government Medical College
Kottayam, Kerala, India

Preface

Primary bone tumours are uncommon, and this has certainly contributed to the scarcity of data about their relative frequency and to the limited understanding of the risk factors. Overall, bone sarcomas account for 0.2% of all malignancies. The age-specific incidence rates of bone sarcomas show a bimodal distribution, with the first peak occurring in the second decade and a second peak occurring in older individuals. Many bone tumours are seen in children and young adults. A misdiagnosis will end up in losing a limb in these patients. Hence, a proper knowledge of these tumours is essential.

Because of the rarity, students are not exposed enough to bone tumours. Only some specialized centres are doing bone onco-surgery. Apart from this, histology of bone tumours, both benign and malignant and also tumour-like lesions is overlapping. Hence, a thorough knowledge regarding clinical presentation, radiological findings and histopathology of various tumours is essential for proper typing and further management of these tumours. Unlike other tumours, ancillary techniques have a limited role in the diagnosis of bone tumours. There are only few monographs on bone tumour pathology which give a comprehensive picture of the lesions.

Significant progress has been made in diagnosis, particularly in staging and treatment of bone tumours. In most centres, limb-sparing surgery has replaced the more radical ablative surgery, with or without preoperative chemotherapy. Prognostication of these tumours and further management depend on the proper grossing and histopathology of these tumours. Reporting post-chemotherapy tumours requires experience and a good knowledge of histological findings. Newer diagnostic modalities like immunohistochemistry, FISH and other molecular techniques are required in tumours like small round cell tumours, malignant lymphoma and metastatic tumours.

Hence, a monograph on bone tumours was planned. First 17 chapters are written by the main author Dr. Jayasree K, and last 2 chapters are written by Dr. Jayasree Geothe and Dr. Sindhu Nair P, respectively, and edited by Dr. Jayasree K.

This book has 19 chapters, which include the structure of the skeleton and a systematic approach to bone tumours. The chapters are divided according to the cell of origin or the predominant matrix produced, for example, osteoid-producing lesions, chondroid tumours or giant cell-rich tumours. This will give the student an idea to approach such lesions. Each tumour is briefly described by subheadings like clinical features, radiology findings, gross, microscopy, differential diagnosis and molecular findings wherever applicable, treatment and prognosis. Both recent and old references are included, which are grouped under each entity. Many differential diagnoses are given as tables. Radiologic and microscopic images are from our own cases as well as the second opinion cases received over many years.

In short, this book offers a comprehensive update on bone tumours and tumour-like conditions with chapters on synovial and odontogenic tumours as well. The book provides the readers a solid foundation of knowledge about bone tumour recognition and evaluation. It is an ideal resource for practicing pathologists and residents in pathology, radiology, orthopaedics and oncology for updating their knowledge on bone tumours and for quick reference. The book emphasizes the need for a multidisciplinary approach for the diagnosis of bone tumours.

Thiruvananthapuram, Kerala, India Jayasree Kattoor
Thiruvananthapuram, Kerala, India Sindhu Nair P
Kulasekharam, Tamil Nadu, India Jayasree Geothe

Acknowledgements

- First of all, I thank God Almighty who has been with me throughout and helped me sail through successfully.
- I am deeply indebted to my teachers for their blessings and support in completing this book:

Dr. K. Krishnan Unni, world-renowned bone tumour pathology expert (former Professor and Chair, Department of Anatomic Pathology, Mayo Clinic, Rochester, MN, USA), for teaching me all about bone tumours and tumour-like conditions.

Professor Malini Thomas, Former Professor and Head, Department of Pathology, Government Medical College, Kozhikode, and Professor Elizabeth K. Abraham, Former Professor and Head, Department of Pathology, Regional Cancer Centre (RCC), Thiruvananthapuram, for teaching the basics of approach to bone tumours.

Professor M. Krishnan Nair (late), Former Director, Regional Cancer Centre (RCC), Thiruvananthapuram, and Professor N. Sreedevi Amma and Professor B. Chandralekha, Former Heads of the Department of Pathology, RCC, Thiruvananthapuram, for giving me the opportunity to go abroad to learn bone tumour pathology and constantly encouraging me throughout my career.

- My special thanks and respect to Dr. A. Vijayalakshmi, Former Professor and Head of Pathology, Government Medical College, Kottayam, for taking pains to read my book fully, for giving valuable suggestions and also for writing foreword for the book in spite of her busy schedule.
- I am extremely thankful to Dr. Rekha A. Nair, Director, Regional Cancer Centre, Thiruvananthapuram, for her valuable support.
- Orthopaedic oncology diagnosis is a multidisciplinary approach. Without the help of orthopaedic surgeons, medical oncologists and radiologists, it is impossible to give a proper diagnosis. I thank all my clinical and radiology colleagues for their constant support.
- I thank the Scientific Review Board and Human Ethics Committee of the Regional Cancer Centre, Thiruvananthapuram, for giving me the permission to publish the book with the illustrations.
- A big thanks to my patients without whom I would not have learned bone tumours and the constant challenge they gave me every day.

- I am grateful to the orthopaedic surgeons, especially late Dr. (Prof.) Gopalakrishnan of SUT Hospital, Thiruvananthapuram, and Dr. Subin Sugath, Aster Medcity, Kochi, for sending their difficult cases for opinion. I am also grateful to the pathologists and clinicians from different parts of the state who had sent cases for second opinions.
- My co-authors Dr. Jayasree Geothe, Professor, Department of Pathology, Sree Mookambika Medical College, Kulasekharam, Tamil Nadu, and Dr. Sindhu Nair P, Associate Professor of Pathology, RCC, Thiruvananthapuram, for their valuable suggestions, contributions and guidance throughout the preparation of the book.
- I am extremely thankful to Professor Heera, Head of Pathology, Government Dental College, Thiruvananthapuram, for the microphotographs of odontogenic tumours, and Dr. Nanda Kachare; Dr. Sreelatha K.N. of Aster labs, Kochi; Dr. Sanjay Gandhi; Dr. Jayanthi Kamashi; and Dr. Jayasree Geothe for gross and microscopic pictures of their cases.
- Thanks to everyone on my publishing team.
- A special thanks to Dr. C.C. Kartha and Dr. Mira Kartha for their valuable suggestions in publishing the manuscript.
- I want to thank all my friends for their encouragement and motivation given to me to fulfil the idea of writing a book during my hard times.
- I owe the completion of the book to all my colleagues including the supporting staff and students of my department for their constant encouragement and timely help.
- Having an idea and turning it into a book is as hard as it sounds. The experience is both internally challenging and rewarding. I am thankful to my family—my late husband Dr. Ramdas Pisharody for his constant encouragement and support throughout my life and my children and grandchildren for patiently supporting me.

Thiruvananthapuram, Kerala, India Jayasree Kattoor

Contents

Abbreviations

ABC	Aneurysmal bone cyst
ALCL	Anaplastic large cell lymphoma
ASPS	Alveolar soft part sarcoma
Ca	Calcium
CB	Chondroblastoma
CMF	Chondromyxoid fibroma
CS	Chondrosarcoma
CT	Computerized tomography
DD	Differential diagnosis
DDCS	Dedifferentiated chondrosarcoma
ECD	Erdheim-Chester disease
EDTA	Ethylene diamine tetraacetic acid
EH	Epithelioid haemangioma
EHE	Epithelioid haemangioendothelioma
ES	Ewing sarcoma
FD	Fibrous dysplasia
FISH	Fluorescent in situ hybridization
FNAC	Fine needle aspiration cytology
FS	Fibrosarcoma
GCRG	Giant cell reparative granuloma
GCT	Giant cell tumour
HPC	Haemangiopericytoma
HPT	Hyperparathyroidism
IHC	Immunohistochemistry
LCH	Langerhans cell histiocytosis
LDH	Lactate dehydrogenase
ML	Malignant lymphoma
MPNST	Malignant peripheral nerve sheath tumour
MRCN	Malignant round cell neoplasm
MRI	Magnetic resonance imaging
NB	Neuroblastoma
NGS	Next-generation sequencing
NOF	Non-ossifying fibroma
OB	Osteoblastoma
OCM	Osteochondromyxoma
OFD	Osteofibrous dysplasia
OF	Ossifying fibroma

OO	Osteoid osteoma
OS	Osteosarcoma
P	Phosphorus
PET	Positron emission tomography
PO4	Phosphate
RANK	Receptor activator of nuclear factor kappa-B
RANKL	Receptor activator of nuclear factor kappa-B ligand
RT-PCR	Real-time polymerase chain reaction
SBC	Simple bone cyst
SCh	Synovial chondromatosis
SHML	Sinus histiocytosis with massive lymphadenopathy
SS	Synovial sarcoma
UPS	Undifferentiated pleomorphic sarcoma
US	Ultrasound

Human Skeletal System

1

Bones, cartilage, ligaments and tendons constitute the human skeletal system. The soft organs of the body are protected and supported by the rigid framework provided by the body. While standing, the long bones of the lower limbs support the trunk. Bones work together with the muscles in body movement. Bones contain the highest amount of calcium than any other organ. Large amounts of calcium salts are seen in the intracellular matrix, the most important being calcium phosphate. Calcium is released from the bones when blood calcium falls below normal. The excess calcium is stored in the bone matrix when blood calcium levels are more than normal. This mechanism of release and storage of calcium is a continuous process.

The formation of blood cells, namely haematopoiesis, occurs in red marrow. As age advances, the red marrow gets replaced largely by yellow marrow for fat storage. In adults, the red marrow is seen only in the spongy bones of the skull, ribs, sternum, clavicles, vertebrae and pelvis. Red blood cells, white blood cells and blood platelets are produced by the red marrow.

1.1 Bone Development

The osteogenesis and ossification are terms used synonymously. The skeletal formation begins in the form of cartilage and connective tissue membranes by the end of 8 weeks of gestation, and then ossification begins. This is continued throughout adulthood. Bone development also occurs for repair of fractures. The growth and remodelling of bones are by the three cell types, namely osteoblasts, osteocytes and osteoclasts.

Intramembranous and endochondral are the two types of ossification.

1.1.1 Intramembranous Ossification

The replacement of connective tissue membranes with bony tissue is called as intramembranous ossification. Examples of bones formed by this type of ossification are flat bones of the skull.

1.1.2 Endochondral Ossification

In endochondral ossification, the bony tissue replaces hyaline cartilage. Majority of the bones in our body are formed in this manner and are called endochondral bones. Hyaline cartilage is formed initially. The perichondrium that surrounds the hyaline cartilage gets vascularized, and osteoblasts infiltrate and change into a periosteum during the third month of gestation. The osteoblasts form a collar of compact bone around the diaphysis. The osteoblasts get into the disintegrating cartilage in the centre of diaphysis, replacing it with spongy bone. This is known as primary ossification centre. Ossification progresses from this centre towards the ends of the

J. Kattoor et al., *Bone Tumors*, https://doi.org/10.1007/978-981-99-4738-6_1

bones. The osteoclasts break down the newly formed spongy bone, and marrow cavity is formed.

The developing bone increases in length by continuous growth of cartilage in the epiphysis. The formation of secondary ossification centre formation in the epiphyses happens after birth. After the formation of secondary ossification, the hyaline cartilage is totally replaced by bone. The cartilage is retained in two sites—articular surface of bone and an area between epiphysis and diaphysis (epiphyseal growth plate).

1.2 Bone Growth

At the epiphyseal plate, bone continues to grow by division of chondrocytes by mitosis. In the region adjacent to the diaphysis, the cartilage cells age and degenerate. The osteoblasts which produce osteoid migrate into the matrix ossifying it to form bone. These osteoblasts become osteocytes in the new bone formed. The cartilage growth continues throughout childhood and the adolescent years. In the early 20s, the cartilage growth gets arrested. The epiphyseal plate gets completely ossified leaving behind a thin epiphyseal line. Bone growth ceases. After this, the bones cannot grow in length. But they continue to increase in thickness. The bone growth is influenced by growth hormone from the anterior pituitary and sex hormones from the ovaries and testes.

1.3 Classification of Bones

The four main types of bones are long, short, flat and irregular.

1.3.1 Long Bones

The long bones have a shaft and two ends. They are hard and strong. Examples are femur, tibia and humerus.

1.3.2 Short Bones

Short bones are cubical in shape. They contain spongy bone covered with a thin compact bone. The bones of the hands and feet are short bones.

1.3.3 Flat Bones

Flat bones are thin, flat and curved. Examples are bones of the cranium.

1.3.4 Irregular Bones

Irregular bones are those which are not included in any of the above three categories classified. They include the vertebrae and some of the bones in the skull, which have surface markings like holes, depression lines or projections that make a specific bone unique.

1.4 Divisions of the Skeleton

The adult human skeleton usually consists of 206 bones. The bones can be divided into two types called axial skeleton and appendicular skeleton. Axial skeleton consists of skull bones, vertebral column, ribs and sternum, whereas the appendicular skeleton consists of limb bones and its girdles (shoulder and pelvic girdles). The bones of the adult human skeleton are listed below (Table 1.1).

1.5 Joints

Joints are the areas where two or more bones meet. The three types of joints are fibrous, cartilaginous and synovial. Joints consist of cartilage, synovial membrane, ligaments, tendons, bursa and meniscus. Cartilage reduces friction, synovial membrane secretes synovial fluid which lubricates the joint and ligaments and tendons control the movements of joint. Bursas are fluid-

Table 1.1 The bones of adult human skeleton

Axial skeleton	Appendicular skeleton
Axial skeleton (80 bones) **Skull (28)** **Cranial bones (8)** • Parietal (2) • Temporal (2) • Frontal (1) • Occipital (1) • Ethmoid (1) • Sphenoid (1) **Facial bones (14)** • Maxilla (2) • Zygomatic (2) • Mandible (1) • Nasal (2) • Palatine (2) • Inferior nasal concha (2) • Lacrimal (2) • Vomer (1) **Auditory ossicles (6)** • Malleus (2) • Incus (2) • Stapes (2) **Hyoid (1)** **Vertebral column (26)** • Cervical vertebrae (7) • Thoracic vertebrae (12) • Lumbar vertebrae (5) • Sacrum (1) • Coccyx (1) **Thoracic cage (25)** • Sternum (1) • Ribs (24)	**Pectoral girdle** • Clavicle (2) • Scapula (2) • Upper extremity **(60)** – Humerus (2) – Radius (2) – Ulna (2) – Carpals (16) – Metacarpals (10) – Phalanges (28) Pelvic girdle • Coxal, innominate or hip bones (2) • Lower extremity (60) – Femur (2) – Tibia (2) – Fibula (2) – Patella (2) – Tarsals (14) – Metatarsals (10) – Phalanges (28)

filled sacs, which give a cushion effect for the joint.

Other classifications of joints or articulations are immovable (synarthroses), slightly movable (amphiarthroses) and freely movable (diarthroses) joints. The sutures in the skull are examples of immovable joints. The ribs connected to the sternum by costal cartilages, the symphysis pubis and the joints between the vertebrae and the intervertebral discs are slightly movable joints. Most of the joints in the body are freely movable joints.

Different types of movable joints are given in Table 1.2.

Table 1.2 Different types of movable joints

- **Ball-and-socket joints**: These, such as the shoulder and hip joints, allow backward, forward, sideway and rotating movements
- **Hinge joints**: Hinge joints, such as in the fingers, knees, elbows and toes, allow only bending and straightening movements
- **Pivot joints**: Pivot joints, such as the neck joints, allow limited rotating movements
- **Gliding or ellipsoidal joints**: Ellipsoidal joints, such as the wrist joint, allow all types of movement except pivotal movements
- **Saddle joint**: This permits movement back and forth and from side to side, but does not allow rotation, such as the joint at the base of the thumb
- **Condyloid joint**: This permits movement without rotation, such as in the jaw or finger joints

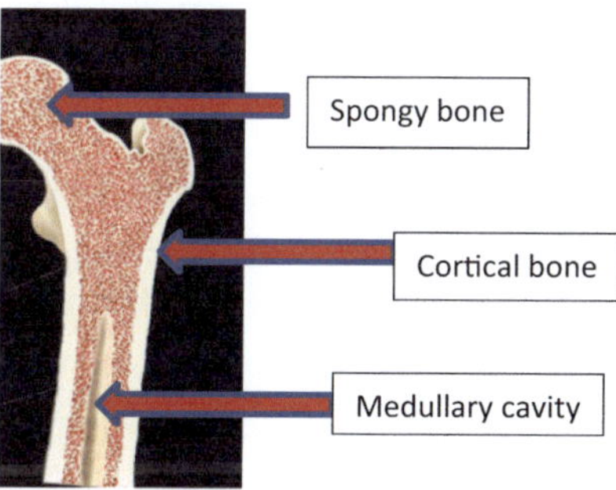

Fig. 1.1 Cortical and cancellous bone and medullary cavity

1.6 Anatomy of Bones

1.6.1 Types of Bones

Bones are of two types [1] (Fig. 1.1):

1. **Cortical bone**: It comprises 80% of the skeleton and is dense or compact. The shape of bone is determined by its outer shell.
2. **Cancellous bone** (spongy, trabecular or marrow bone): This is found within the medullary canal at the ends of long bones.

All bones contain both cortical and cancellous bone [1], but in different proportions. For example, femur is a long tubular bone with shaft (body) composed of cortical bone with marrow mainly containing fat. The cortex becomes thin towards the ends of the femur, and the coarse cancellous bone is the predominant structure here. In the skull, it is mainly cortical bone with inner and outer tables. Within the marrow space called the diploe, only a small amount of cancellous bone is seen.

In the growing child, there is a transverse cartilage plate termed growth plate seen in between epiphysis and metaphysis. We name the parts of bone as epiphysis, metaphysis and diaphysis in relation to the growth plate or the physis.

Epiphysis: The area of the bone that extends from the subarticular bone plate to the base of the growth plate is called epiphysis.

Metaphysis: It is the region from the growth plate facing away from the joint to the area where bone becomes tubular in shape, and it contains cancellous bone.

Diaphysis: The portion of body or shaft of the bone between two metaphyses in a long bone is called diaphysis. It is the area which is important in infections, haematopoietic tumours and malformations of the skeleton.

1.6.2 Bone Marrow

The bone marrow fills the space enclosed by cortical bone called marrow space, and it is supported by a delicate connective tissue framework. There are three types of marrow:

1. **Red marrow**: It is the haematopoietic tissue and is seen in all bones at the time of birth. At the growing age (time of adolescence), the red marrow is mainly seen in axial skeleton like skull, ribs, vertebrae, sternum, scapulae, clavicles, pelvis, proximal humerus and femur. If red marrow is seen in the femoral diaphysis of a man aged 55 years, it is considered pathological and an underlying disease such as leukaemia has to be ruled out.
2. **Yellow marrow**: Microscopically, it is fat tissue and found in the bones of the limbs. Its presence in a normally haematopoietic area like vertebra is abnormal.
3. **Gray or white marrow**: It is fibrous and lacks haematopoietic elements. It is always pathological in areas distant from growth plate in a child and in a non-growing adult bone.

1.6.3 Periosteum

The periosteum is a specialized connective tissue that covers all bones. It can form bone also. It has inner cambium layer and outer fibrous layer. Inner layer is on the surface of bone. Inner layer consists of collagen, fibroblasts and a network of elastic fibres. The outer layer is continuous with soft tissue planes and fascia.

1.6.4 Bone Matrix

Bone tissue is composed of organic matrix (30%) and inorganic matrix consisting of mineralized hydroxyl apatite crystals (60%). 10% of the bones are composed of cells. The organic matrix is constituted mainly by type I collagen. Other constituents are proteins like osteocalcin and osteopontin and 2% lipids and glycosaminoglycans.

1.6.5 Cells of Bone

There are four types of cells (Fig. 1.2):

1. **Osteoprogenitor cell**: This ultimately differentiates into osteoblasts, osteocytes, chondrocytes, adipocytes, myoblasts and fibroblasts. It is a small stellate or spindle-shaped cell, which is not recognized by light microscopy.
2. **Osteoblast:** Osteoblasts are the protein-synthesizing cells that produce osteoid, which gets mineralized to form bone tissue. These

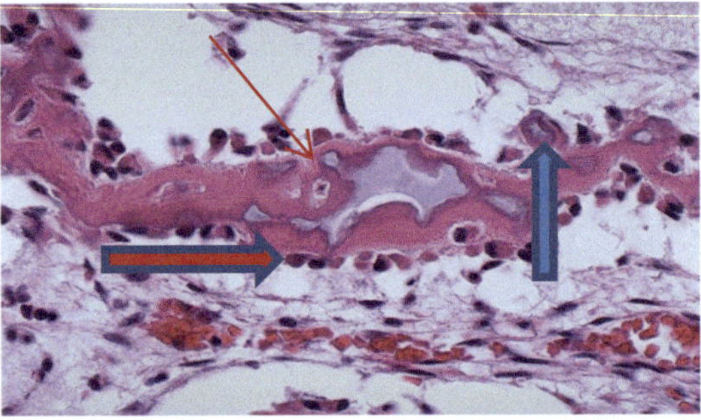

Fig. 1.2 Normal cells, H&E ×250. Broad red arrow—osteoblasts, thin red arrow—osteocytes in lacunae, blue arrow—osteoclast

large mononuclear cells line along the bone surface. Osteoblasts are seen as flattened cells on the surface of bone tissue when they are inactive. The osteoblast produces osteocalcin, contains alkaline phosphatase and has parathyroid receptors. The osteoclastic activity is facilitated by collagenase produced by the osteoblasts. Growth factors produced by osteoblasts like transforming growth factor (TGF), insulin-like growth factor (IGF-1 and IGF-2), platelet-derived growth factor (PDGF), IL-1, and TNF are responsible for the regulation of growth and differentiation of bone.

3. **Osteocyte:** An osteoblast completely embedded in bone matrix is called an osteocyte. They lie in lacunae. The recognition and response to mechanical forces are done by bone cells.
4. **Osteoclast**: The bone resorption is exclusively done by osteoclast. It is a member of the monocyte/macrophage family. Three factors are required for bone resorption—the TNF-related cytokine RANK-ligand (RANKL), the growth factor CSF-1 and the activation of RANK haematopoietic precursor cells. Osteoclasts are multinucleated cells, which are found in Howship lacunae. These lacunae are small depressions found on the surface of bones. The bone resorption by osteoclasts involves integrins which attach the cell to bone.
5. **Bone remodelling unit**: The resorptive action of osteoclasts initiates constant remodelling of bone. Bone remodelling is under the influence of parathormone (PTH) and is initiated by the activation of RANK by its ligand, which results in the cellular changes necessary for bone to be resorbed by the osteoclast [2]. During resorption, certain factors are released, and these in turn recruit osteoblasts to the site and new bone is produced. Thus, the bone remodelling involves replacement of old bone by new bone through the coupling of osteoclasts and osteoblasts [3–5]. This coupling is known as the bone remodelling unit (Fig. 1.3).

1.6.6 Microscopy of Bone

There are two types of bone—lamellar (mature) bone and woven (immature) bone. Both these types can be mineralized or non-mineralized. The non-mineralized bone is termed osteoid [6].

1.6.6.1 Lamellar Bone

This is the mature bone, and it forms the adult skeleton. Lamellar bone (Fig. 1.4) has parallel arrangement of type I collagen fibres (Fig. 1.5) and less number of osteocytes in the matrix. The osteocytes are uniform and lie in lacunae.

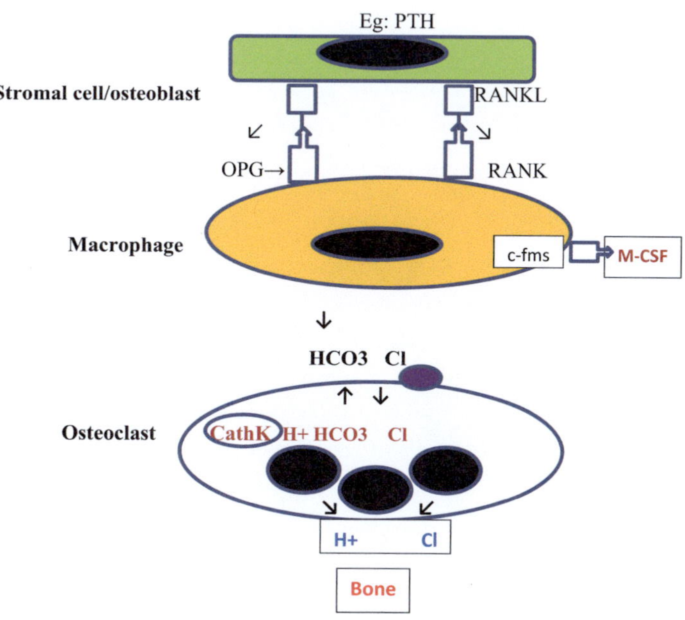

Fig. 1.3 Bone remodelling unit

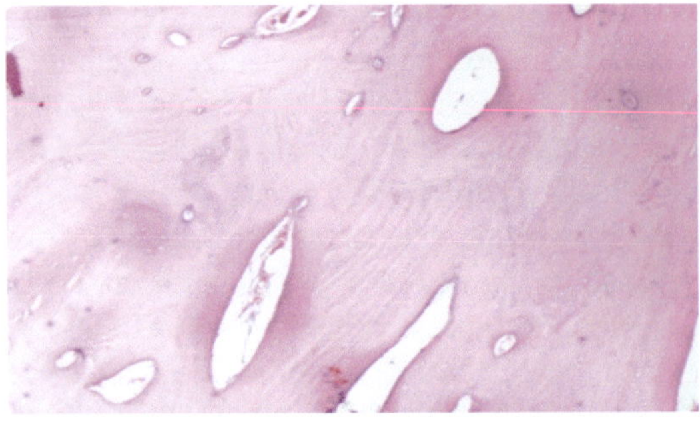

Fig. 1.4 Normal cortical bone, H&E ×400

Lamellar bone is of four types. They are circumferential, concentric (around Haversian canals), interstitial and trabecular (bone seen in the medullary cavity) types.

1.6.6.2 Woven Bone

The three main characteristics of woven bone are irregular arrangement of type I collagen fibres ("woven"), numerous osteocytes and variation in the size and shape of the osteocytes (Fig. 1.6). Woven bone is seen in the foetus. It is also seen

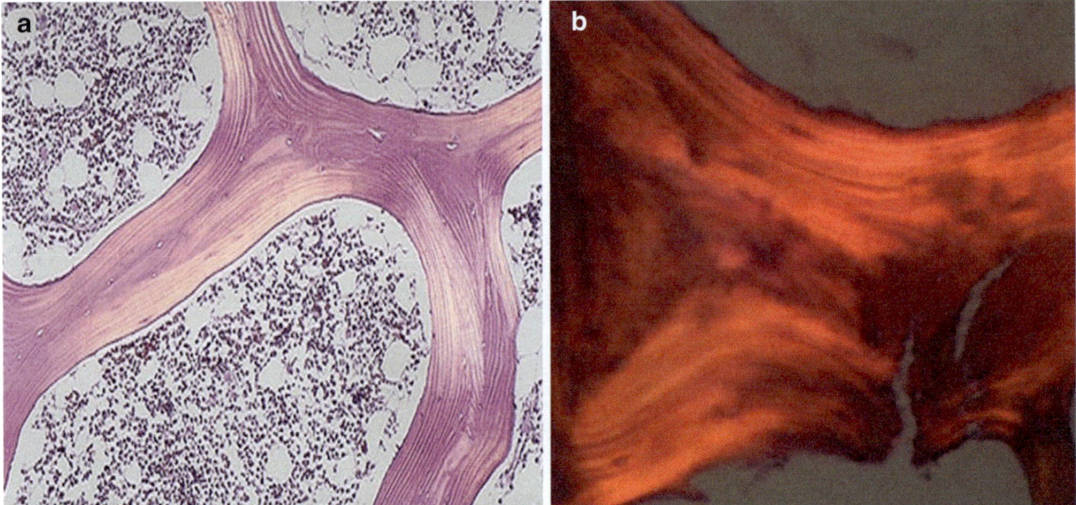

Fig. 1.5 (**a**) Lamellar bone (trabecular bone) with marrow, H&E ×100. (**b**) Normal bone under polarizer-parallel arrangement of collagen, ×400

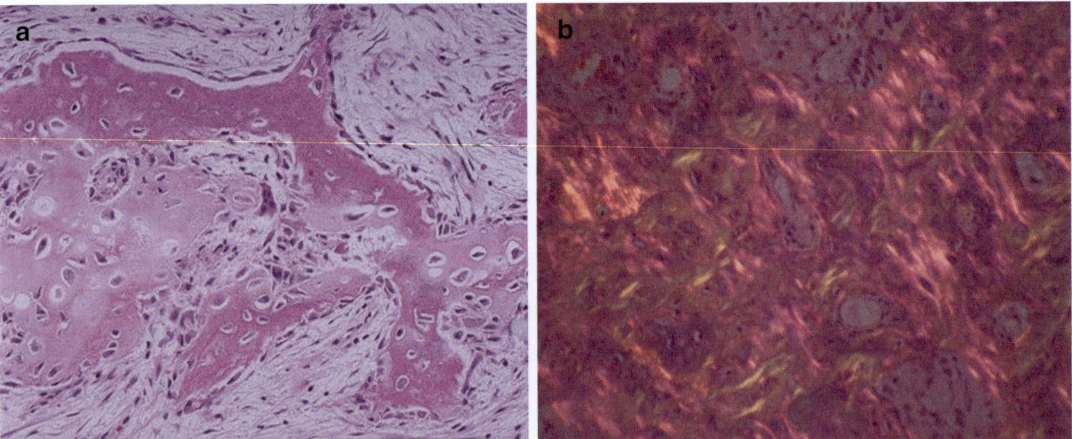

Fig. 1.6 Woven bone: (**a**) immature bone with increased number of osteocytes of varying size, H&E ×250. (**b**) Woven bone under polarizer with irregular arrangement of collagen, ×250

around areas of infections, in tumours and as part of fracture callus. The presence of woven bone in an adult is always pathological.

1.7 Cartilage

Cartilage does not contain blood vessels, nerves or lymphatics. It is a flexible connective tissue. Since it has no nerve supply, it has to depend on diffusion to get nutrients. Hence, healing of damaged cartilage is slow. In some areas in order to give internal strength, cartilage gets calcified. Cartilage also contains organic and inorganic matrix. The organic matrix present in cartilage is different from bone. It contains mainly water (80%). Type II collagen and proteoglycans form rest of the cartilage organic matrix. Water enhances the resilience and lubrication of joints. Proteoglycans contain proteins with polysaccharides, which are called as glycosaminoglycans. The main glycosaminoglycans are chondroitin 4 and chondroitin 6 sulphates and keratin sulphate. 50–90% of the cartilage matrix is chondroitin sulphates. It varies according to the age of the tissue.

1.7.1 Types of Cartilage

There are three types of cartilage (Fig. 1.7):

- **Hyaline cartilage**: This is the most common type of cartilage seen. Freshly, it looks like a glass and hence its name (derived from Greek word hyalos, which means glassy). In H&E sections, it is basophilic. It has fine collagen type II fibres, e.g., articular cartilage, growth plates, costochondral junction, cartilage of trachea and bronchi and nasal cartilage. The cartilage seen in fracture healing and cartilage seen in most of the tumours also belong to this type.
- **Fibrocartilage**: This is hyaline cartilage mixed with a lot of type I and type II collagen fibres. It is flexible and tough due to fibrous tissue and elastic due to cartilaginous tissue. They are seen in intervertebral disc (Fig. 1.8), tendinous and ligamentous insertions, symphysis pubis and temporomandibular joint.
- **Elastic cartilage**: This type of cartilage has a lot of elastic fibres. In H&E sections, it looks like hyaline cartilage. The chondrocytes lie in a thread-like network of elastic fibres. In Verhoeff-Van Gieson stain, elastic fibres stain black. It provides strength and elasticity and maintains shape of the structures. Cartilage found in epiglottis, arytenoid cartilages of larynx and external ear belongs to this group.

1.7.2 Cartilage Cells

- **Chondrocytes**: Chondrocytes are derived from primitive mesenchymal cells. Chondrocytes are formed from the chondroblast with the help of the transcription factor

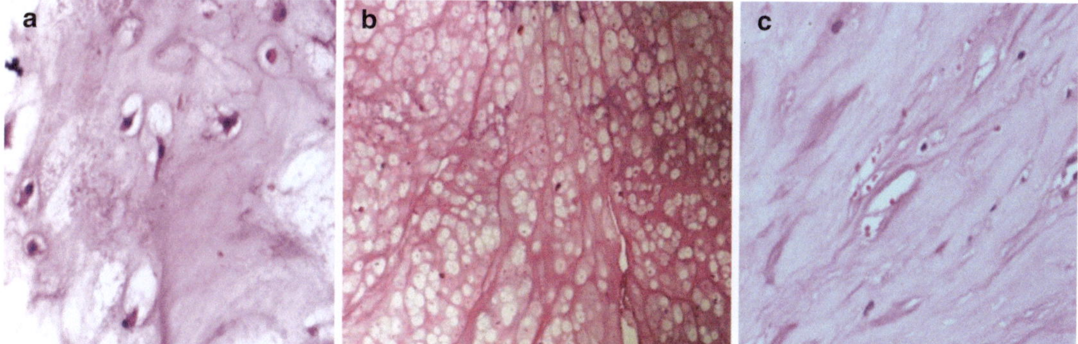

Fig. 1.7 Different types of cartilage: (**a**) hyaline cartilage, H&E ×400. (**b**) Elastic cartilage, H&E ×100. (**c**) Fibrocartilage, H&E ×100

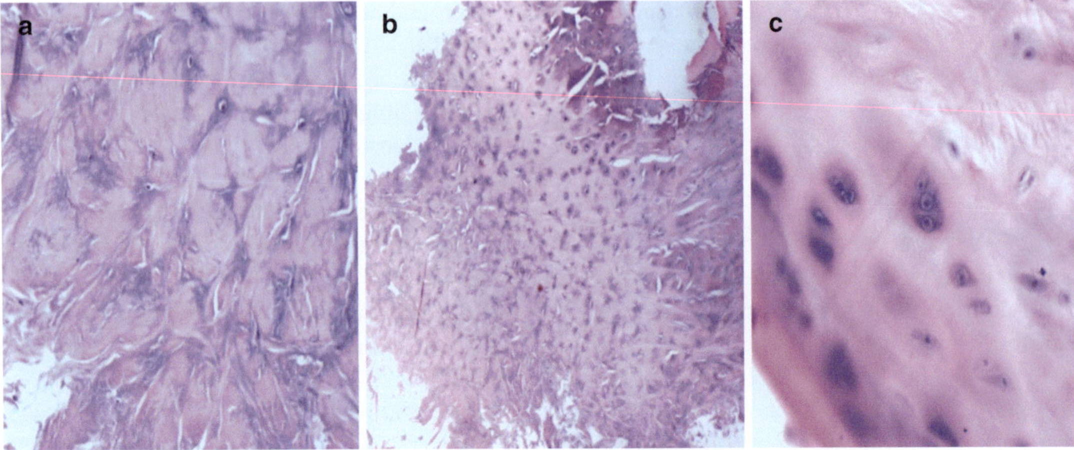

Fig. 1.8 Normal intervertebral disc: (**a**–**c**) fibrocartilage showing a mixture of fibrous and cartilaginous tissue, H&E ×100

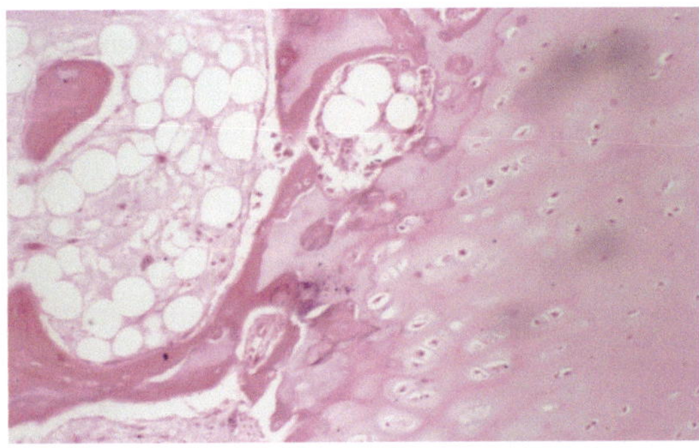

Fig. 1.9 Articular cartilage: normal hyaline cartilage with chondrocytes in columns and underlying trabecular bone and fatty marrow, H&E ×250

SOX9, which is expressed in cartilage neoplasms. Chondroid is tissue resembling cartilage and occurring in adults (pseudocartilage). It is an early form of cartilage occurring in an embryo. Chondroid is pink in colour as osteoid, but it contains chondrocytes in lacunae. If chondrocytes are not prominent, it is difficult to differentiate from osteoid.

- **Chondroblasts**, or perichondrial cells, are mesenchymal progenitor cells, which will form chondrocytes in the growing cartilage matrix. Chondroblasts stain by basic dyes and have euchromatic nuclei. These cells play an important role in the formation of growth plate. The chondrocytes are arranged in vertical rows in a growth plate (Fig. 1.9).
- **The growth plate** is divided into different zones. Sex hormones induce the closure of growth plate. It is early in girls than boys. Due to cessation of formation of new chondrocytes, the entire growth plate gets replaced by bone.

Points to Remember

- 206 named bones
- Appendicular skeleton: pectoral and pelvic girdle
- Axial skeleton: skull and facial bones, flat bones, vertebra
- Bone histology: lamellar (mature) and woven (immature) bone
- Cells of bone: osteoprogenitor, osteoblast, osteocyte, osteoclast
- Cartilage: three types—hyaline, fibro and elastic cartilage
- Cells of cartilage: chondroblast and chondrocyte
- Growth plate: resting zone, proliferative zone, hypertrophic zone and zone of calcification
- Bone marrow: red, yellow and white marrow

References

1. Clarke B. Normal bone anatomy and physiology. Clin J Am Soc Nephrol. 2008;3(Suppl 3):S131–9.
2. Hu H, Hilton MJ, Tu X, Yu K, Ornitz DM, Long F. Sequential roles of hedgehog and Wnt signal-

ing in osteoblast development. Development. 2005;132(1):49–60.
3. Phan A, Xu J, Zheng MH. Interaction between osteoblast and osteoclast: impact in bone disease. Histol Histopathol. 2004;19(4):1325–44.
4. Robling G, Castillo AB, Turner CH. Biomechanical and molecular regulation of bone remodeling. Annu Rev Biomed Eng. 2006;8:455–98.
5. Sims NA, Gooi JH. Bone remodeling: multiple cellular interactions required for coupling of bone formation and resorption. Semin Cell Dev Biol. 2008;19(5):444–51.
6. Florencio-Silva R, da Silva Sasso GR, Sasso-Cerri E, Simões MJ, Cerri PS. Biology of bone tissue: structure, function, and factors that influence bone cells. Biomed Res Int. 2015;2015:421746.

2 Approach to Bone Tumours and Tumour-Like Lesions

2.1 Introduction

Bone lesions and tumours are rare. Hence, they are thought to be one of the difficult lesions/tumours that pathologists encounter. This is due to lack of experience, lack of adequate clinical and radiological data and similarity in the histology of tumours. The pathologist should have basic understanding of radiology images, especially the plain radiograph which is "the gross specimen" for bone tumours.

The morphological findings of certain benign and malignant tumours are overlapping. A team approach is very essential in the diagnosis of bone lesions. A multidisciplinary group consisting of orthopaedic surgeon, radiologist, oncologist and pathologist should work together to diagnose the lesion and decide on proper management.

Systematic approaches to bone tumours include clinical history, physical findings, lab investigations, radiological findings and pathology. A careful evaluation of all these is required for a correct diagnosis [1–4].

2.2 Evaluation of the Patient (Table 2.1)

1. History
2. Physical examination
3. Investigations; laboratory, imaging
4. Biopsy

2.2.1 History

- Age (Tables 2.2 and 2.3)
- Sex (Tables 2.4 and 2.5)
- Location of tumour (Table 2.4)
- Family history
- History of fracture
- History of exposure to chemicals, radiation, chemotherapy, etc.
- Symptoms
  - Pain
  - Swelling
  - History of trauma
  - Neurological symptoms

2.2.2 Physical Examination

- Lump/swelling
- Tenderness
- Effusion of joints
- Deformities
- Regional nodes

2.2.3 Imaging Modalities

- Plain radiograph
- CT scan
- MRI
- Radionuclide scanning
- PET scan

J. Kattoor et al., *Bone Tumors*, https://doi.org/10.1007/978-981-99-4738-6_2

Table 2.1 Approach to evaluation of the bone neoplasm

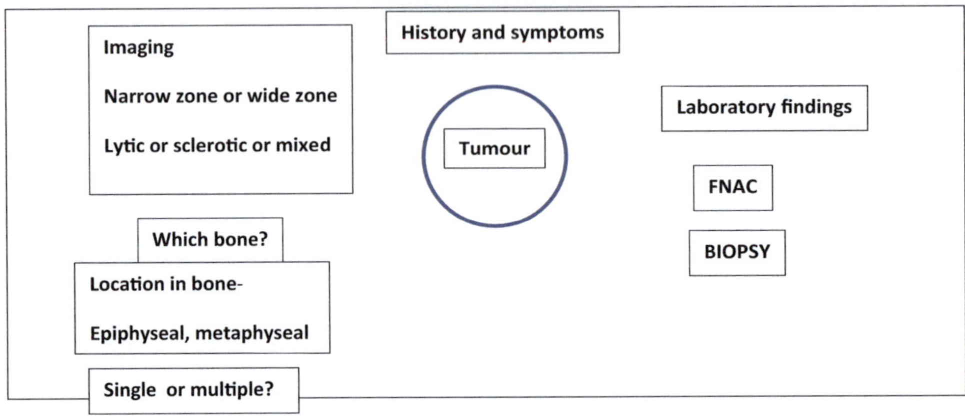

Table 2.2 Age and radiology

Age	Well-defined lytic	Ill-defined lytic	Sclerotic
0–10	LCH, SBC	LCH, ES, OS, Lymphoma/Leukaemia	OS
10–20	NOF, FD, LCH, SBC, ABC, CB, CMF, OB, OO	ES, LCH, OS	OS, OO, OB
20–40	GCT, enchondroma, CS, HPT, OB	GCT	Enchondroma, Osteoma, Bone island, Parosteal OS, Healed lesions
40+	Metastasis, myeloma, geodes	Metastasis, Myeloma, CS	Metastasis, Bone island
All ages	Infection	Infection	Infection

LCH Langerhans cell histiocytosis, *SBC* simple bone cyst, *ES* Ewing's sarcoma, *OS* osteosarcoma, *NOF* non-ossifying fibroma, *FD* fibrous dysplasia, *ABC* aneurysmal bone cyst, *CB* chondroblastoma, *CMF* chondromyxoid fibroma, *OB* osteoblastoma, *OO* osteoid osteoma, *GCT* giant cell tumour, *CS* chondrosarcoma, *HPT* hyperparathyroidism

Table 2.3 Age and histology

Age	Histology
<5	Met NB, LCH, Hamartoma
5–20	NOF, OC, ABC, CB, ES, OS
20–40	GCT, Enchondroma, CS, MFH
>40	CS, Mets, Myeloma, Lymphoma, Secondary OS, Dedifferentiated CS

Table 2.4 Age and location in bone

	<30 years	>30 years
Epiphysis	CB, Infection	Clear Cell CS, GCT, Geode, Infection
Metaphysis	ABC, OS, CMF, NOF, SBC, OC, Enchondroma	Mets, Myeloma, HTP, Enchondroma, CS
Diaphysis	FD, LCH, ES	Mets, Myeloma, Lymphoma

Table 2.5 Sex and bone tumours

Sex	Histology
Male	NOF, OS
Female	GCT, Adamantinoma

A systematic radiologic evaluation is necessary. A plain X-ray should be evaluated first (Figs. 2.1 and 2.2a). CT scan and MRI are useful modalities to determine the extent of lesion, cortical break, soft tissue extension, etc. (Fig. 2.2b). In case of lymphoma, plain X-ray can be apparently normal looking (Fig. 2.2a), but MRI shows abnormal signals (Fig. 2.2b). Sometimes, a nidus of osteoid osteoma is better appreciated on CT scan. Cystic and necrotic components, vascularity and fluid–fluid levels can be determined on MRI with contrast enhancement (Fig. 2.3a, b). Bone scan and PET scan help to determine the multiple bone involvement (Fig. 2.4).

2.2.4 Plain Radiograph

This provides the most useful information about the type of lesion [5–7].

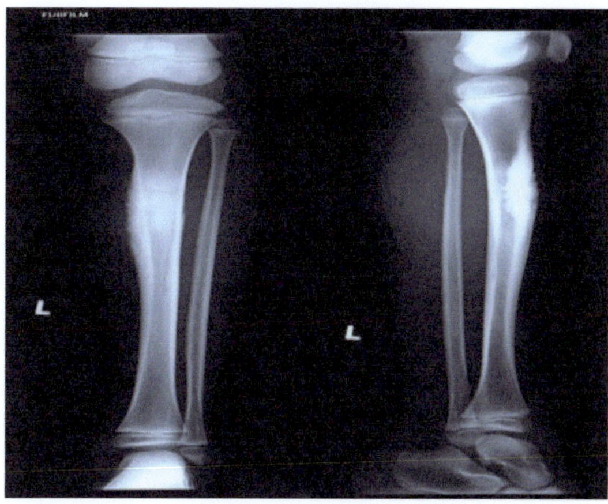

Fig. 2.1 Plain X-ray of osteosarcoma tibia

Information yielded by radiography includes:

(a) Location in the bone
(b) Pattern of bone destruction
(c) Borders and extent of the lesion—zone of transition (ZOT)
(d) Periosteal reaction
(e) Type of matrix
(f) Mono-ostotic or polyostotic

2.2.4.1 Location of Tumour/Lesion in the Bone

The location of tumour, whether it is in the epiphysis, metaphysis or diaphysis, central or cortical, eccentric within the bone or fusiform, on the surface or purely in medullary cavity, etc. can be

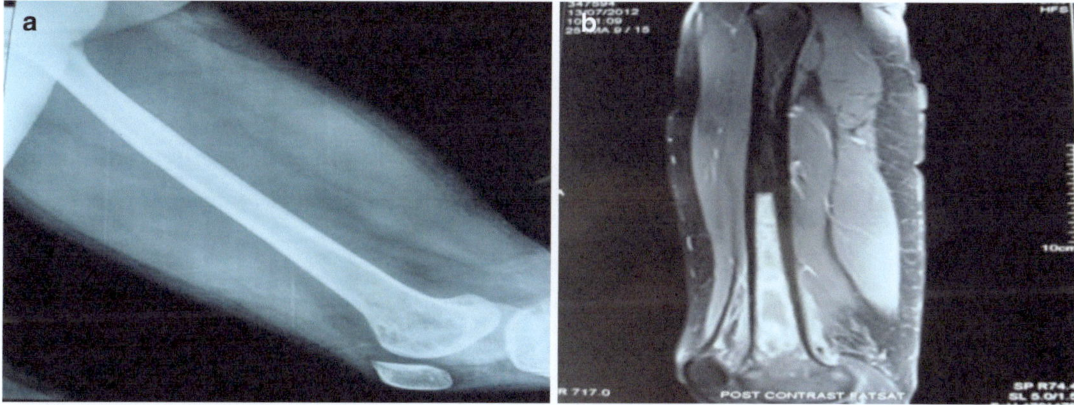

Fig. 2.2 A case of lymphoma bone. (**a**) Plain X-ray apparently normal. (**b**) MRI showing abnormal signals and extent of disease

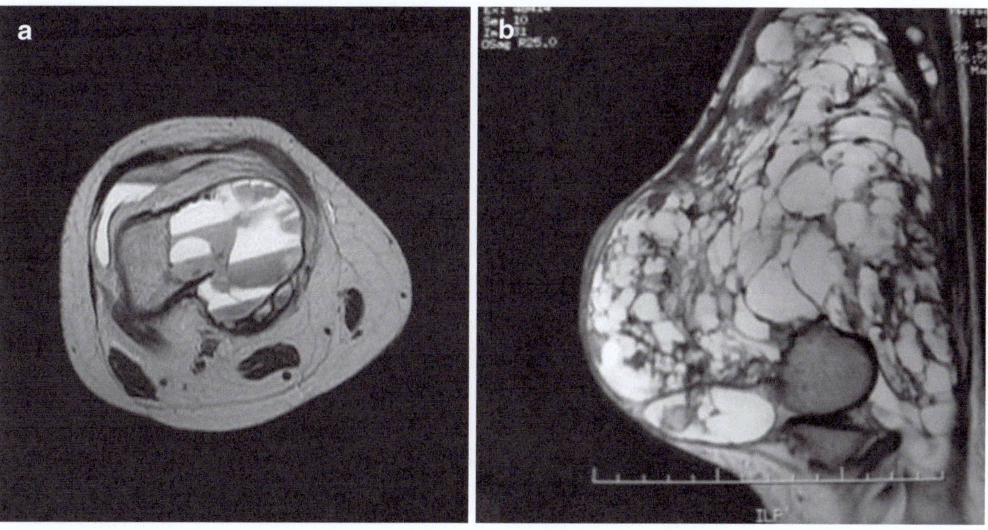

Fig. 2.3 Fluid–fluid level in MRI. (**a**) Fluid level in ABC. (**b**) Fluid level in telangiectatic osteosarcoma

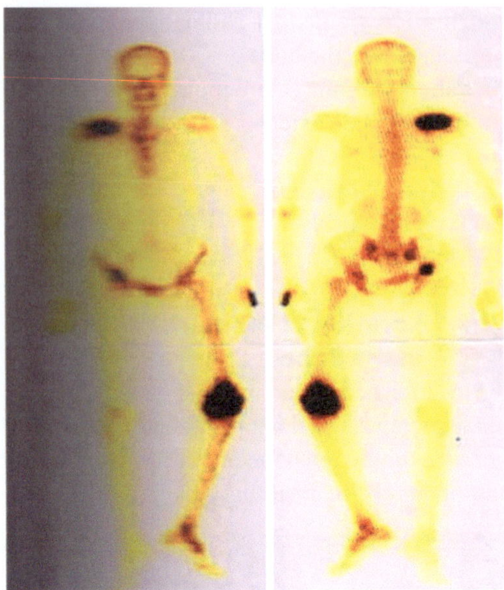

Fig. 2.4 Bone scan showing abnormal localization at the lower end of left femur, right ischium and right scapula in a case of osteosarcoma of femur metastatic to ischium and scapula

determined by plain X-ray. The location of the lesion in the bone—whether it is in the cortex (osteoid osteoma, parosteal osteosarcoma, and adamantinoma) or in the epiphysis (giant cell tumour or chondroblastoma) or is centrally located (simple bone cysts, enchondromas, LCH and Ewing's sarcoma)—can be determined.

Certain tumours have specific site of predilection (Table 2.6). Some other tumours are common in specific locations (Table 2.7).

Epiphyseal tumours: Chondroblastoma, giant cell tumour and clear cell chondrosarcomas are the three common tumours involving epiphysis (Fig. 2.5).

Metaphyseal tumours: There are many tumours, both benign and malignant, which involve the metaphysis. This is especially true in adolescents and young adults because the metaphysis near the growth plate being the growing end in child, tumours are common in this area. Most common benign tumour is non-ossifying fibroma, and most common malignant tumour is osteosarcoma.

Diaphyseal tumours: One of the common tumours in this area are adamantinoma, MFH, Ewing sarcoma, etc. Adamantinoma is cortical in location.

Table 2.6 Predilection of tumours for specific sites in the skeleton

Site	Benign tumours	Malignant tumours
Skull and facial bones	Osteoma, OB, Haemangioma	CS of nasal bone, Mesenchymal CS, Chordoma, Myeloma, Mets, LCH and met NB in children
Jaw bones	FD, GCRG, Myxoma, Ossifying fibroma, Desmoplastic fibroma	OS, Myeloma
Spine	ABC, OB, Haemangioma	Mets, Myeloma, Chordoma
Hands and feet	GCRG, Enchondroma, GCT of tendon sheath, Glomus tumour, Florid reactive periostitis, BPOP, Subungual exostosis, Epidermal cyst	Rare
Long bones	Most of benign tumours	OS, ES, CS, FS, UPS, Angiosarcoma and Adamantinoma
Ribs	FD	CS
Sacrum	GCT	CS, Chordoma
Patella	CB	**Rare**

Table 2.7 Common sites of different tumours

Common site of different lesions
• Parosteal osteosarcoma: posterior aspect of the distal femur • Chondroblastoma: epiphysis of long bones before skeletal maturity • Adamantinoma and osteofibrous dysplasia have a specific predilection for the tibia • Giant cell tumour: extends to articular end of bone • SBC, enchondroma or fibrous dysplasia: always centrally located • Eccentric location is characteristically observed in ABC, CMF, NOF

2.2.4.2 Pattern of Bone Destruction

Bone destruction can be described as geographic, moth-eaten and permeative patterns.

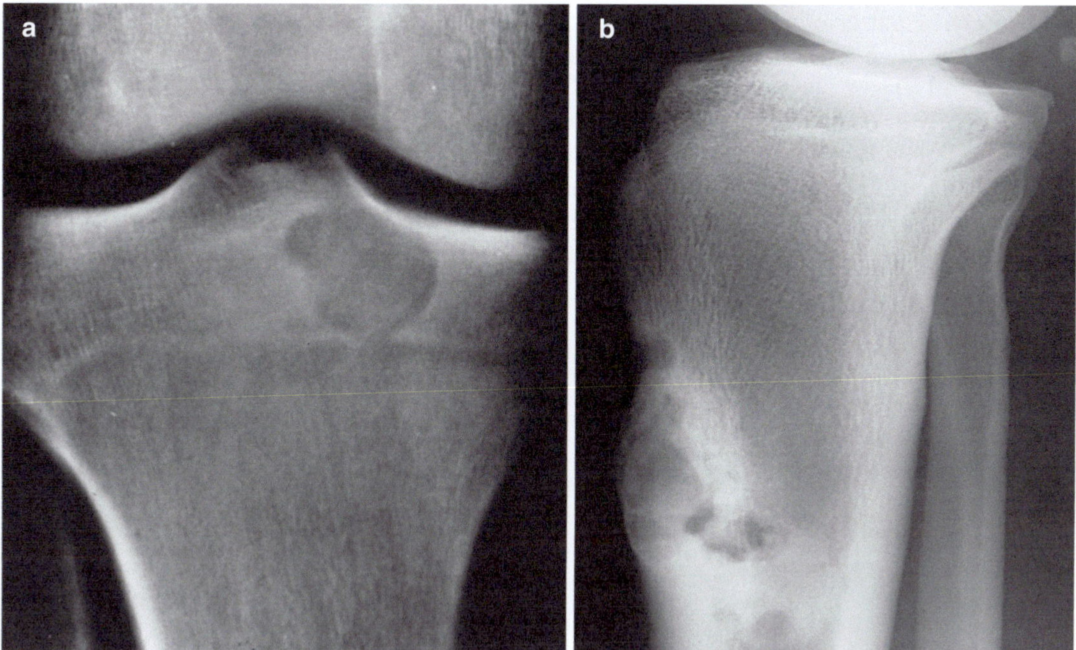

Fig. 2.5 Location of epicentre of lesion usually determines the site of its origin: (**a**) Epiphyseal in chondroblastoma. (**b**) Cortical in non-ossifying fibroma

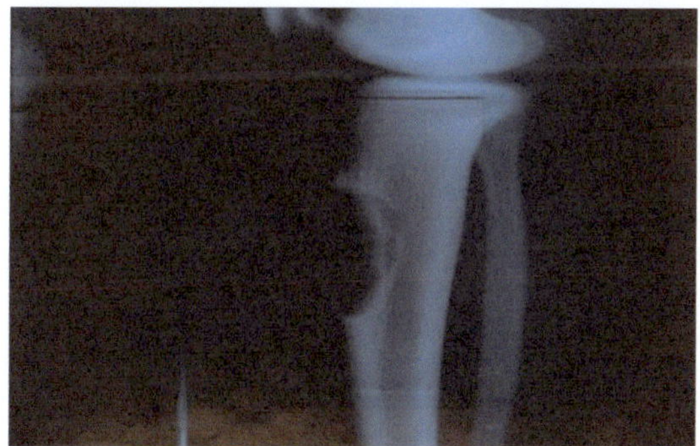

Fig. 2.6 Geographic pattern in non-ossifying fibroma (NOF)

Geographic pattern: In this type, the bone destruction is well-defined lytic with a well-defined margin (Fig. 2.6). Usually, benign tumours with slow growth will have this pattern (e.g. non-ossifying fibroma). A rim of sclerosis may or may not be present.

Moth-eaten pattern: When the bone destruction is multiple with small lytic areas (2–5 mm) separated by normal bone, it is called moth-eaten pattern of bone destruction. It is seen in aggressive tumours, especially malignant tumours. Osteomyelitis and eosinophilic granuloma are other conditions showing this pattern (Fig. 2.7).

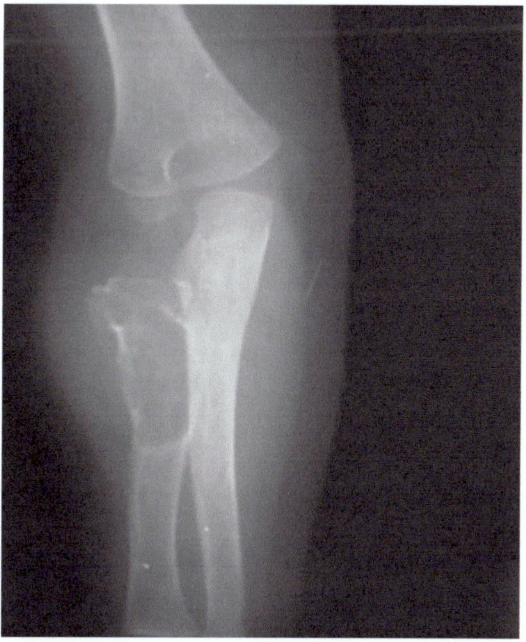

Fig. 2.7 Moth-eaten pattern in LCH

Permeative pattern: A permeative pattern of bone destruction is characterized by diffuse marrow involvement. This pattern is usually seen in rapidly growing tumours. A permeative pattern occurs in malignant tumours such as Ewing sarcoma, malignant lymphoma and osteosarcoma. It can also be seen in some benign conditions like osteomyelitis and LCH (Fig. 2.8).

2.2.4.3 Borders and Extent of the Lesion: Zone of Transition (ZOT)

The type of destruction in the bone provides diagnostic clues. The zone of transition is the margin between abnormal and normal bone margin. A wide ZOT is seen in aggressive lesions like malignant tumours. The lesion is ill circumscribed (Figs. 2.9 and 2.10). Rarely, infection and

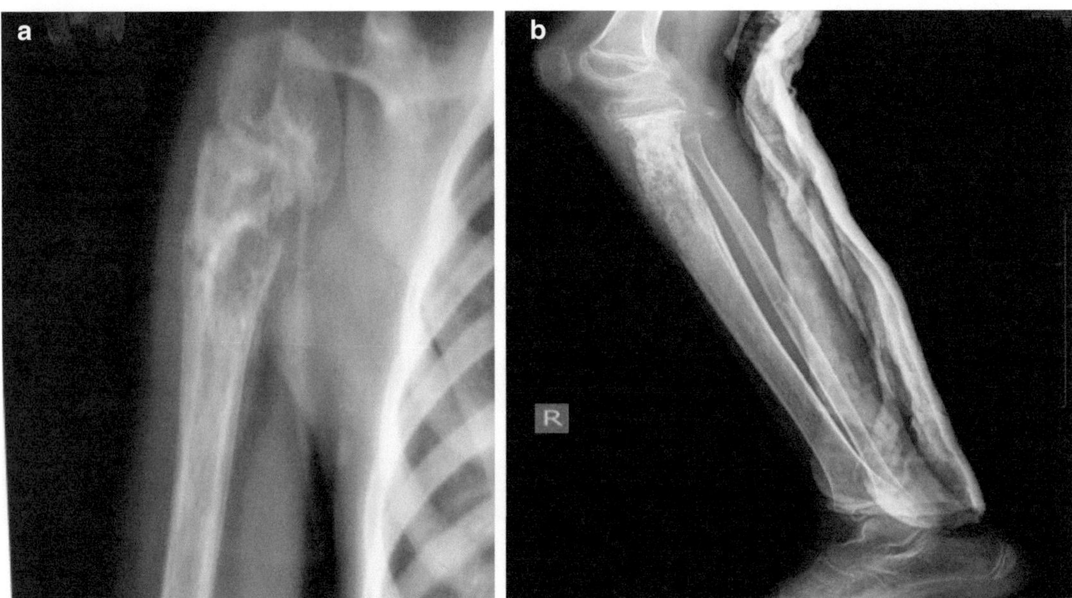

Fig. 2.8 Permeative pattern in (**a**) Ewing sarcoma humerus and (**b**) Malignant lymphoma tibia

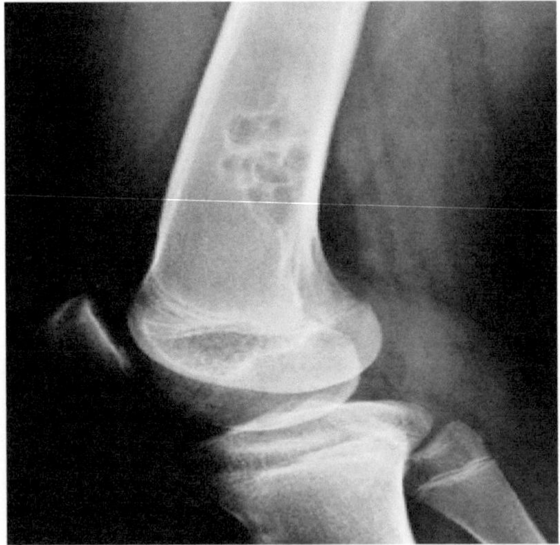

Fig. 2.9 Non-ossifying fibroma with narrow zone of transition

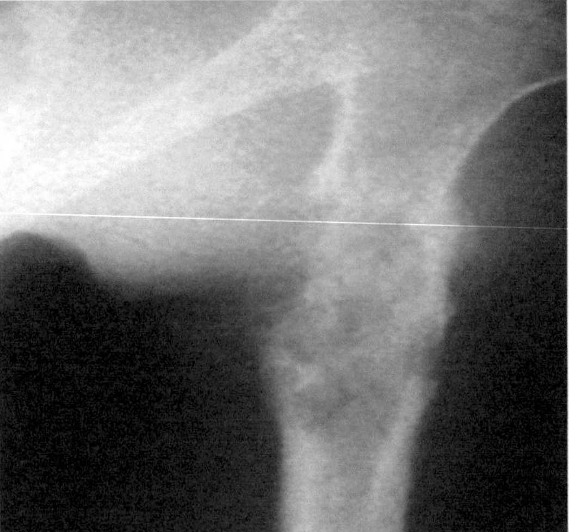

Fig. 2.10 Malignant lymphoma with wide zone of transition

other lesions, such as LCH, can have wide margins. A wide ZOT denotes malignancy. A narrow ZOT (a geographic lesion) is seen in benign lesion (Fig. 2.9). If the lesion has a sclerotic border, the lesion is likely to be benign.

A locally aggressive or malignant tumour shows cortical destruction and soft tissue extension. The calcification within cartilage tumour or ossification within a bone-forming tumour indicates whether the tumour is chondroid or osteoid forming. The interface between the lesion and surrounding bone is very important in determining whether a lesion is benign or malignant. If the lesion is poorly defined, it is more in favour of malignancy. A sclerotic rim denotes a slow-growing benign tumour.

When there are multiple tumours of bone, the commonest diagnoses are metastatic tumours or myeloma, followed by lymphomas and vascular tumours. Presence of lytic lesions in the same bone or in the same geographic area is a feature seen in vascular tumours. Benign multifocal lesions are enchondromatosis, multiple osteochondromas or Langerhans cell histiocytosis (LCH). Among the primary malignant bone tumours, multifocal osteosarcoma and Ewing's sarcoma are the common ones.

2.2.4.4 Periosteal Reaction

The pattern of the periosteal reaction denotes the growth rate of the tumour. The periosteum is thick in slow-growing tumours. Multiple layers of periosteal new bone are formed in fast-growing tumours. The tumour in Ewing sarcoma expands and elevates periosteum gradually and lays down layers of reactive bone (onion-skin appearance) (Figs. 2.11 and 2.12), whereas in osteosarcoma, the periosteum is elevated by the perforating tumour and lays down reactive bone as radiating spicules (Codman triangle and sunray appearance) (Fig. 2.11). In an aggressive lesion, the tumour will be seen on both sides of the cortex before its destruction.

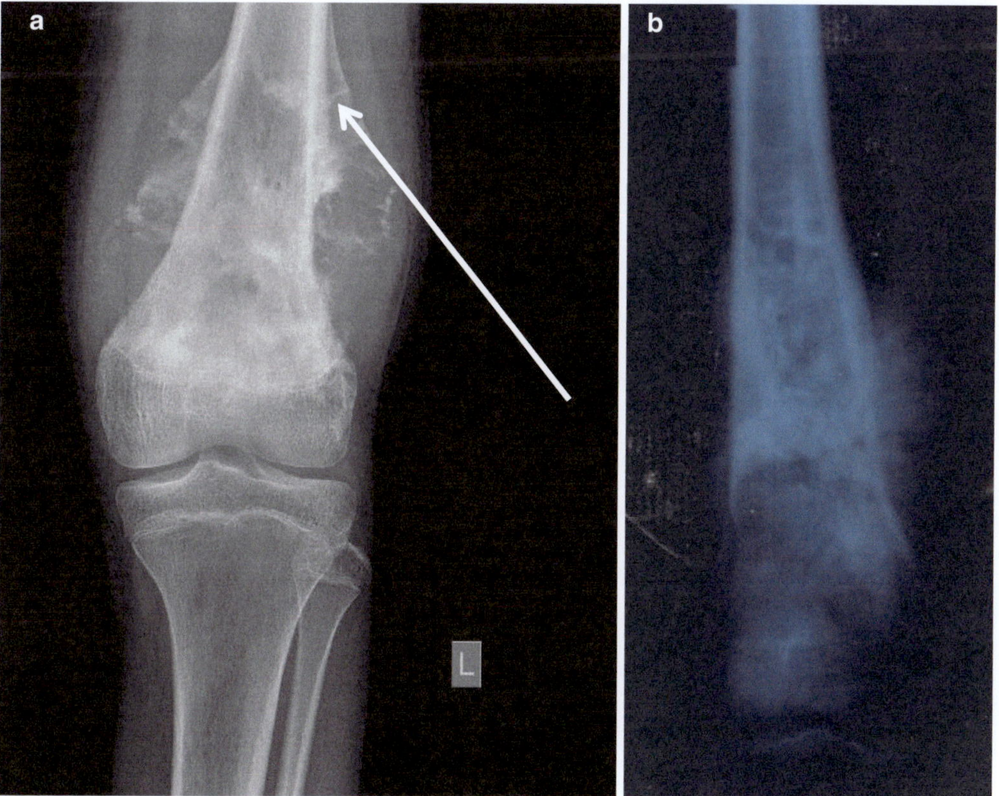

Fig. 2.11 OS: (**a**) Codman's triangle and (**b**) sunray appearance

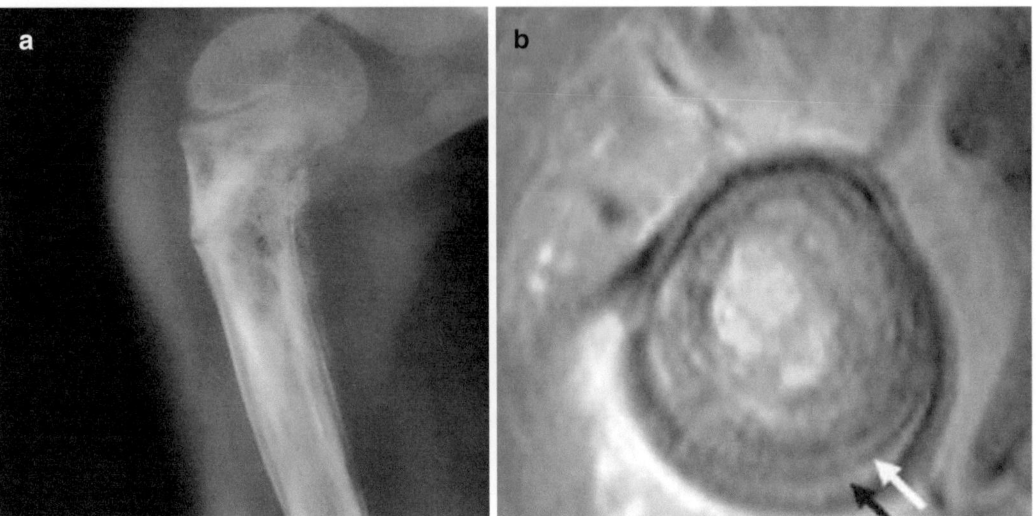

Fig. 2.12 Onion-skin appearance in ES: (**a**) Plain X-ray. (**b**) MRI

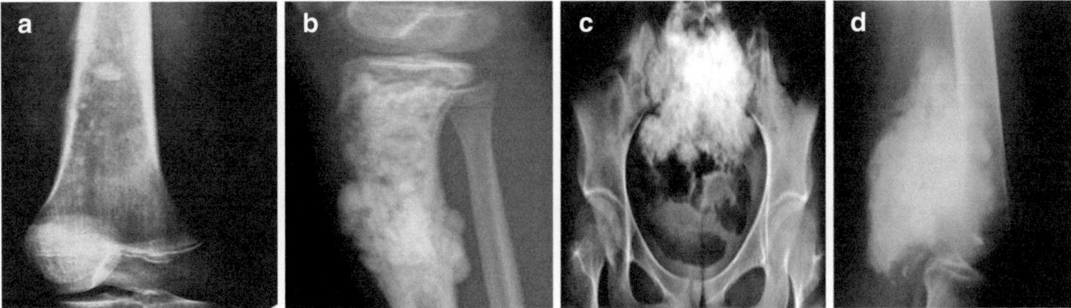

Fig. 2.13 Osteoblastic matrix: (**a**, **b**) cotton wool-like. (**c**) Wisp-like. (**d**) Sclerotic

Periosteal reaction can be categorized as:

Uninterrupted (continuous)—slow growth and usually benign tumour.

Interrupted (discontinuous)—in aggressive lesions.

2.2.4.5 Type of Matrix

The type of material produced by the mesenchymal cells is called matrix. Osteoid, bone, cartilage, myxoid and collagen are the main matrices produced by bone tumours (Figs. 2.13 and 2.14). The calcifications in the tumour matrix point to a chondroblastic process. Fibrous and cartilaginous tissue can be completely lytic. Simple bone cysts and intraosseous ganglion are also lytic without any matrix.

2.2.4.6 Mono-Ostotic or Polyostotic

Some tumours or lesions may involve more than one bone. Common lesions that can have multiple bone involvement are given in Table 2.8 (Figs. 2.15 and 2.16).

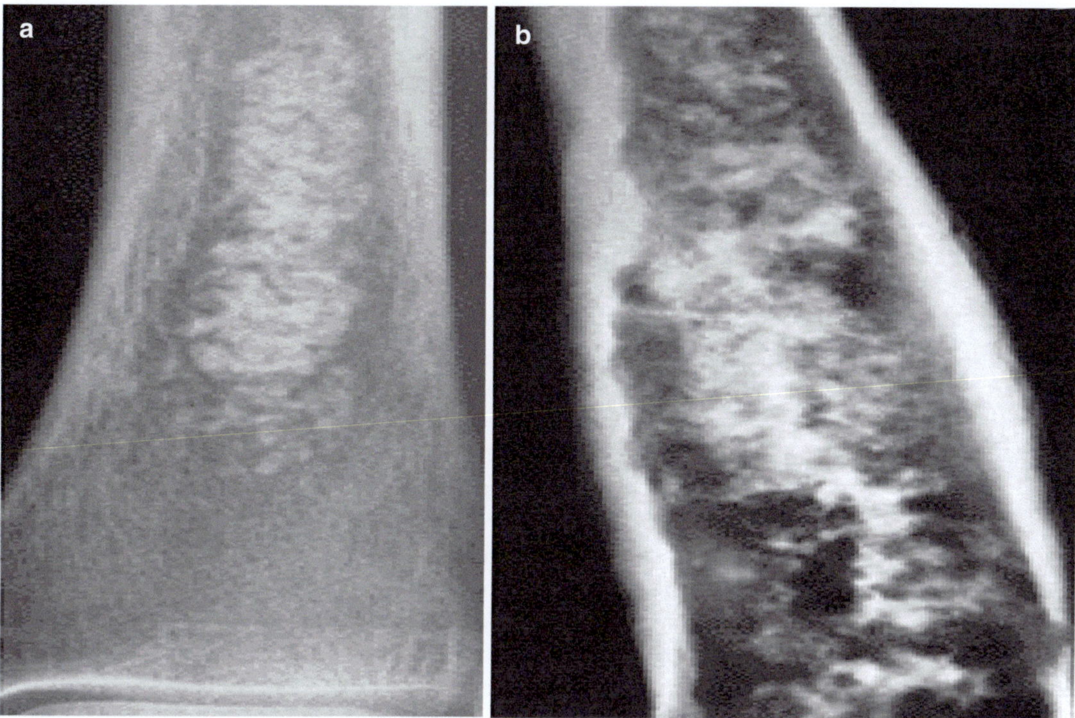

Fig. 2.14 Chondroid matrix: stippled, flocculent, rings and arcs. (**a**) Enchondroma. (**b**) Chondrosarcoma

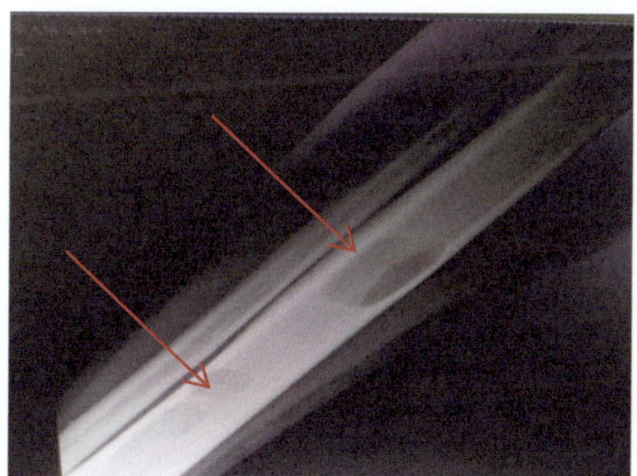

Fig. 2.15 Haemangioma

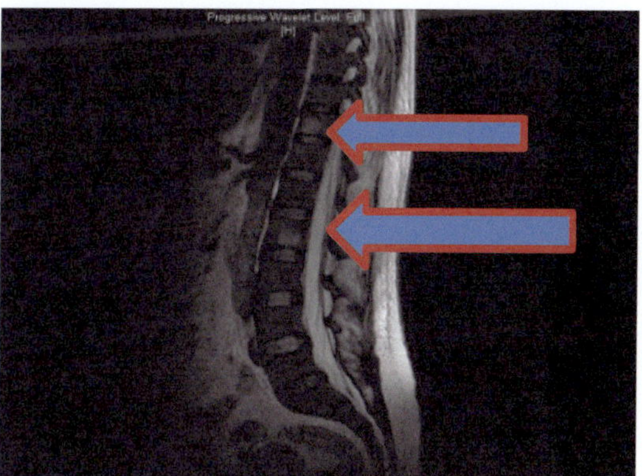

Fig. 2.16 Multiple vertebrae involved multiple lytic lesions in malignant lymphoma

Table 2.8 Polyostotic lesions/tumours

Hereditary exostoses
Enchondromatosis: Ollier and Maffucci
Fibrous dysplasia
Langerhans cell histiocytosis (LCH)
Myeloma
Metastasis
Leukaemia/lymphoma
Vascular tumours
Paget disease
Hyperparathyroidism

2.3 Laboratory Findings and Handling of Specimens

There are certain laboratory findings which are helpful in the diagnosis of certain bone tumours and tumour-like lesions (Table 2.9). Haematolymphoid malignancies are the foremost among this. An increased ESR, serum electrophoresis, presence of urine Bence-Jones proteins (BJPs) and other bio-

Table 2.9 Laboratory findings and bone tumours

Helpful laboratory findings in the evaluation of bone tumours/lesions
• Increased ESR and TC: osteomyelitis, ES • Serum alkaline phosphatase: elevated in OS, fracture, HPT, Paget's disease, blastic metastasis • Serum acid phosphatase: increased in metastatic prostate carcinoma • Serum LDH: elevated in ML • Serum electrophoresis, urine BJP, etc.: in myeloma • Serum ca, P: in HPT, phosphaturic mesenchymal tumour • Serum tumour markers: in case of metastasis to locate primary

chemical findings are seen in cases of plasma cell myeloma. Elevated LDH values are seen in malignant lymphoma. Increased ESR is seen in osteomyelitis and Ewing sarcoma [8]. Serum alkaline phosphatase is elevated in osteosarcoma, Paget's disease, blastic metastasis and hyperparathyroidism. An increased level of acid phosphatase is observed in prostatic carcinoma metastasis. Serum calcium and phosphorus are increased in hyperparathyroidism and phosphaturic mesenchymal tumour. Various serum tumour markers like PSA, CEA, Ca125, Ca19.9, and AFP are useful in the diagnosis of metastatic carcinomas.

2.3.1 Bone Tumour Specimens

Types of specimens received in the lab are fine needle aspiration cytology (FNAC), needle biopsy, curettings, open biopsy and resected specimen. Types of resections include intralesional, marginal, wide and radical.

Fine needle aspiration cytology (FNAC): Cytology is helpful in the diagnosis of certain tumours [9–13]. The diagnosis of primary bone tumours depends on the cellularity of the smear and correlation with radiological findings. In osteosarcomas, it is difficult to recognize osteoid as in biopsy specimen. Hence, only a diagnosis of spindle cell sarcoma or pleomorphic sarcoma will be possible (Fig. 2.17). Similarly, diagnosis of cartilage tumours is difficult by FNA. Benign lesions are difficult to aspirate because of paucicellularity. Usually, cytological diagnosis is given depending on the predominant cells obtained, for example round cell neoplasm, giant cell-rich lesion, chondroid neoplasm, spindle cell sarcoma and pleomorphic sarcoma.

FNAC is particularly useful in the diagnosis of recurrent sarcoma and metastasis of previously diagnosed neoplasms. If adequate radiological and clinical information is available, a diagnosis can be made.

Needle core biopsy: Many tumours can be diagnosed by needle core biopsy if it is representative of the lesion [14]. Correlation with radiological findings increases the diagnostic accuracy. Some people use combined FNA and needle core biopsy for diagnosis. This is because cytological details are better appreciated in FNA or imprint smears (Fig. 2.18). The needle biopsy is likely to have crush artefacts.

Open biopsy: Processing of soft portions of biopsy specimen will facilitate rapid diagnosis. It can be subjected to frozen section (except cortical bone) followed by definitive surgery.

2.3.2 General Handling of Bone Tumour Specimens Before Dissection

While taking biopsy, if there is soft tissue extension of a bone lesion, it should be sampled. Periphery of the lesion is the best for biopsy because it contains the most viable tissue. If there is a suspicion of infection, the biopsy specimen should be sent for culture.

If possible, the specimen should be received fresh in the laboratory. This is especially useful if frozen section is needed or if some histochemical stains are to be done or for molecular studies. Fresh tissue can be sent for microbiological culture. It is good for cytogenetic studies also. If fresh tissue is not required, the specimen is fixed in 10% neutral buffered formalin.

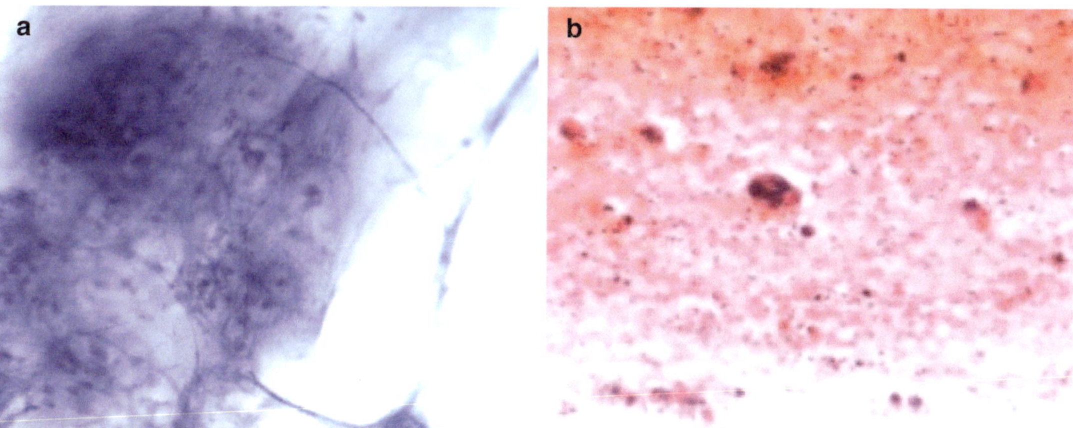

Fig. 2.17 (**a**) FNA: chondroid lesion/neoplasm, PapX100. (**b**) FNA: pleomorphic malignant cells in an osteosarcoma, PapX100

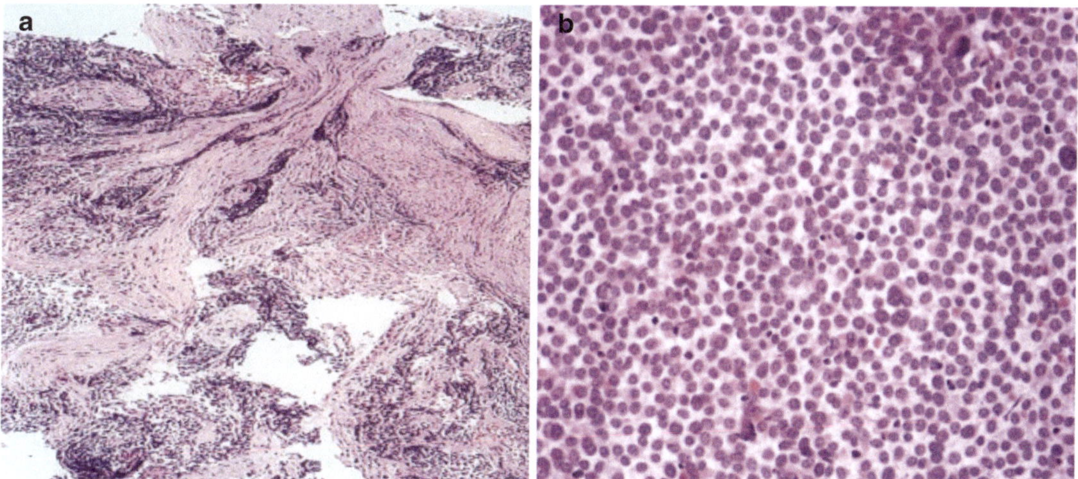

Fig. 2.18 (**a**) Tru-cut biopsy with crush artefact in a small blue round cell tumour, H&E ×40. (**b**) Imprint smear of same case with clear morphology, PapX400

The information required for all bone tumour specimens:

1. Patient and specimen identification details including patient name, age (date of birth), sex, hospital and surgical pathology identification numbers
2. Identification of the type of specimen received, e.g. core needle (closed) biopsy, surgical (open) biopsy, curettage, excision (segmental resection/en bloc), limb salvage, amputation or specific type of resection

2.3.3 Decalcification

Decalcification should be done with strong (e.g. nitric) or weak (e.g. formic) acid solutions before histological processing of most bone tumour specimens. Tissue which is not heavily mineralized should be selected to reduce the time for decalcification. For decalcification, 2–4 mm thick slices are taken from the large specimens. The antigenicity of many common epitopes is retained even after decalcification in strong acid,

Table 2.10 Procedure of decalcification [15]

Decalcification
• Acid decalcification: nitric acid (10% for big specimen) or hydrochloric acid or solution of 20% formic acid (400 mL) and 10% formalin (1600 mL)
• Entire slice is decalcified by suspending the piece of bone on the surface of acid; otherwise, CO_2 will form in 5–6 days.
• **EDTA/formic acid used for preserving molecular elements: IHC, FISH, PCR (nitric acid should not be used)**
• Monitor your specimen frequently: the specimen is "done" when it can be bent easily and a pin penetrates the cortical bone or if the scalpel blade can cut it
• **After decalcification, rinse the section in water before processing. This helps to prevent continued degradation**

but can interfere with molecular tests. Different decalcifying agents and steps are given in Table 2.10.

Bone biopsy should not be immersed in strong acids for a long time [15]. The specimens should be constantly monitored to know the mineralization status. Specimen radiography and chemical tests (calcium oxalate) are the methods used to determine the end point of decalcification. This also helps to decide the plane of resection of specimen with drill/saw. Another easier method is testing with a pin or scalpel. If the pin can penetrate the cortical bone or a scalpel can cut it easily, the specimen decalcification is complete and can be processed in the same way as undecalcified tissue. Before processing, the specimen should be rinsed in water to prevent continued degradation. Over-decalcification will result in difficulty in interpretation [16, 17]. 3–5 μm sections are cut using a standard rotary microtome. In case of larger sections, sledge microtome is used.

2.3.4 Stains

Routinely, haematoxylin–eosin stains are used. PAS (+/– diastase), reticulin, toluidine blue, Alcian blue, Perls, Congo red and Masson-Fontana are some of the special stains used. Stains like RGB trichrome (R—picrosirius red, G—fast green, B—Alcian blue) help in the identification of cartilage, bone and collagen.

2.3.5 Frozen Section

Frozen section is mainly used to assess the resected margins. But it can be used to assess the adequacy of biopsy. Moreover, it provides an opportunity to collect fresh tissue and triage it for culture in cases of suspected infective process and also for molecular studies. Imprint specimens, prepared from the fresh tissues kept in cold storage (−70 °C) of the tissue bank, can be used for future genotypic studies.

The soft tissue or less mineralized tissue should be sampled. If the stain used for frozen section is toluidine blue, it is not suitable for cartilage tumours. If chondroid neoplasm is suspected, H&E stain should be used.

Imprint preparations of tru-cut biopsy give better morphology and thus are useful in the diagnosis of round cell tumours of bone.

2.3.6 Handling of Biopsy and Curettage Specimen

Biopsy specimens are usually obtained by either closed (percutaneous) needle biopsy or open biopsy. Closed needle biopsy is preferable for the initial diagnosis of a bone tumour [14, 18–20]. The risk of dissemination is very low in this method. The main disadvantage of needle biopsy is inadequate material for histological examination. As the tissue obtained by needle biopsy is less, enough material for ancillary tests like IHC, FISH or molecular tests will not be available. If needle biopsy is not sufficient for diagnosis, open biopsy may have to be done. Frozen section is done to make sure that the tissue taken is adequate.

Core needle biopsy specimens, if properly fixed, may be decalcified overnight. If molecular studies are anticipated, a chelating agent like EDTA may be used for decalcification. If the core is large (>5 mm), it can be cut into two pieces. For ancillary studies, at least three cores of tissue should be taken. For rapid diagnosis, soft areas should be separated and processed first.

If the curetted specimen is large, about 1 section per cm is recommended. Specimens are first fixed in formalin overnight followed by decalcification.

2.3.7 Handling of Amputation and Segmental Resection Specimen

Amputation or segmental resection specimen is usually received fresh from the theatre. It should be grossed immediately so that the tumour tissue is exposed to ensure proper fixation. The fixative should be adequate. The specimen is washed gently to remove the bone dust. Bone dust can produce artifacts in the microscopic sections. Before dissecting an amputation or large segmental resection specimen, the preoperative diagnosis, radiology images and history of any neoadjuvant chemotherapy should be reviewed [21]. The steps of grossing of resected specimen are given in Table 2.11.

After taking measurements, the soft tissue margins are inked. Usually, surgeons send suspicious margins separately. Serially section the soft tissue, and look for soft tissue tumour nodules. All representative soft tissue margins should be submitted. If soft tissue extension is identified, dissect that area and keep this in continuity with bone. All soft tissues up to periosteum are removed. Samples should be taken from previous surgical sites or biopsy tracts to look for tumour implantation.

Table 2.11 Grossing of resection specimen

Grossing of resection specimen
• Slab radiographed for specimen radiograph • Surgical tissue margins taken—medial, lateral, anterior, posterior (as well as osteotomy transverse slice) • If tumour destroyed or breached periosteum, the margin sampled with a scalpel or knife • Cut uninvolved bone sagittally or coronally to look for foci of tumour or other lesions and major joints should be examined • Full slab of tumour blocked and marked • Additional blocks from macroscopically abnormal areas of bone, not included in slab • Previous incision site and biopsy tract • Proximal bone resection margin • LN if any • Major vessels at soft tissue amputation site

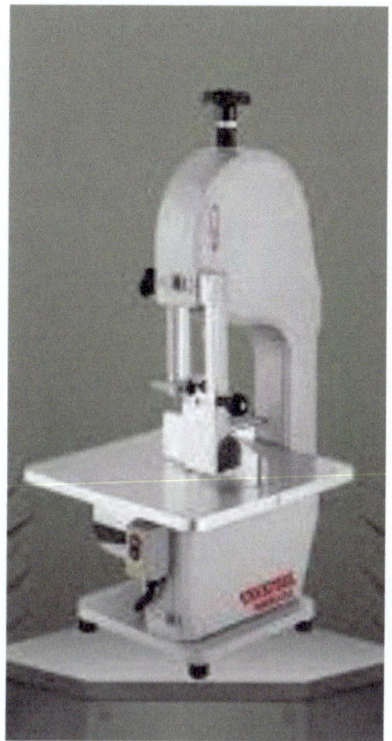

Fig. 2.19 Bone-cutting machine

Usually, surgeon will send cut-end marrow separately, which was evaluated by frozen section. Bone has to be cut longitudinally with band saw through the middle of the marrow cavity (Fig. 2.19). A coronal plane cut is given to make it anterior and posterior half (Fig. 2.20). Cut surface should be washed with a brush under running tap water to remove bone dust. In case of pelvic and scapular bone, bone is cut obliquely and the cut should go through the joint (hip or shoulder).

Fix the specimen for further 24 h. A thin slice of cut is made parallel to the initial cut at 5 mm thickness. The section should be selected such that it is through the greatest extent of tumour covering any cortical defects. Following overnight fixation, completely immerse the full-face bone section in decalcifying acid (8–48 h, depending on the specimen). Slab is radiographed. The surgical tissue margins should be taken. If tumour has destroyed periosteum, the margin is taken using a scalpel or knife. Serial sections of the specimen are cut and looked for any tumour nodules or skip lesions. The joints are examined for tumour invasion.

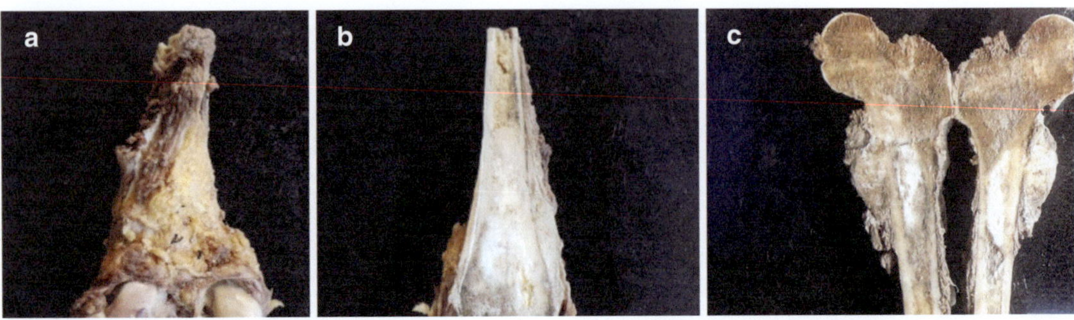

Fig. 2.20 Gross specimen of osteosarcoma: (**a**) specimen after removing soft tissue. (**b**, **c**) Bisected specimen with tumour and involved soft tissue

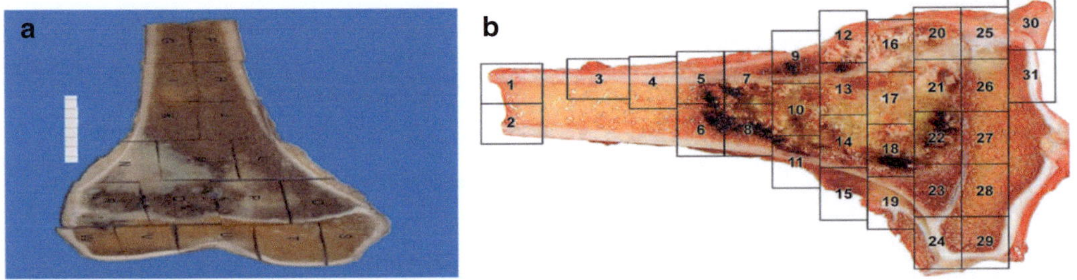

Fig. 2.21 (**a**, **b**) Cut half of gross specimen of osteosarcoma marked as grids of the entire cut surface

Full slab of tumour should be blocked and marked (Fig. 2.21). Additional blocks are taken from macroscopically abnormal areas of bone like previous incision site and biopsy tract. Proximal bone resection margin, lymph nodes if any and major vessels at amputation site should also be sampled. A photograph of the slab is taken, and the bits are marked on the paper. This helps in calculating the extent of tumour necrosis. The gross description and histopathology report formats are given in Tables 2.12 and 2.13, respectively.

2.3.8 Grading of Bone Sarcomas

Most bone sarcomas may be graded. Grading of a tumour is done in comparison to its normal counterpart. The tumours which do not resemble the normal counterpart are high grade. The important criteria for grading are cellularity, nuclear grade and necrosis. Some use three-tier grading of low, intermediate and high grades. Others use two-tier grading of low and high grade. Grading is most useful in chondrosarcomas and angiosarcomas for predicting prognosis. In osteosarcomas, most are high grade. The low grades are the low-grade central and parosteal osteosarcomas. Most small cell tumours are uniformly undifferentiated, and they are always high grade. Hence, they are not graded. Prognosis cannot be predicted by the grade in some tumours, e.g. adamantinoma and chordoma. Previously, grading of giant cell tumours of bone was done. Now they are not graded because the prognosis cannot be predicted. See Table 2.14.

Staging of bone tumours: The Enneking staging system is used. The grade of the tumour, local extent and presence or absence of metastasis are taken for staging [26–28]. Staging by the Musculoskeletal Tumor Society is the staging by grade of neoplasm. Staging is important for treatment and assessing prognosis. See Table 2.15.

Table 2.12 Gross description format

Gross description
• Type and side (left/right) of amputation or bone resection • The dimensions of the resection specimen • The gross presence or absence of exposed tumour in bone or soft tissue of the specimen • The presence, position and dimensions of attached skin and the presence of biopsy sites and surgical scars • The anatomical site and location of the tumour within bone (i.e. whether the lesion is in the epiphysis, metaphysis or diaphysis of a long bone and whether located in the medulla, in the cortex or on the surface of the bone) • Dimensions of the tumour (in centimetres) • Extent of bone, and soft tissue (including joint) involvement • The presence or absence of necrosis (approximate percentage) and other descriptive characteristics (e.g. colour, calcification, hardness, gritty, haemorrhagic and cystic) should be noted • The presence or absence of chemotherapy or radiotherapy effect • Involvement or invasion of major structures (e.g. nerve, major blood vessels) • Presence of satellite lesions of tumour away from the main tumour mass • Presence of lymph nodes and description of cut surface of the nodes • Relation of the tumour to the resection margins; the distance (in centimetres) should be measured
In addition, a record should be kept of whether tissue has been submitted for frozen section, cytogenetics, molecular genetic analysis and other investigations

Table 2.13 Histopathological reporting of bone tumours [22, 23]

Histological reporting of primary bone tumours
• Tumour type (and subtype) according to WHO histological classification • Tumour grade (if relevant) • Morphological and cytological description of the tumour; this may include details of the mitotic count and degree of pleomorphism • Tumour necrosis (presence or absence and percentage necrosis in the resection specimen) [24] • Extent of local tumour spread, in particular whether the tumour involves specific anatomical components or compartments (e.g. medullary cavity, cortex, joint, extra-osseous soft tissues) • Status of resection margins with regard to involvement by tumour • Results of cytogenetic/molecular genetic investigations (if available)

Table 2.14 Grading of bone sarcomas (WHO 2020) [25]

• Grade I—Low grade – Parosteal OS – Low-grade central OS – Clear cell CS – OFD like adamantinoma • Grade II—Intermediate grade – Periosteal OS – Classical adamantinoma • Grade III—High grade – Conventional OS – ES – Dedifferentiated CS, mesenchymal CS – PD and dedifferentiated chordoma – Angiosarcoma – Undifferentiated pleomorphic sarcoma	Variable grading Conventional CS LMS Malignant GCT

Table 2.15 Staging of bone tumours [29, 30]

• Tumours with no metastasis: All low grade—Stage I All high grade: Stage II • If confined to bone: Low grade—Stage IA High grade: Stage IIA • If ST involved: Low grade—Stage IB High grade: Stage IIB • Tumour with metastasis: Stage III

2.4 Ancillary Investigations

2.4.1 Immunohistochemistry

Immunohistochemistry does not have much role in the diagnosis of bone tumours, except in certain tumours like round cell neoplasms, chordomas, vascular tumours and metastatic carcinomas [31]. To locate the primary site, immunohistochemistry is very useful in secondary malignant tumours of bone. Expression of epithelial markers (EMA, CK) may point to a diagnosis of metastatic carcinoma (Fig. 2.22b). Further workup for the site of origin or primary can be determined by doing IHC tests with PSA, TTF1, ER, PR, GATA3, CD10 and thyroglobulin antibodies. In children, NB84a, synaptophysin and chromogranin are useful in the diagnosis of metastatic neuroblastoma. Epithelial markers are positive in some primary bone tumours like osteofibrous dysplasia, adamantinoma and chordoma. Podoplanin and CK are positive in adamantinoma and CK, S100 and brachyury in chordomas. Factor 8-related antigen, CD31, CD34, ERG and FLI1 are useful for vascular tumours. Recently, FOSB1 has been used to differentiate osteoblastoma from osteosarcoma. MDM2 and CDK4 are useful in differentiating low-grade osteosarcomas from its benign mimickers. Similarly, H3.3G34W is a very sensitive marker for giant cell tumour of bone and H3F3B for chondroblastomas. SOX9 is used to identify chondroid tumours especially mesenchymal CS and chondromyxoid fibroma.

In the diagnosis of malignant round cell tumours of bone in children and young adults, a panel of markers is essential for proper typing (Table 2.16). Commonly used markers are CD99, FLI1 and NKX2.2 for Ewing's sarcoma (Fig. 2.22a); desmin and myogenin for rhabdomyosarcoma; SOX9 for mesenchymal chondrosarcoma; LCA, Tdt and other lymphoma-specific markers for lymphoblastic lymphoma; and synaptophysin and chromogranin for metastatic neuroblastoma (Fig. 2.22c). Langerhans cells can be identified using antibodies like CD1a and langerin.

In adults, monoclonal kappa or lambda light-chain restriction helps in the diagnosis of myeloma or plasmacytoma. When malignant lymphoma is suspected, LCA, CD3, CD20 and

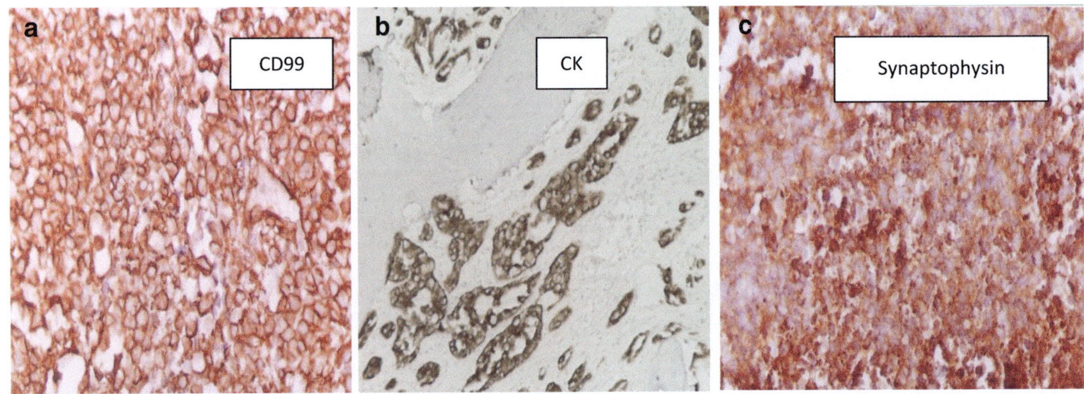

Fig. 2.22 IHC: (**a**) Ewing sarcoma, CD99X400. (**b**) Metastatic carcinoma, cytokeratin ×100. (**c**) Metastatic neuroblastoma, synaptophysin ×250

Table 2.16 IHC of malignant round cell neoplasm

	CD99	Synaptophysin	Desmin	LCA	SOX9	Tdt
ES	95%	20%	–	–	–	–
NB mets	–	95%	–	–	–	–
ARMS	20%	–	80%	–	–	–
LL	92%	–	–	90%	–	100%
Mes CS	80–100%	–	–	–	++	–

ES Ewing's sarcoma, *NB* neuroblastoma, *ARMS* alveolar rhabdomyosarcoma, *LL* lymphoblastic lymphoma, *Mes CS* mesenchymal chondrosarcoma

CD30 may be done as an initial panel. If synovial sarcoma or leiomyosarcoma is suspected, TLE-1, BCl2 and CK are used for the former and at least two smooth muscle markers like SMA and H-caldesmon for the latter.

2.4.2 Molecular Genetic Analysis

In bone tumours, the main problem for molecular analysis is the availability of DNA or RNA from the biopsy specimen (7) [15]. Ideal tissue for this is fresh frozen tissue. But most of the tumours of bone need decalcification. For molecular analysis, decalcification with weak acids like formic acid or chelating agents like EDTA gives good results [32]. To identify genetic abnormalities, FISH or RT-PCR is commonly employed. Examples are EWSR1 for Ewing's sarcoma (Fig. 2.23), CIC and BCOR for newly described undifferentiated round cell sarcomas (Table 2.17) and t (11; 14) for Burkitt lymphoma. MDM2 amplification by FISH is very useful to differentiate low-grade osteosarcoma from its benign mimickers (Fig. 2.24). Molecular markers are useful in the diagnosis of tumours other than round cell sarcomas also (Table 2.18).

2.4.3 Other Ancillary Investigations

Flow cytometry is not routinely done for bone tumours [25]. Aneuploidy is more prevalent in high-grade malignant tumours.

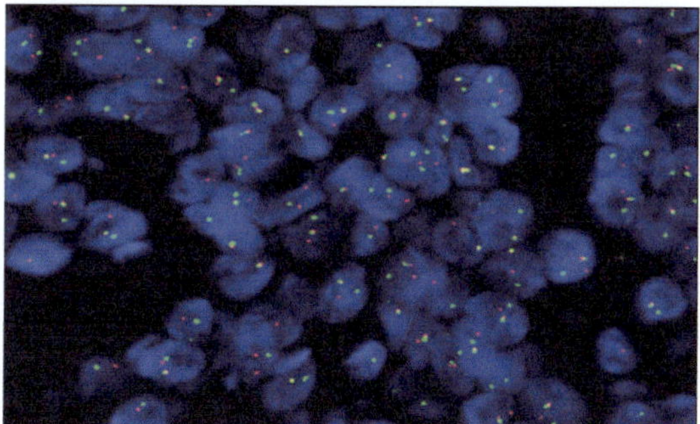

Fig. 2.23 FISH for EWSR1: Break-apart probe for one fused signal of red and green and break-apart signal of one green and one red in most of the cells

Table 2.17 Molecular markers in small round cell tumours of bone [7, 33, 34]

Molecular markers in round cell tumours of bone	
Ewing sarcoma	EWSR1/FUS-ETS family members
EWSR1-non-ETS-rearranged round cell sarcomas	EWSR1-NFATc2 EWSR1-SP3 EWSR1-SMARCA5 EWSR1-PATZ1
CIC-rearranged round cell sarcomas	CIC-DUX4 CIC-FOXO4 CIC-NUTM1
BCOR-rearranged round cell sarcomas	BCOR-CCNB3 BCOR-MAML3 ZC3H7B-BCOR
Non-Hodgkin lymphoma/ leukaemia	Depending on subtype
Synovial sarcoma	SS18-SSX
Mesenchymal chondrosarcoma	HEY1-NCOA2
Extraskeletal myxoid chondrosarcoma	EWSR1-NR4A3 TAF15-NR4A3 TFG-NR4A3 TCF12-NR4A3
Myoepithelial tumour	EWSR1-POU5F1 EWSR1-PBX1 EWSR1-ZNF444

Electron microscopy (EM) is also not routinely done for bone tumour diagnosis. It can help in confirmation of the diagnosis of some bone tumours, for example Birbeck granules in Langerhans cell histiocytosis (LCH) or cytoplasmic glycogen in Ewing's sarcoma [42, 43]. But IHC has replaced electron microscopy in most cases.

NGS is the process by which the exact order of nucleotides within a DNA molecule is determined. Distinct point mutations in H3F3A and H3F3B are detected in GCT and chondroblastoma, respectively. Rearrangements in GRM1 are observed in CMF. Others are FOS rearrangements in epithelioid haemangioma and WWTR1-CAMTA1 fusion in EHE. These are useful in the differential diagnosis of vascular tumours of bone.

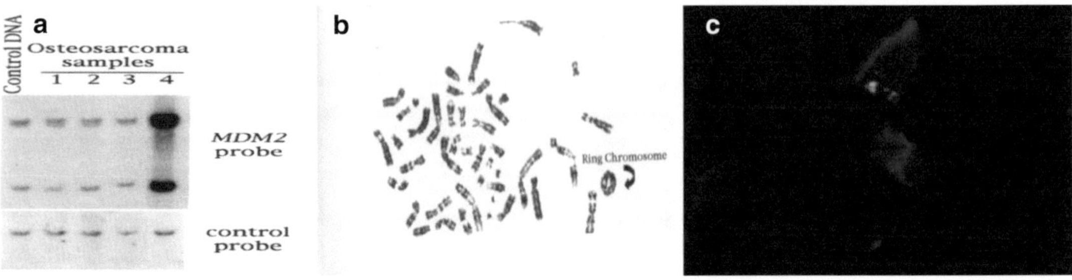

Fig. 2.24 (**a**) MDM2 amplification in parosteal osteosarcoma. (**b**) Ring chromosome in low-grade osteosarcoma. (**c**) MDM2 amplification by FISH: amplified green coloured signals

Table 2.18 Role of molecular markers in other bone tumours [35–41]

- **OS**: Rb or p53 mutations, MDM2 gene amplification in low-grade OS (absence of these in OB)
- **OB and OO**: Rearrangement **of FOS**
- **CB**: H3.3 B mutation (H3F3B)
- **CS**: Chromosome 1 and 7 aberrations (absent in enchondroma), **IDH1 and IDH2 mutations (except clear cell and mesenchymal CS)**
- **OC**: Biallelic inactivation of EXT 1 and 2 genes
- **Mesenchymal CS**: Recurrent gene fusion of HEY1 and NCOA2
- **Chordoma**: Brachyury—**R**eliable diagnostic marker and major susceptibility gene in familial chordoma
- **PD chordoma**: SMARCB1 deletion
- **GCT**: H3.3A(H3F3A) mutation
- **ABC**: USP6 gene rearrangement
- **EH**: FOS or FOSB gene rearrangement
- **EHE**: WWTR1-CAMTA1 fusion in 90–100% and YAP1-TFE3 fusion in <5%
- **NOF**: KRAS and FGFR1 mutation (>80%)
- **FD**: Activating missense mutation of GNAS
- **LCH**: MAPK pathway mutations (>85%)
- **ECD**: BRAF mutation (>50–60%)

OS osteosarcoma, *OB* and *OO* osteoblastoma and osteoid osteoma, *CB* chondroblastoma, *CS* chondrosarcoma, *OC* osteochondroma, *PD* poorly differentiated, *GCT* giant cell tumour, *ABC* aneurysmal bone cyst, *EH* epithelioid haemangioma, *EHE* epithelioid haemangioendothelioma, *NOF* non-ossifying fibroma, *FD* fibrous dysplasia, *LCH* Langerhans cell histiocytosis, *ECD* Erdheim-Chester disease

Points to Remember

- Clinical examination: detailed history, physical examination, laboratory findings
- Radiology: location of tumour (which bone is involved), site in the bone involved (epiphysis, metaphysis or diaphysis), type of destruction, presence and appearance of matrix, periosteal reaction, soft tissue involvement, multifocality
- FNAC: mainly for recurrence and metastasis diagnosis. Rarely for primary diagnosis after correlating with radiology
- Biopsy: needle, open, resection
- Decalcification: nitric acid, hydrochloric acid, formic acid. For molecular studies, EDTA is the best
- Grossing and reporting
- Ancillary tests: immunohistochemistry, FISH, molecular tests

References

1. Flanagan AM, Lindsay D. A diagnostic approach to bone tumours. Pathology. 2017;49(7):675–87.
2. DeYoung BR. Diagnosing bone lesions: a practical non-pathology centric formulaic approach. Semin Diagn Pathol. 2014;31:1–9.
3. Gerrand C, Athanasou N, Brennan B, et al. UK guidelines for the management of bone sarcomas. Clin Sarcoma Res. 2016;6(7):1–21.

4. Weatherby RP, Unni KK. Practical aspects of handling orthopaedic specimens in surgical pathology laboratory. Pathol Annu. 1982;17:1–31.
5. Neyaz Z, Gadodia A, Gamanagatti S, Mukhopadhyay S. Radiographical approach to jaw lesions. Singap Med J. 2008;49(2):165–76.
6. Ritchie DA, Davies AM. Imaging studies in bone neoplasia. In: Helliwell T, editor. Pathology of bone and joint neoplasms. Philadelphia: WB Saunders; 1999. p. 106–28.
7. Suster D, Suster S. Genetic characteristics and molecular diagnostics of bone tumors. J Cancer Metastasis Treat. 2021;7:8. https://doi.org/10.20517/2394-4722.2020.119.
8. Cravern RD. Laboratory evaluation of pediatric bone and soft tissue tumors. Orthop Clin N Am. 1996;27:461–71.
9. Bommer KK, Ramzy I, Mody D. Fine-needle aspiration biopsy in the diagnosis and management of bone lesions: a study of 450 cases. Cancer. 1997;81:148–56.
10. Kilpatrick SE, Cappellari JO, Bos GD, Gold SH, Ward WG. Is fine-needle aspiration biopsy a practical alternative to open biopsy for the primary diagnosis of sarcoma? Experience with 140 patients. Am J Clin Pathol. 2001;115:59–68.
11. Kilpatrick SE, Ward WG, Chauvenet AR, Gold SH. The role of fine-needle aspiration biopsy in the initial diagnosis of pediatric bone and soft tissue tumours: an institutional experience. Mod Pathol. 1998;11:923–8.
12. Layfield LJ, Dodd LG. Fine needle aspiration of bone and joint neoplasms. In: Helliwell T, editor. Pathology of bone and joint neoplasms. Philadelphia: WB Saunders; 1999. p. 129–56.
13. Willen H. Fine needle aspiration in the diagnosis of bone tumours. Acta Orthop Scand Suppl. 1997;273:47–53.
14. Roitman PD, Farfalli GL, Ayerza MA, et al. Is needle biopsy clinically useful in preoperative grading of central chondrosarcoma of the pelvis and long bones? Clin Orthop Relat Res. 2017;475:808–14.
15. Unni KK, Inwards CY, Bridge JA, Kindblom LG, Wold LE. AFIP atlas of tumour pathology; 4th series, fascicle 2: tumours of the bones and joints. Washington, DC: AFIP; 2005.
16. Alers JC, Krijtenburg PJ, Vissers KJ, et al. Effect of bone decalcification procedures on DNA in situ hybridization and comparative genomic hybridization. EDTA is highly preferable to a routinely used acid decalcifier. J Histochem Cytochem. 1999;47:703–10.
17. Athanasou NA, Quinn J, Heryet A, Woods CG, McGee JO. Effect of decalcification agents on the immunoreactivity of cellular antigens. J Clin Pathol. 1987;40:874–8.
18. Skrzynski MC, Biermann JS, Montag A, Simon MA. Diagnostic accuracy and charge-savings of outpatient core needle biopsy compared with open biopsy of musculoskeletal tumors. J Bone Jt Surg Am. 1996;78-A:644–9.
19. Stoker DJ, Cobb JP, Pringle JA. Needle biopsy of musculoskeletal lesions. A review of 208 procedures. J Bone Jt Surg Br Vol. 1991;73B:498–500.
20. Welker JA, Henshaw RM, Jelinek J, Schmookler BM, Malawer MM. The percutaneous needle biopsy is safe and recommended in the diagnosis of musculoskeletal masses. Outcomes analysis of 155 patients at a sarcoma referral centre. Cancer. 2000;89:2677–81.
21. Bharat R, Shantveer U, Jayasree K, Jambhekar Nirmala A, Pradyumn S, Vinita P, Satish R, Nishat A. Grossing and reporting of bone tumor specimens in surgical oncology: rationale with current evidence and recent updates. Indian J Cancer. 2021;58(3): 326–35.
22. Abdul-Karim FW, Bauer TW, Kilpatrick SE, Raymond KA, Siegal GP. Recommendations for the reporting of bone tumours. Hum Pathol. 2004;35:1173–8.
23. National Comprehensive Cancer Network (NCCN). NCCN clinical practice guidelines in oncology. https://www.nccn.org/professionals/physician_gls/pdf/aml.pdf. Accessed 20 Feb 2019.
24. Coffin CM, Lowichik A, Zhou H. Treatment effects in pediatric soft tissue and bone tumours: practical considerations for the pathologist. Am J Clin Pathol. 2055;123:75–90.
25. WHO Classification of Tumours Editorial Board. WHO Classification of tumours. In: Soft tissue and bone tumours, vol. 3. 5th ed. IARC; 2020. p. 337–44.
26. Enneking WF, Spanier SS, Goodman MA. A system for the surgical staging of musculoskeletal sarcoma. Clin Orthop. 1980;153:106–20.
27. Enneking WF. A system of staging musculoskeletal neoplasms. Clin Orthop. 1986;204:9–24.
28. Heck RK, Peabody TD, Simon MA. Staging of primary malignancies of bone. CA Cancer J Clin. 2006;56:366–75.
29. American Joint Committee on Cancer Bone. In: Greene FL, Page DL, Fleming ID, et al., editors. AJCC cancer staging manual. New York: Springer; 2002.
30. Edge SB, Byrd DR, Carducci MA, Compton CC, Fritz AG, Greene FL, Trotti A. AJCC cancer staging manual. New York: Springer; 2009. p. 7.
31. Sailaja M, Satish Rao I. Utility of immunohistochemistry in the diagnosis of bone tumors. J Med Sci Res. 2014;2(2):84–90.
32. Reineke T, Jenni B, Abdou MT, et al. Ultrasonic decalcification offers new perspectives for rapid FISH, DNA, and RT-PCR analysis in bone marrow trephines. Am J Surg Pathol. 2006;30:892–6.
33. Ladanyi M. The emerging molecular genetics of sarcoma translocations. Diagn Mol Pathol. 1995;4:214–9.
34. Williams A, Mangham DC. RT-PCR for the detection of translocations in bone and soft tissue tumours in formalin-fixed paraffin-embedded tissues. Methods Mol Biol. 2011;688:257–68.
35. Amary MF, Bacsi K, Maggiani F, et al. IDH1 and IDH2 mutations are frequent events in central chondrosarcoma and central and periosteal chondromas

but not in other mesenchymal tumours. J Pathol. 2011;224:334–43.
36. Amary MF, Damato S, Halai D, et al. Ollier disease and Maffucci syndrome are caused by somatic mosaic mutations of IDH1 and IDH2. Nat Genet. 2011;43:1262–5.
37. Damato S, Alorjani M, Bonar F, et al. IDH1 mutations are not found in cartilaginous tumours other than central and periosteal chondrosarcomas and enchondromas. Histopathology. 2012;60:363–5.
38. Feugeas O, Guriec N, Babin-Boilletot A, Marcellin L, Simon P, Babin S, Thyss A, Hofman P, Terrier P, Kalita C, Brunat-Mentigny M, Patricot LM, Oberling F. Loss of heterozygosity of the Rb gene is a poor prognostic factor in patients with osteosarcoma. J Clin Oncol. 1996;14:467–72.
39. Hung J, Anderson R. p53: function, mutations and sarcomas. Acta Orthop Scand. 1997;68(Suppl 273):68–73.
40. Jäger M, Westhoff B, Portier S, et al. Clinical outcome and genotype in patients with hereditary multiple exostoses. J Orthop Res. 2007;25:1541–51.
41. Jennes I, de Jong D, Mees K, et al. Breakpoint characterization of large deletions in EXT1 or EXT2 in 10 multiple osteochondromas families. BMC Med Genet. 2011;12:85.
42. Hirohata K, Morimoto K. Ultrastructure of bone and joint diseases. Excerpta Medica; 1971.
43. Roessner A, Grundmann E. Electron microscopy in bone tumor diagnosis. Curr Top Pathol. 1982;71:153–99.

3 Primary Bone Tumours

Primary bone tumours are very rare. The overall frequency of bone tumours is unknown. Benign tumours outnumber malignant tumours (approximately 10,000:1). The benign tumours are usually detected incidentally. Bone sarcomas form 0.2% of all invasive cancers. Majority of bone sarcomas occur in the first three decades of life. The bone sarcomas have two peaks of age distribution—first peak in patients with 10–20 years of age and second peak in 60–70-year age group. The benign bone tumours occur more frequently in males, whereas the bone sarcomas occur in males and females in a ratio of 1:0.7 (Dorfman Cancer 1995). Most bone tumours arise around knee especially benign tumours because this is the area where maximum growth occurs in a child.

Benign and malignant bone tumours are part of many genetic syndromes like Ollier disease, Maffucci syndrome, multiple hereditary osteochondromas, bilateral retinoblastoma, Li-Fraumeni syndrome, Gardner's syndrome, Mazabraud syndrome, McCune-Albright syndrome, neurofibromatosis and diaphyseal medullary stenosis.

A variety of bone lesions like bone infarction, Paget disease, radiation injury, chronic osteomyelitis and preceding trauma can lead on to the development of sarcoma. Pre-existing bone tumours like enchondromatosis, osteochondroma, rarely fibrous dysplasia and simple bone cysts can undergo malignant transformation. Recently, sarcomas have been reported to occur near orthopaedic implants.

3.1 Syndromes Associated with Bone Tumours

Various syndromes are associated with bone tumours [1]. Many of them are associated with osteosarcoma [2]. Table 3.1 gives the syndromes that are associated with osteosarcoma along with other components of the syndrome and their mode of inheritance.

Another group of syndromes are associated with either enchondromas or osteochondromas, which is given in Table 3.2.

Fibrous dysplasia, especially polyostotic type, is also associated with Mazabraud and McCune-Albright syndromes (Table 3.3). Some syndromes are associated with giant cell lesions of bone (Table 3.4).

3.2 Classification

Primary bone tumours are classified based on the normal cell or tissue of origin. They are chondrogenic tumours, osteogenic tumours, hematopoietic tumours, giant cell tumour, fibrogenic tumours, histiocytic tumours, notochordal tumours and vascular tumours.

There is a small group of tumours, which lack a normal counterpart, but with consistent and distinctive clinicopathologic features: for example, Ewing sarcoma and other round cell sarcomas, adamantinoma, and Langerhans cell histiocytosis (LCH).

J. Kattoor et al., *Bone Tumors*, https://doi.org/10.1007/978-981-99-4738-6_3

Table 3.1 Syndromes associated with osteosarcoma

Syndromes associated with osteosarcoma	Mode of inheritance	Gene involved
• Bloom syndrome: growth deficiency, immunodeficiency, early development of cancer including osteosarcoma • Li-Fraumeni syndrome: early onset of various malignancies including osteosarcomas and soft tissue sarcomas • Mazabraud syndrome sporadic; polyostotic fibrous dysplasia, osteosarcoma, intramuscular myxoma • McCune-Albright syndrome: polyostotic fibrous dysplasia, osteosarcoma, endocrine disorders, skin pigmentation • Familial Paget disease: early-onset Paget disease, osteosarcoma • Retinoblastoma: osteosarcoma, soft tissue sarcomas • Rothmund-Thomson syndrome: Poikiloderma, sparse hair, small stature, skeletal abnormalities, increased risk of cancer including osteosarcoma • Familial expansile osteolysis: osteosarcoma	Autosomal recessive Autosomal dominant Sporadic Sporadic Autosomal dominant Autosomal dominant Autosomal recessive Autosomal recessive	BLM TP53 CHEK2 Mutation in GNAS1 gene Mutation in GNAS1 gene TNFRSF11A Germline mutation of RB1 tumour suppressor gene RECQL4 mutation

Table 3.2 Syndromes associated with enchondromas and osteochondromas

Syndrome	Mode of inheritance	Genes involved
• Maffucci syndrome multiple enchondromas, chondrosarcoma, haemangioma, spindle cell haemangioma, angiosarcoma • Ollier disease multiple enchondromas • Multiple osteochondromas (osteochondromatosis)	Sporadic/autosomal dominant Sporadic/autosomal dominant Autosomal dominant	– Mutation of PTHR1 gene Mutation in Ext gene

Table 3.3 Syndromes associated with fibrous dysplasia

- Mazabraud syndrome sporadic: polyostotic fibrous dysplasia, osteosarcoma, intramuscular myxoma
- McCune-Albright syndrome sporadic: polyostotic fibrous dysplasia, osteosarcoma, endocrine disorders, skin pigmentation

Table 3.4 Syndromes associated with giant cell lesions of bone

- Noonan syndrome 1: giant cell lesions of small bones, granular cell tumours
- Noonan syndrome 4: embryonal RMS, granular cell tumours, giant cell tumour of small bones, pigmented villonodular tenosynovitis
- Neurofibromatosis type 1: neurofibromas, MPNST, GIST, giant cell lesions of bone (central), RMS, glomus tumours
- Craniofaciocutaneous syndrome

The widely used classification is the WHO classification (Table 3.5).

3.3 Staging

The **staging** used for bone tumours is TNM staging [3]. TNM staging is based on tumour size, lymph node status and spread to different parts of the body. According to the stage, treatment is decided. Grade of the tumour is also taken into account while staging. **TNM** stands for **T**umour**,** **N**ode **and** **M**etastasis. This is the most commonly used staging system. This staging is used for sites like extremities, trunk (chest and ribs), skull bones and face bones. For the staging for pelvis and spine tumours, use different T (size) stages.

Table 3.5 The WHO 2020 classification of bone tumours [4]

WHO 2020 classification of bone tumours with ICD-O codes
Chondrogenic tumours
Benign
9213/0 Subungual exostosis
9212/0 Bizarre parosteal osteochondromatous proliferation
9221/0 Periosteal chondroma
9220/0 Enchondroma
9210/0 Osteochondroma
9230/0 Chondroblastoma NOS
9241/0 Chondromyxoid fibroma
9211/0 Osteochondromyxoma
Intermediate (locally aggressive)
9220/1 Chondromatosis NOS
9222/1 Atypical cartilaginous tumour
Malignant
9222/3 Chondrosarcoma, grade 1
9220/3 Chondrosarcoma, grade 2
9220/3 Chondrosarcoma, grade 3
9221/3 Periosteal chondrosarcoma
9242/3 Clear cell chondrosarcoma
9240/3 Mesenchymal chondrosarcoma
9243/3 Dedifferentiated chondrosarcoma
Osteogenic tumours
Benign
9180/0 Osteoma NOS
9191/0 Osteoid osteoma NOS
Intermediate (locally aggressive)
9200/1 Osteoblastoma NOS
Malignant
9187/3 low-grade central osteosarcoma
9180/3 Osteosarcoma NOS
Conventional osteosarcoma
Telangiectatic osteosarcoma
Small cell osteosarcoma
9192/3 Parosteal osteosarcoma
9193/3 Periosteal osteosarcoma
9194/3 High-grade surface osteosarcoma
9184/3 Secondary osteosarcoma
Fibrogenic tumours
Intermediate (locally aggressive)
8823/1 Desmoplastic fibroma
Malignant
8810/3 Fibrosarcoma NOS
Vascular tumours of bone
Benign
9120/0 Haemangioma NOS
Intermediate (locally aggressive)
9125/0 Epithelioid haemangioma
Malignant
9133/3 Epithelioid haemangioendothelioma NOS
9120/3 Angiosarcoma
Osteoclastic giant cell-rich tumours
Benign
9260/0 Aneurysmal bone cyst
8830/0 Non-ossifying fibroma

Table 3.5 (continued)

WHO 2020 classification of bone tumours with ICD-O codes
Intermediate (locally aggressive, rarely metastasizing)
9250/1 Giant cell tumour of bone NOS
Malignant
9250/3 Giant cell tumour of bone, malignant
Notochordal tumours
Benign
9370/0 Benign notochordal tumour
Malignant
9370/3 Chordoma NOS
Chondroid chordoma
9370/3 Poorly differentiated chordoma
9372/3 Dedifferentiated chordoma
Other mesenchymal tumours of bone
Benign
Chondromesenchymal hamartoma of chest wall
Simple bone cyst
8818/0 Fibrous dysplasia
Osteofibrous dysplasia
8850/0 Lipoma NOS
8880/0 Hibernoma
Intermediate (locally aggressive)
9261/1 Osteofibrous dysplasia-like adamantinoma
8990/1 Mesenchymoma NOS
Malignant
9261/3 Adamantinoma of long bones
Dedifferentiated adamantinoma
8890/3 Leiomyosarcoma NOS
8802/3 Pleomorphic sarcoma, undifferentiated
Bone metastases
Haematopoietic neoplasms of bone
9731/3 Plasmacytoma of bone
9591/3 Malignant lymphoma, non-Hodgkin, NOS
9650/3 Hodgkin disease NOS
9680/3 Diffuse large B-cell lymphoma NOS
9690/3 Follicular lymphoma NOS
9699/3 Marginal zone B-cell lymphoma NOS
9702/3 T-cell lymphoma NOS
9714/3 Anaplastic large cell lymphoma NOS
9727/3 Malignant lymphoma, lymphoblastic, NOS
9687/3 Burkitt lymphoma NOS
9751/1 Langerhans cell histiocytosis NOS
9751/3 Langerhans cell histiocytosis, disseminated
9749/3 Erdheim-Chester disease
Rosai-Dorfman disease

Points to Remember

- Primary bone tumours are rare
- Benign-to-malignant ratio is approximately 10,000:1
- Syndromes associated with bone tumours
- Classification of bone tumours: new—WHO 2020
- TNM staging of bone tumours

References

1. Gnoli M, Ponti F, Sangiorgi L. Tumor syndromes that include bone tumors: an update. Surg Pathol Clin. 2017;10(3):749–64.
2. Alessandro G, Calvert George T, Randall RL, Jones Kevin B, Lisa C-A, Stephen L, Schiffman JD. At-risk populations for osteosarcoma: the syndromes and beyond. Sarcoma. 2012;2012:152382. https://doi.org/10.1155/2012/152382.
3. American Joint Committee on Cancer. TNM staging of bone tumours in American joint committee on cancer. Bone. In: AJCC cancer staging manual. 8th ed. New York: Springer; 2017. p. 471–86.
4. WHO Classification of Tumours Editorial Board. WHO Classification of tumours. In: Soft tissue and bone tumours, vol. 3. 5th ed. IARC; 2020.

4 Cartilage Tumours

Cartilage tumours can be benign or malignant [1]. The WHO classification of cartilage tumours is given below.

Cartilage Tumours: 2020 WHO CLASSIFICATION [160]

Benign

Subungual exostosis

Bizarre parosteal osteochondromatous proliferation (BPOP)

Periosteal chondroma

Enchondroma

Osteochondroma

Chondroblastoma NOS

Chondromyxoid fibroma (CMF)

Osteochondromyxoma

Intermediate (locally aggressive)

Synovial Chondromatosis

Atypical cartilaginous tumour

Malignant

Conventional chondrosarcoma grade 1, 2 and 3

Periosteal chondrosarcoma

Clear cell chondrosarcoma

Mesenchymal chondrosarcoma

Dedifferentiated chondrosarcoma

4.1 Benign Cartilage Tumours

Benign cartilage tumours are of two types—those with foetal type cartilage, and those with more mature hyaline type cartilage. The foetal type occurs in children and young adults. The common foetal type tumours are chondroblastoma and chondromyxoid fibroma. These tumours are well defined with sclerotic margins. Mature type comprises osteochondroma, enchondroma, osteochondromyxoma, subungual exostosis and bizarre parosteal osteochondromatous proliferation (BPOP or Nora's lesion).

4.1.1 Subungual Exostoses

These are painful projections from the distal phalanges, under the nail bed [15], usually less than 1 cm in size [7, 8, 10]. They occur after injury to the site. It is a type of myositis and is also called Dupuytren exostosis [21]. The proliferating fibrocartilaginous tissue resembles callus. A recent study has shown a consistent chromosomal rearrangement suggesting that they are true neoplasms [20, 22].

4.1.1.1 Clinical

Presenting complaints are pain and swelling [13]. Ulceration and infection may be present. Majority of these lesions occur in the nail bed of big toe [12, 18]. They occur in second and third decades.

4.1.1.2 Radiology

Subungual exostoses appear as outgrowth of bone projecting from distal phalanx.

4.1.1.3 Microscopy

A gradual maturation from spindle cells, cartilage to bone, as seen in callus or myositis ossificans can be seen (Fig. 4.1).

J. Kattoor et al., *Bone Tumors*, https://doi.org/10.1007/978-981-99-4738-6_4

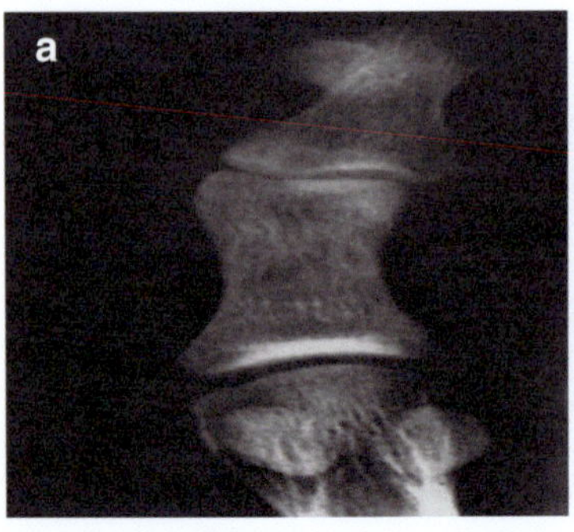

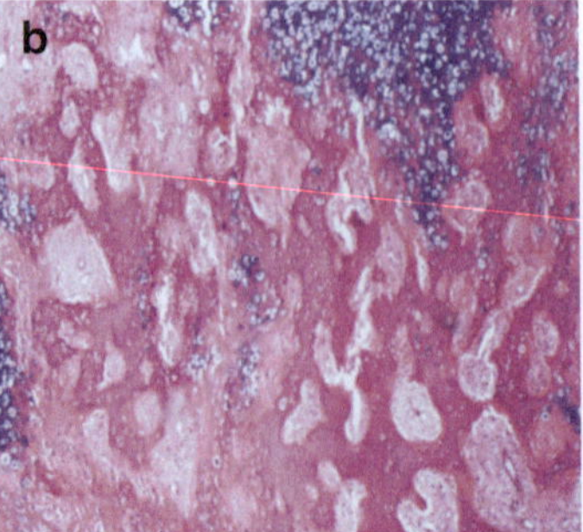

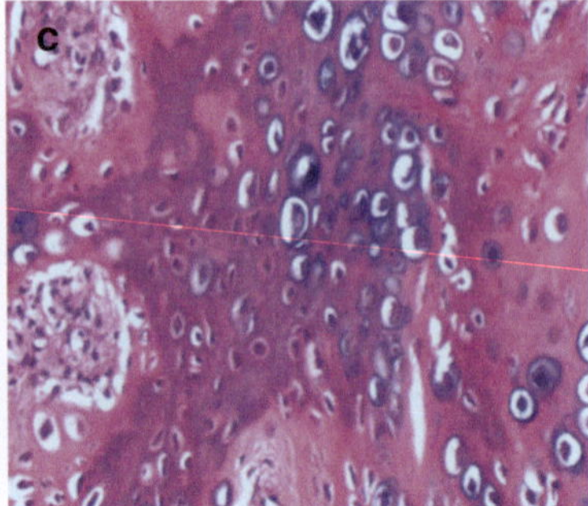

Fig. 4.1 (**a**, **b**) Subungual exostosis in a 10-year-old boy. (**a**) Plain X-ray of sclerotic lesion involving terminal phalanx of big toe. (**b**) Cartilaginous cap and osseous trabeculae in the nail bed, H&E ×100. (**c**) Cartilage can be hypercellular and may show atypia, H&E ×400

4.1.1.4 Differential diagnosis

It includes BPOP, subungual osteochondroma [7, 14, 16], subungual haematoma [11], and subungual osteogenic melanoma. Overlying epithelium will show melanoma in case of subungual melanoma, which helps in differentiation.

4.1.1.5 Molecular

These lesions show t(X; 6) (q24–q26; q15–q25) translocation involving COL12A1 gene on chromosome 6 [20, 22].

4.1.1.6 Treatment and prognosis

Simple excision is the treatment. It can be done as an OP procedure [9, 17, 19]. The disease is benign in nature. Local recurrence can occur.

4.1.2 Bizarre Parosteal Osteochondromatous Proliferation (BPOP or Nora Lesion)

Nora lesion [27] (bizarre parosteal osteochondromatous proliferation) was named after the pathologist who first described this lesion in 1983. It is a form of reactive periostitis [27]. Some consider this as a true neoplasm, but others do not. Recurrent cytogenetic abnormalities which are different from subungual exostoses are described.

4.1.2.1 Clinical

They are seen on the surface of bone as an exophytic growth. The lesion is clinically benign [24, 25].

4.1.2.2 Radiology

Small bones of the hands and feet are commonly affected, especially hands [28]. It is seen rarely in long bones. Unlike osteochondroma, they lack continuity with the cortex [23]. No unmineralized soft tissue mass is seen [29].

4.1.2.3 Pathology

A mixture of bone, cartilage and spindle cells is seen in different proportions. Cartilage is present at the periphery as a cap or is seen in lobules (Fig. 4.2). Cartilage is hypercellular, and the chondrocytes are large in size [28]. The blue tinctorial quality of the bone in routine sections is helpful in diagnosis.

4.1.2.4 DD

Subungual exostosis, osteochondroma, parosteal osteosarcoma and fibro-osseous pseudotumour of digits are the main differentials.

4.1.2.5 Molecular

Cytogenetic abnormalities described are t (1; 17) (q32; q21), inv. (7) and inv. (6).

4.1.2.6 Treatment and Prognosis

Simple excision is the line of treatment. 50% of cases have recurrence [26]. They are benign tumours with no capacity for metastasis.

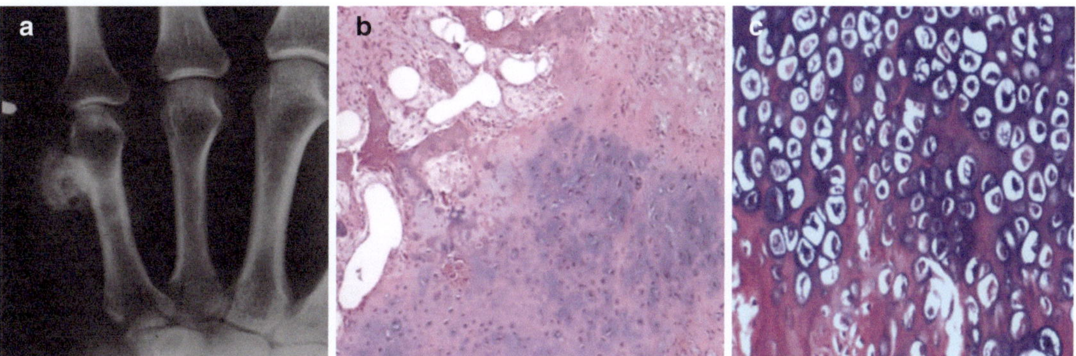

Fig. 4.2 BPOP: (**a**) On the surface of proximal phalanx of ring finger, mature bone attached to cortex and fluffy calcifications towards periphery. (**b**) Disorganized cartilage and bone known as blue bone is a characteristic feature, H&E ×100. (**c**) Proliferation of chondrocytes, H&E ×400

4.1.3 Enchondroma and Periosteal Chondroma

Chondromas are benign hyaline cartilage neoplasms [32]. Those tumours which are within the medullary cavity of bone are known as enchondromas. The tumours on the surface are called periosteal chondromas. Rarely, lesions are partly intramedullary and partly on the surface. They are called enchondroma protuberans. Enchondromas can affect any bone. They are commonly seen in the small bones of the hands and feet, and the long bones like humerus, femur and tibia. Chondroma is the most common tumour of the small bones of hands and feet. Enchondroma rarely affects flat bones and is extremely rare in craniofacial bones. This may be due to membranous ossification of skull bones.

4.1.3.1 Clinical

Enchondromas are painless and asymptomatic. There is a wide age distribution. It is more common in females. They are usually detected incidentally. In long bones, onset of pain and rapid increase in size are considered signs of malignant transformation. Lesions may be solitary or multiple (Maffucci syndrome and Ollier disease) [41]. Multiple lesions usually occur in younger age group, and incidence of malignant transformation is common in these syndromes (25% of cases) [40, 42]. Soft tissue chondromas are rare. If purely chondroid, it occurs in hands and feet. Rarely, large chondromas occur in the dura mater in the falx cerebri. Somatic mutations of IDH1/IDH2 (isocitrate dehydrogenase genes) are found in 50% of enchondromas and 90% of cases with multiple enchondromatosis [31, 39]. A mutant PTH/PTHrP type I receptor (PTHR1) is identified in enchondromatosis [34].

4.1.3.2 Radiology

They are metadiaphyseal, small (<5 cm) and well-demarcated tumours (Fig. 4.3). In hands and feet, there is expansion of the bone, and they are sometimes associated with a pathological fracture. Pathological fracture associated with chondroid lesion in a long bone is more likely to be chondrosarcoma. The pattern of mineralization is referred to as popcorn or ring-like calcification. Calcification not evident in plain X-ray can be appreciated in CT scan. Increased scalloping of the inner margins of the bone by the tumour indicates aggressive nature of the tumour. Unless there is a fracture, cortical destruction is absent in enchondromas. MRI is helpful in confirming the lack of permeation and cortical involvement. The cortex is thinned in chondromas of small bones. This should not be taken as a sign of malignancy [33].

Periosteal chondromas are small, 2–3 cm in size. Since it is on the surface of bone, it causes saucerization of the cortex (Fig. 4.5a). A sclerotic margin can be seen, and it is well demarcated. On bone scan, enchondromas are hot.

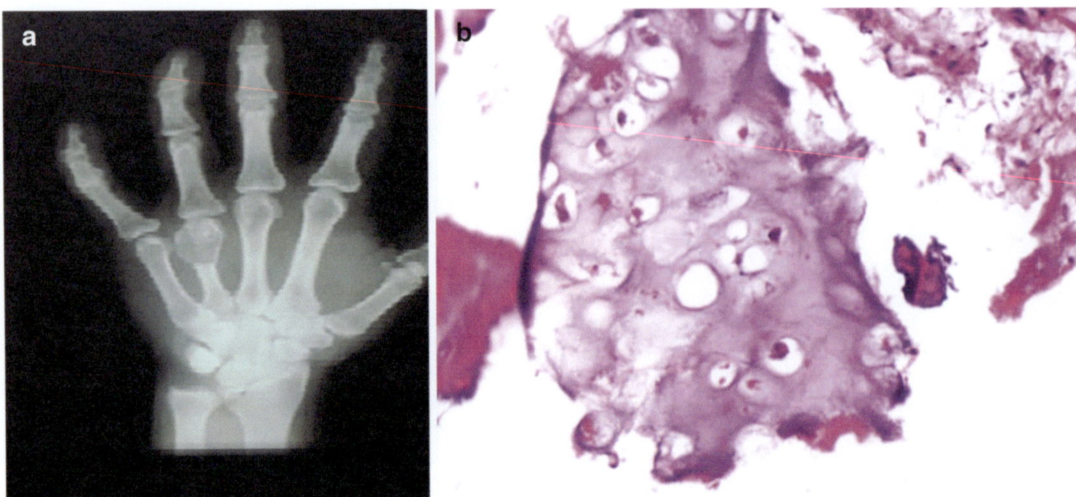

Fig. 4.3 Enchondroma in metacarpal bone in a 34-year-old male: (**a**) Expansile lytic lesion. Tumour is seen abutting the cortex, but not destroying it. (**b**) Hyaline cartilage tumour with enlarged chondrocytes lying loosely in the medullary cavity, H&E ×250

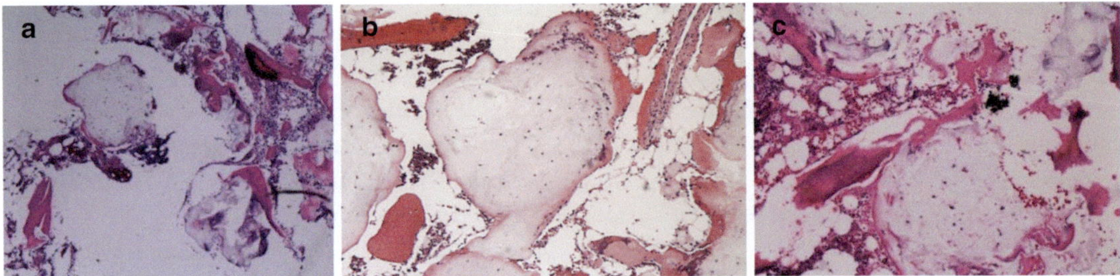

Fig. 4.4 Enchondroma humerus: (**a**) Loose clusters of grade I hyaline cartilage in marrow space, H&E ×40. (**b**, **c**) Encasement of tumour in enchondroma, H&E ×100

4.1.3.3 Pathology

Gross: It is well circumscribed, lobulated with glistening cut surface. A myxoid watery appearance indicates malignancy.

Microscopy: In enchondromas, hyaline cartilage is seen as lobules, which lie loosely in marrow cavity (Fig. 4.4b). The lobules will lie in the marrow without destroying or entrapping medullary bone (Fig. 4.4). Cortical destruction and soft tissue extension in the absence of a fracture are signs of malignancy. The cartilage is usually hypocellular. But the cartilage can be cellular with pleomorphism in enchondromas of small bones of hands and feet and in periosteal chondroma. Even myxoid change can be observed. This should not be mistaken for malignancy. If the chondroid neoplasm of small tubular bone is malignant, it will be obvious in plain X-ray. If bone is entrapped or the tumour permeates through the cortex, the diagnosis is chondrosarcoma.

Periosteal chondroma and **soft tissue chondromas** show clustering of chondrocytes, which is a feature of benign tumours (Fig. 4.5c). Myxoid change and cytologic atypia can be seen (Fig. 4.5d). Soft tissue chondromas have elongated grooved nuclei similar to chondroblastoma. 15% of the soft tissue tumours show osteoclastic giant cells. Double-nucleated cells are common. It should not be mistaken as a feature of malig-

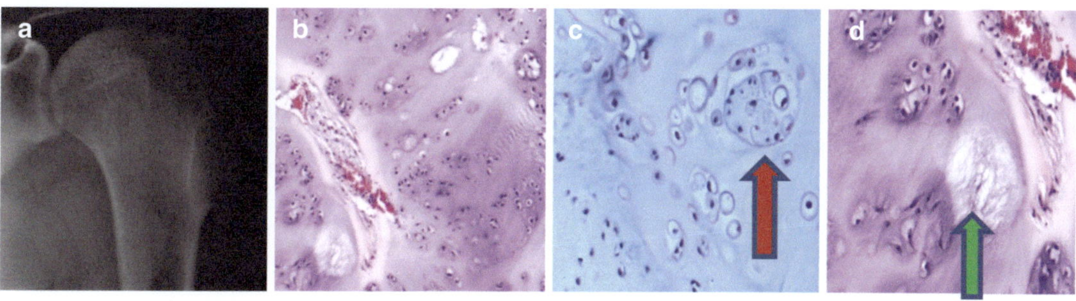

Fig. 4.5 (**a**) Plain X-ray showing well-demarcated lytic surface lesion at metaphysis of humerus with a sclerotic border (saucerization). (**b**) Periosteal chondroma with mild increase in cellularity, H&E ×100. (**c**) Clustering of chondrocytes in periosteal chondroma (red arrow), H&E ×250. (**d**) Myxoid change in periosteal chondroma (green arrow), H&E ×250

nancy. Sometimes, several nuclei may be seen in a lacuna. Necrosis, atypia and mitosis are absent.

4.1.3.4 Differential Diagnosis

- Grade I chondrosarcomas: this will be discussed under chondrosarcoma [32, 33, 37].
- Secondary or peripheral chondrosarcoma: periosteal chondromas are often confused with secondary and peripheral chondrosarcoma. Radiologically sclerotic margin, small size of the lesion and sharp circumscription indicate benign nature of the tumour. Clustering of chondrocytes, lack of myxoid change and permeation are helpful features to distinguish from sarcoma.
- Fracture or recent injury can show active fibrocartilaginous proliferation. This should not be mistaken for malignant disease. The appearance may simulate dedifferentiated chondrosarcoma.

4.1.3.5 Treatment and Prognosis

Both enchondromas and periosteal chondromas are benign tumours. If the lesion needs to be removed, enchondromas are treated by curettage followed by cement or bone graft. Periosteal chondromas usually do not require resection. If resected, they generally do not recur. Chondromas of small tubular bone require treatment because they can cause pathological fracture.

4.1.4 Enchondroma Protuberans

This is extremely rare (less than 1% of enchondromas). It is an eccentric protuberation—exophytic enchondroma with a small intramedullary component.

4.1.4.1 Radiology

It protrudes from the surface of bone and resembles soft tissue chondroma. MRI is helpful in the diagnosis. A complete thin periosteal shell with low intensity on MRI is seen at the periphery of the lesion, suggesting a benign diagnosis.

4.1.4.2 DD

Osteochondroma, periosteal chondroma and soft tissue chondromas are the main differentials. Histologically, it is an enchondroma with less cellular grade I hyaline cartilage. If it is misinterpreted as soft tissue extension, a wrong diagnosis of chondrosarcoma may be given. Radiology correlation helps in differentiation.

4.1.5 Enchondromatosis (Multiple Chondromas)

Multiple chondromas occur due to dysplasia of bone [38]. This causes failure of normal endochondral ossification and proliferation, which in

Table 4.1 Common syndromes of enchondromatosis

	Ollier	Maffucci	Metachondromatosis (OC+ enchondromas)
Age	Early childhood	At birth or early childhood	Childhood, regress by adulthood
Mode of inheritance	Nonhereditary	Nonhereditary	Hereditary: autosomal dominant PTPN11 gene mutation
Clinical	Metaphysis of long bones Deformity Pathological #	Small and long tubular bones Bilateral Cavernous and spindle haemangioma	Hands, feet, femur, tibia, pelvis Asymptomatic
Risk of other tumours	Glioma and juvenile granulosa cell tumour	Angiosarcoma astrocytoma Pituitary adenoma Adenocarcinoma of pancreas	Nil
Risk of malignancy	**5–50% chance**	**53%**	**Low**

turn results in formation of cartilaginous masses in the bone and adjacent regions. In addition, it causes bowing and shortening of bones.

Enchondromatosis is a heterogeneous group of diseases. The most important among them are Ollier disease, Maffucci syndrome and metachondromatosis (Table 4.1). Somatic mosaic mutations of IDH1 and IDH2 are seen in both Ollier and Maffucci syndromes [31]. Ollier disease [41] is unilateral with multiple bone involvement. When associated with angiomas of soft tissue, it is called Maffucci syndrome. Spindle cell haemangiomas are common [39]. Cavernous and other types of haemangiomas are also described. In 25% of patients with Ollier disease, chondrosarcomas develop by 40 years of age [36, 42]. The incidence of malignancy is higher in Maffucci syndrome [30]. Enchondromas located in the pelvis have the highest risk of developing malignancy [40]. Sporadic cases are common. Rarely, familial cases with autosomal dominant inheritance can be seen. They can also have gliomas and juvenile granulosa cell tumours.

The bones involved are expansile and popcorn type of calcification is seen as in chondroma. Sometimes, massive calcifications of chondroid lesions are seen in metadiaphyseal regions of long bones. The cartilage in multiple chondromas is cellular with lobular architecture. The chondrocytes are oval without cytologic atypia. Slight myxoid change can be seen (Fig. 4.23). Sarcoma arising in these syndromes is usually chondrosarcoma (Fig. 4.23c). But osteosarcoma and chondroid chordoma are reported. Sudden increase in size of one of the lesions, associated with pain, is a sign of malignant transformation.

A favourable response to radiotherapy is reported in chondrosarcoma developing in Ollier disease [35].

4.1.6 Osteochondromas (OC) [43–60]

Osteochondroma is the most common benign cartilage lesion, which is seen on the surface of bone. Bony projection with a cartilaginous cap is seen. The outgrowth can be either sessile or pedunculated. It is usually located at the metaphyseal region of long bones [57, 59]. In osteochondromas, the cortex of the underlying bone and the marrow cavity it encloses is continuous with that of the osteochondroma.

4.1.6.1 Clinical

30% of benign bone tumours are osteochondromas. They are asymptomatic. They are detected incidentally, and hence the exact incidence is unknown for these tumours. Osteochondromas can be solitary or multiple. Multiple lesions are usually hereditary.

They have an autosomal dominant inheritance [46]. Both sporadic and familial lesions show alterations of EXT genes [45].

4.1.6.2 Radiological features

Osteochondromas are seen mainly in the metaphysis of long bones (Fig. 4.6a, b). They are rarely located in short bones, phalanges, iliac wings (Fig. 4.6c) or vertebrae. CT scan shows continuity of the marrow between the lesion and the underlying bone. The thickness of the cap is better assessed by MRI (less than 1.5 cm). The cap thickness decreases with age [49].

4.1.6.3 Pathology

If removed intact, they project from the surface of bone as a stalk. It consists of cortical bone with inner medulla and a cartilage cap. To assess the cap thickness, it should be cut perpendicular to the cartilage cap. Malignancy should be ruled out if the cap thickness is greater than 2 cm.

Microscopically, the cartilage is hyaline cartilage with trabecular bone, fat and normal marrow particles. The cartilage shows an arrangement resembling a physis (growth plate), with columnar arrangement of chondrocytes (Fig. 4.7). At the junction of the cartilage and bone, endochondral ossification can be seen. Infarction in the lesion can show worrisome morphological features [47]. But radiology correlation helps in establishing the correct diagnosis. If there is a fracture or infarct, the adjacent areas show sec-

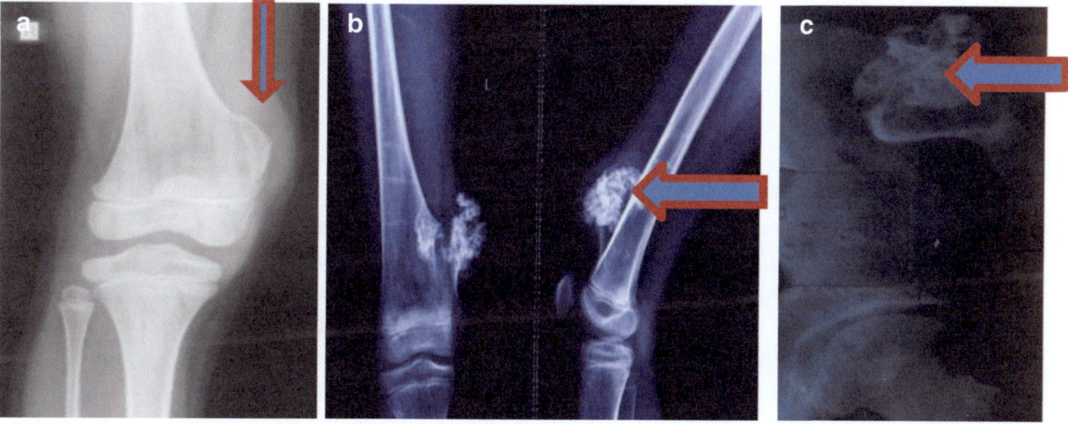

Fig. 4.6 OC: Plain X-ray: (**a**) sessile OC with broad base—femur lower end. (**b**) Pedunculated OC in an 11-year-old boy—lower end of femur. A stalk and cartilaginous cap. (**c**) Pedunculated OC of iliac bone

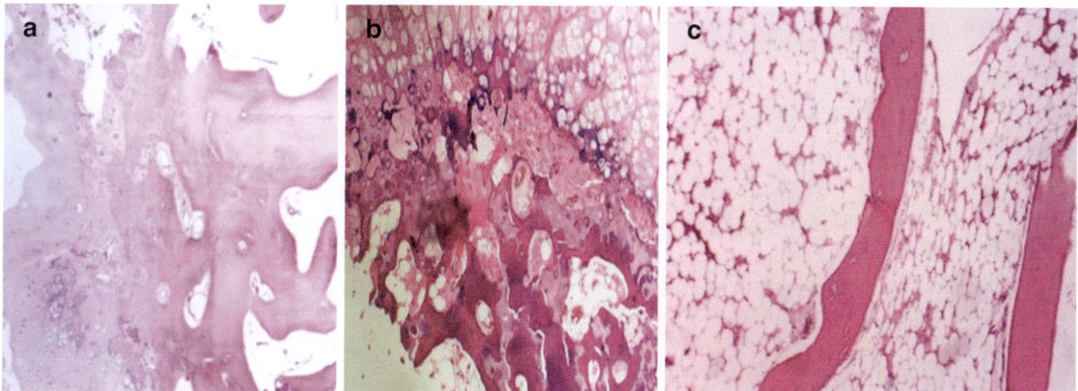

Fig. 4.7 Osteochondroma: (**a**, **b**) cartilaginous cap with endochondral ossification-like appearance. Note the columnar arrangement of chondrocytes, H&E ×40. (**c**) Underlying bone with marrow, H&E ×100

ondary changes (necrosis and repair). Rarely, a secondary chondrosarcoma can develop from osteochondroma [43, 44, 48]. The features are more than 2 cm thickness of cartilage cap, myxoid change of cartilage and evidence of infiltration into the adjacent soft tissues. Liquefaction of matrix, increased cellularity and loss of columnar arrangement of cartilage are other useful features to suggest malignancy. If atypical cartilage fills the low-power view in a section of osteochondroma, malignancy should be ruled out. This indirectly denotes that the cartilage cap is thick and abnormal.

4.1.6.4 Differential Diagnosis

- Parosteal osteosarcoma: Shows bland spindle cell proliferation between bony spicules. In osteochondromas, marrow is seen between bony spicules. Cartilage cap in osteosarcoma lacks the columnar arrangement and shows mild atypia.
- BPOP or Nora's lesion: These lesions mainly involve small bones of hands and feet, whereas OCs occur in long bones. The BPOP has no continuity with the cortex, but OC has continuity with the cortex.
- Other less important differential diagnoses are **osteophytes**, **subungual exostosis** and **secondary chondrosarcoma**.

4.1.6.5 Molecular

- Loss of EXT1 (exostosis gene): Del(8)(q24.1) [48]
- Increased BCl2 and PTH LH: higher if there is malignant transformation

4.1.6.6 Treatment and prognosis

Osteochondromas are benign tumours. When they cause mechanical or cosmetic problems or compression of nerves or vessels, they are excised. If they are not excised completely, they may recur.

4.1.7 Osteochondromatosis (Multiple Hereditary Exostoses)

15% of osteochondromas are multiple [46] (Fig. 4.8) with autosomal dominant inheritance. 90% of these patients have germline mutations in the tumour suppressor gene EXT1 or EXT2 [45]. Shortening of the ulna and displacement of the radius can be seen in some cases. The fibula also may be shortened. The risk of malignancy developing in multiple exostoses is unknown. It varies from less than 1–27.3% in various studies.

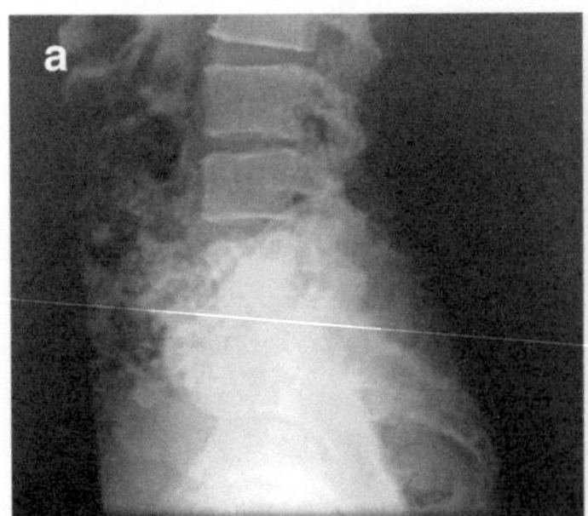

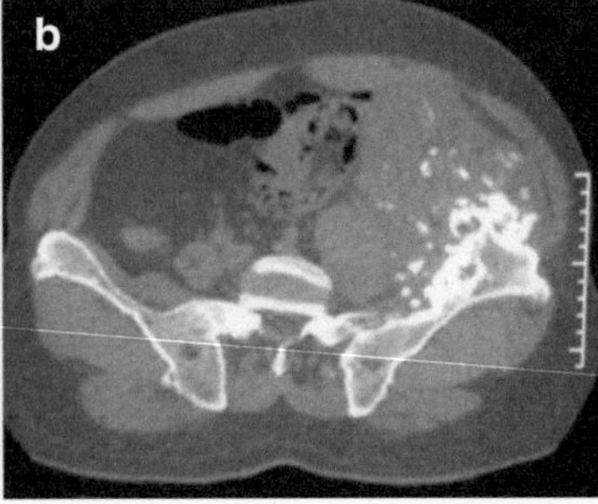

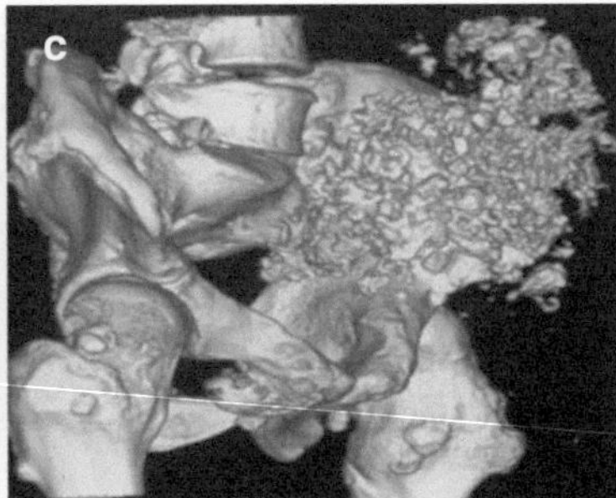

Fig. 4.8 Osteochondromatosis in a 46-year-old man. Two of his brothers also had osteochondromatosis. He developed chondrosarcoma in one of the swellings. (**a**) Plain X-ray. (**b**) MRI showing multiple OCs. (**c**) 3-dimensional CT picture

Recent increase in size associated with pain in previous osteochondroma should arouse suspicion of progressive disease. 18-FDG PET scan can help in the differentiation of benign and malignant osteochondromas [49]. Conventional chondrosarcomatous transformation is the most common malignant transformation seen in osteochondroma [43, 44, 47, 48] (Fig. 4.9). But osteosarcoma [50, 51] and dedifferentiated chondrosarcomas have also been reported.

Histologically, if the cartilage is occupying one low-power field, it is a worrisome feature and should suspect malignant transformation (Fig. 4.10). Usually, thickness of cartilage is >2 cm in these cases.

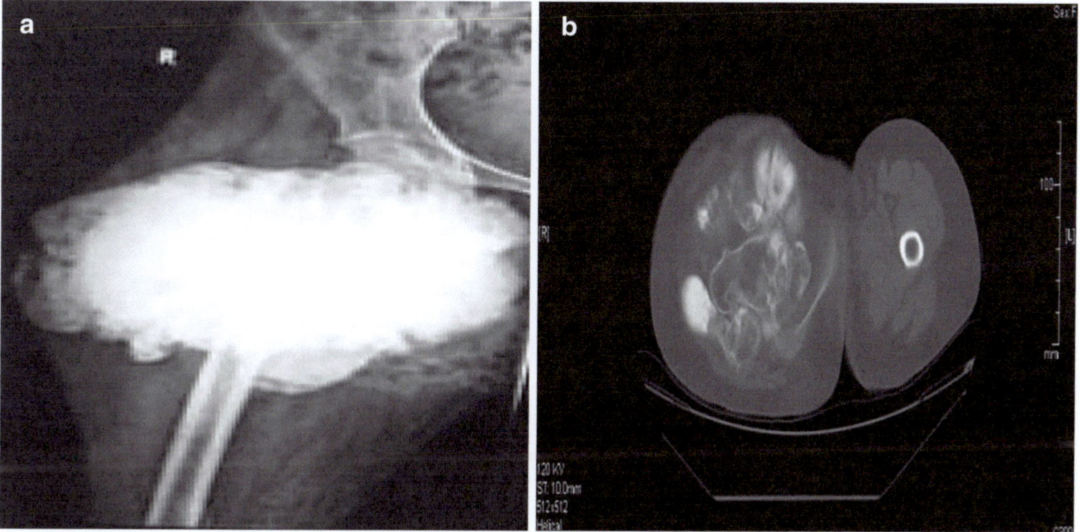

Fig. 4.9 Chondrosarcoma arising in osteochondroma in a 21-year-old female. (**a**) Plain X-ray. (**b**) MRI

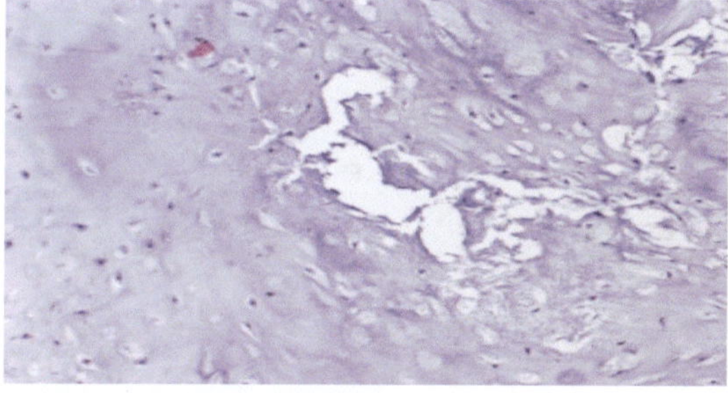

Fig. 4.10 OC: low-power view showing atypical cartilage only. An evidence that thickness of cartilage is >2 cm and malignant transformation should be suspected. H&E ×100

4.1.8 Chondroblastoma (CB)

Chondroblastoma is a tumour of epiphyses and apophyses of skeletally immature patients [53, 65]. It rarely occurs in older patients and unusual locations [59–61]. Most tumours are seen in long bones [74]. It is also described in short bones, flat bones, vertebrae and craniofacial skeleton [64, 74]. Majority of cases occur around knee-proximal tibia and distal femur. Other preferred sites are upper humerus, calcaneum, talus [52, 66], patella and temporal bone [62]. It constitutes >50% of benign tumours of patella.

4.1.8.1 Clinical

The patients present with pain, limping, stiffness or effects due to tumour [81]. Tinnitus and progressive loss of hearing are the complaints in temporal bone lesions. Some patients may present with oncogenic osteomalacia. FGF 23 can be positive in chondroblastoma [83]. This is a phosphatonin produced by tumours causing osteomalacia.

4.1.8.2 Radiological features

The lesions are lytic, epiphyseal, small (generally less than 5 cm) and sharply demarcated with a sclerotic rim (Figs. 4.11 and 4.12). Giant chondroblastomas are described which can be mistaken for malignancy [81]. They can occur at any centre of ossification like greater trochanter. When the lesion involves epiphysis and metaphysis adjacent to epiphyseal plate (both sides of epiphyseal plate), it is diagnostic of chondroblastoma. In flat bones, there will be expansion of bone and periosteal reaction. Mineralized matrix or a aneurysmal cyst like changes may be seen in a few cases [68]. In the pelvic bone, it usually arises in triradiate cartilage [74]. Peritumoural oedema is seen in MRI and should not be mistaken for permeation.

4.1.8.3 Pathology

Microscopically, the characteristic cell is the chondroblast. Cells are oval with well-defined cytoplasmic borders, moderate pink or pale cytoplasm and oval nucleus showing a prominent longitudinal groove (coffee bean appearance) (Fig. 4.13). Osteoclasts may be present throughout the lesion. An immature pink chondroid matrix is usually seen (Fig. 4.14). Calcification around the degenerating tumour cells, classically described as "chicken wire" calcification, may be seen (Figs. 4.15 and 4.16). Even though common, this is not pathognomonic of chondroblastoma. Such calcification can be seen in other conditions like osteosarcoma also. Atypia of the stromal cells can be mistaken for malignancy. Some people call these tumours aggressive chon-

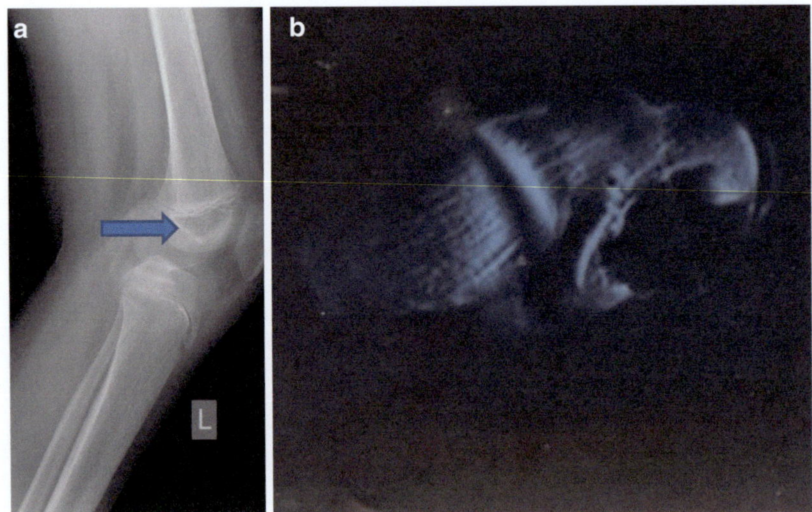

Fig. 4.11 CB: (**a**) Plain X-ray of lower end of femur in the epiphysis with a sclerotic border. (**b**) Lateral view of 3D CT showing well-defined lytic area

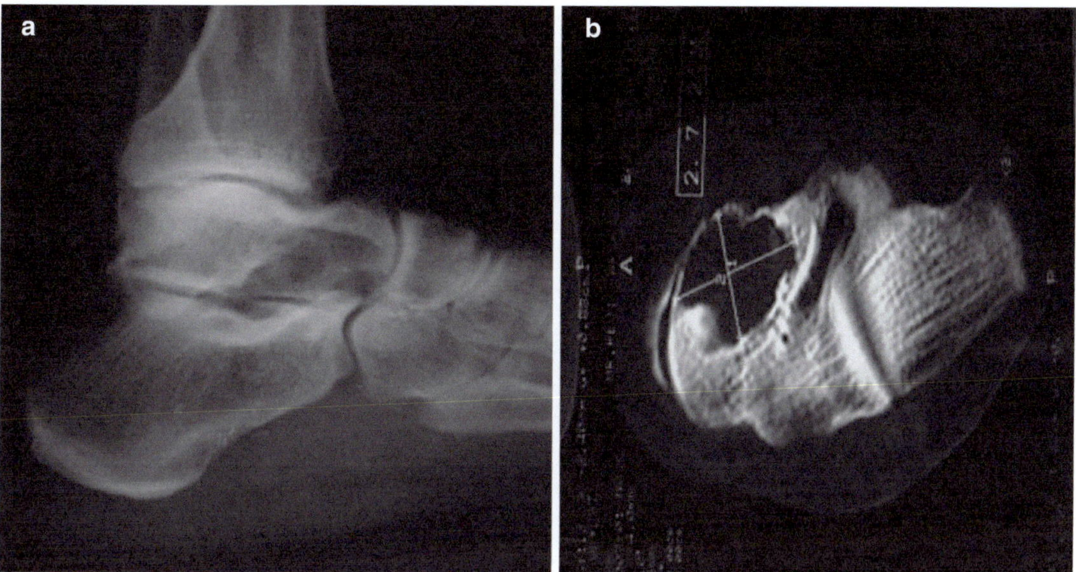

Fig. 4.12 CB talus. (**a**) Plain X-ray showing lytic lesion with sclerotic border. (**b**) 3D CT of same case

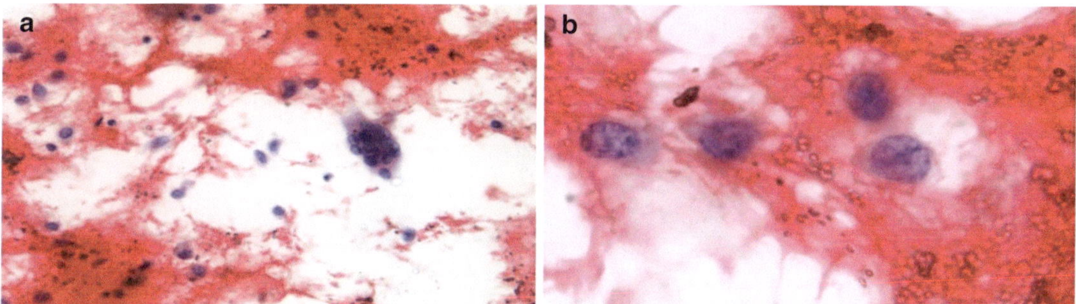

Fig. 4.13 FNAC from a case of CB. (**a**) Low power: chondroblasts and osteoclastic giant cells, PapX40. (**b**) High power showing chondroblasts with convoluted nuclei, Pap X250

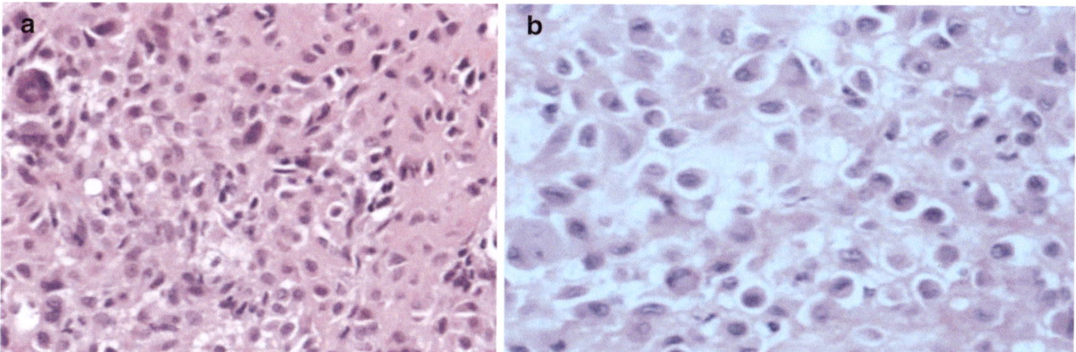

Fig. 4.14 CB: (**a**) Low power with chondroblasts, chondroid matrix and osteoclastic giant cells, H&E ×100. (**b**) Chondroblasts with abundant eosinophilic cytoplasm and convoluted nuclei with nuclear grooves, H&E ×400

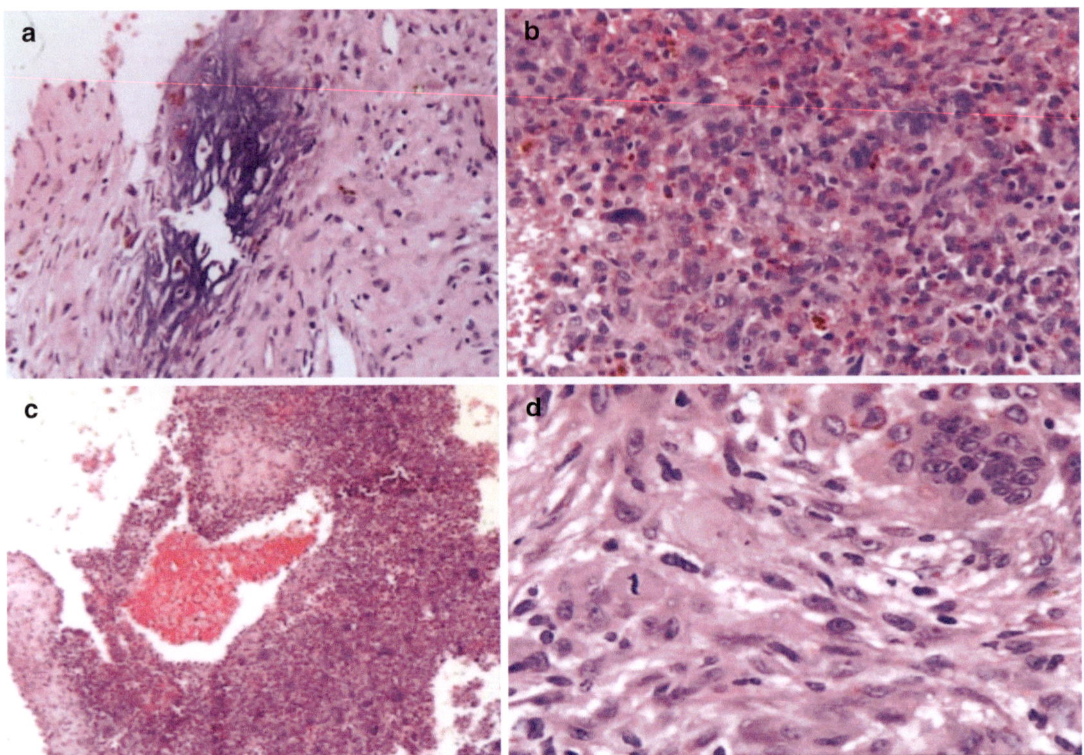

Fig. 4.15 CB in temporal bone in a 36-year-old male. This tumour recurred three times. (**a**) Chicken wire calcification, H&E ×100. (**b**) Haemosiderin laden cells, H&E ×250. (**c**) Secondary ABC with blood-filled space, H&E ×40. (**d**) Fibroblasts in the stroma of cyst wall and scattered giant cells, H&E ×250

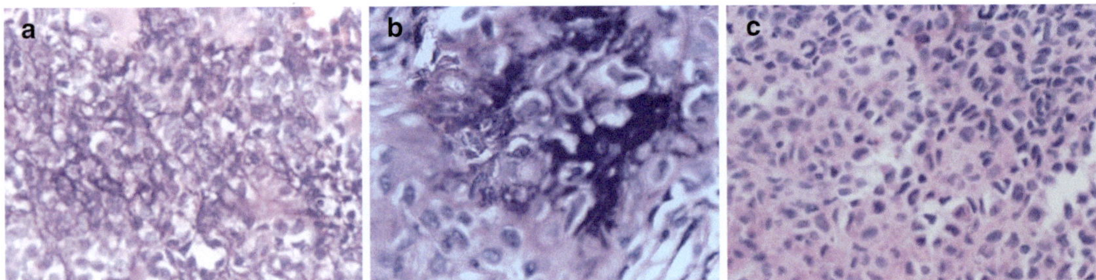

Fig. 4.16 CB vertebra. (**a**) Chicken wire calcification in CB—individual cells surrounded by calcification, H&E ×100. (**b**) H&E ×400. (**c**) Chondroblasts and chondroid matrix, H&E ×100

droblastomas [67, 79]. Presence of a few typical mitoses is not uncommon. Hemosiderin deposition can be present in temporal bone tumours. Secondary aneurysmal bone cyst formation is common [68] (Fig. 4.17). This must be kept in mind while grossing tumours with aneurysmal bone cyst-like areas. A search for focal solid areas should be done so that the primary lesion is not missed. USP6 gene translocations are absent. The chondroblasts are usually positive for S-100 protein, SOX9 and vimentin. H3F3B mutations have been described in chondroblastomas [55, 57, 72]. IHC for H3.3K 36M is a specific and sensitive marker for CB.

Malignant chondroblastoma [76, 78] is a recently introduced terminology for those chon-

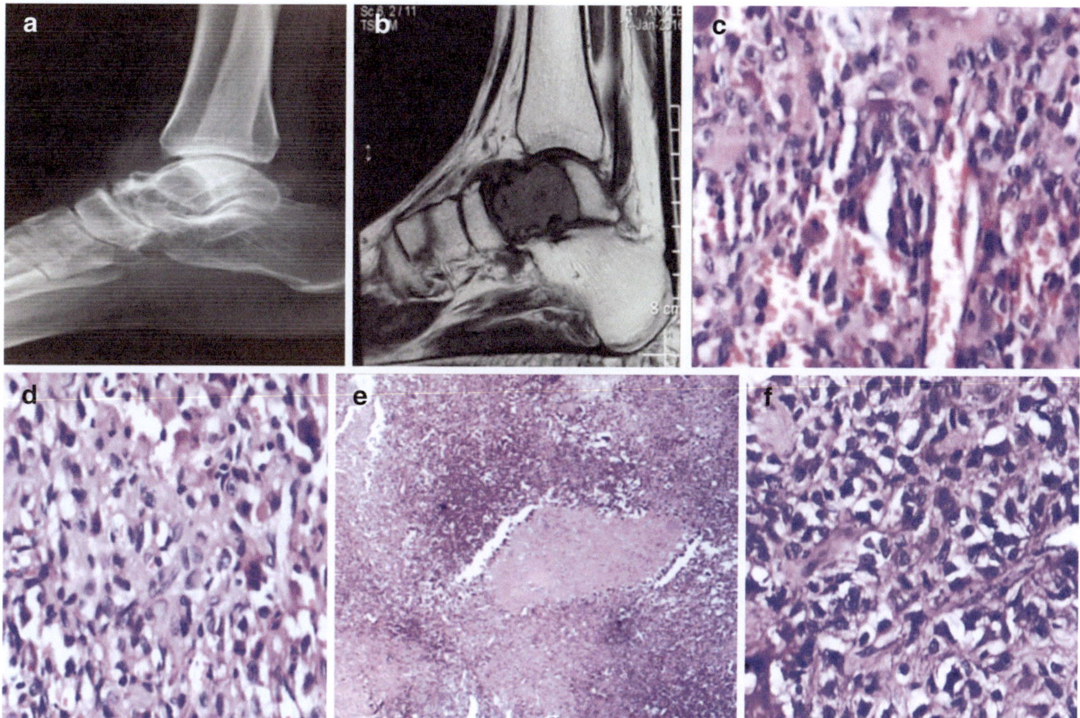

Fig. 4.17 Male 17 years, well-defined lytic lesion talus. (**a**, **b**) X-ray and MRI showing well-defined lytic lesion. (**c**, **d**) Cells with atypia and ABC like changes, H&E ×250. (**e**, **f**) Second biopsy showing chondroblasts and matrix. (**e**) Chondroid matrix H&E ×40. (**f**) Chondroblasts with mild atypia, H&E ×250. Radiology correlation helped in differentiation from osteosarcoma in this case

droblastomas with cytologic atypia and permeative growth. These tumours are positive for H3K36M by IHC. Malignant chondroblastoma occurs in older individuals, and mean age is 52 years. They are described in unusual sites like scapula and vertebra. Those tumours lacking H3F3B K36M mutation are designated as chondroblastoma-like osteosarcoma. Chondroblastoma-like osteosarcoma occurs in younger patients (<20 years), and they produce tumour osteoid. No mutations in H3F3A/H3F3B are seen in osteosarcomas.

4.1.8.4 Differential Diagnosis

The differential diagnosis mainly includes other epiphyseal tumours like giant cell tumour of bone and clear cell chondrosarcoma [75]. Other DDs are chondroblastic osteosarcomas and chondromyxoid fibroma.

1. Giant cell tumour: In GCT, the nuclei of mononuclear cells in giant cell tumour resemble nuclei in osteoclastic giant cells. Nuclear grooves are absent. They are positive for histiocytic markers. The characteristic chondroid matrix of chondroblastoma is absent in giant cell tumour. Giant cell tumours occur in skeletally mature patients. IHC for H3.3G34W is a sensitive and specific marker for GCT. Calcification is uncommon in GCT.
2. Chondroblastic osteosarcoma: OSs are usually metaphyseal, and the cells are high-grade cartilage cells in lobules with peripheral cellular areas and spindling of cells. Osteoid may or may not be present.
3. Chondromyxoid fibroma: Chondroblastomas can show areas resembling CMF. The site of involvement of CMF is usually metaphyseal.
4. Chondrosarcoma [63].

4.1.8.5 Cytogenetics and Molecular Diagnostic Pathology

Structural abnormalities of chromosomes 5 and 8 and H3F3B alterations on chromosome 17 are seen in >95% of cases [55, 57, 72]. IDH1 and IDH2 mutations are not seen in chondroblastomas.

4.1.8.6 Treatment and Prognosis

Chondroblastomas are benign tumours. They are treated by intralesional or marginal procedures like curettage. Percutaneous radiofrequency ablation is given for small lesions [54, 58, 73, 77]. Yang et al. tried mTOR inhibitors and reported positive effects [84]. Large lesions at the weight-bearing surfaces are at an increased risk of articular collapse and recurrence [64, 65]. Some chondroblastomas can metastasize to lung [69–71, 82]. Rarely, rib [56], skin or soft tissue metastases are reported [82]. But they are amenable to treatments like metastasectomy.

4.1.9 Chondromyxoid Fibroma (CMF)

Chondromyxoid fibroma is a rare tumour. They occur in the second or third decade. It is composed of chondroid, myxoid and myofibroblastic components.

4.1.9.1 Clinical

Tibia is the most common site. It can also arise in flat bones (25%) predominantly in ilium. In the small bones of hands and feet, the most common site is metatarsal bones. Other sites are ulna [85] and skull base [87]. Like chondroblastoma, oncogenic malacia can be seen as a paraneoplastic syndrome. FGF 23 is found in some tumours [88].

4.1.9.2 Radiological Features

These tumours are sharply defined, eccentric and located in the metaphysis (Fig. 4.18). The small bones of the hands and feet can show expansion of bone with focal cortical break. The calcified matrix if present can be seen on CT scans.

4.1.9.3 Pathology

The tumour is seen as lobules of spindle cells in a myxoid stroma (Fig. 4.19). The lobules are cellular at the periphery, and the central portion is paucicellular (Fig. 4.20). This lobulation may not be evident in needle biopsy, and radiology correlation is mandatory in those cases (Fig. 4.21). It is well demarcated, and no infiltrative pattern is seen (Fig. 4.20a). Osteoclastic giant cells can be noted (Fig. 4.20f). Chondroblastoma-like areas may be seen (Fig. 4.20d, e). Mitotic activity is sparse. Secondary aneurysmal bone cyst formation is seen in some cases. Calcification is present in one-third of tumours (Fig. 4.19d). Well-developed hyaline cartilage is focally present (around 20%) in these tumours.

4.1.9.4 Differential Diagnosis

- Chondroblastoma: Usually, chondroblastomas are epiphyseal tumours, whereas CMF is

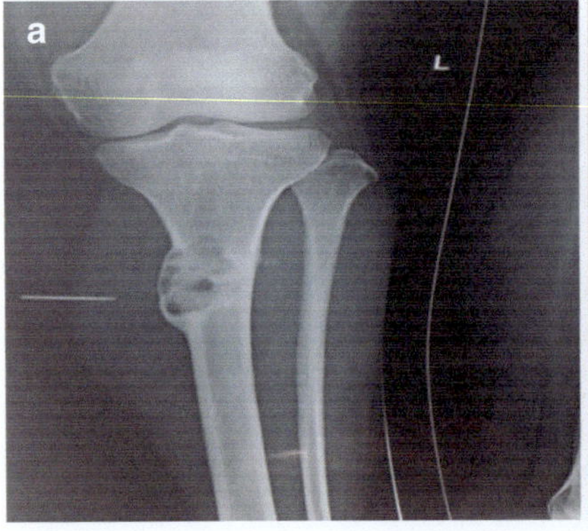

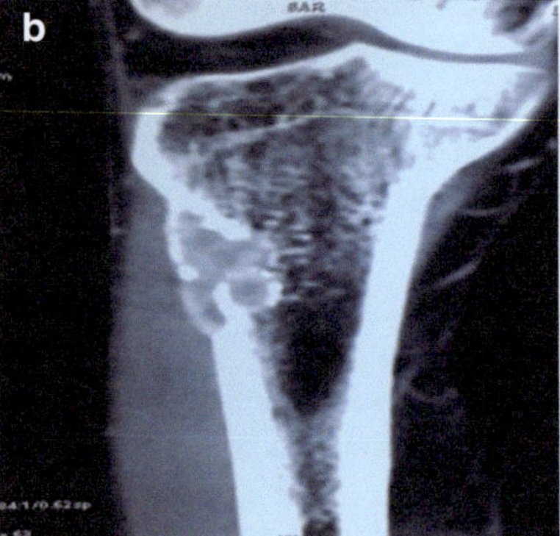

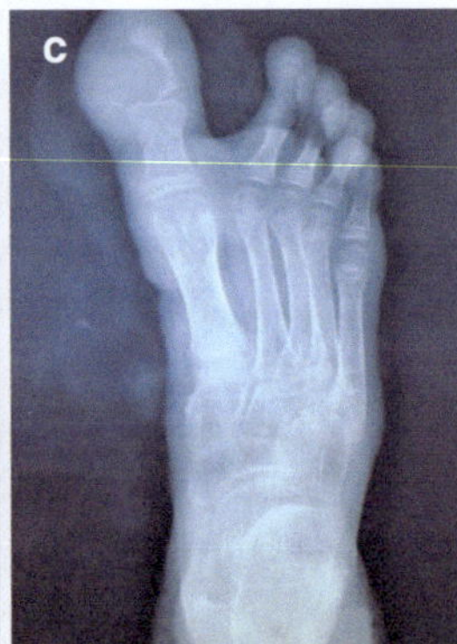

Fig. 4.18 CMF: (**a**) Metaphyseal eccentrically placed lesion with sclerotic border in plain X-ray. (**b**) MRI confirms narrow zone of transition. (**c**) Lytic lesion terminal phalanx of big toe

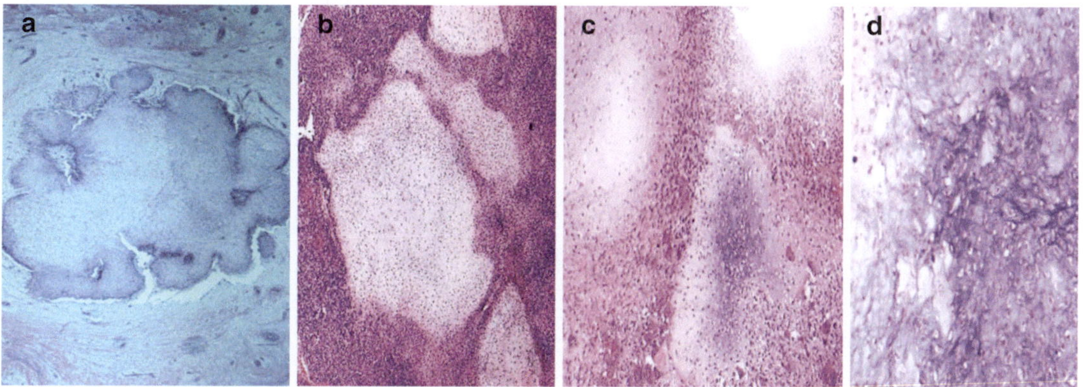

Fig. 4.19 CMF: (**a**, **b**) Lobulated appearance of CMF, H&E ×40. (**c**) CMF with cellular periphery and central hypocellular areas, H&E ×100. (**d**) Calcification, H&E ×100

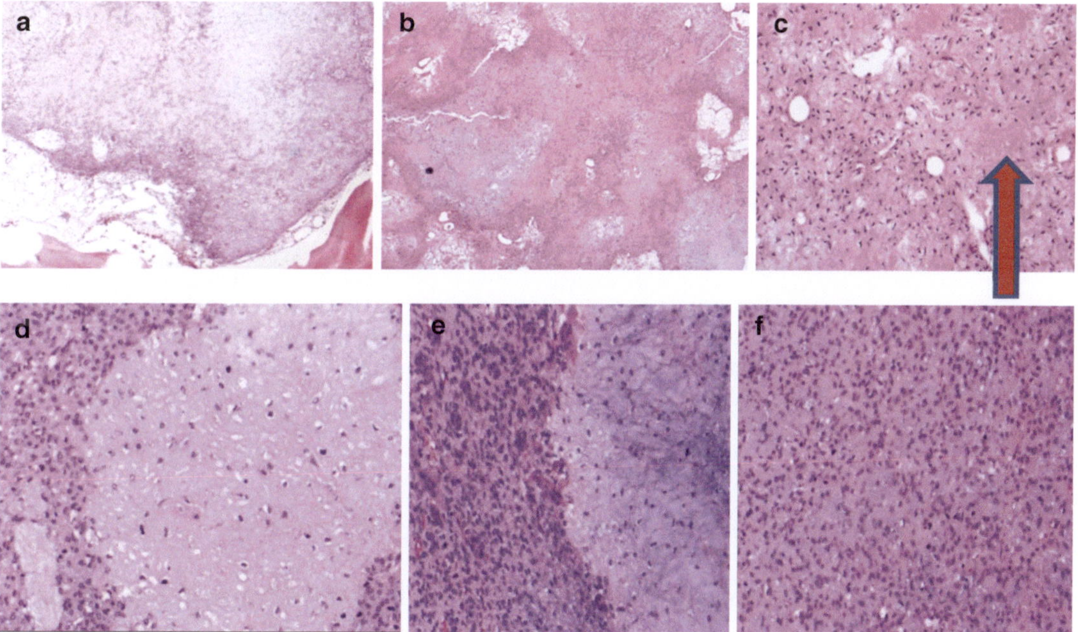

Fig. 4.20 CMF: (**a**) Bone with well-defined tumour, H&E ×40. (**b**) Lobules with cellular periphery and central hypocellular area, H&E ×100. (**c**) Red arrow showing hypocellular area, H&E ×250. (**d**) Chondroid area resembling chondroblastoma, H&E ×250. (**e**, **f**) Cellular periphery with osteoclastic giant cells and central myxoid hypocellular area, H&E ×250

metaphyseal. But there are overlaps between these two entities. Both are benign tumours.

- CMF like osteosarcoma [86]: The lesion has to be differentiated from a chondromyxoid fibroma like osteosarcoma, which is a low-grade osteosarcoma. Osteosarcoma is cellular with nuclear atypia, at least focally. The lobulated growth pattern seen in CMF is absent in OS, and it is seen in diffuse pattern. OS shows permeation of pre-existing bony spicules and soft tissue extension. Extensive liquefaction of stroma is also a worrisome feature.

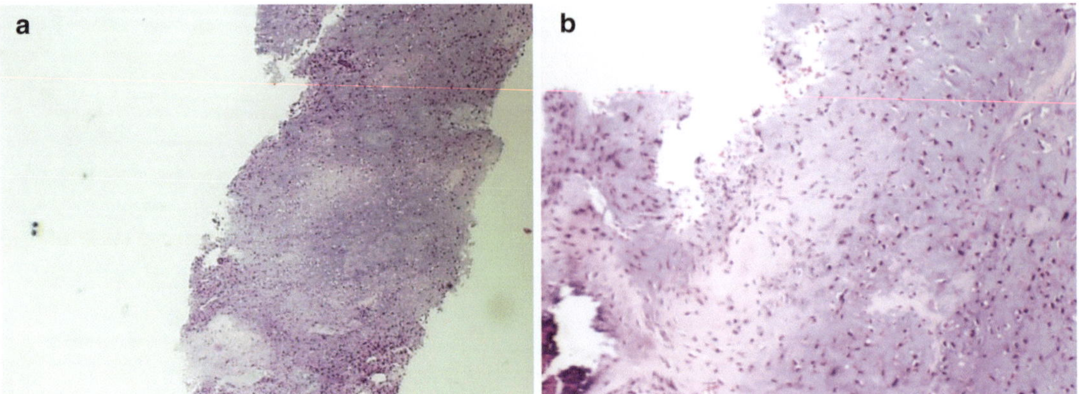

Fig. 4.21 CMF: In needle biopsy, it is difficult to see lobulation with peripheral cellular and central paucicellular areas. Radiology correlation is mandatory in these cases. (**a**) Needle biopsy showing cellular and hypocellular areas, H&E ×40. (**b**) Stellate cells in chondromyxoid background. H&E ×100

Table 4.2 Differentiating features between CMF and CS

Differentiation of CMF from CS		
	CMF	CS
Age	Second and third decades	Older age group
Sites	Long bones—metaphysis	Flat bones Long bones—diaphysis
Radiology	Sharply circumscribed, lobulated, eccentric and osteolytic Chondroid type of calcification rare	Poorly circumscribed, cortical destruction, soft tissue mass Chondroid type of calcification common
Low power appearance	Lobulated, circumscribed with cellular periphery and central hypocellular	Haphazard arrangement Hypercellular throughout
Myxoid change	Cystic or liquefactive change unusual	Cystic and liquefactive change common
Cells	Stellate or spindle cells. Hyaline cartilage cells rare	Hyaline cartilage cells with multinucleation and pleomorphism
Osteoclastic giant cells	Present at the periphery of lobules	Not seen
Permeation of pre-existing bone	Absent	Present

- Chondrosarcoma: Differentiation from CS is given in Table 4.2.
- Myxoma is another differential diagnosis, which usually occurs in jaw bones. Myxoma lacks the lobular growth pattern of chondromyxoid fibroma.

4.1.9.5 Molecular

Translocations: t (6; 9) and t (7; 12).
Rearrangement of Chr 6 at q13 and q25.

4.1.9.6 Treatment and Prognosis

Chondromyxoid fibromas are benign tumours. They are treated by curettage. CMF has excellent prognosis with a recurrence rate of 15%.

4.1.10 Osteochondromyxoma (OMX)

Osteochondromyxoma is an extremely rare bone tumour [115]. It is seen associated with 1% Carney complex cases. It is also called Carney bone tumour. This was first described by J. Aidan Carney in 1985. It is a combination of myxomas, spotty pigmentation and endocrine overactivity. Myxomas of heart, skin and breast; multiple endocrine neoplasms; psammomatous melanotic schwannomas; pigmented mucosal and skin lesions; Sertoli cell tumours; pituitary adenomas that secrete growth hormones; and ductal adenomas of breast are other components of this complex. At least two of these clinical criteria or one criterion with a family history of CNC/PRKARIA

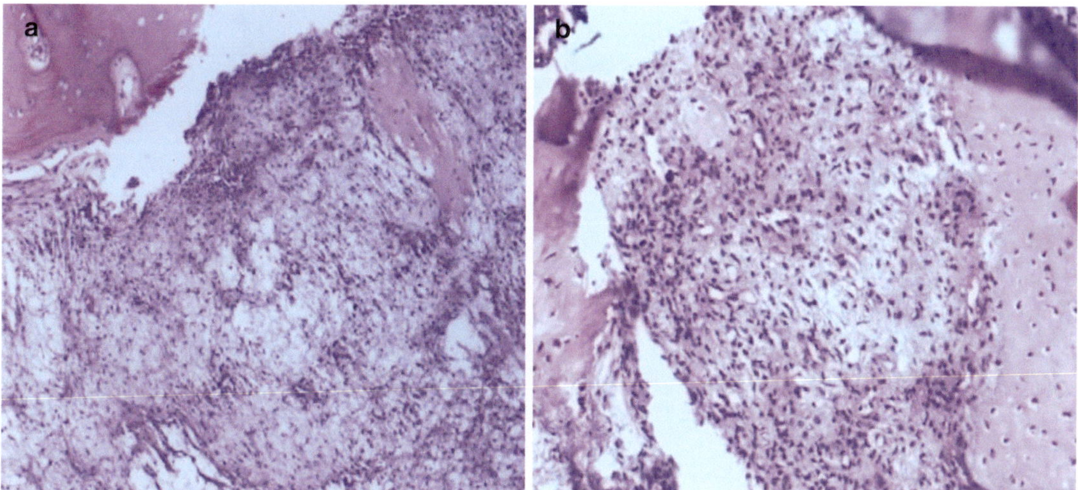

Fig. 4.22 Osteochondromyxoma. (**a**) Myxoid areas with stellate cells and hyaline band, H&E ×40. (**b**) Chondroblast-like cells and myxoid areas with clear cells, H&E ×100

mutation should be there to diagnose this disease.

4.1.10.1 Clinical

The common sites are nasal region, tibia and radius. It can occur at any age. Usually, it presents before 2 years of age and is also reported at birth. It presents as painless mass with symptoms related to oedema and mass effect or nasal obstruction leading to breastfeeding difficulties.

4.1.10.2 Radiology

It is well circumscribed but can be destructive and mineralized (Fig. 4.22a).

4.1.10.3 Pathology

Grossly, they are well-circumscribed bony or cartilaginous, calcified white mass eroding bone and sometimes extending to soft tissue. Histologically, lobules of hyaline cartilage admixed with osteoid and hyalinized bands are seen. It resembles BPOP morphologically. However, blue tinctorial quality of bone seen in BPOP is absent in OMX. Cells are polygonal or stellate with cytoplasmic vacuolation with occasional inclusion bodies. They are seen around myxochondroid areas (Fig. 4.22b). Chondroblast and osteoblast-like cells are commonly seen (Figs. 4.22c and 4.23) with small foci of adipocytes. Rarely, nuclear atypia is noted. Cells are positive for PAS and colloidal iron.

4.1.10.4 IHC

Cells are positive for vimentin and rarely for S100 protein.

4.1.10.5 Molecular

Carney complex carries an autosomal dominant trait with 100% penetrance. It is associated with mutations in 17q24 in the gene PRKARIA (CNC1) and in 2q31 in the gene PDE11A.

4.1.10.6 Treatment and Prognosis

Complete excision is the treatment. It has got a good prognosis. Recurrences can occur if the excision is not complet.

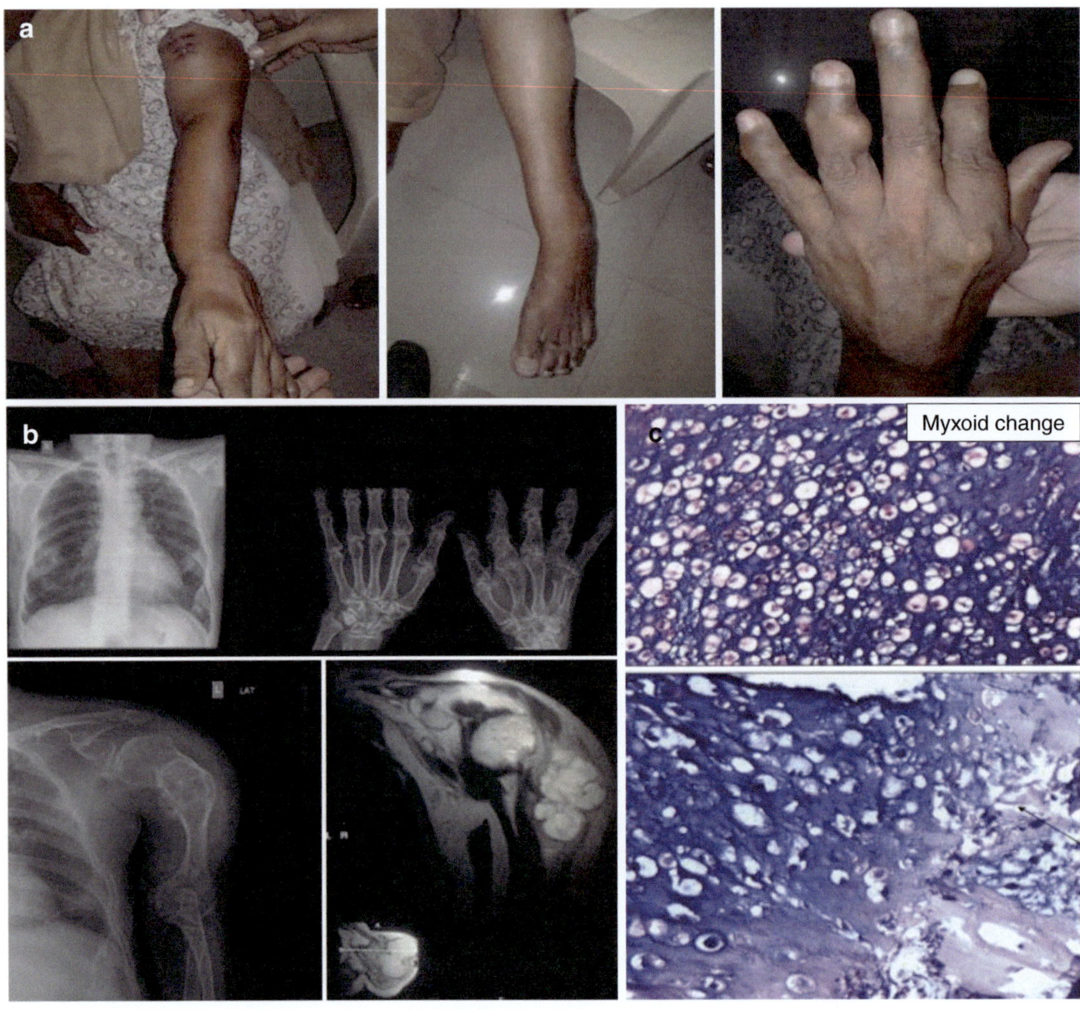

Fig. 4.23 Chondrosarcoma in Ollier disease in a 38-year-old female. (**a**) Clinical photograph of swellings in the upper arm and hands. (**b**) Radiographs of enchondromas involving ribs, hands, left arm and shoulder. (**c**) Biopsy showing hypercellularity and myxoid change, H&E ×250

4.2 Intermediate (Locally Aggressive) Tumours

In this group, synovial chondromatosis and atypical cartilaginous tumour are included.

4.2.1 Synovial Chondromatosis

Synovial chondromatosis is discussed in the chapter on synovial tumours (Chap. 18).

4.2.2 Atypical cartilaginous tumour/grade I chondrosarcoma (ACT/CS 1)

The common hyaline cartilage tumours within the intramedullary cavity are benign enchondromas and malignant chondrosarcomas. Chondrosarcomas are of three grades. Distinction of grade I chondrosarcomas and enchondromas requires clinical and radiological correlation [97]. This difficulty was dealt with by a new ter-

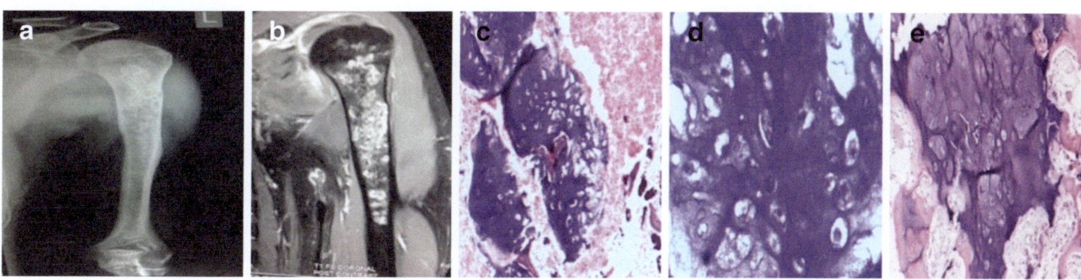

Fig. 4.24 Atypical cartilaginous tumour of humerus. (**a**) Plain X-ray showing lesion in humerus with stippled calcification, endosteal scalloping and irregular thickening of cortex. (**b**) MRI showing the extent of lesion (>5 cm) with no definite cortical destruction. (**c**) Hyaline cartilage and blood, H&E ×40. (**d**) Increased cellularity with open chromatin and small nucleolus, H&E ×400. (**e**) Entrapment between bony spicules, H&E ×250

minology, atypical cartilaginous tumour/grade I chondrosarcoma in WHO 2013 [141], which is similar to the WHO classification of atypical lipomatous tumour/well-differentiated liposarcoma. This modification places atypical cartilaginous tumour/grade I chondrosarcoma into an intermediate (locally aggressive) category. Tumours of appendicular skeleton are termed ACT, and those of axial skeleton (scapula, pelvis, etc.) are termed chondrosarcoma grade I [100]. Similar to the terminology of atypical lipomatous tumour, the terminology of atypical cartilaginous tumour is used for tumours of appendicular skeleton. Chondrosarcoma grade I terminology is used for the same tumour in axial skeleton such as pelvis, scapula and base of skull.

4.2.2.1 Radiology

In this, the lesion is intraosseous with a size of 5 cm, cortical deep scalloping without cortical break is observed and soft tissue involvement is rare. There is enhancement on dynamic gadolinium chelate-enhanced MRI [5] within seconds, which is absent in enchondroma. Radiologically, it closely mimics enchondroma.

4.2.2.2 Pathology

There are many overlapping features between ACT and enchondroma [100]. The most important diagnostic feature is entrapment of pre-existing lamellar bone. There is absence of encasement also in ACT. Another feature favouring ACT is more than 20% myxoid change of matrix. On small biopsy, this distinction is very difficult, and one has to correlate with clinical and radiological findings. Localization of tumour is also important. These tumours have abundant hyaline cartilage matrix. Increased cellularity with irregular distribution, small condensed nuclei and double-nucleated cells with absence of mitoses and severe nuclear atypia, in the medulla of long bone, favour ACT (Fig. 4.24), whereas the same findings in small bones of hands and feet or in a patient with enchondromatosis favour enchondroma. The features of ACT are given in Table 4.3.

Table 4.3 Features of atypical cartilaginous tumour

Atypical cartilaginous tumour
• Locally aggressive hyaline cartilage neoplasm
• Tumours in appendicular skeleton: ACT
• Tumours of axial skeleton: CS grade I
• Cortical scalloping without frank full-thickness cortical destruction visible on plain X-ray
• Enhancement within seconds on gadolinium contrast MRI
• Presence of entrapment of bone
• >20% myxoid change, ↑ cellularity, irregular distribution, binucleation, open chromatin and visible nucleoli
• IDH1 and IDH2 mutations+
• Conservative treatment: appendicular skeleton—curettage, axial skeleton—resection

4.2.2.3 Treatment and Prognosis

These tumours are treated by surgical curettage and followed up closely. Radical treatment is not given. They are locally aggressive tumours. Local recurrence is seen in 7–11% of tumours. They never metastasize. 10-Year survival rate is 83–95%. Recurrent tumours can transform to higher grade.

4.3 Malignant

4.3.1 Chondrosarcoma (CS)

4.3.1.1 Conventional CS

Chondrosarcomas (CSs) are malignant hyaline cartilage tumours. They are second common sarcomas of bone in adults [112]. Chondrosarcomas can be central or peripheral. Central chondrosarcomas arise de novo, whereas the peripheral chondrosarcomas arise commonly within a pre-existing osteochondroma. Another classification of CS is conventional (75–85%) and less common subtypes like clear cell chondrosarcoma, dedifferentiated chondrosarcoma and mesenchymal chondrosarcoma. The recent WHO classification (2020) includes chondrosarcoma of axial skeleton (CS grade I), and chondrosarcomas grade II and III under malignant category [115].

Secondary chondrosarcomas [44] arise in osteochondromas especially in the multiple, familial type. They are also seen in Ollier disease and Maffucci syndrome. Chondrosarcomas can develop de novo in soft tissues and in teratomas. In the joints, CS can be secondary to synovial chondromatosis.

Chondrosarcomas usually occur in adults, mostly in fourth, fifth and sixth decades. Patients with secondary chondrosarcomas are younger—in third and fourth decades. In the second decade, one has to rule out chondroblastic osteosarcoma when malignant cartilage is seen. Rarely, chondrosarcomas can occur in children [117].

More than two-thirds of CS occur in the trunk and the upper ends of humerus and femur [94]. The most commonly involved sites are the proximal femur, bones of the pelvis [108] (particularly the ilium) and proximal humerus. Other sites are distal femur, ribs, tibia and metacarpal and metatarsal bones. Spine, skull base and craniofacial bones are rare sites [109]. In the maxillary region, nasal bone is the preferred site. CS can occur in the base of the skull, where it is difficult to differentiate from chondroid chordomas [109]. CSs of small bones of hands and feet are extremely rare. Chondroid tumours of cricoid and sternum usually show malignant behaviour and are diagnosed as chondrosarcomas even if they are benign looking [102, 112].

Clinical

CS is a slow-growing tumour, with swelling and pain being presenting symptoms. Pathologic fracture may be the presenting symptom in some patients. When CS arises in osteochondromas or enchondromatosis, sudden increase in size associated with pain is the presenting complaint. Inadequately treated cases have a history of multiple recurrences. The interval between treatment and recurrence can be 5–10 years. When a mass cannot be palpated, the diagnosis may be difficult especially CS of innominate bone or acetabulum.

Radiology

Chondrosarcomas are large tumours usually more than 5 cm in size (Fig. 4.25). 75% of cases show characteristic mineralization on plain X-ray (Fig. 4.26). Calcification not evident on plain X-ray can be visualized on computerized tomograms [103] (CT scan). Areas of lucency in an otherwise calcified lesion indicate malignancy. Cortical abnormalities like destruction and soft tissue extension (40%) can be seen in the majority of cases (Fig. 4.27). About 20% of cases show expansion of bone and cortical thickening. Periosteal new bone formation is unusual. In small bones of hands and feet, there should be cortical destruction and extension to soft tissue to call a cartilage tumour as malignant [120] (Fig. 4.32). Vertebral lesions are seen in the body

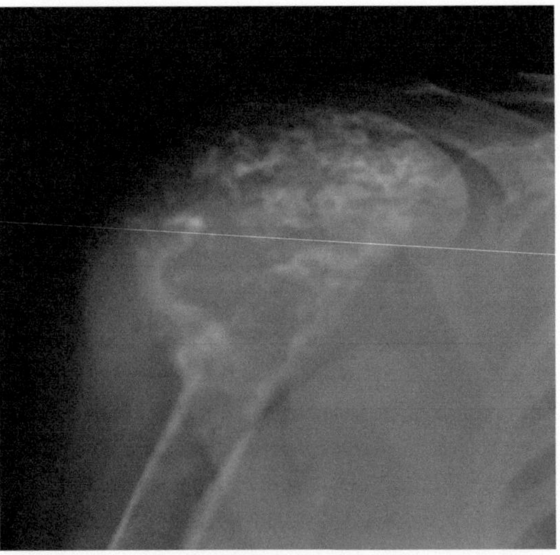

Fig. 4.25 CS humerus: plain X-ray

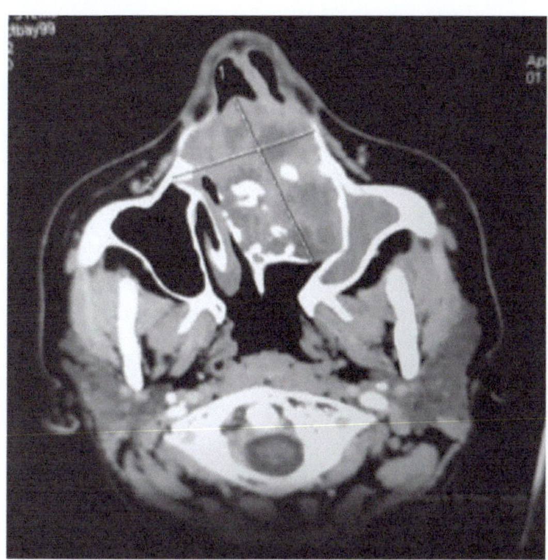

Fig. 4.26 MRI of CS of nasal bone with cortical destruction and soft tissue extension. Chondroid type of calcification can be seen

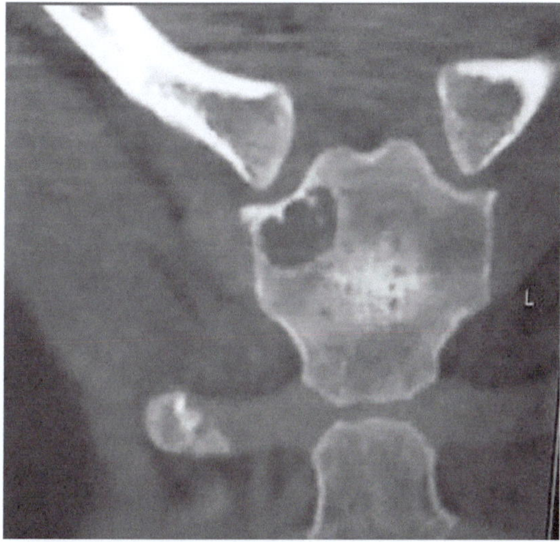

Fig. 4.27 CS sternum

of vertebra (Fig. 4.28). In the skull bones [109], nasal bone is the common site for CS (Fig. 4.29). Another skull bone is clivus, where chondroid chordomas are more common than CS (Fig. 4.30). In some cases, cortical destruction may not be evident. The bone may show expansion with characteristic calcification (Fig. 4.31). Endosteal scalloping which is more than two-thirds of cortical thickness is suggestive of malignancy [100].

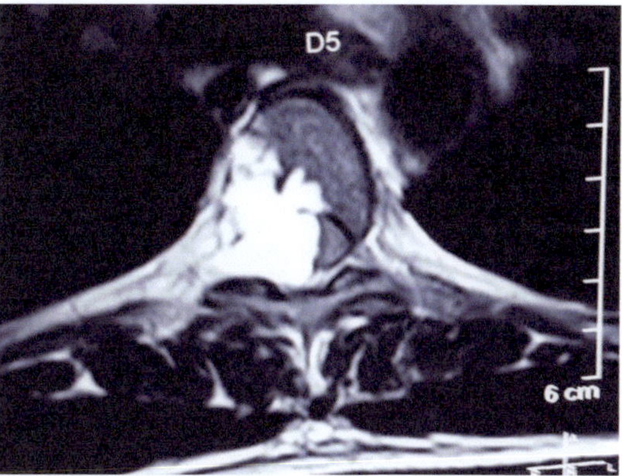

Fig. 4.28 CS of vertebra: body of vertebra and pedicle involved by tumour

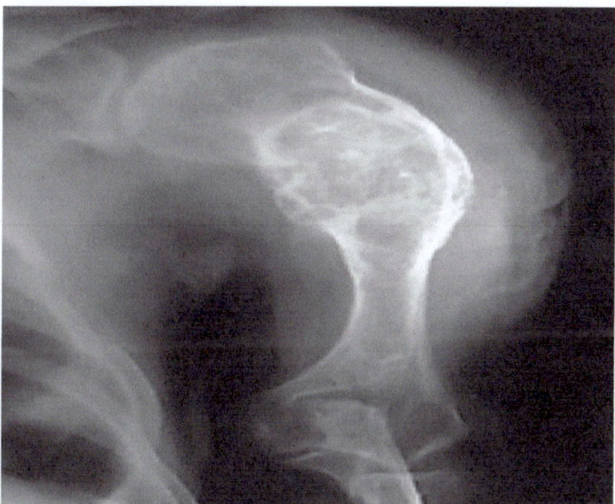

Fig. 4.29 CS in Ollier disease

Marked uptake on bone scan is another feature to suggest malignancy [96].

In osteochondromas, thickness of cartilage cap is important to call it benign or malignant (Fig. 4.9). Thickness can be better assessed by CT scan and MRI [5, 98]. Thickness of cap >2 cm is indicative of malignancy. A large soft tissue mass associated with irregular deposits of calcification is characteristic of malignancy. Areas of lysis are also suggestive of secondary chondrosarcoma.

Pretherapeutic tumour SUV obtained by FDG PET [4, 6] imaging with a cut-off value of 4 combined with grading seems to be a useful parameter for predicting relapse rates in chondrosarcoma patients [96, 107, 122].

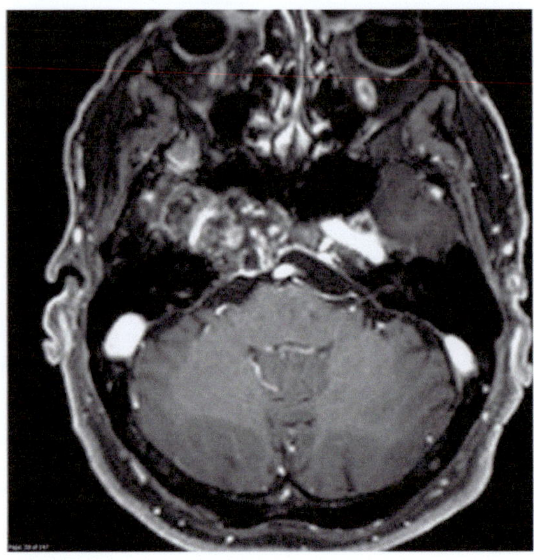

Fig. 4.30 (**a**, **b**) CS base of skull—MRI

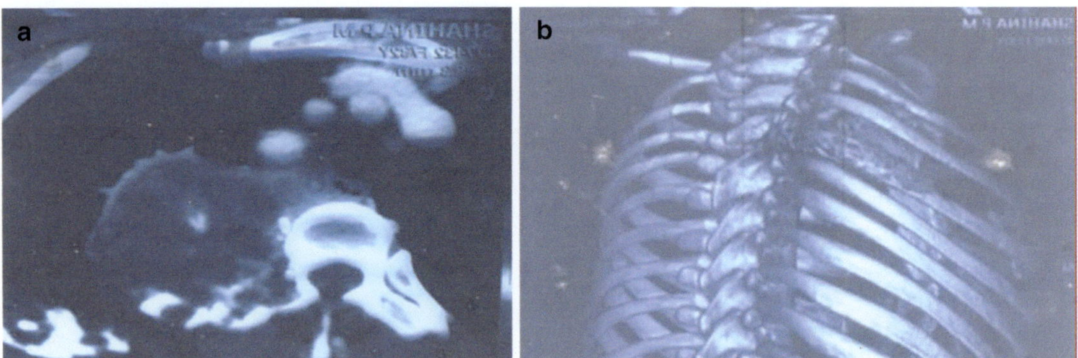

Fig. 4.31 (**a**, **b**) CS rib

Pathogenesis

More than 50% of CS has IDH1 and IDH2 mutations [89, 116]. Complex karyotypes and aneuploidy are seen in grade II and III chondrosarcomas [91, 110]. In tumour progression, alterations of p53 [2] and RB1 pathways are seen [118]. Hedgehog signalling [111] and mTOR [93] signalling pathways have been identified in central CS. This is useful for new treatment options. BCL2 plays an important role in the chemoresistance of CS [114].

Gross: Chondrosarcomas are usually greater than 5 cm in size (Fig. 4.33). They usually show cortical destruction and soft tissue extension. Cut surface will be nodular and glistening. The centres of lobules will be cystic or necrotic with myxoid quality. Foci of calcification may be noted.

In CS arising in osteochondroma, the cartilaginous cap is irregularly thickened to more than 2 cm. Cartilaginous masses of more than 3–4 cm are indicative of malignancy.

Pathology

The difficulty of borderline cartilage lesions was first described by Dahlin in 1956. Recently, the term atypical cartilaginous tumour has been used for grade I CS of appendicular skeleton [94].

Differentiating enchondroma and grade I CS is impossible on small biopsy [97, 100]. They are composed of hyaline cartilage with variable cel-

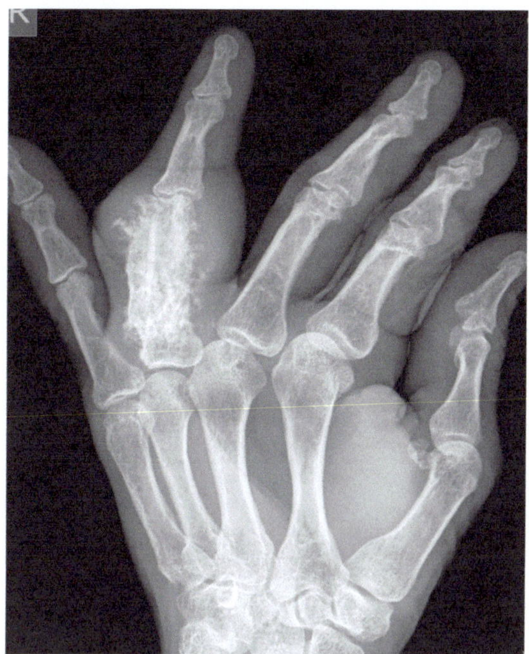

Fig. 4.32 CS ring finger. Lesion has extended to the soft tissue after destroying cortex. In small bones, make sure that the cortical destruction is definite. Do not mistake fracture caused by enchondroma with cortical destruction

lularity in lobules separated by fibrocollagenous tissue (Fig. 4.34). Chondrosarcomas tend to permeate the marrow cavity and entrap bony trabeculae (Fig. 4.35a). This is the most important feature to call it malignant. Formation of a soft tissue mass is another definite feature of malignancy in a cartilage tumour arising in the medullary cavity (Fig. 4.35b). CS permeates the pre-existing bony trabeculae and fills the marrow cavities. This is called entrapment. When there is presence of tumour on three sides of pre-existing trabecular bone of medullary cavity, it is called entrapment. This is different from encasement pattern of enchondromas (deposition of bone surrounding tumour).

The important worrisome features on histology in a needle biopsy are myxoid change, increased cellularity (Fig. 4.36) and necrosis (Table 4.4). Myxoid change is dissolution (liquefaction) of matrix partially into strings or chords (Fig. 4.37). If myxoid change is marked, the matrix is lost and an empty space is seen. Necrosis of cartilage is seen as chondrocytes with pink nuclei (Fig. 4.38b). Mitotic figures are

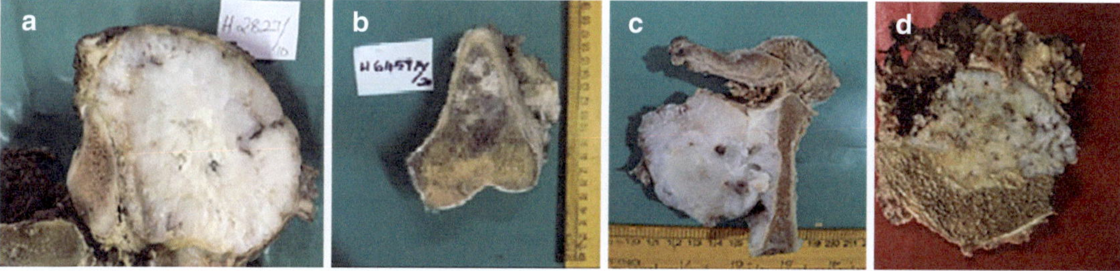

Fig. 4.33 (**a**) Gross specimen of CS of pelvis—nodular glistening cut surface. (**b**) CS of femur with areas of haemorrhage and necrosis. (**c**) CS ilium. (**d**) CS sacrum

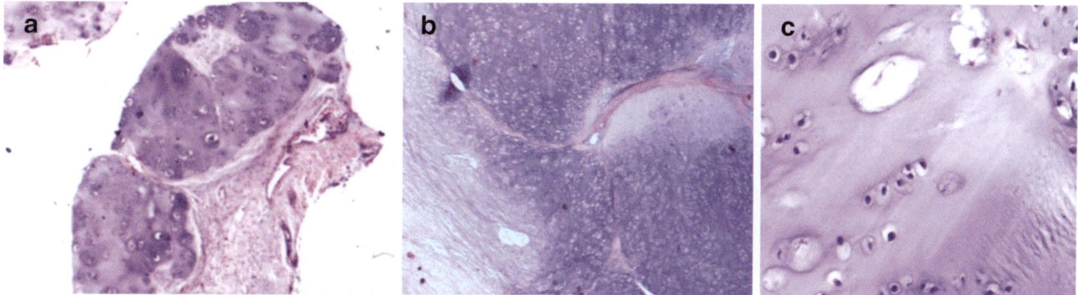

Fig. 4.34 (**a**) Hyaline cartilage in lobules, H&E ×40. (**b**) Lobules with increased cellularity separated by fibrous septa, H&E ×100. (**c**) Chondrocytes in chords, H&E ×250

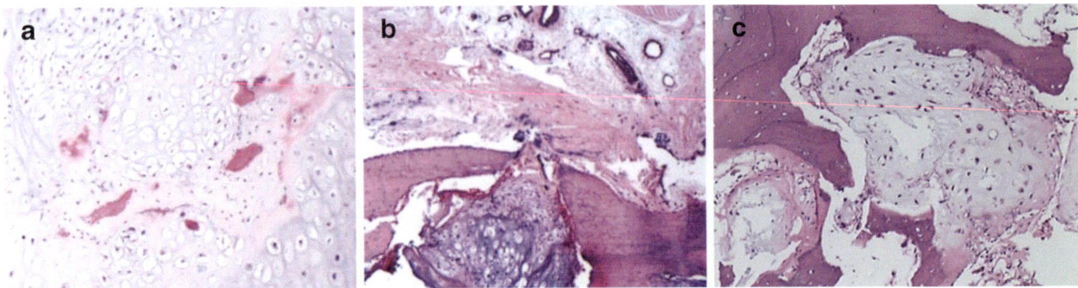

Fig. 4.35 (**a**) Entrapment of tumour in CS, H&E ×100. (**b**) CS permeating soft tissue, H&E ×100. (**c**) Permeation of cartilage between pre-existing bony trabeculae. The cartilage is embraced by bony spicules without intervening fat or marrow, H&E ×250

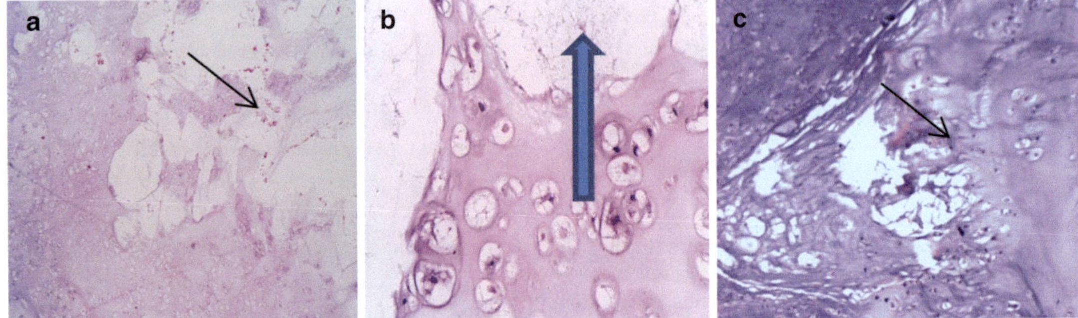

Fig. 4.36 (**a**) Myxoid change—liquefaction of chondroid matrix (arrows), H&E ×100. (**b**) Atypical chondrocytes with pleomorphism and myxoid change (arrow), H&E ×250. (**c**) Liquefaction of hyaline stroma, H&E ×100

Table 4.4 Worrisome features of malignancy in cartilage tumours

Sudden increase in size associated with pain
Size more than 5 cm
Cartilage cap more than 1.5 cm in a case of osteochondroma
Myxoid change of hyaline cartilage
Cellular atypia
Permeation of bony spicules

unusual in chondrosarcomas [98]. But its presence indicates malignant transformation. Double nucleation or multinucleation can be seen (Fig. 4.38a).

In case of secondary CS in osteochondroma, if cartilage fills a low-power field, one should suspect malignant change. The columnar arrangement of chondrocytes towards the base is lost when malignancy arises in osteochondromas. Nodules of cartilage separated from the main mass of the tumour and permeating soft tissues are evidence of chondrosarcoma.

A correlation between clinical and radiological findings is essential to confidently diagnose malignancy in hyaline cartilage neoplasm of low grade. In high-grade tumours, difficulty is differentiating between chondrosarcoma and chondroblastic osteosarcoma [104]. Clinical scenario along with radiological findings is very essential. A high-grade malignant hyaline cartilage tumour in a young patient is most likely to be chondroblastic osteosarcoma.

Grading in CS

Grading is important in chondrosarcomas. Dahlin was the first to grade chondrosarcomas [112]. They are graded from grade I to III (Fig. 4.39). There can be interobserver vari-

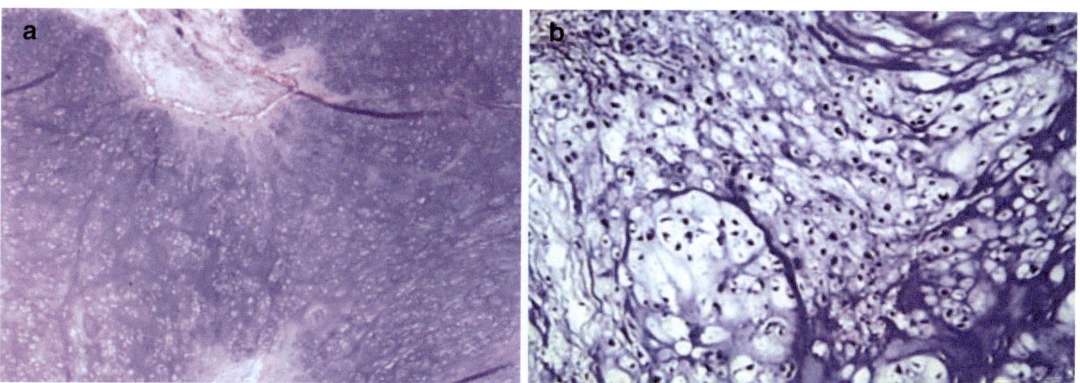

Fig. 4.37 CS—increased cellularity. (**a**) H&E ×100. (**b**) H&E ×250

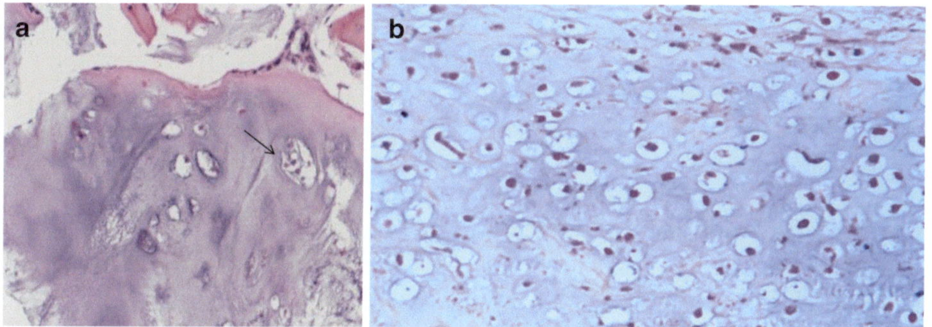

Fig. 4.38 (**a**) CS—multinucleation (arrow), H&E ×250. (**b**) Necrosis in CS. Nuclei are pink in colour, H&E ×250

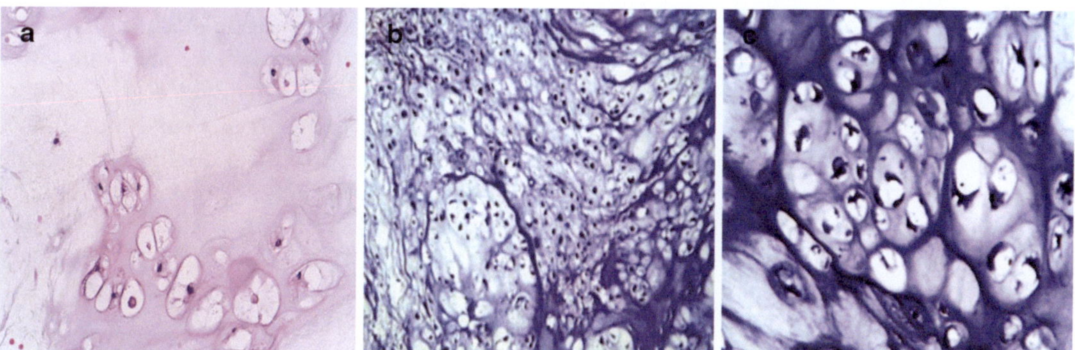

Fig. 4.39 (**a**) CS grade I, H&E ×100. (**b**) CS grade II, H&E ×100. (**c**) CS grade III, H&E ×400

ability in grading [3]. Majority of chondrosarcomas are either grade I or II (about 90%), and grade III chondrosarcomas account for less than 10%. The term grade I chondrosarcomas is given for axial skeleton tumours [102, 124].

Grade I CS has an increased degree of cellularity and cytologic atypia than enchondroma. The cartilage cells are small with round nuclei in abundant hyaline cartilage matrix. Occasional binucleate chondrocytes are present. Mitoses are absent.

Table 4.5 Differentiating enchondroma and CBOS from CS

	Enchondroma	CS	CBOS
Age	>30	>40	<20
Size	<3 cm	>5 cm	Any size
Bone	Appendicular and small bones of hands and feet	Axial	Appendicular
Site of bone	Medullary cavity	Irregular expansion with cortical scalloping and thickening	Metaphysis
Cortical destruction	–	+	+
ST extension	–	+	+
Periosteal reaction	–	–	+
Permeation of bone	–	+	+
Grade of cartilage	1	1, 2 or rarely 3	3
Spindling of cells	–	–	Present towards periphery of lobules
IDH1 or IDH2 mutation	+	+	–

Grade II chondrosarcomas are more cellular. They have enlarged vesicular or hyperchromatic nuclei and less chondroid matrix than ACT/CS1 tumours. Mitoses are present. The nuclei of chondrocytes are enlarged, vesicular or hyperchromatic. Approximately 10–15% of cases have metastatic potential.

Grade III chondrosarcomas are highly cellular. The nuclei are pleomorphic, and mitoses can be easily detected. At the periphery of the tumour nodules, the cells may show spindling. Chondroid matrix shows higher degree of liquefaction (myxoid change). These tumours have high metastatic potential.

DD

1. Enchondroma
2. Chondroblastic OS (see Table 4.5) [117, 127]
3. CMF
4. Exuberant callus
5. Cellular disc material

Treatment and Prognosis

En bloc resection is the primary line of treatment [106]. Radiotherapy and chemotherapy do not have much role in CS. Radiotherapy [105] and chemotherapy [101, 103, 114] are given for unresectable or recurrent tumours [95, 113]. Anti-oestrogen therapy has been tried recently [101]. mTOR inhibitors are thought to be of benefit in a subset of cases [93].

After surgery, 5-year survival rates for grade II and grade III chondrosarcomas are >90% and >75%, respectively [90, 92].

4.3.2 Variants of Chondrosarcoma

4.3.2.1 Periosteal Chondrosarcoma

Periosteal CSs are difficult to differentiate from periosteal chondromas. But periosteal chondromas are usually less than 5 cm, and radiographs show well-defined lesion [120, 122]. Periosteal chondrosarcomas are very large and ill defined. Histologically, they show invasion to adjacent soft tissue. Adequate local resection is the treatment for these tumours. They have a good prognosis even if the tumour is high grade [121, 123]. Histological grading is not used at this location. IDH1 and IDH2 mutations are seen in periosteal CS as in conventional CS [119, 120].

4.3.2.2 Clear Cell Chondrosarcoma (CCCS)

Clear cell CS is a rare type of chondrosarcoma, which has unusual clinical and histological features. In 1976, Unni et al. [149] described this tumour. It accounts for 0.4–2.5% of all CS. These tumours have a tendency to occur in the ends of long bones. It extends to articular cartilage [151].

Clinical

They are slow-growing tumours with long duration of symptoms. Most of the tumours involved thc epiphyseal region. Involvement of metaphysis and diaphysis is extremely uncommon. Proximal femur and humerus are the common locations.

Radiology

They are seen as well-defined lytic lesions in the epiphysis and resemble chondroblastoma (Fig. 4.40a). In larger lesions, the lesion may destroy the cortex and extend to soft tissue. Chondroid type of calcification can be seen. Chondroblastoma is a close differential diagnosis because of the location.

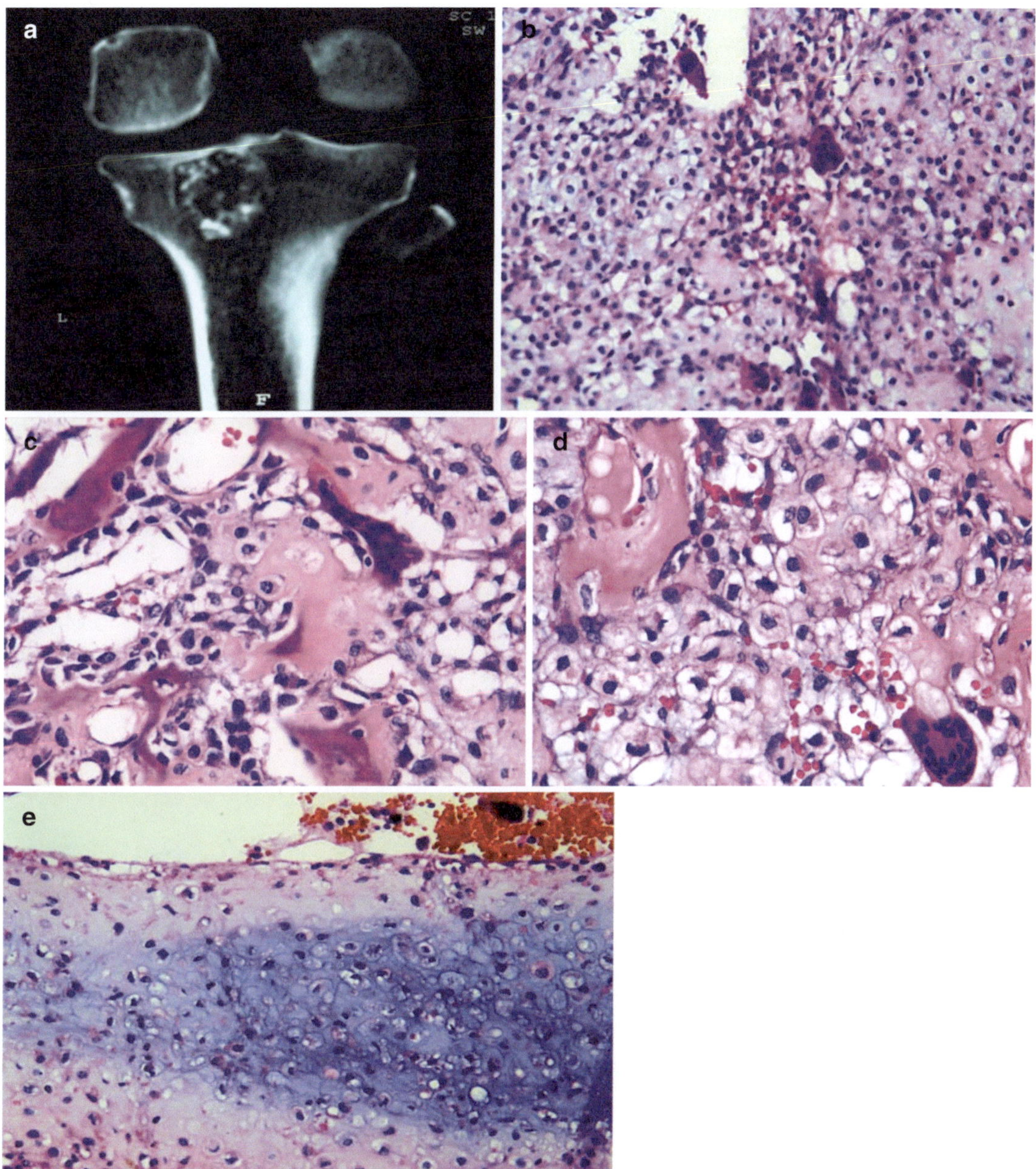

Fig. 4.40 CCC. (**a**) CT scan showing epiphyseal lytic lesion with mineralization. (**b**) Clear cells admixed with OCGCs, H&E ×250. (**c**) Central calcifying osteoid, H&E ×400. (**d**) Well-defined cell borders with clear cytoplasm, H&E ×400. (**e**) Conventional CS-like area, H&E ×250

Pathology

Grossly, the lesion may be cystic with mural nodule, solid gelatinous blue-like ordinary chondrosarcoma or fleshy grey white with or without calcification.

Microscopy is quite different from usual chondrosarcoma. Clear cell CSs are lobulated with cells having clear cytoplasm admixed with osteoclastic giant cells and thin-walled capillaries. The centre of the lobule shows new bone formation, and this finding may be mistaken for bone-forming neoplasm (Fig. 4.40). Occasionally, bone formation can be extensive and is mistaken for osteoblastoma. Cells have clear or pink cytoplasm, central vesicular nuclei and a single nucleolus. 50% of the tumours show conventional chondrosarcomatous areas. Rarely, dedifferentiated clear cell CSs are reported. Immunohistochemistry is of little value. The cells are positive for S100 (Fig. 4.41), Runx2, SOX9 and sometimes cytokeratins. BCL2 expression is high. No cytogenetic abnormalities are identified in CCC. IDH1/IDH2 seen in conventional CS is not seen in CCC.

Differential diagnosis

Other clear cell tumours like metastatic clear cell renal carcinoma are an important differential diagnosis. Clinical history and immunohistochemistry will help in differentiation. Other less important differential diagnoses are osteoblastoma, osteosarcoma involving epiphysis, chondroblastoma and other giant cell-rich lesions.

Treatment and prognosis

This involves surgical excision with negative margins, which is usually curative. Five-year survival rate is almost 100%, and 10-year survival rate is 89%. In patients with positive resected margins, recurrence and metastasis can occur. Metastasis occurs to other bones and lungs, even decades after initial diagnosis. Hence, long-term follow-up is necessary [150].

4.3.2.3 Mesenchymal CS

Mesenchymal chondrosarcoma is one of the rarest of bone sarcomas (2–4% of all CSs) with a bimorphic growth pattern consisting of islands of more or less differentiated cartilage admixed with a small cell malignancy frequently associated with a haemangiopericytomatous pattern [136, 141]. About 1/3 of cases occur in soft tissue [142, 148].

Clinical

Young adults are usually affected, i.e. second and third decades [136, 138]. Any bone may be involved. Majority of cases are reported in jaw bones [146], followed by spine, ilium and ribs. Involvement of skull bones is extremely rare [144]. Among the extraskeletal sites, meninges are reported to be a preferred site of involvement. Pain and swelling are the main symptoms. Around 15% of cases have metastasis at the time of presentation.

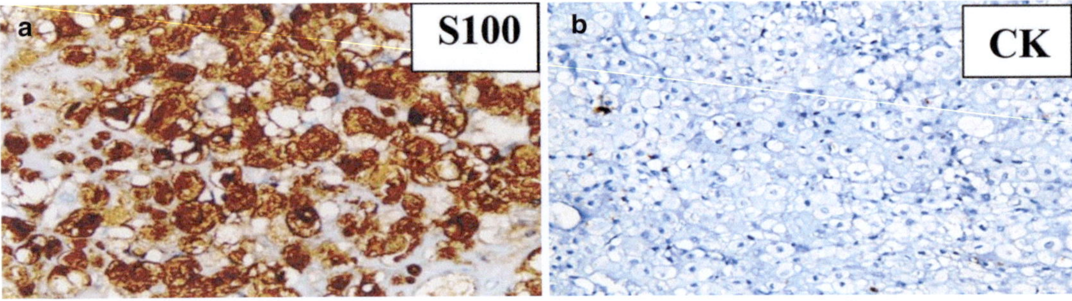

Fig. 4.41 IHC of CCCS. (**a**) S100 showing diffuse and strong cytoplasmic and nuclear positivity ×400. (**b**) Cytokeratin is negative, ×250

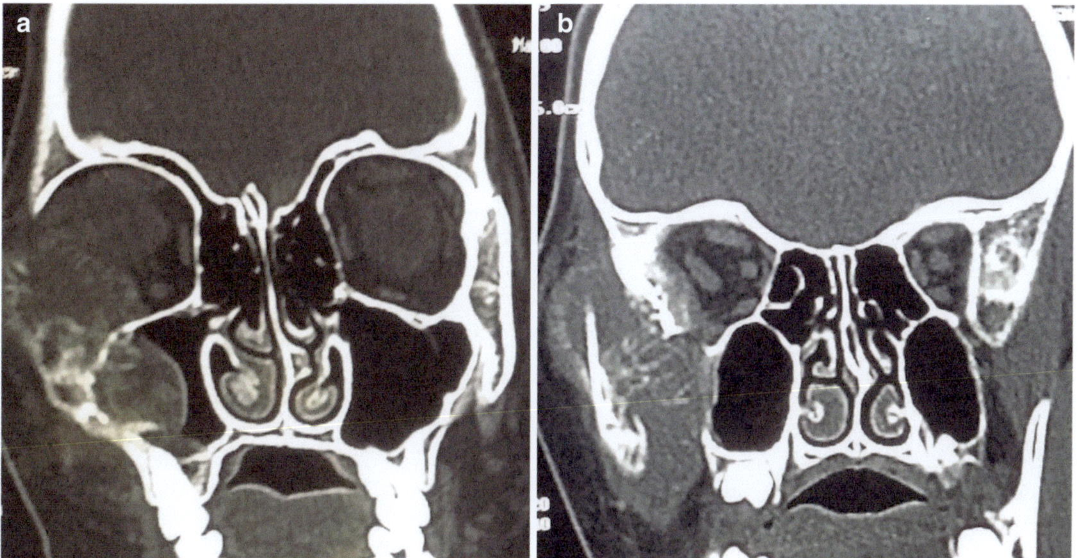

Fig. 4.42 (**a**) Mesenchymal CS of maxilla. (**b**) Mesenchymal CS of skull bone

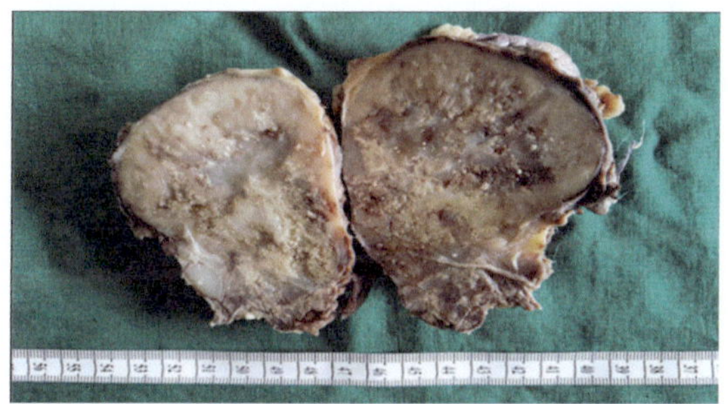

Fig. 4.43 Gross picture of mesenchymal CS of pelvis. Bluish chondroid area with solid grey-white granular cut surface

Radiology

They are lytic and destructive with mottled calcifications (Fig. 4.42). Involved bone is expansile with cortical destruction and soft tissue extension. Tumours of soft tissue also show chondroid type of calcification.

Microscopy

Mesenchymal chondrosarcoma consists of two distinct elements—malignant small round cells and islands of cartilage (Fig. 4.43). Some tumour has small inconspicuous islands of cartilage. Cartilage is usually low-grade hyaline cartilage. The nuclei of small cells are usually round, but may be oval or even spindle shaped. Cytoplasm is scanty, and nuclei have usually dense chromatin. One of the characteristic features is thin-walled vessels giving a haemangiopericytomatous pattern (Fig. 4.44c). Sometimes, the tumour can have an alveolar pattern or spindle cells with herringbone pattern. Islands of cartilage may undergo calcification or ossification (Fig. 4.45).

IHC

S100 is usually positive in chondroid islands, and small cells can be positive for CD99. They are characteristically negative for FLI1. SOX9 (transcription factor) has been shown to be helpful in differentiating from other small cell malignancies (Fig. 4.44e) [147]. Aberrant EMA, desmin, myogenin and MyoD1 positivity has been described. GFAP, SMA and cytokeratin are negative. NKX3.1 is considered as a reliable marker for mesenchymal chondrosarcoma (Fig. 4.44d) [135, 143, 144]. But a recent study has shown that it can be negative in mesenchymal chondrosarcoma [137]. Hence, SOX9 is a better marker to differentiate from other small round cell tumours of bone.

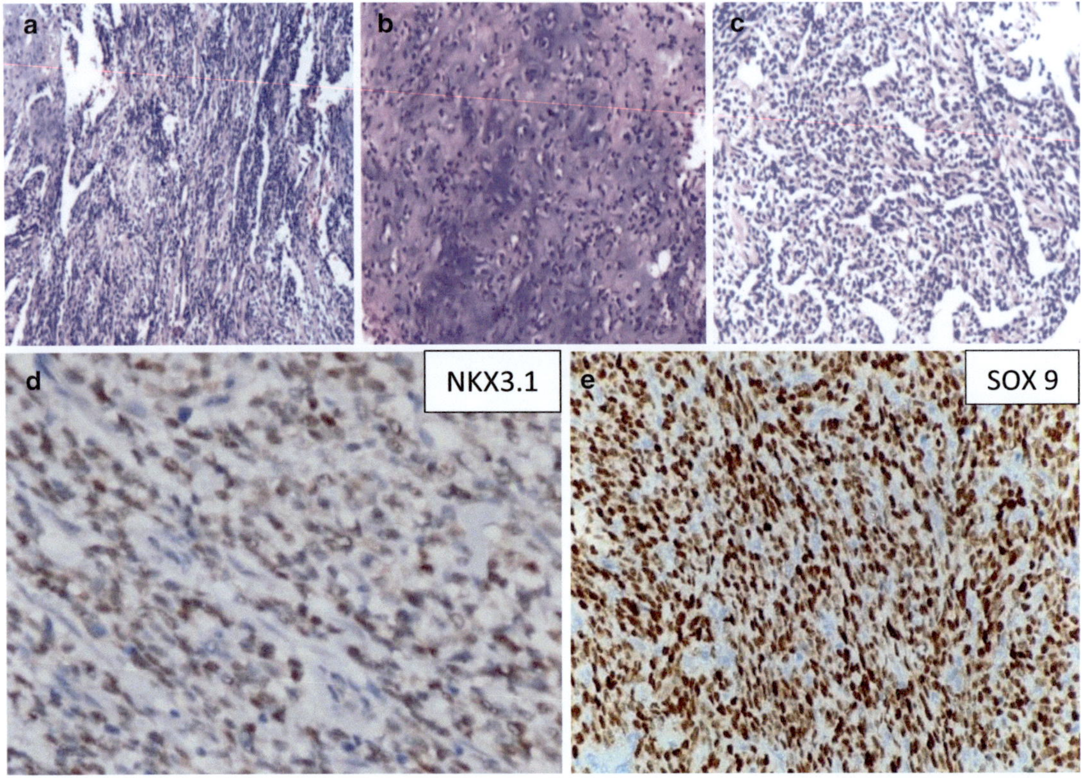

Fig. 4.44 Mesenchymal CS of skull bone in an 8-year-old female. (**a**) Mixture of small round cells and chondroid areas, H&E ×40. (**b**) Chondroid area, H&E ×100. (**c**) Haemangiopericytoma pattern of blood vessels, H&E ×100. (**d**) NKX3.1 shows diffuse nuclear positivity, ×100. (**e**) SOX9 is diffusely strongly positive

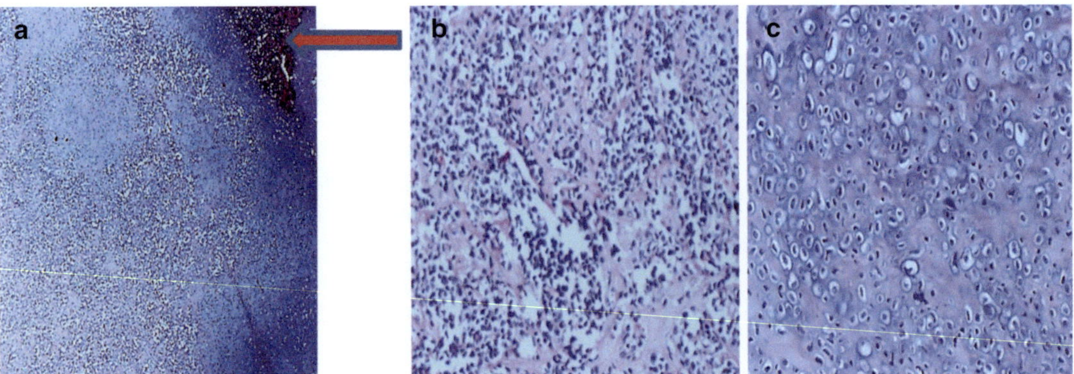

Fig. 4.45 Mesenchymal CS of maxilla. (**a**) Small round cells and calcified chondroid matrix (red arrow), H&E ×100. (**b**) Small round cells with hyperchromatic nuclei, H&E ×100. (**c**) Atypical cartilage, H&E ×100

Molecular

Recurrent HEY1-NCOA2 rearrangement is seen in almost all mesenchymal CS [147]. A Robertsonian translocation involving chromosomes 13 and 21 [der (13; 21) (q10; q10)] is reported in mesenchymal chondrosarcoma [145]. IDH1/IDH2 mutations are not identified.

DD

Differential diagnosis includes other small cell malignancies especially when chondroid islands

Table 4.6 Differentiating features between mesenchymal CS and Ewing sarcoma

	Mesenchymal CS	Ewing sarcoma
Haemangiopericytoma-like vascular pattern	Present	Absent
Nuclei	Hyperchromatic round, oval or spindle	Vesicular round
Cartilage	Present	Absent
IHC	SOX9+, CD99+, FLI1+/−, NKX3.1+	NKX2.2+, CD99+, FLI1+
Cytogenetics	Recurrent HEY1-NCOA2 rearrangement	EWSR1+

are inconspicuous. Needle biopsy may show only small round cell areas, which are mistaken for Ewing sarcoma. Typical nuclear characteristics and HPC pattern help in diagnosis (Table 4.6).

Treatment and prognosis

Mesenchymal CS is treated by wide resection [140]. Radiation is given for local control. Adjuvant chemotherapy is given for metastatic disease. A 5-year survival rate of 42–55% has been reported. Craniofacial primaries are thought to have a better prognosis than other skeletal primaries. Metastasis usually involves lungs. Other visceral organs and skeleton can be involved. Some patients present with disseminated metastasis, but others survive for decades. A long-term follow-up is mandatory since metastasis after 20 years has been reported. Metastatic disease at the time of diagnosis carries a poor outcome [139].

4.3.2.4 Dedifferentiated CS (DDCS)

Dahlin and Beabout in 1971 described dedifferentiated CS [128]. Dedifferentiated chondrosarcoma (DDCS) is a high-grade sarcoma without cartilaginous differentiation adjacent to a well-differentiated grade I CS. The transition from low-grade cartilaginous area to high-grade sarcoma without chondroid differentiation is abrupt. DCS occurs in approximately 10% of all chondrosarcomas.

Clinical

Usually, it is a disease of older adults (peak incidence in the sixth decade). Pain and swelling are present in almost all cases. Sometimes, there will be a history of sudden increase in size of an existing mass present for years [132]. It can arise in pre-existing osteochondroma [133].

Radiology

There will be conventional CS or enchondroma-like area and adjacent destructive aggressive component with cortical destruction and soft tissue extension [125, 129].

Pathogenesis

Both conventional and dedifferentiated CS show identical TP53 and IDH mutations [124, 127].Pathology

Grossly, the cartilaginous component is small and may be overlooked (Fig. 4.46). The aggressive fleshy tumour destroys the cartilage precursor. Cortical destruction and soft tissue extension will be present. Some DDCSs have small fleshy component.

Microscopically, there is an abrupt transition of low-grade hyaline cartilage to high-grade sarcomatous component (Fig. 4.47). Rarely, low-grade and high-grade areas mingle each other. The high-grade component can be osteosarcoma (Fig. 4.48), fibrosarcoma or undifferentiated sarcoma. Rhabdomyosarcomas (Fig. 4.49) and angiosarcomas are also described. The low-grade component is grade I in 75% and grade II in 25%. IDH1 and IDH2 mutations are present in 50–70%.

DD

A high-grade (grade III) conventional chondrosarcoma has to be distinguished from this tumour because it shows spindle cell morphology, especially at its periphery.

Treatment and prognosis

Treatment is radical surgery followed by chemotherapy according to dedifferentiated component [130]. The prognosis is poor, and most patients present with metastatic disease. 5-Year survival rate is less than 25% [126]. Older age, axial

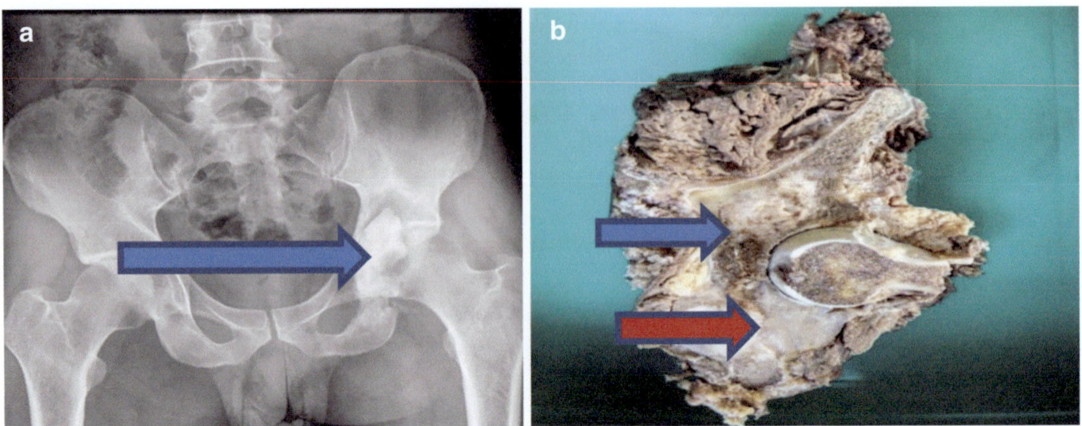

Fig. 4.46 DDCS of acetabulum. (**a**) Plain X-ray densely mineralized growth. (**b**) Gross cut surface: red arrow—low-grade cartilage, blue arrow—high-grade tumour

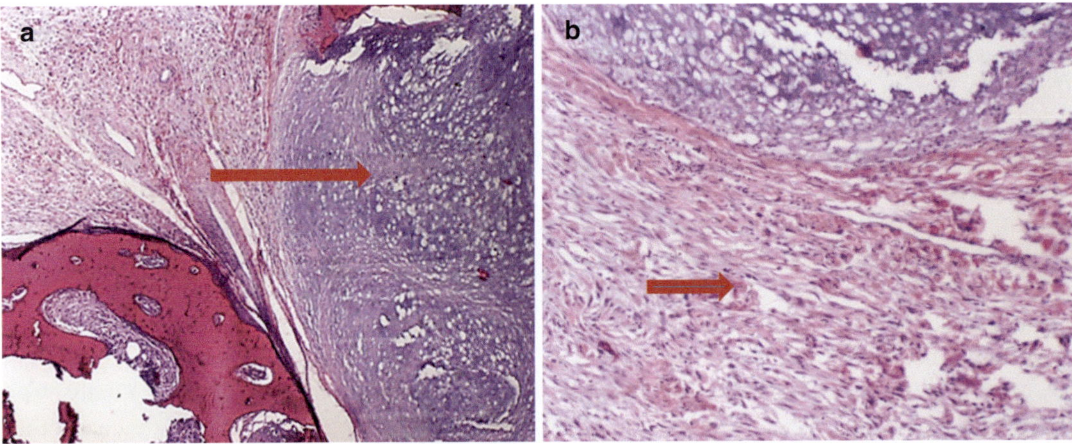

Fig. 4.47 DDCS: (**a**) Low-grade cartilage, H&E ×100 (red arrow). (**b**) Abrupt transition to high-grade sarcoma (red arrow), H&E ×250

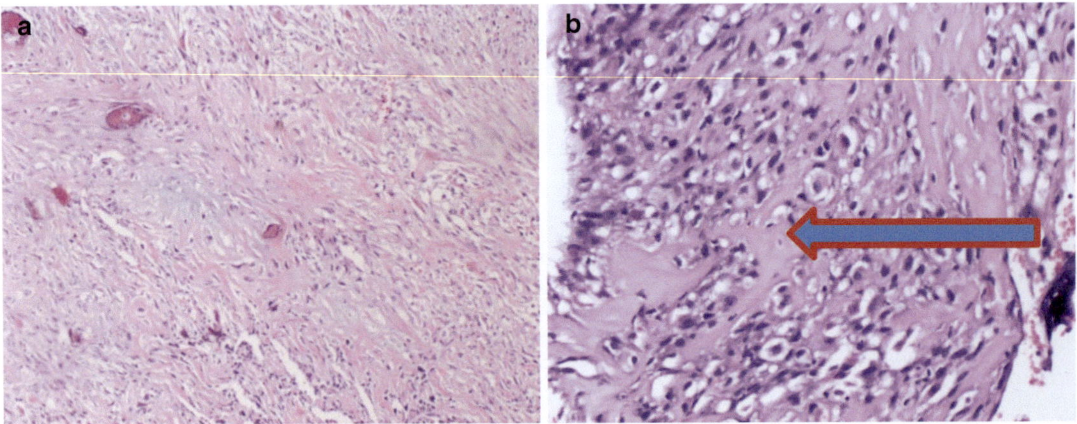

Fig. 4.48 DDCS with osteosarcoma. (**a**) Osteosarcomatous component, H&E ×100. (**b**) Osteoid (blue arrow), H&E ×250

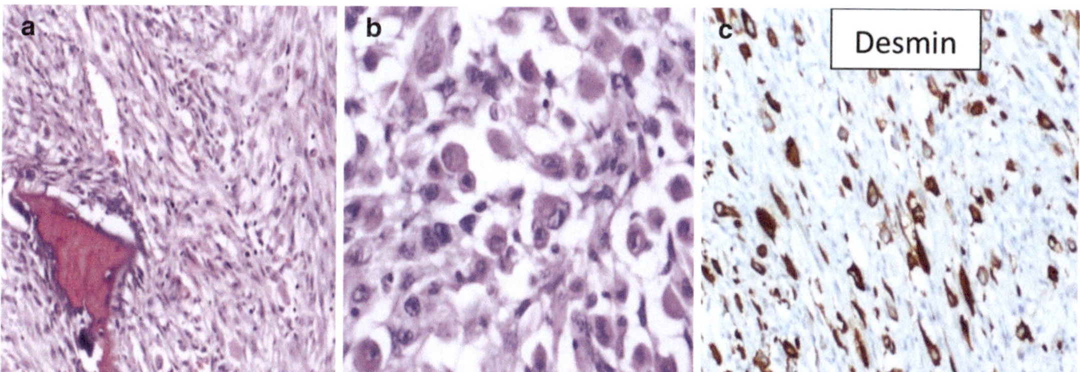

Fig. 4.49 Rhabdomyosarcoma (RMS) in DDCS with rhabdomyoblast. (**a**) Bone with RMS, H&E ×40. (**b**) Rhabdomyoblasts, H&E ×400. (**c**) Desmin, ×250

tumours, presence of fracture and positive resected margins are poor prognostic factors. If the tumour volume of dedifferentiated component is high (>50% of tumour volume), the prognosis is poor. If the high-grade sarcoma is undifferentiated, it carries a worse outcome [131, 134].

4.3.3 Myxoid CS of Bone (MCS)

Extraskeletal myxoid chondrosarcoma (EMCS) was originally described by Enzinger and Shiraki in 1972. Myxoid chondrosarcoma of bone is rare compared to its soft tissue counterpart [152]. Hence, the WHO has not included this entity under bone tumours. Some studies have shown that myxoid chondrosarcomas are not of chondroid origin [163].

4.3.3.1 Clinical

They have been reported in ribs, manubrium, scapula, proximal humerus, distal femur and pelvis [152, 154]. Metastasis from EMCS to bone is more common than primary MCS of bone.

4.3.3.2 Radiology

MCS presents as an intramedullary mass with cortical destruction and soft tissue extension. The typical calcifications characteristic of conventional chondrosarcoma are usually absent [158].

4.3.3.3 Pathology

Primary osseous myxoid chondrosarcomas morphologically resemble their soft tissue counterparts. The cells are arranged in lobules. The nuclei are round to oval with hyperchromatic/granular chromatin. Cells are arranged in chord-like or lace-like pattern, resembling chordoma. Hence, some call it chordoid sarcoma [157]. A prominent extracellular myxoid background is present (Fig. 4.50). Hypercellular foci may be seen.

4.3.3.4 IHC

Immunohistochemical staining for S100 is negative or focally positive. SOX9, NSE, synaptophysin, P63 and PGP9.5 are focally positive [156]. Collagen II and aggrecan are usually absent in MCS. Electron microscopy shows neurosecretory granules. Cytogenetic study demonstrates EWSR1 rearrangement (EWS-NR4A3) [153]. It is usually absent in conventional chondrosarcoma [164].

4.3.3.5 DD

Myxoid chondrosarcoma of pelvic region should be differentiated from chordoma, metastatic carcinoma and myxopapillary ependymoma. IHC will help in differentiation.

4.3.3.6 Treatment and prognosis

Excision with negative margins is the treatment. These tumours can recur and metastasize [155].

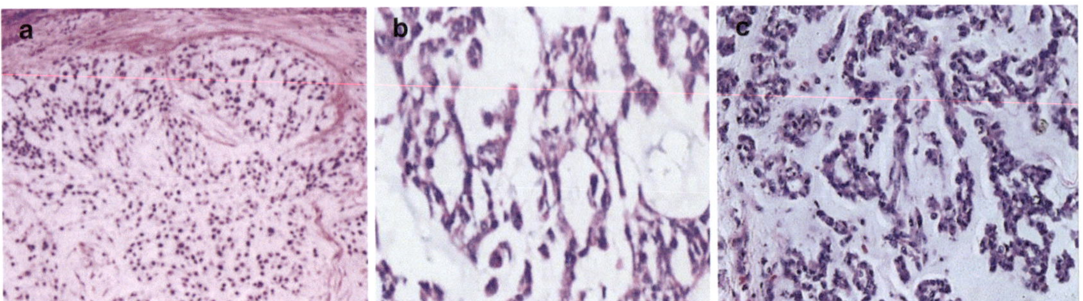

Fig. 4.50 Myxoid chondrosarcoma. (**a**) Lobules of cells arranged in chords in a myxoid stroma, H&E ×100. (**b**) Chords of cells in myxoid matrix, H&E ×100. (**c**) Chordoid appearance, H&E ×100

4.4 Other Chondroid Lesions Mistaken for Neoplasm

4.4.1 Exuberant Callus

A healing fracture can be very cellular without an orderly arrangement. They can have many mitotic figures. Later maturation of these resolves the problem. Certain diseases like osteogenesis imperfecta [161–165] and some neurological problems can cause exuberant callus, which may be mistaken for malignancy [160, 166]. The orderly maturation and radiologic correlation will render a correct diagnosis (Fig. 4.51).

Increased size of **costochondral junction**, the hyaline cartilage which connects ribs to the sternum, can occur in certain diseases [167]. This should not be mistaken for a tumour of hyaline cartilage. The diseases are

1. Autosomal recessive hypophosphataemic bone disease
2. Autosomal recessive spondyloepimetaphyseal dysplasia
3. Dyggve–Melchior–Clausen syndrome
4. Shwachman-Diamond syndrome 1
5. Spondylometaphyseal dysplasia, A4 type
6. Symphalangism-brachydactyly syndrome
7. Vitamin D hydroxylation-deficient rickets, type 1b
8. Vitamin D-dependent rickets, type 1

4.4.2 Intervertebral Disc

The intervertebral disc is a highly organized matrix seen between the vertebrae. A combination of genetic and environmental factors and normal variations in genes related to the body's immune function may cause intervertebral disc disease [168]. This can lead to disc degeneration and herniation. Aging, obesity, chronic inflammation and driving for a long time are other risk factors for the development of disc disease. Degenerated intervertebral disc can be mistaken for a tumour (Fig. 4.52).

Points to Remember

- Correlate with radiology before signing out cartilage tumours.
- Normal costochondral junction, intervertebral disc and articular cartilage should not be mistaken for tumours.
- Worrisome features for cartilage tumours are recent onset of pain, sudden increase in size of an existing tumour, size >5 cm, myxoid change of matrix, bi/multinucleation, and high-grade nuclei.
- Suspect malignancy when cartilage cap size is >2 cm in osteochondroma.
- In case of grade III cartilage tumour in young adults and children, always rule out chondroblastic osteosarcoma.

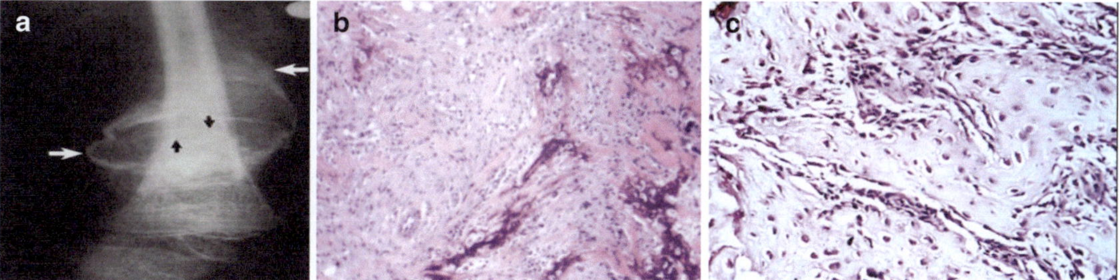

Fig. 4.51 (**a**) X-ray showing multiple fractures and callus in renal osteodystrophy. (**b**) Exuberant callus with orderly maturation, H&E ×100. (**c**) Cellular cartilage in callus, H&E ×250. It should not be mistaken for chondroblastic osteosarcoma or chondrosarcoma

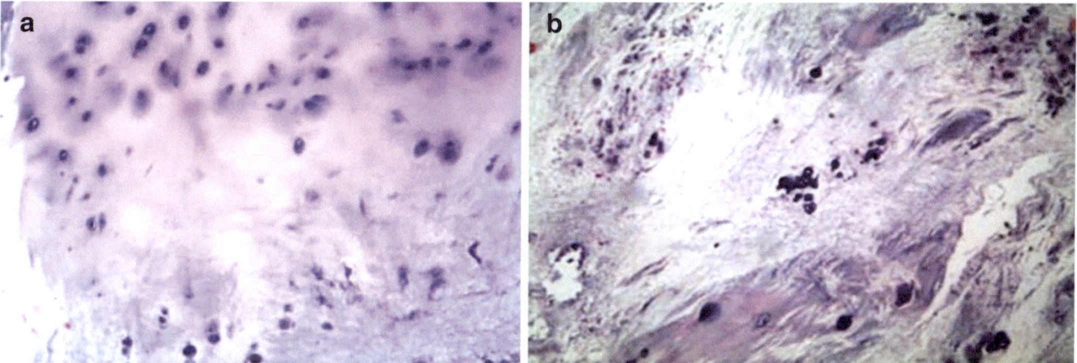

Fig. 4.52 (**a**, **b**) Degenerated disc material. This was mistaken for chondrosarcoma, H&E ×100

References

1. Brien EW, Mirra JM, Kerr R. Benign and malignant cartilage tumors of bone and joint: their anatomic and theoretical basis with an emphasis on radiology, pathology and clinical biology. I. The intramedullary cartilage tumors. Skelet Radiol. 1997;26:325.
2. Coughlan B, Feliz A, Ishida T, et al. p53 expression and DNA ploidy of cartilage lesions. Hum Pathol. 1995;26:620.
3. Eefting D, Schrage YM, Geirnaerdt MJ, et al. Assessment of interobserver variability and histologic parameters to improve reliability in classification and grading of central cartilaginous tumors. Am J Surg Pathol. 2009;33:50.
4. Feldman F, Van Heertum R, Saxena C, Parisien M. 18FDG-PET applications for cartilage neoplasms. Skelet Radiol. 2005;34:367.
5. Geirnaerdt MJ, Bloem JL, Eulderink F, et al. Cartilaginous tumors: correlation of gadolinium-enhanced MR imaging and histopathologic findings. Radiology. 1993;186:813.
6. Lee FY, Yu J, Chang SS, et al. Diagnostic value and limitations of fluorine-18 fluorodeoxyglucose positron emission tomography for cartilaginous tumors of bone. J Bone Jt Surg Am. 2004;86-A:2677.

Subungual Exostosis

7. Bostanci S, Ekmekçi P, Ekinci C, Akçaboy B, Gürgey E. Subungual osteochondroma: a case report. Dermatol Surg. 2001;b27:591–3.
8. Cohen HJ, Frank SB, Minkin W, Gibbs RC. Subungual exostoses. Arch Dermatol. 1973;107:431–2.
9. DaCambra MP, Gupta SK, Ferri-de-Barros F. A novel management strategy for subungual exostosis. BMJ Case Rep. 2013;2013:bcr2013200396. https://doi.org/10.1136/bcr-2013-200396.

10. Fikry T, Dkhissi M, Harfaoui A, Adil A, Haddoun A, Zryouil B. Subungual exostosis: a retrospective study of 28 cases. Acta Orthop Belg. 1998;64:35–40.
11. Grisafi PJ, Lombardi CM, Sciarrino AL, Rainer GF, Buffone WF. Three select subungual pathologies: subungual exostosis, subungual osteochondroma, and subungual hematoma. Clin Podiatr Med Surg. 1989;6:355–64.
12. Guarneri C, Guarneri F, Risitano G, Lentini M, Vaccaro M. Solitary asymptomatic nodule of the great toe. Int J Dermatol. 2005;44:245–7.
13. Ippolito E, Falez F, Tudisco C, Balus L, Fazio M, Morrone A. Subungual exostosis. Histological and clinical considerations on 30 cases. Ital J Orthop Traumatol. 1987;13:81–7.
14. Kim S, Park K, Son S. Subungual osteochondroma presenting as verruca vulgaris in a 6-year-old boy. Pediatr Dermatol. 2007;24:584–5.
15. Landon GC, Johnson KA, Dahlin DC. Subungual exostoses. J Bone Jt Surg Am. 1979;61:256–9.
16. Lee SK, Jung MS, Lee YH, Gong HS, Kim JK, Baek GH. Two distinctive subungual pathologies: subungual exostosis and subungual osteochondroma. Foot Ankle Int. 2007;28:595–601.
17. Letts M, Davidson D, Nizalik E. Subungual exostosis: diagnosis and treatment in children. J Trauma Acute Care Surg. 1998;44:346–9.
18. DaCambra MP, Gupta SK, Ferri-de-Barros F. Subungual exostosis of the toes: a systematic review. Clin Orthop Relat Res. 2014;472:1251–9.
19. Oliveira AS, Picoto AS, Verde SF, Martins O. Subungual exostosis: treatment as an office procedure. J Dermatol Surg Oncol. 1980;6:555–8.
20. Storlazzi C, Wozniak A, Panagopoulos I, Sciot R, Mandahl N, Mertens F, Debiec-Rychter M. Rearrangement of the COL12A1 and COL4A5 genes in subungual exostosis: molecular cytogenetic delineation of the tumor-specific translocation t (X; 6)(q13–14; q22). Int J Cancer. 2006;118:1972–6.
21. Suga H, Mukouda M. Subungual exostosis. Ann Plast Surg. 2005;55:272–5.
22. Zambrano E, Nosé V, Perez-Atayde AR, Gebhardt M, Hresko MT, Kleinman P, Richkind KE, Kozakewich HP. Distinct chromosomal rearrangements in subungual (Dupuytren) exostosis and bizarre parosteal osteochondromatous proliferation (Nora lesion). Am J Surg Pathol. 2004;28(8):1033–9.

BPOP

23. Dhondt E, Oudenhoven L, Khan S, et al. Nora's lesion, a distinct radiological entity? Skelet Radiol. 2006;35(7):497–502.
24. Gruber G, Giessauf C, Leithner A, et al. Bizarre parosteal osteochondromatous proliferation (Nora lesion): a report of 3 cases and a review of the literature. Can J Surg. 2008;51(6):486–9.
25. Flint JH, McKay PL. Bizarre parosteal osteochondromatous proliferation and periosteal chondroma: a comparative report and review of the literature. J Hand Surg. 2007;32(6):893–8.
26. Joseph J, Ritchie D, MacDuff E, Mahendra A. Bizarre parosteal osteochondromatous proliferation: a locally aggressive benign tumor. Clin Orthop Relat Res. 2011;469(7):2019–27.
27. Nora FE, Dahlin DC, Beabout JW. Bizarre parosteal osteochondromatous proliferations of the hands and feet. Am J Surg Pathol. 1983;7:245e50.
28. Barrera-Ochoa S, Lluch A, Gargallo-Margarit A, Perez M, Bizarre RV. Parosteal osteochondromatous proliferation (Nora's lesion) of the hand: a report of two atypical cases. Case Rep Med. 2012;2012:453560. https://doi.org/10.1155/2012/453560.
29. Torreggiani WC, Munk PL, Al-Ismail K, et al. MR imaging features of bizarre parosteal osteochondromatous proliferation of bone (Nora's lesion). Eur J Radiol. 2001;40(3):224–31.

Enchondroma and Enchondromatosis

30. Albregts AE, Rapini RP. Malignancy in Maffucci's syndrome. Dermatol Clin. 1995;13:73.
31. Amary MF, Damato S, Halai D, et al. Ollier disease and Maffucci syndrome are caused by somatic mosaic mutations of IDH1 and IDH2. Nat Genet. 2011;43:1262.
32. Flemming DJ, Murphey MD. Enchondroma and chondrosarcoma. Semin Musculoskelet Radiol. 2000;4:59.
33. Geirnaerdt MJ, Hermans J, Bloem JL, et al. Usefulness of radiography in differentiating enchondroma from central grade 1 chondrosarcoma. AJR Am J Roentgenol. 1997;169:1097.
34. Hopyan S, Gokgoz N, Poon R, et al. A mutant PTH/PTHrP type I receptor in enchondromatosis. Nat Genet. 2002;30:306.
35. Le A, Ball D, Pitman A, et al. Chondrosarcoma of bone complicating Ollier's disease: report of a favourable response to radiotherapy. Australas Radiol. 2003;47:322.
36. Liu J, Hudkins PG, Swee RG, Unni KK. Bone sarcomas associated with Ollier's disease. Cancer. 1987;59:1376.
37. Mirra JM, Gold R, Downs J, Eckardt JJ. A new histologic approach to the differentiation of enchondroma and chondrosarcoma of the bones. A clinicopathologic analysis of 51 cases. Clin Orthop Relat Res. 1985;201:214–37.
38. Pannier S, Legeai-Mallet L. Hereditary multiple exostoses and enchondromatosis. Best Pract Res Clin Rheumatol. 2008;22:45.
39. Pansuriya TC, van Eijk R, d'Adamo P, et al. Somatic mosaic IDH1 and IDH2 mutations are associated with enchondroma and spindle cell hemangioma in

Ollier disease and Maffucci syndrome. Nat Genet. 2011;43:1256.
40. Schwartz HS, Zimmerman NB, Simon MA, et al. The malignant potential of enchondromatosis. J Bone Jt Surg Am. 1987;69:269.
41. Silve C, Jüppner H. Ollier disease. Orphanet J Rare Dis. 2006;1:37.
42. Verdegaal SH, Bovée JV, Pansuriya TC, et al. Incidence, predictive factors, and prognosis of chondrosarcoma in patients with Ollier disease and Maffucci syndrome: an international multicenter study of 161 patients. Oncologist. 2011;16:1771.

Osteochondroma and Osteochondromatosis

43. Ahmed AR, Tan TS, Unni KK, et al. Secondary chondrosarcoma in osteochondroma: report of 107 patients. Clin Orthop Relat Res. 2003;411:193–206.
44. Altay M, Bayrakci K, Yildiz Y, et al. Secondary chondrosarcoma in cartilage bone tumors: report of 32 patients. J Orthop Sci. 2007;12:415.
45. Bovée JV, Cleton-Jansen AM, Wuyts W, et al. EXT-mutation analysis and loss of heterozygosity in sporadic and hereditary osteochondromas and secondary chondrosarcomas. Am J Hum Genet. 1999;65:689.
46. Bovée JV. Multiple osteochondromas. Orphanet J Rare Dis. 2008;3:3.
47. de Andrea CE, Kroon HM, Wolterbeek R, et al. Interobserver reliability in the histopathological diagnosis of cartilaginous tumors in patients with multiple osteochondromas. Mod Pathol. 2012;25:1275.
48. de Andrea CE, Reijnders CM, Kroon HM, et al. Secondary peripheral chondrosarcoma evolving from osteochondroma as a result of outgrowth of cells with functional EXT. Oncogene. 2012;31:1095.
49. Feldman F, Vanheertum R, Saxena C. 18Fluoro-deoxyglucose positron emission tomography evaluation of benign versus malignant osteochondromas: preliminary observations. J Comput Assist Tomogr. 2006;30:858.
50. Lamovec J, Spiler M, Jevtic V. Osteosarcoma arising in a solitary osteochondroma of the fibula. Arch Pathol Lab Med. 1999;123:832–4.
51. Pierz KA, Womer RB, Dormans JP. Pediatric bone tumors: osteosarcoma Ewing's sarcoma, and chondrosarcoma associated with multiple hereditary osteochondromatosis. J Pediatr Orthop. 2001;21:412.

Chondroblastoma

52. Angelini A, Arguedas F, Varela A, Ruggieri P. Chondroblastoma of the foot: 40 cases from a single institution. J Foot Ankle Surg. 2018;57(6):1105–9.
53. Ramappa AJ, Lee FY, Tang P, Carlson JR, Gebhardt MC, Mankin HJ. Chondroblastoma of bone. J Bone Jt Surg. 2000;82-A(8):1140–5.
54. Tins B, Cassar-Pullicino V, McCall I, Cool P, Williams D, Mangham D. Radiofrequency ablation of chondroblastoma using a multi-tined expandable electrode system: initial results. Eur Radiol. 2006;16(4):804–10.
55. Behjati S, Tarpey PS, Presneau N, et al. Distinct H3F3A and H3F3B driver mutations define chondroblastoma and giant cell tumor of bone. Nat Genet. 2013;45:1479–82.
56. Birch PJ, Buchanan R, Golding P, Pringle JA. Chondroblastoma of the rib with widespread bone metastases. Histopathology. 1994;25:583–5.
57. Chen M, Klein M. Hameed, histone H3K36M mutation and trimethylation patterns in chondroblastoma. Histopathology. 2019;74(2):291–9.
58. Xie C, Jeys L, James SL. Radiofrequency ablation of chondroblastoma: long-term clinical and imaging outcomes. Eur Radiol. 2015;25(4):1127–34.
59. Suneja R, Grimer RJ, Belthur M, Jeys L, Carter SR, Tillman RM, Davies AM. Chondroblastoma of bone: long-term results and functional outcome after intralesional curettage. J Bone Jt Surg Br. 2005;87(7):974–8.
60. Dahlin DC, Ivins JC. Benign chondroblastoma. A study of 125 cases. Cancer. 1972;30:401–13.
61. Springfield DS, Capanna R, Gherlinzoni F, Picci P, Campanacci M. Chondroblastoma. A review of 70 cases. J Bone Jt Surg. 1985;67(5):748–55.
62. Demirhan H, et al. Temporal bone localized chondroblastoma. J Craniofac Surg. 2015;26(8):e689–90.
63. Dhandra S, et al. Atypical giant chondroblastoma mimicking chondrosarcoma. J Cancer Res Ther. 2015;11(3):660.
64. Konishi E, Nakashima Y, Mano M, Tomita Y, Kubo T, Araki N, Morii E, Yoshikawa H, Haga H, Toguchida J, Ueda T, Osawa M, Hoshi M, Inoue T, Aono M, Yanagisawa A. Chondroblastoma of extra-craniofacial bones: clinicopathological analyses of 103 cases. Pathol Int. 2017;67(10):495–502.
65. Sailhan F, Chotel F, Parot R. Chondroblastoma of bone in a pediatric population. J Bone Jt Surg. 2009;91(9):2159–68.
66. Xu H, Nugent D, Monforte HL, Binitie OT, Ding Y, Letson GD, Cheong D, Niu X. Chondroblastoma of bone in the extremities: a multicenter retrospective study. J Bone Jt Surg. 2015;97(11):925–31.
67. Huvos AG, Higinbotham NL, Marcove RC, O'Leary P. Aggressive chondroblastoma. Review of the literature on aggressive behavior and metastases with a report of one new case. Clin Orthop Relat Res. 1977;126:266–72.
68. Crim JR, Gold RH, Mirra JM, Eckardt J. Case report 748: chondroblastoma of the femur with an aneurysmal bone cyst. Skelet Radiol. 1992;21(6):403–5.
69. Jambhekar NA, Desai PB, Chitale DA, Patil P, Arya S. Benign metastasizing chondroblastoma: a case report. Cancer. 1998;82:675–8.

70. Joshi DD, Anderson PM, Matsumoto J, et al. Metastatic chondroblastoma with elevated creatine kinase and paraneoplastic neurologic autoimmunity. J Pediatr Hematol Oncol. 2003;25:900–4.
71. Kunze E, Graewe T, Peitsch E. Histology and biology of metastatic chondroblastoma. Report of a case with a review of the literature. Pathol Res Pract. 1987;182:113–23.
72. Lu C, Ramirez D, Hwang S, et al. Histone H3K36M mutation and trimethylation patterns in chondroblastoma. Histopathology. 2019;74(2):291–9. https://doi.org/10.1111/his.13725.
73. Christie-Large M, Evans N, Davies AM, James SL. Radiofrequency ablation of chondroblastoma: procedure technique, clinical and MR imaging follow up of four cases. Skelet Radiol. 2008;37(11):1011–7.
74. Laitinen MK, Stevenson JD, Evans S, Abudu A, Sumathi V, Jeysb LM, Parry MC. Chondroblastoma in pelvis and extremities—a single centre study of 177 cases. J Bone Oncol. 2019;17:100248.
75. de Silva MV, Reid R. Chondroblastoma: varied histologic appearance, potential diagnostic pitfalls, and clinicopathologic features associated with local recurrence. Ann Diagn Pathol. 2003;7(4):205–13.
76. Papke DJ, Hung YP, Schaefer IM, Bredella MA, Charville GW, Reith JD, Fletcher CDM, Nielsen GP, Hornick JL. Clinicopathologic characterization of malignant chondroblastoma: a neoplasm with locally aggressive behavior and metastatic potential that closely mimics chondroblastoma-like osteosarcoma. Mod Pathol. 2020;33(11):2295–306.
77. Suneja R, Grimer RJ, Belthur M, Jeys L, Carter SR, Tillman RM, Davies AM, Lalam RK, Cribb GL, Tins BJ, Cool WP, Singh J, Tyrrell PN, Cassar-Pullicino VN. Image guided radiofrequency thermo-ablation therapy of chondroblastomas: should it replace surgery? Skelet Radiol. 2014;43(4):513–22.
78. Rodgers WB, Mankin HJ. Metastatic malignant chondroblastoma. Am J Orthop (Belle Mead NJ). 1996;25:846–9.
79. Viswanathan S, Jambhekar NA, Merchant NH, Puri A, Agarwal M. Chondroblastoma of bone—not a benign disease: clinico-pathologic observations on 60 cases. Indian J Pathol Microbiol. 2004;47(2):198–201.
80. Seline PC, Jaskierny DJ. Cutaneous metastases from a chondroblastoma initially presenting as unilateral palmar hyperhidrosis. J Am Acad Dermatol. 1999;40(2 Pt 2):325–7.
81. Sindhu Nair P, Jayasree K, Nair SG, Venugopal M. Clinico pathological analysis of chondroblastoma: a tertiary care centre experience. EC Orthop. 2020;11(1):01–8.
82. Wirman JA, Crissman JD, Aron BF. Metastatic chondroblastoma: report of an unusual case treated with radiotherapy. Cancer. 1979;44:87–93.
83. Liu YJ, Wang W, Yeh J, Wu Y, Mantilla JG, Fletcher CD, Ricciotti RW, Chen EY. Calcified chondroid mesenchymal neoplasms with FN1-receptor tyrosine kinase gene fusions including FGFR2, FGFR1, MERTK, NTRK1, and TEK: a molecular and clinicopathologic analysis. Mod Pathol. 2021;34:1373–83.
84. Yang X, Yang ZJ, Liu FX, Zeng K, Qian MQ, Chen G, et al. Inhibition of mTOR and HIF pathways diminishes chondro-osteogenesis and cell proliferation in chondroblastoma. Tumour Biol. 2013;34(5):3111–9.

Chondromyxoid Fibroma

85. Abdelwahab IF, Klein MJ. Surface chondromyxoid fibroma of the distal ulna: unusual tumor, site, and age. Skelet Radiol. 2014;43:243–6.
86. Chow LT, Lin J, Yip KM, et al. Chondromyxoid fibroma-like osteosarcoma: a distinct variant of low-grade osteosarcoma. Histopathology. 1996;29:429–36.
87. Keel SB, Bhan AK, Liebsch NJ, Rosenberg AE. Chondromyxoid fibroma of the skull base: a tumor which may be confused with chordoma and chondrosarcoma. A report of three cases and review of the literature. Am J Surg Pathol. 1997;21:577–82.
88. Suryawanshi P, Agarwal M, Dhake R, et al. Phosphaturic mesenchymal tumor with chondromyxoid fibroma-like feature: an unusual morphological appearance. Skeletal Radiol. 2011;40:1481–5.

Chondrosarcoma

89. Rosenberg AE, Nielsen GP, Keel SB, Renard LG, Fitzek MM, Munzenrider JE, Liebsch NJ, Amary MF, Bacsi K, Maggiani F, et al. IDH1 and IDH2 mutations are frequent events in central chondrosarcoma and central and periosteal chondromas but not in other mesenchymal tumours. J Pathol. 2011;224:334–43.
90. Angelini A, Guerra G, Mavrogenis AF, et al. Clinical outcome of central conventional chondrosarcoma. J Surg Oncol. 2012;106:929.
91. Bovée JV, Hogendoorn PC, Wunder JS, Alman BA. Cartilage tumours and bone development: molecular pathology and possible therapeutic targets. Nat Rev Cancer. 2010;10:481.
92. Bauer HC, Brosjö O, Kreicbergs A, Lindholm J. Low risk of recurrence of enchondroma and low-grade chondrosarcoma in extremities. 80 patients followed for 2–25 years. Acta Orthop Scand. 1995;66:283.
93. Bernstein-Molho R, Kollender Y, Issakov J, et al. Clinical activity of mTOR inhibition in combination with cyclophosphamide in the treatment of recurrent unresectable chondrosarcomas. Cancer Chemother Pharmacol. 2012;70:855.
94. Björnsson J, McLeod RA, Unni KK, et al. Primary chondrosarcoma of long bones and limb girdles. Cancer. 1998;83:2105.

95. Bovée JV, Cleton-Jansen AM, Taminiau AH, Hogendoorn PC. Emerging pathways in the development of chondrosarcoma of bone and implications for targeted treatment. Lancet Oncol. 2005;6:599.
96. Brenner W, Conrad EU, Eary JF. FDG PET imaging for grading and prediction of outcome in chondrosarcoma patients. Eur J Nucl Med Mol Imaging. 2004;31:189.
97. Crim J, Scmidt R, Layfield L, Hanrahan C, Manaster BJ. Can imaging criteria distinguish enchondroma from grade 1 chondrosarcoma? Eur J Radiol. 2015;84:2222–30.
98. Douis H, Singh L, Saifuddin A. MRI differentiation of low-grade from high-grade appendicular chondrosarcoma. Eur Radiol. 2014;24:232–40.
99. Evans HL, Ayala AG, Romsdahl MM. Prognostic factors in chondrosarcoma of bone: a clinicopathologic analysis with emphasis on histologic grading. Cancer. 1977;40:818.
100. Frisch CD, Inwards CY, Lalich IJ, Carter JM, Neff BA. Atypical cartilaginous tumor/chondrosarcoma, grade 1, of the mastoid in three family members: a new entity. Laryngoscope. 2016;126(9):E310–3. https://doi.org/10.1002/lary.25802. Epub 2015 Dec 15.
101. Grifone TJ, Haupt HM, Podolski V, Brooks JJ. Immunohistochemical expression of estrogen receptors in chondrosarcomas and enchondromas. Int J Surg Pathol. 2008;16:31.
102. Hogendoorn PCW, Bovee JM, Nielsen GP. Chondrosarcoma (grades I–III), including primary and secondary variants and periosteal chondrosarcoma. In: Fletcher CDM, Bridge JA, Hogendoorn PCW, Mertens F, editors. World Health Organization classification of tumours of soft tissue and bone, vol. 5. 4th ed. Lyon: IARC; 2013. p. 264.
103. Italiano A, Mir O, Cioffi A, et al. Advanced chondrosarcomas: role of chemotherapy and survival. Ann Oncol. 2013;24:2916.
104. Kerr DA, Lopez HU, Deshpande V, et al. Molecular distinction of chondrosarcoma from chondroblastic osteosarcoma through IDH1/2 mutations. Am J Surg Pathol. 2013;37:787.
105. Krochak R, Harwood AR, Cummings BJ, Quirt IC. Results of radical radiation for chondrosarcoma of bone. Radiother Oncol. 1983;1:109.
106. Leerapun T, Hugate RR, Inwards CY, et al. Surgical management of conventional grade I chondrosarcoma of long bones. Clin Orthop Relat Res. 2007;463:166.
107. Murphey MD, Walker EA, Wilson AJ, et al. From the archives of the AFIP: imaging of primary chondrosarcoma: radiologic–pathologic correlation. Radiographics. 2003;23:1245.
108. Pring ME, Weber KL, Unni KK, Sim FH. Chondrosarcoma of the pelvis. A review of 64 cases. J Bone Jt Surg Am. 2001;83-A:1630.
109. Rosenberg AE, Nielsen GP, Keel SB, Renard LG, Fitzek MM, Munzenrider JE, Liebsch NJ. Chondrosarcoma of the base of the skull: a clinicopathologic study of 200 cases with emphasis on its distinction from chordoma. Am J Surg Pathol. 1999;23(11):1370–8.
110. Sandberg AA, Bridge JA. Updates on the cytogenetics and molecular genetics of bone and soft tissue tumors: chondrosarcoma and other cartilaginous neoplasms. Cancer Genet Cytogenet. 2003;143:1–31.
111. Tiet TD, Hopyan S, Nadesan P, et al. Constitutive hedgehog signaling in chondrosarcoma upregulates tumor cell proliferation. Am J Pathol. 2006;168:321.
112. Unni KK, Inwards CY, Bridge JA, Kindblom LG, Wold LE. AFIP atlas of tumour pathology; 4th series, fascicle 2: tumours of the bones and joints. Washington, DC: AFIP; 2005.
113. van Maldegem AM, Gelderblom H, Palmerini E, et al. Outcome of advanced, unresectable conventional central chondrosarcoma. Cancer. 2014;120:3159.
114. van Oosterwijk JG, Herpers B, Meijer D, et al. Restoration of chemosensitivity for doxorubicin and cisplatin in chondrosarcoma in vitro: BCL-2 family members cause chemoresistance. Ann Oncol. 2012;23:1617.
115. WHO Classification of Tumours Editorial Board. WHO Classification of tumours. In: Soft tissue and bone tumours, vol. 3. 5th ed. IARC; 2020.
116. Yen KE, Bittinger MA, Su SM, et al. Cancer-associated IDH mutations: biomarker and therapeutic opportunities. Oncogene. 2010;29:6409–17.
117. Young CL, Sim FH, Unni KK, McLeod RA. Chondrosarcoma of bone in children. Cancer. 1990;66:1641.
118. de Jong Y, Ingola M, Briaire-de Bruijn IH, et al. Radiotherapy resistance in chondrosarcoma cells; a possible correlation with alterations in cell cycle related genes. Clin Sarcoma Res. 2019;9:9.

Periosteal Chondrosarcoma

119. Bovée JV, Cleton-Jansen AM, Kuipers-Dijkshoorn NJ, et al. Loss of heterozygosity and DNA ploidy point to a diverging genetic mechanism in the origin of peripheral and central chondrosarcoma. Genes Chromosomes Cancer. 1999;26:237.
120. Cleven AH, Zwartkruis E, Hogendoorn PC, et al. Periosteal chondrosarcoma: a histopathological and molecular analysis of a rare chondrosarcoma subtype. Histopathology. 2015;67:483.
121. Goedhart LM, Ploegmakers JJ, Kroon HM, et al. The presentation, treatment and outcome of periosteal chondrosarcoma in The Netherlands. Bone Jt J. 2014;96-B:823.
122. Chaabane S, Bouaziz MC, Drissi C, Abid L, Ladeb MF. Periosteal chondrosarcoma. Am J Roentgenol. 2009;192(1):W1–6.

123. Papagelopoulos PJ, Galanis EC, Mavrogenis AF, et al. Survivorship analysis in patients with periosteal chondrosarcoma. Clin Orthop Relat Res. 2006;448:199.

Dedifferentiated Chondrosarcoma

124. Bovée JV, Cleton-Jansen AM, Rosenberg C, et al. Molecular genetic characterization of both components of a dedifferentiated chondrosarcoma, with implications for its histogenesis. J Pathol. 1999;189:454.
125. Dickey ID, Rose PS, Fuchs B, et al. Dedifferentiated chondrosarcoma: the role of chemotherapy with updated outcomes. J Bone Jt Surg Am. 2004;86-A:2412.
126. Grimer RJ, Gosheger G, Taminiau A, et al. Dedifferentiated chondrosarcoma: prognostic factors and outcome from a European group. Eur J Cancer. 2007;43:2060.
127. Grote HJ, Schneider-Stock R, Neumann W, Roessner A. Mutation of p53 with loss of heterozygosity in the osteosarcomatous component of a dedifferentiated chondrosarcoma. Virchows Arch. 2000;436:494.
128. Inwards C, Hogendoorn PCW. Dedifferentiated chondrosarcoma. In: Fletcher CDM, Bridge JA, Hogendoorn PCW, Mertens F, editors. WHO classification of tumours of soft tissue and bone. 4th ed. Lyon: IARC; 2013. p. 269.
129. Littrell LA, Wenger DE, Wold LE, et al. Radiographic, CT, and MR imaging features of dedifferentiated chondrosarcomas: a retrospective review of 174 de novo cases. Radiographics. 2004;24:1397.
130. Mitchell AD, Ayoub K, Mangham DC, et al. Experience in the treatment of dedifferentiated chondrosarcoma. J Bone Jt Surg Br. 2000;82:55.
131. Röpke M, Boltze C, Neumann HW, et al. Genetic and epigenetic alterations in tumor progression in a dedifferentiated chondrosarcoma. Pathol Res Pract. 2003;199:437.
132. Staals EL, Bacchini P, Bertoni F. Dedifferentiated central chondrosarcoma. Cancer. 2006;106:2682.
133. Staals EL, Bacchini P, Mercuri M, Bertoni F. Dedifferentiated chondrosarcomas arising in preexisting osteochondromas. J Bone Jt Surg Am. 2007;89:987.
134. Strotman PK, Reif TJ, Kliethermes SA, et al. Dedifferentiated chondrosarcoma: a survival analysis of 159 cases from the SEER database (2001–2011). J Surg Oncol. 2017;116:252.

Mesenchymal Chondrosarcoma

135. Yoshida KI, Machado I, Motoi T, Parafioriti A, Lacambra M, Ichikawa H, Kawai A, Antonescu CR, Yoshida A. NKX3-1 is a useful immunohistochemical marker of EWSR1-NFATC2 sarcoma and mesenchymal chondrosarcoma. Am J Surg Pathol. 2020;44:719.
136. Cesari M, Bertoni F, Bacchini P, et al. Mesenchymal chondrosarcoma. An analysis of patients treated at a single institution. Tumori. 2007;93:423.
137. Chen W, Hornick JL, Fletcher CDM. NKX3.1 immunoreactivity is not identified in mesenchymal chondrosarcoma: a 25-case cohort study. Histopathology. 2021;78(2):334–7.
138. Dantonello TM, Int-Veen C, Leuschner I, et al. Mesenchymal chondrosarcoma of soft tissues and bone in children, adolescents, and young adults: experiences of the CWS and COSS study groups. Cancer. 2008;112:2424.
139. Frezza AM, Cesari M, Baumhoer D, et al. Mesenchymal chondrosarcoma: prognostic factors and outcome in 113 patients. A European musculoskeletal oncology society study. Eur J Cancer. 2015;51:374.
140. Huvos AG, Rosen G, Dabska M, Marcove RC, Mesenchymal chondrosarcoma. A clinicopathologic analysis of 35 patients with emphasis on treatment. Cancer. 1983;51:1230.
141. Nakashima Y, de Pinieux G, Ladanyi M. Mesenchymal chondrosarcoma. In: Fletcher CDM, Bridge JA, Hogendoorn CDW, Mertens F, editors. WHO classification of tumours of soft tissue and bone. 4th ed. Lyon: IARC; 2013. p. 271.
142. Nakashima Y, Unni KK, Shives TC, et al. Mesenchymal chondrosarcoma of bone and soft tissue. A review of 111 cases. Cancer. 1986;57:2444.
143. Ramanayake N, Vargas AC, Talbot J, Bonar F, Wong DD, Wong D, Mahar A, Karim R, Luk PP, Selinger C, Sioson L, Gill AJ, Maclean F. NKX3.1 immunohistochemistry is highly specific for the diagnosis of mesenchymal chondrosarcomas: experience in the Australian population. Pathology. 2021;53(6):705–12.
144. Rushing EJ, Armonda RA, Ansari Q, Mena H. Mesenchymal chondrosarcoma: a clinicopathologic and flow cytometric study of 13 cases presenting in the central nervous system. Cancer. 1996;77:1884.
145. Sainati L, Scapinello A, Montaldi A, Bolcato S, Ninfo V, Carli M, Basso G. A mesenchymal chondrosarcoma of a child with a reciprocal translocation (11;22)(q24;q12). Cancer Genet Cytogenet. 1993;71:144–7.
146. Vencio EF, Reeve CM, Unni KK, Nascimento AG. Mesenchymal chondrosarcoma of the jaw bones: clinicopathologic study of 19 cases. Cancer. 1998;82:2350.
147. Wang L, Motoi T, Khanin R, et al. Identification of a novel, recurrent HEY1-NCOA2 fusion in mesenchymal chondrosarcoma based on a genome-wide screen of exon-level expression data. Genes Chromosomes Cancer. 2012;51:127.
148. Xu J, Li D, Xie L, et al. Mesenchymal chondrosarcoma of bone and soft tissue: a systematic review of 107 patients in the past 20 years. PLoS One. 2015;10:e0122216.

Clear Cell Chondrosarcoma

149. Carthy EF, Hogendoorn PCW. Clear cell chondrosarcoma. In: Fletcher CDM, Bridge JA, Hogendoorn PCW, Mertens F, editors. World Health Organization classification of tumours of soft tissue and bone. 4th ed. Lyon: IARC; 2013. p. 273.
150. Donati D, Yin JQ, Colangeli M, et al. Clear cell chondrosarcoma of bone: long time follow-up of 18 cases. Arch Orthop Trauma Surg. 2008;128:137.
151. Itälä A, Leerapun T, Inwards C, et al. An institutional review of clear cell chondrosarcoma. Clin Orthop Relat Res. 2005;440:209.

Myxoid Chondrosarcoma

152. Antonescu CR, Argani P, Erlandson RA, et al. Skeletal and extraskeletal myxoid chondrosarcoma: a comparative clinicopathologic, ultrastructural, and molecular study. Cancer. 1998;83:1504.
153. Brody RI, Ueda T, Hamelin A, et al. Molecular analysis of the fusion of EWS to an orphan nuclear receptor gene in extraskeletal myxoid chondrosarcoma. Am J Pathol. 1997;150:1049.
154. Demicco EG, Wang WL, Madewell JE, et al. Osseous myxochondroid sarcoma: a detailed study of 5 cases of extraskeletal myxoid chondrosarcoma of the bone. Am J Surg Pathol. 2013;37:752.
155. Drilon AD, Popat S, Bhuchar G, et al. Extraskeletal myxoid chondrosarcoma: a retrospective review from 2 referral centers emphasizing long-term outcomes with surgery and chemotherapy. Cancer. 2008;113:3364.
156. Goh YW, Spagnolo DV, Platten M, et al. Extraskeletal myxoid chondrosarcoma: a light microscopic, immunohistochemical, ultrastructural and immuno-ultrastructural study indicating neuroendocrine differentiation. Histopathology. 2001;39:514.
157. Kilpatrick SE, Inwards CY, Fletcher CD, et al. Myxoid chondrosarcoma (chordoid sarcoma) of bone: a report of two cases and review of the literature. Cancer. 1997;79:1903.
158. Shapeero LG, Vanel D, Couanet D, et al. Extraskeletal mesenchymal chondrosarcoma. Radiology. 1993;186:819.

Osteochondromyxoma

159. Carney JA, Boccon-Gibod L, Jarka DE, Tanaka Y, Swee RG, Unni KK, Stratakis CA. Osteochondromyxoma of bone: a congenital tumor associated with lentigines and other unusual disorders. Am J Surg Pathol. 2001;25(2):164–76.

Exuberrant Callus

160. Binesh F, Sobhan M, Moghadam RN, et al. Exuberant callus formation misdiagnosed as osteosarcoma: a case report. Chin Ger J Clin Oncol. 2013;12:137–9.
161. Dobrocky I, Seidl G, Grill F. MRI and CT features of hyperplastic callus in osteogenesis imperfecta tarda. Eur Radiol. 1999;9:665–8.
162. Brusin JH. Osteogenesis imperfecta. Radiol Technol. 2008;79(6):535–51.
163. Kutsumi K, Nojima T, Yamashiro K, et al. Hyperplastic callus formation in both femurs in osteogenesis imperfecta. Skelet Radiol. 1996;25:384–7.
164. Cheung MS, Glorieux FH, Rauch F. Natural history of hyperplastic callus formation in osteogenesis imperfecta type V. J Bone Miner Res. 2007;22:1181–6.
165. Ramirez N, Vilella FE, Colon M, Flynn JM. Osteogenesis imperfecta and hyperplastic callus formation in a family: a report of three cases and a review of the literature. J Pediatr Orthop B. 2003;12:88–96.
166. Vieira RL, Amaral DT, Jesus-Garcia FR, Saraiva G, Fernandes AR, Resnick D. Hyperplastic callus formation in osteogenesis imperfecta type V mimicking osteosarcoma: 4-year follow-up with resolution. Skelet Radiol. 2006;35:402–5.

Costochondral Junction

167. Guttentag AR, Salwen JK. Keep your eyes on the ribs: the spectrum of normal variants and diseases that involve the ribs. Radiographics. 1999;19(5):1125–42.

Intervertebral Disc

168. Rutges JPHJ, Duit RA, Kummer JA, Bekkers JEJ, Oner FC, Castelein RM, Dhert WJA, Creemers LB. A validated new histological classification for intervertebral disc degeneration. Osteoarthr Cartil. 2013;21(12):2039–47.

5 Osteogenic Tumours

5.1 Terminology

1. **Osteoid**: Extracellular material produced by the osteoblasts, largely type I collagen (Fig. 5.1)

2. **Bone**: Same tissue after calcium salts have been deposited.

3. **Lamellar bone (trabecular bone)**: Mature bone—concentric layers of collagen in parallel arrays (Fig. 5.2a)

4. **Woven bone**: Woven bone or immature bone is with increased number of osteocytes and haphazard arrangement of collagen fibres in osteoid matrix. Its presence in adults is always pathological (Fig. 5.2b).

5. **Reactive osteoid**: Benign cells producing osteoid (Fig. 5.3). For example, ABC, GCT, and callus.

6. **Malignant (tumour) osteoid**: Malignant cells surrounding osteoid or malignant cells producing osteoid (Fig. 5.4).

Osteogenic tumours of the bone consist of a spectrum of entities, ranging from benign lesions to frankly malignant, with many histologic variations.

Osteogenic Tumours: WHO 2020 Classification [152]

Benign

Osteoma

Osteoid osteoma

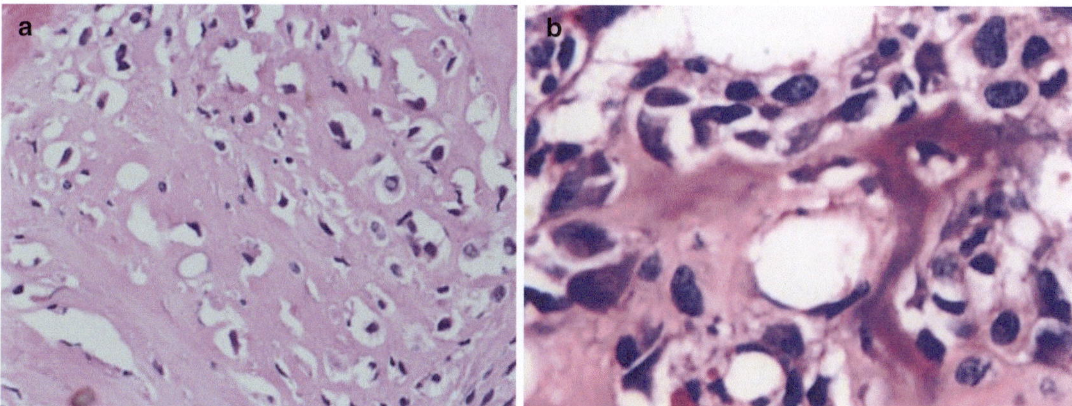

Fig. 5.1 (**a**) Osteoid without calcification, H&E ×250. (**b**) Calcifying osteoid, H&E ×400

J. Kattoor et al., *Bone Tumors*, https://doi.org/10.1007/978-981-99-4738-6_5

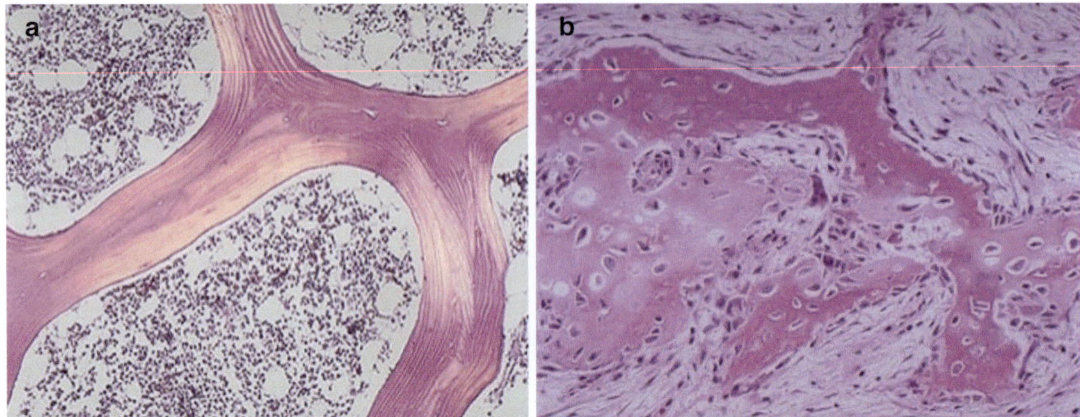

Fig. 5.2 (**a**) Trabecular or lamellar bone—concentric layers of collagen in parallel arrays and less number of osteocytes, H&E ×100. (**b**) Woven bone (immature bone)—haphazard placement of collagen fibres in the osteoid matrix. Increased number of osteocytes, H&E ×250

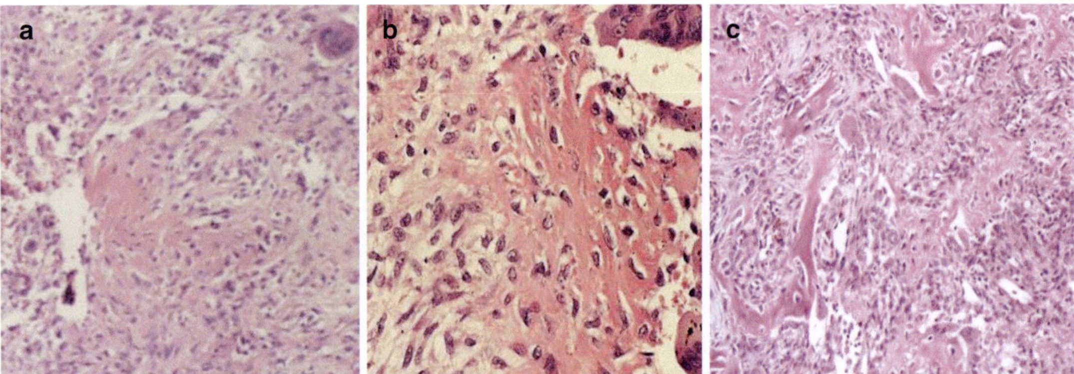

Fig. 5.3 Reactive osteoid. (**a**) Benign cells producing osteoid in aneurysmal bone cyst, H&E ×100. (**b**) Fracture callus, H&E ×250. (**c**) In giant cell tumour, H&E ×100

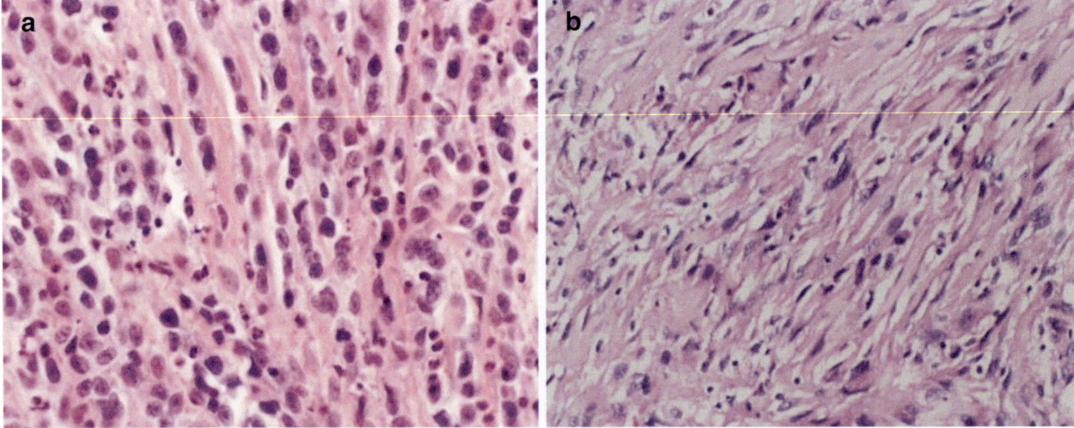

Fig. 5.4 (**a**) Osteoid produced by malignant cells in osteosarcoma in lace-like pattern, H&E ×250. (**b**) Pleomorphic malignant cells producing osteoid, H&E ×100

Intermediate (locally aggressive)
 Osteoblastoma
Malignant
 Osteosarcoma
 Low-grade central osteosarcoma
 Osteosarcoma NOS
  Conventional osteosarcoma
  Telangiectatic osteosarcoma
  Small cell osteosarcoma
 Parosteal osteosarcoma
 Periosteal osteosarcoma
 High-grade surface osteosarcoma
 Secondary osteosarcoma

5.2 Benign and Intermediate Osteoid-Producing Tumours

5.2.1 Osteoma

Osteomas are benign surface tumours consisting of cortical bone. If it occurs in medullary cavity, it is called bone island.

5.2.1.1 Clinical

Osteomas usually occur in bone formed by membranous ossification. Common sites are skull and facial bones [1, 2, 5, 36] and jaw bones [29, 41]. They are slow-growing tumours and usually asymptomatic. Sometimes, it can cause pain and headache. Gigantic osteomas are described.

5.2.1.2 Radiology

They are dense and sclerotic (ivory-like appearance), occurring on the surface of the bone. Multiple osteomas occur in Gardner's syndrome. On bone scan, it shows mild uptake and can mimic a blastic metastasis. Gigantic osteoma of the mandible has been reported [49].

Reactive changes from trauma and infection can show osseous overgrowth. Similarly, some tumours near the surface of bone like haemangioma, lipoma and dural meningioma can show osteomatous growth mimicking osteomas. An old osteochondroma with involuted cartilage cap can mimic osteoma.

Parosteal osteoma of long bones is extremely rare. One has to rule out parosteal osteosarcoma if unmineralized soft tissue mass is detected on the surface of long bones.

5.2.1.3 Pathology

These tumours are well circumscribed, broadly attached to the surface of the bone. Histologically, they are composed of mature lamellar/cortical bone (Fig. 5.5). The marrow spaces may show fibrous and vascular stroma, mimicking the appearance of osteoblastoma. Any spindle cell proliferation as seen in parosteal osteosarcoma is absent in osteoma and will rule out this entity.

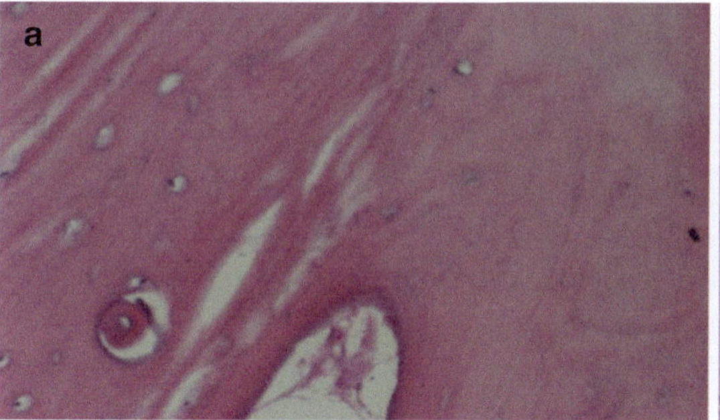

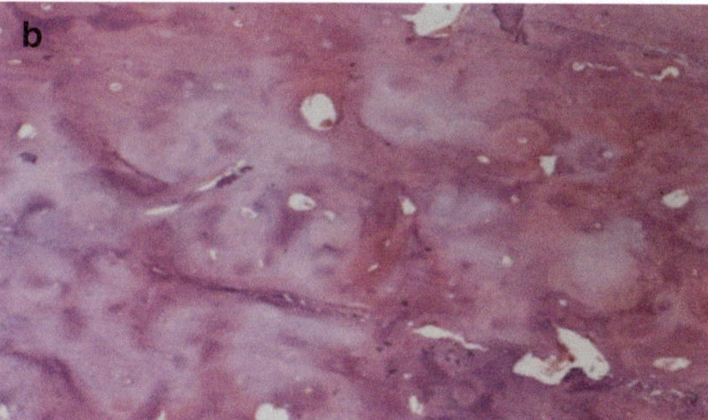

Fig. 5.5 Osteoma. (**a**, **b**) Cortical bone with scattered osteocytes, H&E ×400

5.2.1.4 Treatment

Symptomatic cases are excised. Asymptomatic cases do not require treatment.

5.2.2 Osteoid Osteoma (OO)

Osteoid osteoma is a benign neoplasm of small size with an osteoblastic round mass in the centre called as nidus [7, 8]. The nidus is surrounded by a sclerotic bone. The surrounding sclerosis is a reactive process, which disappears when the nidus is removed. The disease usually occurs in the first two decades with a male predominance [11, 13]. The common bones involved are femur and tibia. The proximal femur, especially the neck of femur, is the most common site [8]. Other rare sites are arch of vertebra [42], skull bones, phalanges of hands and tarsal bone [27].

5.2.2.1 Clinical

These tumours present as pain of gradually progressing severity, which is present for weeks to years. The pain is more at night, interfering with sleep [25]. Sometimes, pain may present as referred pain well away from tumour, thus causing delay in diagnosis. In vertebral lesions, the pain resembles disc prolapse clinically [24, 32]. The pain is typically relieved by salicylates. High levels of prostaglandins in the lesion are implicated to cause pain (PGE2, PGI2 and COX2), and this explains why aspirin relieves pain [26, 40]. The patient will have dysfunction resulting in limp, and atrophy of muscles of affected extremity is common.

5.2.2.2 Radiology

The nidus may appear as a rounded area of sclerosis with a halo of lucency around it [7]. Sometimes, cortical thickening, with or without central lytic area, may be seen. Most of the cases are diagnosed on plain radiographs. In difficult cases, CT scan usually helps in diagnosis [20]. CT combined with MRI also helps in localizing nidus, especially in the spine [16, 28]. Multiple osteoid osteomas attached like a bead and elongated in appearance on radiology are described [10]. Multicentric osteoid osteomas can occur in children [50].

5.2.2.3 Pathology

OO is usually less than 1.5 cm. To distinguish from OB, the cut-off limit of size is 2 cm. Sometimes, microscopy in both osteoid osteomas and osteoblastomas is similar. Both have a nidus surrounded by sclerotic bone (Fig. 5.6a). The nidus consists of interlacing network of woven bone (immature bone) with or without calcification and fibrovascular stroma in between. The osteoid/woven bone is rimmed by osteoblasts.

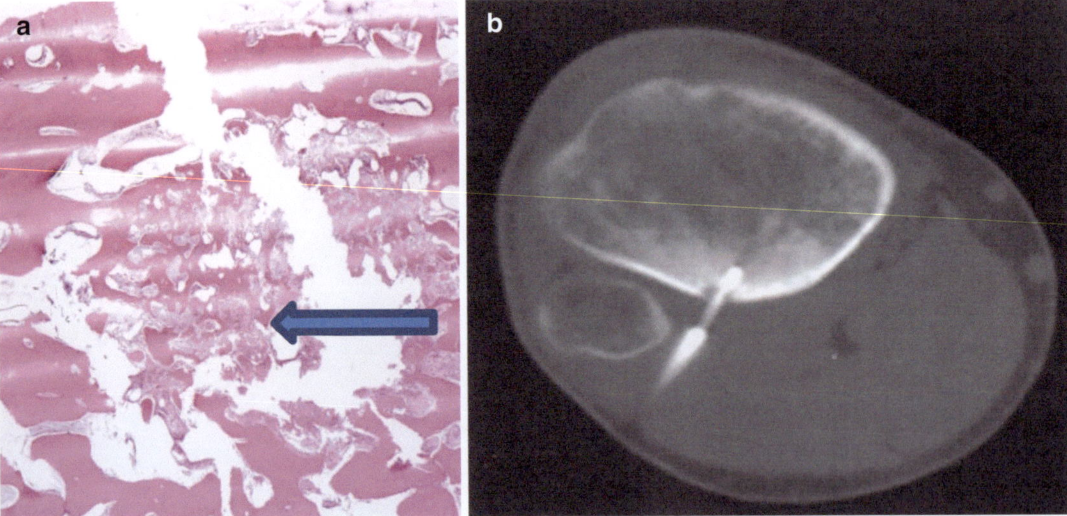

Fig. 5.6 Osteoid osteoma. (**a**) Nidus of osteoid osteoma (arrow)and surrounding sclerotic bone, H&E ×40. (**b**) CT-guided radio ablation of nidus

Clear-cut cartilage is unusual in this tumour. When the tissue is received in fragments, the distinction of nidus surrounded by sclerotic bone is difficult. In case the treatment is radio ablation, histopathologic examination is not possible. Fragments of necrotic bone will be seen.

5.2.2.4 Molecular Findings

Both OO and OB show rearrangement of FOS [12].

5.2.2.5 Treatment and Prognosis

Earlier, these tumours were treated with excision [4]. Now it has changed dramatically in the last two decades. Now majority undergo thermablation/radiofrequency ablation under CT guidance [20, 43, 44, 48] (Fig. 5.6b). Most of the patients experience relief of symptoms. Complete removal of nidus results in cure [24]. If complete removal is not possible, it will recur [52]. If surgery is difficult, treatment with nonsteroidal anti-inflammatory drugs gives great pain relief [21, 26, 32]. Progression of osteoid osteoma to osteoblastoma is reported [6].

5.2.3 Osteoblastoma (OB)

OB is a large lesion previously known as giant osteoid osteoma [41]. The osteoblastic nature of the tumour resembles morphologically to that of osteoid osteoma [45]. They are more than 2 cm in size, and the most common site is posterior elements of vertebra [19, 60]. Most of these tumours (>40%) occur either in vertebra or in sacrum. Some osteoblastomas are locally aggressive neoplasms [22, 39].

5.2.3.1 Clinical

It occurs in younger patients, predominantly in the first three decades of life [8, 34]. It is more common in males. Apart from spine and sacrum, they also occur in long bones, mandible, maxilla and ribs [8, 45]. They are also reported in tarsals, carpals, phalanges of the hand and clavicle [14, 17]. According to the location, progressive pain, local swelling, gait disturbances or neurologic symptoms are the usual complaints [51]. Systemic symptoms are described, namely fever and weight loss [38]. This is said to be due to exaggerated immune response to the neoplasm. Rarely, OB can be observed in association with oncogenic phosphaturic syndrome [53].

5.2.3.2 Radiology

Features of osteoblastomas may be similar to those of osteoid osteoma, but the size will be more than 2 cm. The appearance is quite variable and may be nonspecific. They are lytic with surrounding sclerosis. In 25% of cases, features suggestive of a malignant neoplasm are seen (Fig. 5.7). In the vertebra, osteoblastoma usually results in the expansion of posterior elements [42] (Fig. 5.8). Fifty percent show ossification radiographically. Mandibular lesions (cementoblastoma) are "ossified", surrounded by a lucent halo, and located near a tooth root. If associated with secondary ABC, fluid–fluid levels are seen in CT and MRI.

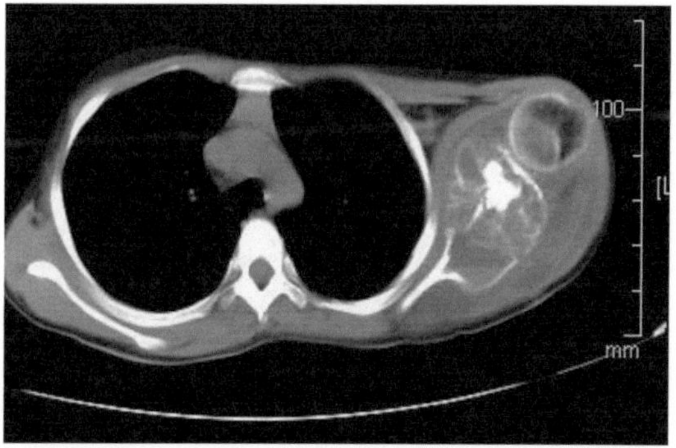

Fig. 5.7 MRI of osteoblastoma of scapula in an 8-year-old girl

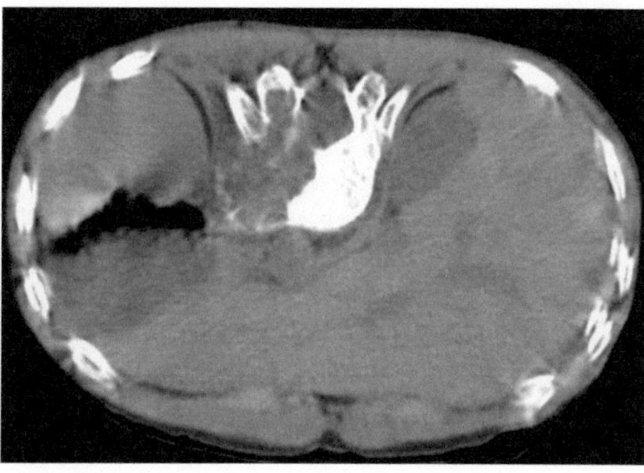

Fig. 5.8 MRI of osteoblastoma of vertebra in an 11-year-old boy

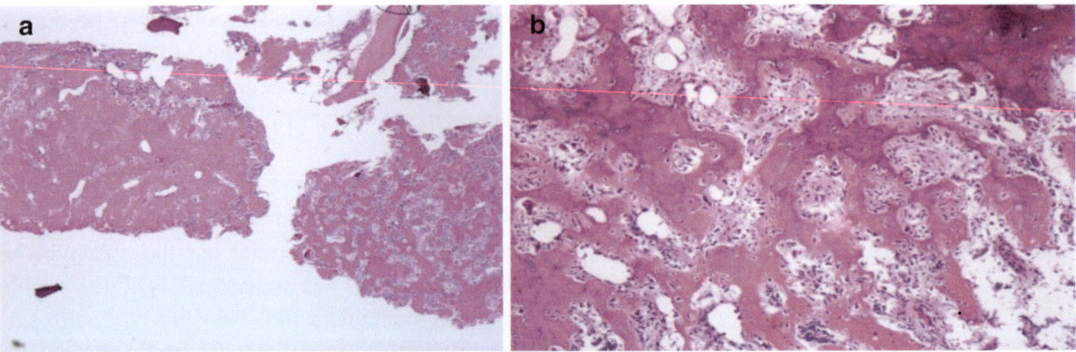

Fig. 5.9 Osteoblastoma. (**a**) Abundant osteoid and fibrovascular stroma. Difficult to differentiate from osteoblastic osteosarcoma. Cells are obscured by matrix. (**b**) Calcifying woven bone and fibrovascular stroma

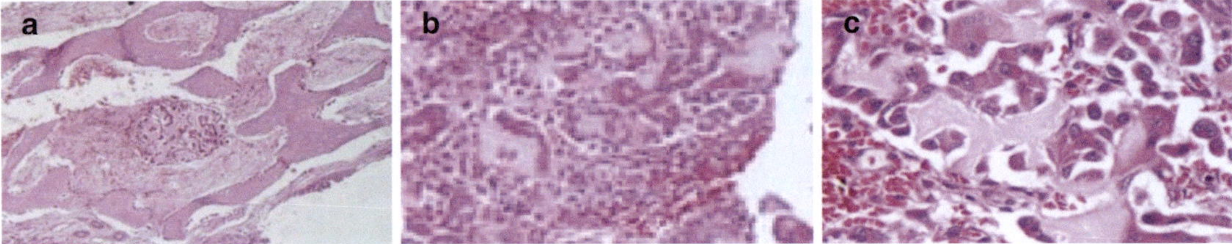

Fig. 5.10 Epithelioid osteoblastoma. (**a**) Multiple foci, H&E ×100. (**b**, **c**) Osteoid with plump epithelioid osteoblasts, H&E ×250

5.2.3.3 Pathology

Grossly, the lesional tissue is haemorrhagic and reddish in colour. The tissue is granular and friable in quality. In excised specimen, the tumour shows sharp circumscription at its periphery. Blood-filled cystic spaces are present if associated with secondary ABC.

Microscopically, osteoblastomas are composed of interlacing network of bony trabeculae in a loose fibrovascular stroma (Fig. 5.9). The periphery of the lesion is well circumscribed, but the osteoid may merge with the adjacent normal bone at the periphery. Some osteoblastomas have immature bone matrix with or without calcification, whereas others have appearance of mature bony trabeculae. The bone and osteoid seams are lined by single-layered osteoblasts. Sometimes, these osteoblasts are plump and appear atypical [18]. Osteoclastic giant cells can be seen scattered throughout the lesion. Epithelioid osteoblasts are also seen. In some cases, the osteoid may be quite fine and "lace-like" as is seen in osteosarcoma, but cartilaginous differentiation is unusual. But few cases may show islands of cartilage maturing into bone giving a chondro-osteoid appearance. Mitotic figures may be identified and may be quite numerous, but atypical mitoses are not present. 10% of cases show secondary aneurysmal bone cyst formation. This may mimic malignancy clinically due to rapid growth (Fig. 5.12). Necrosis is unusual in osteoblastoma without pathologic fracture.

Epithelioid osteoblastomas are described [15]. They can be multifocal with nodules of epithelioid osteoblasts, and this may mimic permeation of bony trabeculae [54] (Fig. 5.10). This will give false impression of osteosarcoma or metastatic carcinoma. Dorfman and Weiss sug-

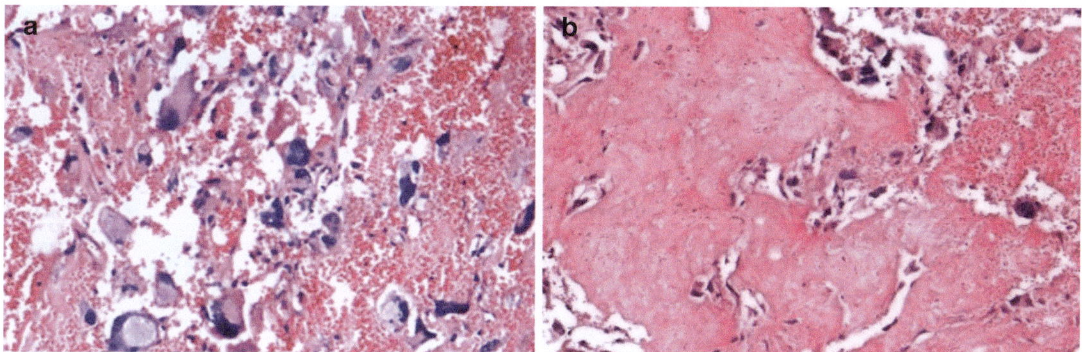

Fig. 5.11 (**a**, **b**) OB with bizarre smudged nuclei (formerly called as pseudosarcomatous osteoblastoma), H&E ×250

gested that epithelioid osteoblast indicates aggressive behaviour [19, 30]. But other authors have not found any correlation between morphology of osteoblasts and its clinical behaviour. Hence, the terminology aggressive and malignant osteoblastoma is no longer used.

Bizarre, pleomorphic nuclei can be seen in some osteoblastomas. These nuclei are large, pleomorphic and hyperchromatic but do not have crisp nuclear features. They resemble cells of ancient schwannoma or post-radiation nuclei. They were termed **pseudosarcomatous osteoblastomas** [9, 33, 39] (Figs. 5.11 and 5.12). But this terminology is not used now.

5.2.3.4 IHC

To differentiate from osteosarcoma, FOSB staining is found to be good. SATB2 will be positive in OB and OS.

5.2.3.5 Molecular

FOS gene rearrangement is seen in OB, similar to osteoid osteomas [12]. An unbalanced translocation with loss of short arm of chromosome 17 is reported in osteoblastoma [37].

5.2.3.6 DD

1. Osteoid osteoma [31]. The differentiating features are given in Table 5.1.
2. Osteoblastic osteosarcoma [3, 16, 35]

5.2.3.7 Treatment and Prognosis

Small lesions are treated by intralesional curettage +/− cryotherapy and bone grafting. Large tumours are treated by en bloc resection with internal fixation or bone grafting [23]. Prognosis is good. Rarely, recurrences are seen in patients treated with curettage. Rare cases of malignant transformation are reported [46, 47].

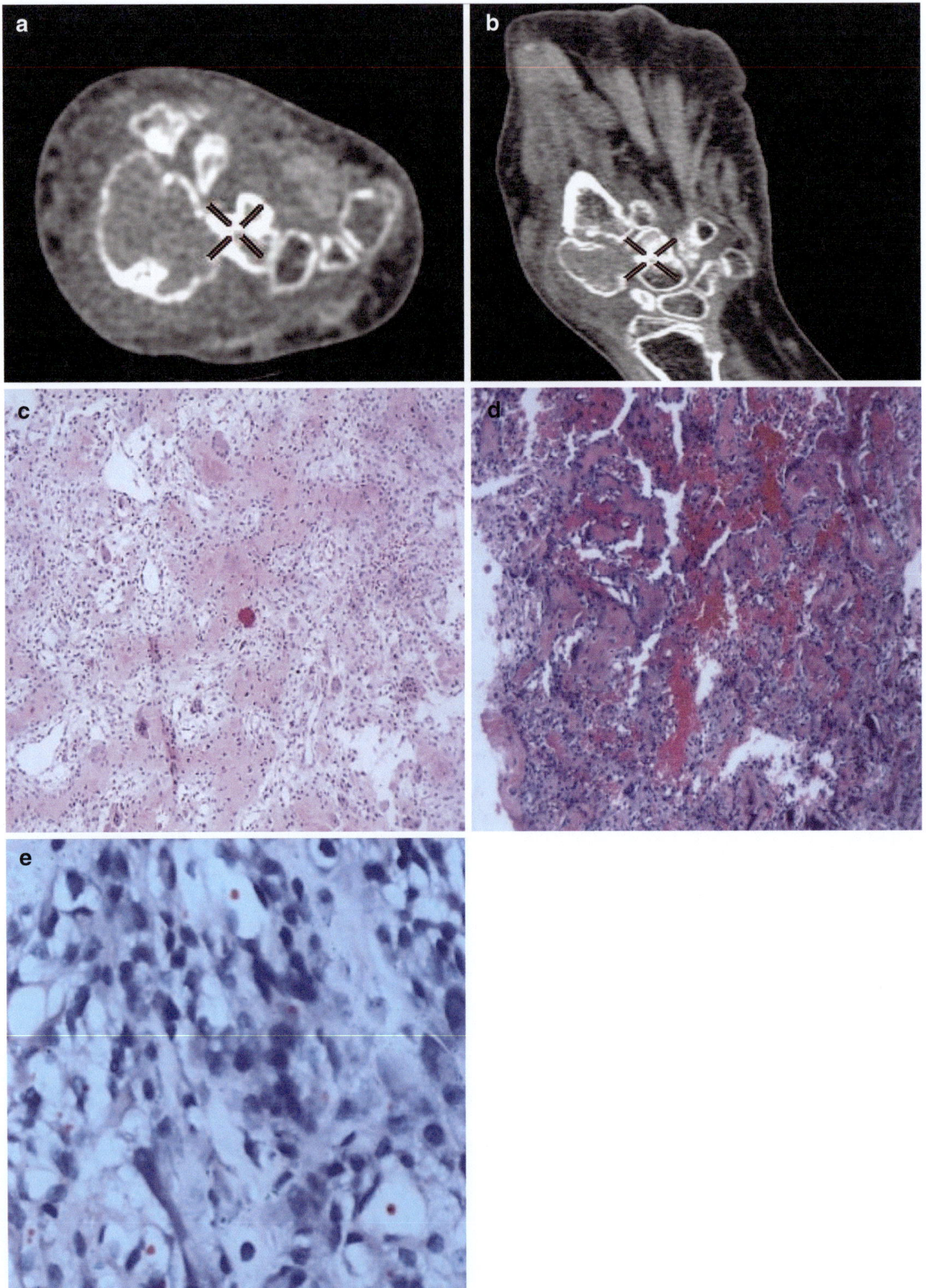

Fig. 5.12 (**a**, **b**) MRI of a rapidly enlarging wrist mass of a 13-year-old girl with cortical break. (**c**) OB—woven bone with loose fibrovascular stroma, H&E ×40. (**d**) With ABC like changes, H&E ×100. (**e**) Areas of nuclear atypia mimicking malignancy. H&E ×250. Cortical break and rapid enlargement were due to ABC like changes

Table 5.1 Differentiating features of osteoid osteoma and osteoblastoma

	Osteoid osteoma	Osteoblastoma
Incidence	10% of benign tumours	3% of benign tumours
Size	<2 cm (typically <1.5 cm)	>2 cm (average, 3.5–4.0 cm)
Site	>50% in long bone diaphysis	>35% in posterior elements of spine
Location	Proximal femur, tibia diaphysis	Spine, proximal humerus, hip
Symptoms	Nocturnal pain, relieved by NSAIDS	Dull ache, not relieved by NSAIDS
Natural history	Self-limited	Progressive
Histology	Benign appearance. No growth potential, central nidus	Benign appearance Localized growth Nidus with aggressive potential

5.3 Malignant tumours-Osteosarcoma

Osteosarcoma is a malignant osteoid-producing tumour. It also produces chondroid and fibrous tissue in variable proportions. 80% of osteosarcomas are conventional type [109]. Osteoid is abundant in osteoblastic type and minimal in some other types. It can be minimal and sometimes not detected in a small biopsy. The pattern of osteoid deposition is also different. It can be lace-like or filigree pattern (Fig. 5.13a) or dense eosinophilic (Fig. 5.13b) or calcifying (Fig. 5.13c). If radiology and clinical scenario are typical of osteosarcoma, one is justified in giving a diagnosis of osteosarcoma, even if osteoid is not very evident. This difficulty is mainly encountered in fibroblastic and telangiectatic variants.

Osteosarcomas are the most common primary bone sarcoma [102]. It is most common in the second decade. Children and adolescents are affected, and there is a male predilection for the disease. Another peak of incidence is seen in older age group [82]. But these are mainly secondary osteosarcomas occurring in patients with Paget disease, previous irradiation, bone infarct, chronic osteomyelitis and dedifferentiation in chondrosarcomas, chordomas or secondary malignancy in giant cell tumour. There is an increased incidence of osteosarcoma in genetic syndromes like Li-Fraumeni syndrome (TP53) [100], hereditary retinoblastoma (TP53 and RB1) [87], Bloom syndrome (BLM-[RECQL3]), Werner syndrome (WRN) and Rothmund-Thomson syndrome (RECQL4) (Table 5.2).

The metaphysis of long bones is the site of predilection. Areas around knee-lower end of femur and upper end of tibia are the most common locations. It is because this is the growing region in children and adolescents. Other common sites are upper end of humerus, lower end of radius and lower end of tibia. In the jaw bones, most of them occur in the mandible. Skull bone and small bones of hands and feet are very rarely involved. In the older age group, osteosarcomas occur mainly in the axial skeleton [82].

5.3.1 Clinical

Pain and swelling are the most common symptoms [56, 80, 90]. It is rare to find a patient without symptoms. Hence, if a child or adolescent complains of pain, it should not be ignored. Pathological fracture is unusual. Swelling or pain in a patient with Paget disease, flare-up of symptoms in a patient who had irradiation for a benign bone lesion and rapid progression of disease in chondrosarcoma should arouse suspicion of development of aggressive sarcoma like osteosarcoma.

5.3.2 Radiology

Tumours may be completely lytic or completely sclerotic or a mixture of both. There is a wide zone of transition, which is evident on MRI scan. The osteosarcomas push the periosteum resulting in cortical destruction and extension to adjacent soft tissue. This type of periosteal reaction is

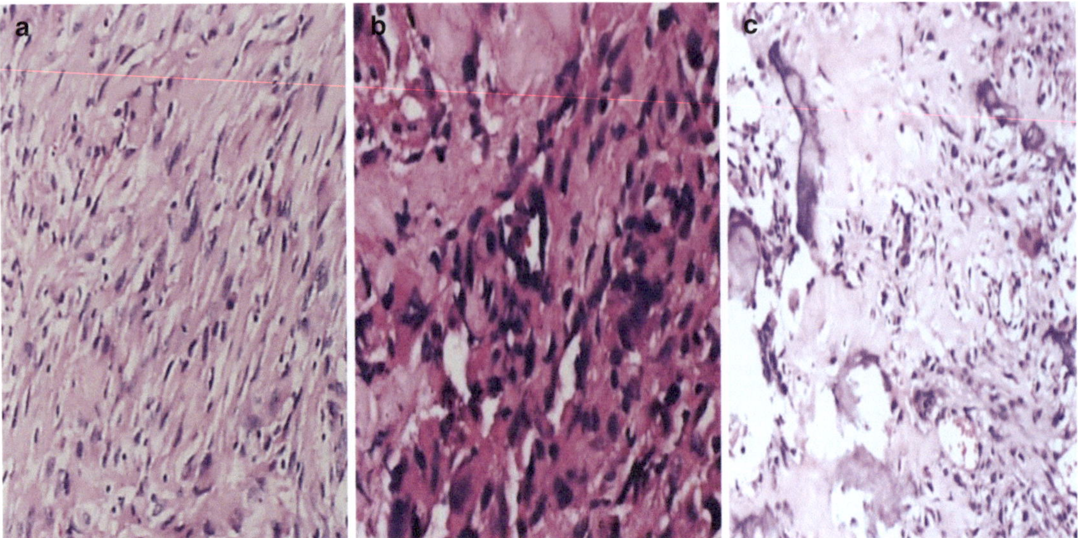

Fig. 5.13 Osteoid in osteosarcoma. (**a**) Filigree (lace-like) osteoid, H&E ×100. (**b**) Abundant dense osteoid, H&E ×250. (**c**) Calcifying osteoid, H&E ×100

Table 5.2 Genetic syndromes associated with OS

Syndrome	Mutation
Rothmund-Thomson syndrome	8q24.3
Bloom	15q26.1
Werner	8p11
Li-Fraumeni	17p13
B/L retinoblastoma	13q14

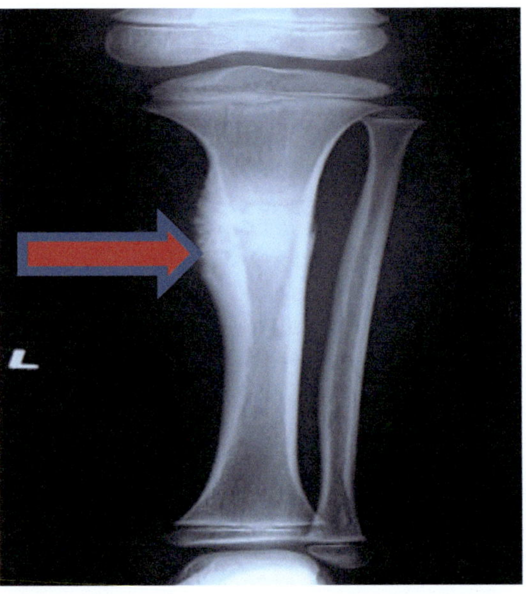

Fig. 5.14 Plain X-ray of metadiaphyseal OS in a 9-year-old boy with Codman triangle and sunray appearance of new bone formation

common in osteosarcoma and may result in a classic "Codman triangle" [75]. New bone formation perpendicular to the surface of bone results in classical "sunray" appearance (Fig. 5.14). When an osteosarcoma produces sufficient calcifying osteoid, it will be visible on plain X-ray (Fig. 5.15). Even if there is plenty of osteoid production as seen in osteoblastic osteosarcoma, it does not produce radio density if it is completely uncalcified. Plain radiograph is the best for diagnosing osteosarcoma. CT and MRI are mainly used to assess the extent of disease prior to surgery (Fig. 5.16). Cortical irregularities, mineralization, presence of fracture and neurovascular involvement are better appreciated in CT scan. Bone scan is done to diagnose multiple bone involvement, metastases to other bones and intraosseous tumour extension. Vascular anatomy can be seen in angiography. This is helpful for preoperative planning in patients with tumours where vascular anatomic abnormalities are seen, for example, proximal tibia or shoulder girdle. Positron emission tomography (PET) scans are done to detect metastatic lesions. X-ray of the chest is done as an initial workup because lung is the most common metastatic site. Sometimes, radiological appearance of osteosarcomas can

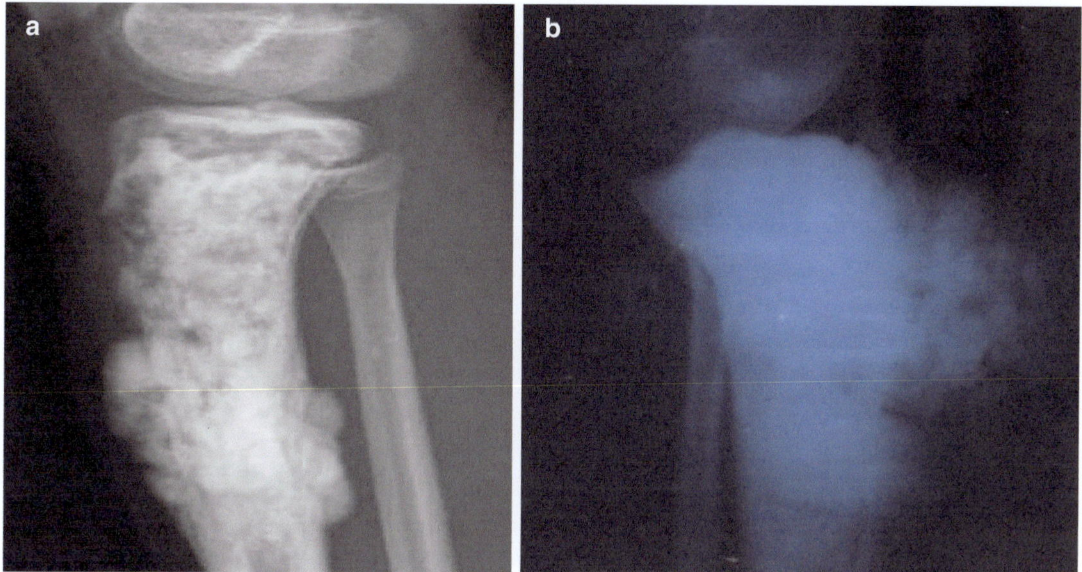

Fig. 5.15 Different types of matrix in OS: (**a**, **b**) Fluffy matrix in OS

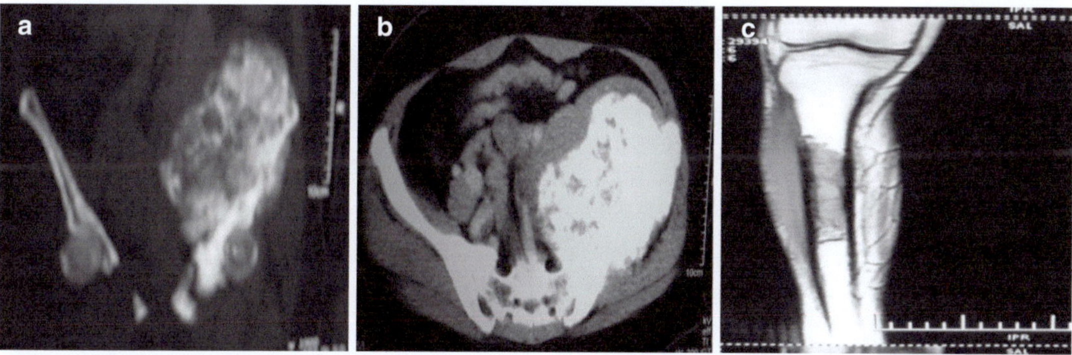

Fig. 5.16 MRI of OS of pelvis. (**a**, **b**) Huge mass ilium with soft tissue extension. (**c**) MRI of diaphyseal OS in a 25-year-old male

mimic other tumours like Ewing sarcoma or Langerhans cell histiocytosis (Fig. 5.17).

5.3.3 Pathology

Grossing of different types of specimens is given in Chap. 2.

Grossly, conventional osteosarcomas are large fleshy or firm (Fig. 5.18) with cortical destruction and soft tissue extension (Fig. 5.20). They are present at the metaphysis but can extend to diaphysis and epiphysis (Fig. 5.19). Cartilaginous foci may be evident macroscopically. Areas of necrosis, cyst formation and haemorrhage are commonly seen in the soft tissue. Periosteal elevation and Codman triangle can be appreciated in the gross resected specimen.

Microscopy shows varying pattern according to the predominant pattern of growth [96]. In needle biopsy, accuracy of diagnosis may be less compared to open biopsy.

Conventional OS shows a mixture of osteoblastic, chondroblastic and fibroblastic areas. In a needle biopsy, one type of cell may be prominent. Even though there is no prognostic significance for these types, there can be diagnostic difficulties due to overlapping morphological features between benign, malignant and tumour-like lesions.

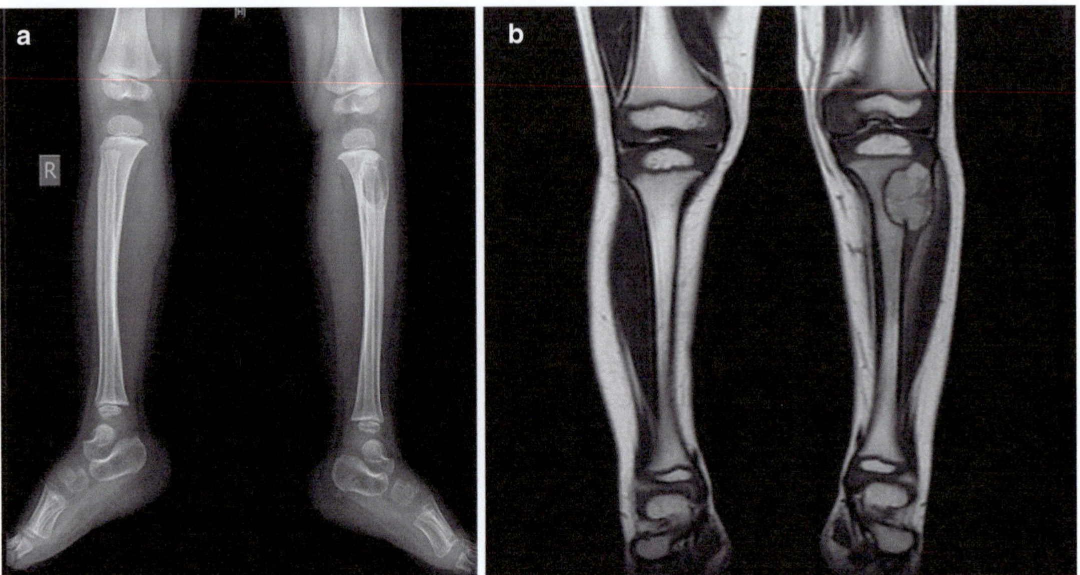

Fig. 5.17 OS in a 2-year-old boy mimicking LCH of upper end of left tibia. (**a**) X-ray showing lytic expansile lesion without periosteal reaction. (**b**) MRI showing expansile lesion without significant periosteal reaction

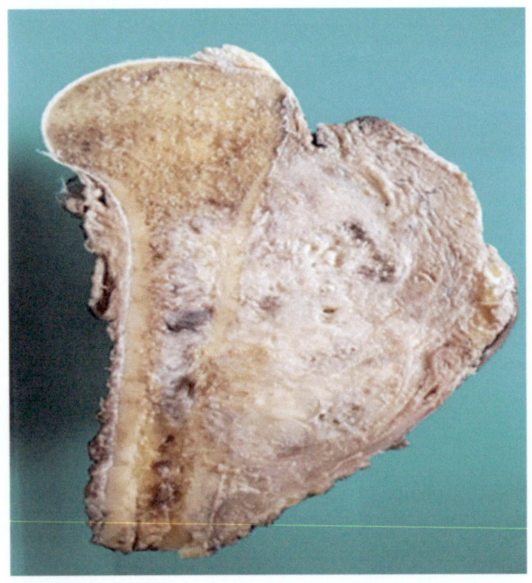

Fig. 5.18 Gross specimen of OS: OS of upper femur with glistening cut surface

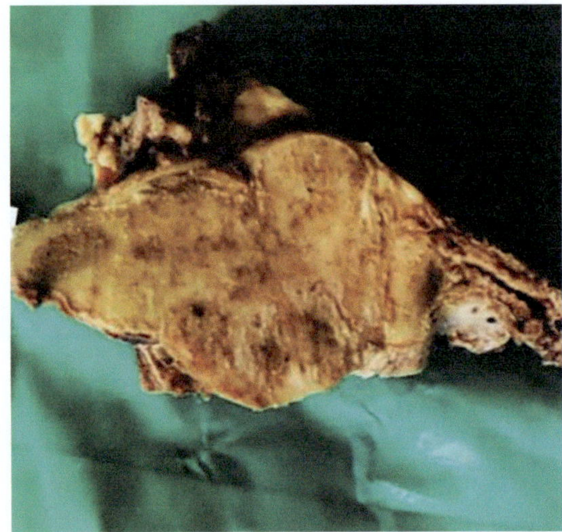

Fig. 5.19 OS of rib. Expansile growth chondroblastic areas

5.3.4 Immunohistochemistry

Commonly, positive markers are SATB2, osteocalcin, osteonectin, RUNX2, S100 and CD99 [84]. Osteosarcomas are also positive for CK and EMA [92]. FOS which is positive in osteoid osteoma and osteoblastoma is negative in osteosarcoma. SATB2 is a very sensitive marker for osteoblastic differentiation. SATB2 is usually negative in Ewing sarcoma. Since osteosarcomas have heterogeneous cell types, the immunohistochemical findings are also heterogeneous [84]. Ezrin and Galectin-1 are novel IHC markers to differentiate chondroblastic osteosarcoma from chondrosarcoma, where both are negative in the latter [81, 106].

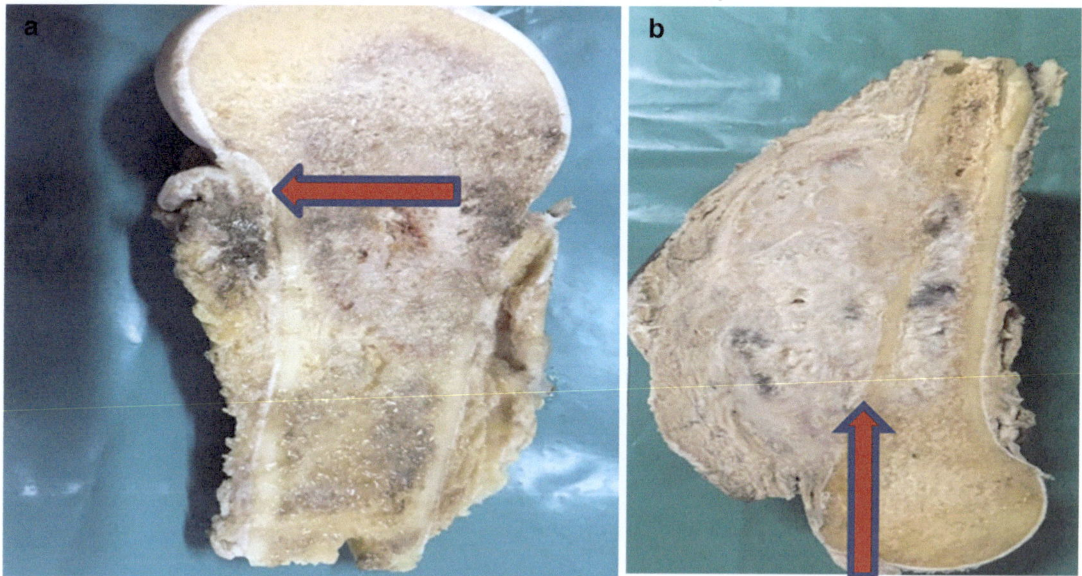

Fig. 5.20 (**a**) OS with cortical destruction. (**b**) OS with predominant soft tissue component

5.3.5 Molecular

Acquiring chromosomal instability is thought to be the most important reason for osteosarcoma development [60]. This leads to both intertumoural and intratumoural heterogeneity. Complex karyotypes are seen in paediatric osteosarcomas [64, 67]. Various numerical and structural alterations are seen. TP53 inactivation is the most common mutation seen in OS (>90%). IDH1 and IDH2 mutations are absent, which helps to differentiate chondroblastic osteosarcoma from chondrosarcoma [72] (Fig. 5.20).

5.3.6 Grading of Osteosarcoma

Majority of osteosarcomas are high grade [108]. Grade I or low-grade osteosarcomas are parosteal osteosarcoma and low-grade central osteosarcomas. Periosteal osteosarcoma because of its location behaves in a less aggressive manner. Hence, it is considered as intermediate grade. Similarly, jaw bone osteosarcomas also behave as intermediate grade with locally aggressive nature. More than 90% of osteosarcomas are high grade [56].

5.3.7 Morphological Subtypes

The importance of morphological subtypes is that it mimics other bone tumours or tumour-like lesions of bone morphologically. This causes diagnostic difficulty.

5.3.7.1 Low-Grade Central Osteosarcoma (LGCOS)

LGCOS is a rare type of osteosarcoma (1–2%). This was described by Unni et al. in 1977 [117]. They are difficult to distinguish from benign bone lesions [112, 113]. They can arise from bone infarct [114]. They are slow growing with low metastatic rate and have a good prognosis with prolonged survival after treatment.

Clinical

Metaphysis of femur and tibia are the common sites. Jaw, axial bones and small bones of hands and feet are rarely affected. The symptoms may be present for a long time (average of more than 2 years).

Radiology

They are lytic with varying amounts of thick and coarse trabeculations or with densely sclerotic areas or mixed lytic and sclerotic. Cortical

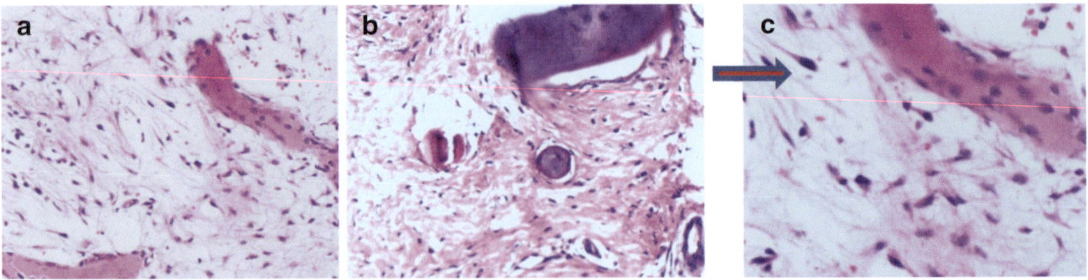

Fig. 5.21 Low-grade central osteosarcoma. (**a**, **b**) Loose spindle cells permeating bony spicules, H&E ×100. (**c**) Scattered atypical cells (arrow), H&E ×250

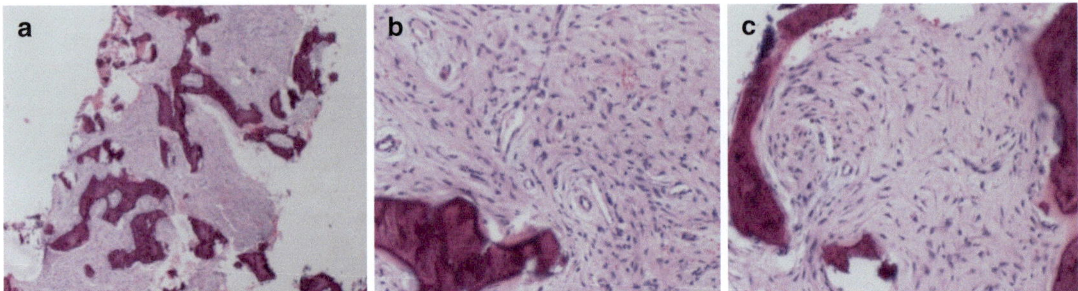

Fig. 5.22 Low-grade OS of tibia in a 20-year-old male. (**a**) Permeation of spindle cells in between pre-existing bone, H&E ×40. (**b**, **c**) Proliferating low-grade spindle cells permeating bony spicules resembling desmoplastic fibroma. Nuclei show mild atypia, H&E ×100

destruction and soft tissue extension are observed on CT scan or MRI.

Pathology

This is a rare variant of osteosarcoma, which is often mistaken for benign tumour because of the bland appearance of cells. Spindle cells are arranged loosely in a heavy collagenous background, with bone or osteoid production (Fig. 5.21). The osteoid production can be minimal, and the predominant spindle cell component can mimic desmoplastic fibroma or low-grade fibrosarcoma. The tumour may mimic parosteal osteosarcoma or fibrous dysplasia. In rare cases, the tumour may mimic the appearance of osteoblastoma. Sometimes, it shows low cellularity with dense sclerotic bone with cement lines in mosaic pattern as in sclerotic phase of Paget disease (Fig. 5.22). Host bone permeation will be present (Fig. 5.21a, b). This is an important clue that it is malignant. Sometimes, cortical destruction and soft tissue extension can be seen. One has to search for atypical cells (Fig. 5.21c). These tumours show low mitotic activity. 10–30% of cases progress to high grade, and then it is called dedifferentiation and requires adjuvant chemotherapy. Hence, thorough sampling is mandatory.

IHC

Immunohistochemically, both murine double-minute type 2 (MDM2) and cyclin-dependent kinase 4 (CDK4) are positive [115].

Molecular

Amplification of MDM2/CDK4 [116] by molecular testing is more reliable in differentiation from benign mimickers. But some cases lack MDM2 amplification. Conventional karyotyping can show ring chromosome. Since conventional osteosarcoma lacks MDM2 amplification, presence of amplification helps to differentiate dedifferentiated LGCOS from conventional OS.

Table 5.3 Differentiating features between low-grade OS and fibrous dysplasia

	Low-grade central OS	Fibrous dysplasia
Radiology	Metaphyseal destructive	Diaphyseal well-defined lytic with ground-glass appearance
Type of bone	Trabecular	Woven
Cells	Elongated cells with atypia	Oval cells without atypia
Permeation	+	–
IHC: MDM2/CDK4	+	–
Cytogenetics: Ring chromosome [gain of 12q(13;15)]	Present	Absent
Molecular	MDM2 amplification	Gsp mutations (GNAS mutation)

DD

These tumours are difficult to differentiate from benign fibro-osseous lesions, especially fibrous dysplasia (Table 5.3). The permeation of cells between pre-existing host trabeculae is the most important diagnostic feature of LGCOS. Immunohistochemical stains MDM2 and CDK4 are used to differentiate them from their benign mimics.

Treatment and Prognosis

Wide excision with negative margins is the line of treatment [115]. Local recurrence occurs in those cases with inadequate excision and with possible dedifferentiation to high-grade sarcoma. A combination of surgery and chemotherapy is given when there is dedifferentiation (foci of high-grade transformation in central low-grade osteosarcoma). LGCOS has got a good prognosis. Prognosis is poor when there is dedifferentiation.

5.3.7.2 Conventional Osteosarcoma (COS)

COS is a mixture of **osteoblastic, chondroblastic and fibroblastic** cells, and depending on the predominant component, they are called osteoblastic OS, chondroblastic OS or fibroblastic OS. Distinguishing each variant is important while differentiating from its morphological mimics [96].

It has no prognostic importance, and treatment is same for all types. In all forms of osteosarcoma, tumour cells permeate bony trabeculae, filling the marrow space. Cells are pleomorphic, round, epithelioid or spindle shaped. Mitotic activity is easily found in all forms of conventional osteosarcoma. In a needle biopsy, it is difficult to see many mitotic figures. In these situations, a clinico-radiological correlation will be required. Haemorrhage and necrosis are also frequent.

Tumour cells produce eosinophilic osteoid matrix (malignant osteoid). But in a needle biopsy, one may have to search for osteoid especially in certain morphological subtypes like fibroblastic or giant cell-rich osteosarcomas. Histologically, osteoid is a dense, pink, refractile, amorphous intercellular material. It is difficult to identify osteoid from other eosinophilic extracellular materials like collagen, fibrin and amyloid. Nonosseous collagen is seen as a linear, fibrillar intercellular material, which is compressed between neoplastic cells. Osteoid is glassy in appearance, which arborizes in between cells and arch with a small bulge. It may show focal calcification. Osteoid thickness can vary in different tumours. The thinnest osteoid is termed as "filigree" osteoid. Lace-like calcification around individual cells (chicken wire calcification), similar to chondroblastoma, can be seen.

Osteoblastic OS: In osteoblastic osteosarcoma (OBOS), there will be large amounts of osteoid, and the cells are seen as small and pyknotic embedded in between the matrix. The atypia may be minimal (Fig. 5.23). This is known as "normalization". Sometimes, the matrix is so abundant that it is difficult to identify the cells. In such situations, the only feature for malignancy will be permeation of pre-existing bony trabeculae. The osteoid gets calcified and forms disorga-

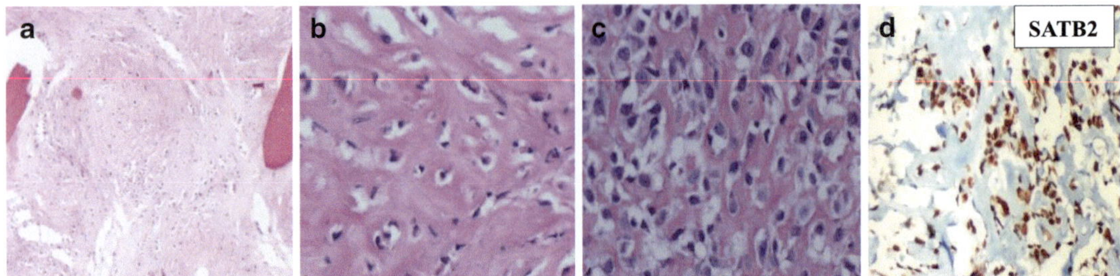

Fig. 5.23 Osteoblastic osteosarcoma. (**a**) Abundant matrix (osteoid) and scanty cells showing permeation of bony spicules—a sign of malignancy, H&E ×40. (**b**) Scattered cells and predominant matrix. Atypia of the cells is difficult to appreciate. Radiology correlation is essential for diagnosis, H&E ×250. (**c**) Cellular atypia can be appreciated, H&E ×250. (**d**) SATB2 is a reliable marker for osteoblasts, ×100

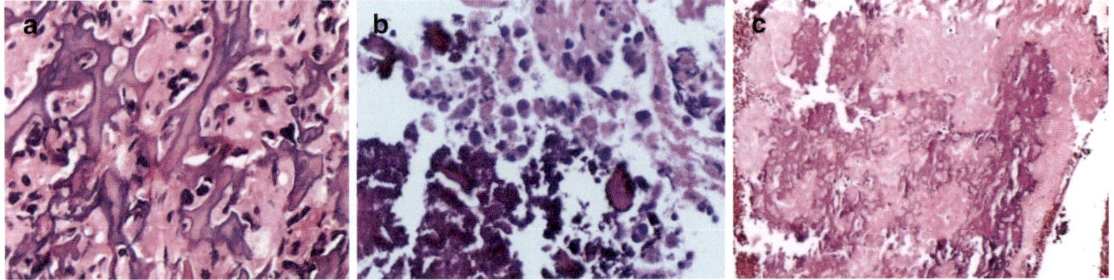

Fig. 5.24 Osteosclerotic OS. (**a–c**) Dense sclerosis of the matrix with calcifications and scattered malignant cells, H&E ×100

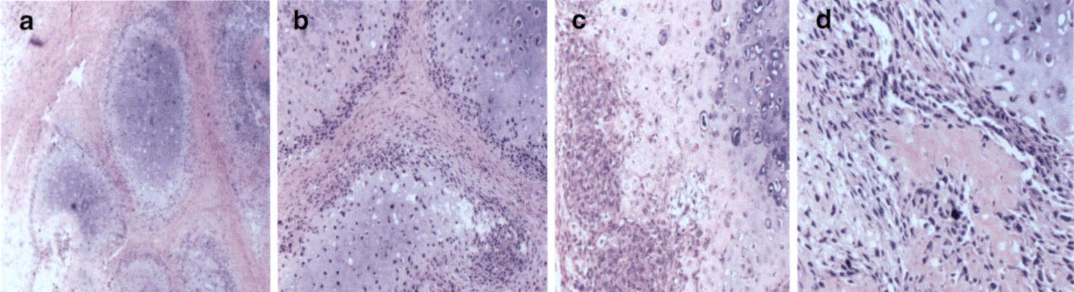

Fig. 5.25 Chondroblastic osteosarcoma of mandible in a 37-year-old male. (**a**) Hyaline cartilage tumour in lobules, H&E ×40. (**b**) Cellular spindle cell area towards the periphery of lobules, H&E ×100. (**c**) Osteoid in the cellular area, H&E ×100. (**d**) High-grade (grade III) cartilage, H&E ×250

nized trabeculae. The amount of osteoid, woven bone and calcified bone varies from tumour to tumour. Sometimes, the trabeculae have pagetoid appearance with cement lines. Osteoid is the prominent matrix in osteoblastic osteosarcoma. It can be lace-like (filigree pattern) or dense osteoid or sclerotic (bone formation) (Fig. 5.24).

Chondroblastic osteosarcoma (CBOS) produces chondroid matrix. It is usually high-grade cartilage (grade III hyaline cartilage) in lobules (Fig. 5.25). The clue to diagnosis is spindling with increased cellularity of cells towards the periphery of lobules (Fig. 5.25b). Osteoid/chondroid matrix can be seen in this area (Figs. 5.25c and 5.26). When high-grade cartilage is seen in a young patient or in jaw tumours (where cartilage tumours are practically absent), one has to consider/rule out chondroblastic osteosarcoma.

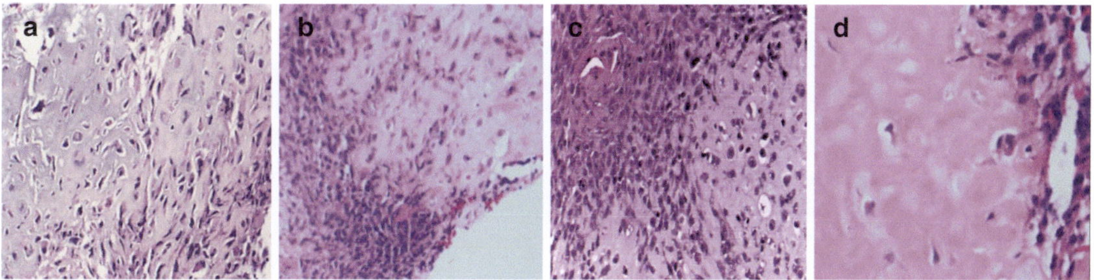

Fig. 5.26 (**a**, **b**) Chondroblastic osteosarcoma with high-grade hyaline cartilage, H&E ×100. (**c**) Cellular periphery with spindling of cells, H&E ×250. (**d**) Chondroid matrix, H&E ×400

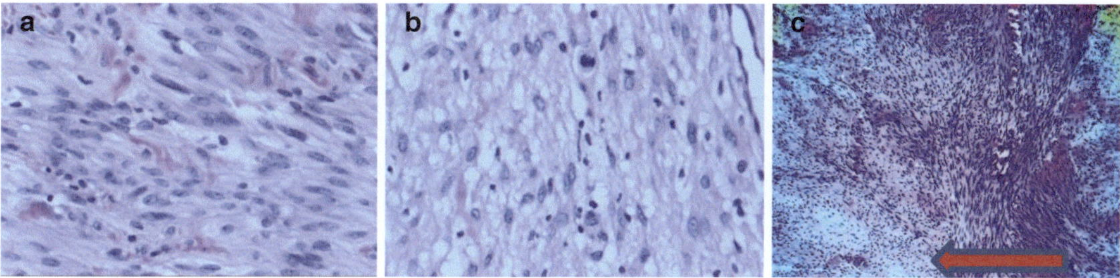

Fig. 5.27 Fibroblastic osteosarcoma. (**a**, **b**) Spindle cell sarcoma resembling fibrosarcoma, H&E ×250. (**c**) It is difficult to see tumour osteoid. One has to search for it (red arrow), H&E ×250

Fibroblastic osteosarcoma (FBOS) resembles fibrosarcoma. Fibroblastic osteosarcomas are common in less-than-5-year age group. Careful search may show lace-like osteoid. In needle biopsy, it is difficult to see osteoid. In such cases, if clinical and radiological findings strongly favour osteosarcoma, one is justified in giving a diagnosis of fibroblastic osteosarcoma (Fig. 5.27).

5.3.7.3 Telangiectatic Osteosarcoma (TAEOS)

TAEOS forms 2.5–12% of all OS. In 1903, the term malignant bone aneurysm was used by Gaylord to refer this lesion. Large haemorrhagic or necrotic cavities constitute the majority of the tumour volume (90% or more). This may cause a resemblance to aneurysmal bone cyst [98]. In telangiectatic osteosarcoma, the cyst walls are thick, and it shows high-grade malignant cells that produce osteoid. Osteoid may not be evident on a needle biopsy. The clinical features of telangiectatic osteosarcoma are similar to that of conventional osteosarcoma.

Radiology

TAEOS is metaphyseal and is usually purely lytic in plain X-ray (Fig. 5.28a). It has a wide zone of transition. TAEOS is difficult to differentiate from ABC radiologically. These lesions are known to appear radiographically similar. CT scan can be with or without fluid levels (Fig. 5.28b).

Pathology

Grossly, TAEOS is a haemorrhagic, cystic mass filled with blood clots (bag of blood) (Fig. 5.28b). Solid areas or bony fragments are not seen. Histologically, low-power view will resemble aneurysmal bone cyst (ABC) (Fig. 5.29a). But the higher magnification of cyst wall will show high-grade malignant cells with or without osteoid (Fig. 5.29b). Increased number of osteoclastic giant cells and increased number of atypical mitosis are seen (Fig. 5.29c).

5.3.7.4 Small Cell Osteosarcoma (SCOS)

Small cell OS is an extremely rare variant of OS (1–2%) with histologic features similar to Ewing

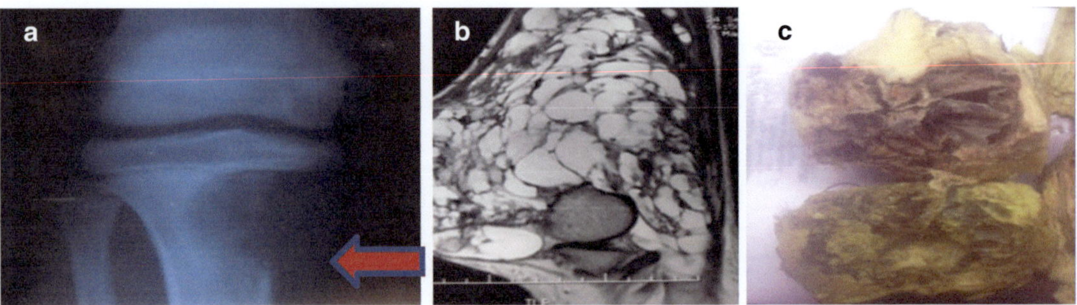

Fig. 5.28 (**a**) Plain X-ray of telangiectatic OS in a 15-year-old boy resembling ABC. (**b**) MRI showing fluid–fluid levels. (**c**) Gross picture of TAEOS consisting of multiple cysts containing haemorrhagic material

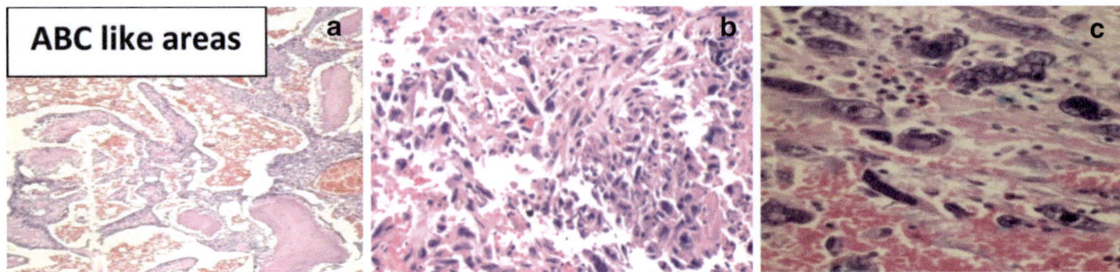

Fig. 5.29 Telangiectatic osteosarcoma. (**a**) At low power, it resembles aneurysmal bone cyst, H&E ×100. (**b**) Malignant cells in cyst wall, H&E ×250. (**c**) High power of cyst wall showing high-grade malignant cells. Osteoid may or may not be present, H&E ×400

Table 5.4 Malignant round cell tumours of bone

Ewing sarcoma
Malignant lymphoma and leukaemia
Small cell OS
Mesenchymal CS
Metastatic neuroblastoma

sarcoma [118, 121]. Radiologically, it is similar to COS, but rarely it can be purely lytic and resemble Ewing sarcoma. The cells are small and have round hyperchromatic nuclei, similar to Ewing sarcoma and other round cell tumours of bone (Table 5.4). However, the presence of calcifying osteoid by tumour cells confirms the diagnosis of OS. But one has to search thoroughly to find calcifying osteoid (Fig. 5.30) and spindling of cells. Pink osteoid-like material is present in many cases of Ewing sarcoma. Immunohistochemical profile is similar to Ewing sarcoma. But FLI1 is usually negative in OS, and SATB2 is positive [119]. Its differentiation from Ewing sarcoma is given in Table 5.5.

Molecular: Recent studies have shown EWSR1-CREB3L1 fusion transcript in small cell osteosarcoma [120, 122].

5.3.7.5 Other Unusual Morphological Variants

There are many histological variants of osteosarcoma resembling other primary tumours of bone. They are given in Table 5.6.

Giant Cell-Rich OS

Giant cell-rich osteosarcoma (GCR OS) is a rare histological pattern seen in osteosarcoma [71, 101]. It is located in the metaphysis of long bones. But this type is reported in the diaphysis of long bones [95] and jaw bones [88]. Grossly, these tend to be a fleshy or haemorrhagic mass. Histologically, there is presence of plenty of benign osteoclast-like giant cells. The mononuclear cells are markedly atypical and pleomorphic, and the giant cells are not distributed uniformly [89] (Fig. 5.31). The mononuclear

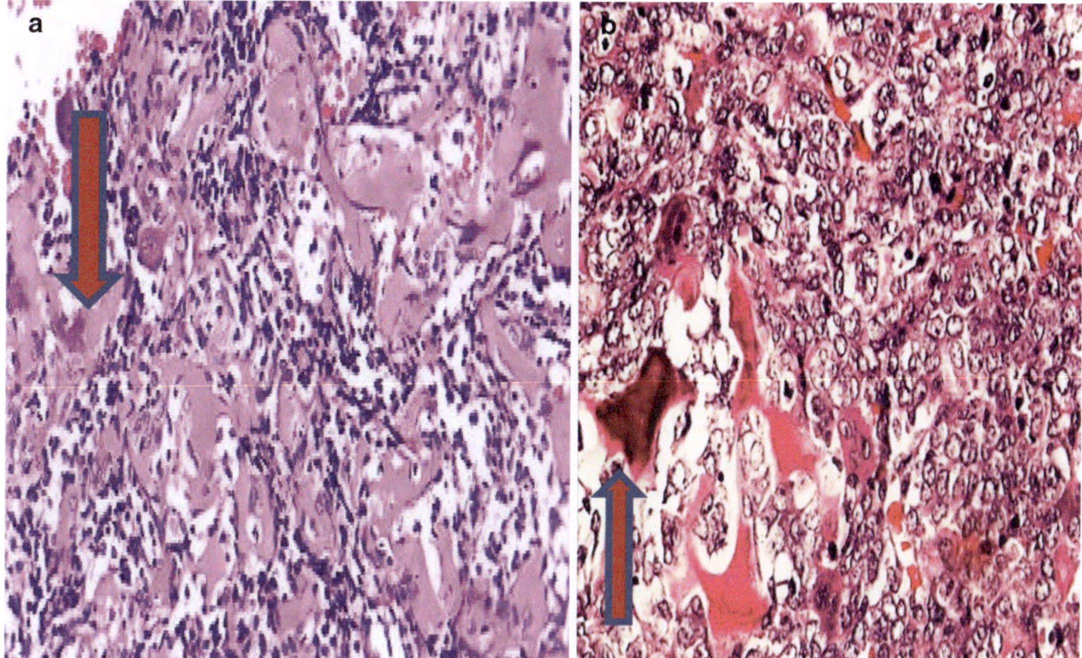

Fig. 5.30 Small cell osteosarcoma. (**a**, **b**) Small round malignant cells resembling Ewing sarcoma with eosinophilic matrix and calcifying osteoid (arrow), H&E ×100. The diagnosis of osteosarcoma is justified, only if calcifying osteoid is present. Sometimes, molecular study may be required for proper typing

Table 5.5 Differentiation of small cell OS from Ewing sarcoma

	Small cell OS	Ewing sarcoma
Light microscopy	Osteoid+ (calcifying)	Osteoid−
IHC [119]	Vim+, NSE+, CD99+, SAT B2+	Vim+, NSE+, CD99+, FLI 1+, NKX 2.2+
EM	Less glycogen, more developed organelles, early osteoid formation	Glycogen ++, Paucity of organelles
Cytogenetics	**EWS-FLI 1 usually negative**	**EWS-FLI 1+/ EWSR1+**

Table 5.6 Unusual histological forms of osteosarcoma

1. Giant cell-rich osteosarcoma
2. Epithelioid osteosarcoma
3. Osteosarcoma resembling osteoblastoma
4. Chondromyxoid fibroma-like osteosarcoma
5. Chondroblastoma-like osteosarcoma
6. Clear cell osteosarcoma
7. Malignant fibrous histiocytoma-like osteosarcoma (rich in tumour giant cells)

cells are seen as sheets without giant cells in many areas. This should arouse suspicion, and one has to search for atypical mitosis. Osseous matrix production is variable. The prognosis of GCR OS is similar to conventional osteosarcoma. Cutaneous metastasis of giant cell-rich osteosarcoma is reported [70]. Some of these tumours have shown molecular markers like H3F3A or H3F3B p.Gly 34 mutation as seen in primary malignant giant cell tumour. Hence, some authors are considering these tumours as primary malignant giant cell tumours [107, 110]. In the jaw bones, MDM2/CDK4 amplification is reported in giant cell-rich type [88]. For treatment, denosumab and bisphosphonates are tried for this subtype as in giant cell tumour of bone [71, 101].

Differential Diagnosis

- Giant cell tumour of bone
- Malignancy in giant cell tumour of bone

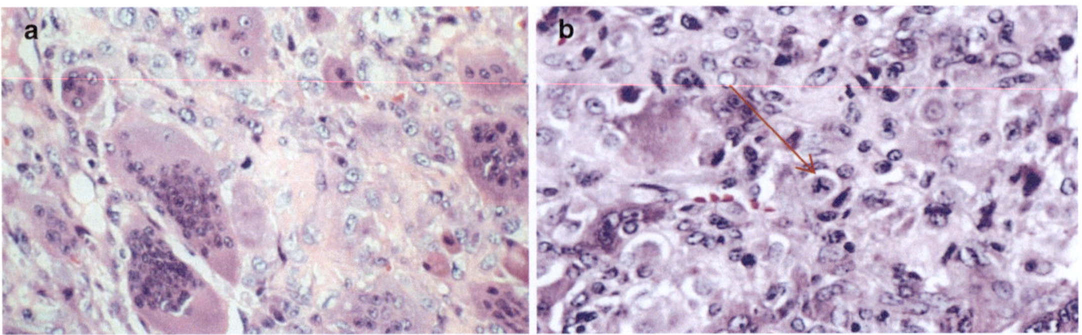

Fig. 5.31 Giant cell-rich osteosarcoma. (**a**) Numerous osteoclastic giant cells mimicking giant cell tumour, H&E ×250. (**b**) Stromal cell atypia and atypical mitosis (red arrow) are the clue to diagnosis, H&E ×400

Table 5.7 Differentiating points of giant cell tumour and giant cell-rich osteosarcoma

	GC-rich OS	GCT
Age	<20	20–40
Site	Metaphysis	Epiphysis
Distribution of giant cells	Haphazard	Uniform
Stromal cells	Highly atypical	No/minimal atypia
Mitosis	Plenty including atypical	No atypical mitosis
Osteoid	Malignant osteoid	Reactive osteoid
Degenerative changes: histiocytes, cholesterol clefts	Not common	Common
IHC	SATB2++H3F3A+/–	RANK-L++ H3F3A++
Molecular	Gain of chr 1, loss of chr 9, 10, 13, 17 and long arm of chr 6	Telomeric associations

It is very difficult to differentiate GCR OS from giant cell tumour because stromal cells of giant cell tumour can also show moderate atypia. Clinical and radiological findings like age below 20 years and metaphyseal location may to some extent help in diagnosis (Table 5.7). The points for differentiation include paucity of giant cells, haphazard distribution of giant cells and marked atypia of stromal cells with prominent mitosis including **atypical mitosis**. Osteoid can be seen in giant cell tumour especially towards periphery and also if there is secondary aneurysmal bone cyst formation. H3F3A IHC may also not be helpful because giant cell-rich osteosarcomas can be positive for this marker, and research is going in the direction whether these tumours are basically primary malignant GCT.

Epithelioid OS

Epithelioid OS is another morphologic variant with large polyhedral epithelioid cells [85, 97]. It should not be mistaken for metastatic carcinoma. Attempted glandular pattern and papillary pattern may be seen. True gland formations are extremely unusual (Fig. 5.32). Cytokeratin can be positive in osteosarcoma. SATB2 helps in differentiating from metastatic carcinoma.

Osteoblastoma-Like OS

In osteoblastoma-like OS, cells are less pleomorphic, and rimming of woven bone may be seen. But a destructive growth pattern with permeation of pre-existing bony trabeculae will be present [62] (Fig. 5.33). This pattern is seen more often in post-radiation osteosarcomas.

Chondromyxoid Fibroma-Like OS

Chondromyxoid fibroma-like OS is a low-grade osteosarcoma [69]. It closely resembles CMF [69]. It is commonly seen in jaw bones and is rare in extremities. Radiology shows aggressive features suggesting malignancy. Haphazard arrangement of spindle cells in a chondromyxoid stroma is seen. It is very difficult to differentiate from CMF on small biopsy. Presence of osteoid, permeation of pre-existing bony trabeculae and aggressive radiology help in differentiation from CMF [111] (Fig. 5.34).

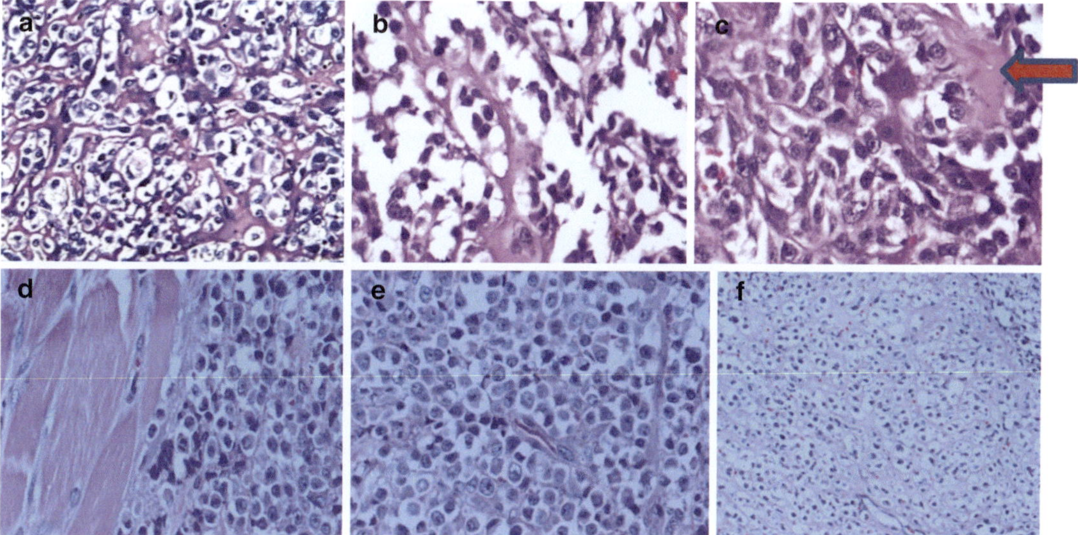

Fig. 5.32 Epithelioid osteosarcoma resembling metastatic carcinoma with lace-like osteoid. (**a**) Nesting pattern of cells, H&E ×100. (**b**) Epithelioid cells in attempted acinar pattern, H&E ×250. (**c**) Tumour osteoid (arrow). IHC and radiology correlation may be required in needle biopsy to rule out metastatic carcinoma, H&E ×400. (**d**) OS resembling melanoma with prominent nucleolus infiltrating muscle, H&E ×100. (**e**) Plasmacytoid cells in OS, H&E ×250. (**f**) Lace-like osteoid in epithelioid OS, H&E ×100

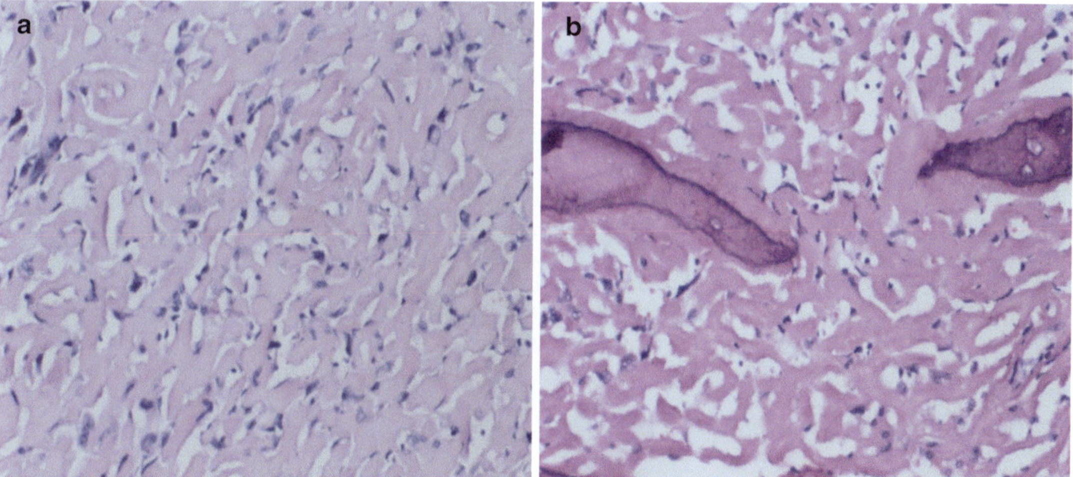

Fig. 5.33 Osteoblastoma-like OS. (**a**) Abundant osteoid, H&E ×100. (**b**) Permeation of tumour in between pre-existing bony trabeculae is the clue for malignancy, H&E ×400

Chondroblastoma-Like OS

Chondroblastoma-like OS is a very rare morphological variant of OS [86]. The tumour occurs in lower extremities. Radiology findings are usually consistent with malignancy. Morphologically, it resembles chondroblastoma with folded or grooved nuclei and pale cytoplasm. They show osteoid production. The clues to differentiate from chondroblastoma are non-epiphyseal location, older age, osteoid production by tumour cells, pleomorphism with atypical mitosis and permeation of bony trabeculae (Fig. 5.35). Recently, malignant chondroblastoma has been described as mainly occurring in axial skeleton in older age group. They harbour H3F3B mutation similar to chondroblastoma, which is absent in chondroblastoma-like osteosarcoma.

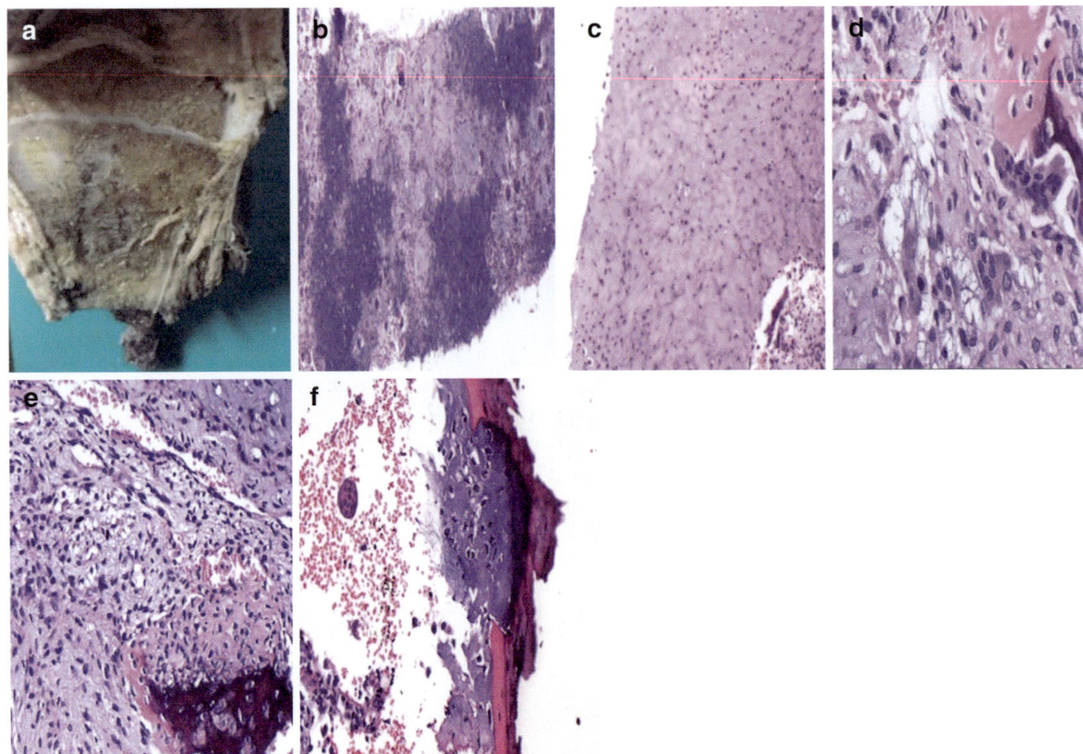

Fig. 5.34 CMF-like OS in tibia in a 13-year-old girl. (**a**) Gross specimen showing metaphyseal growth (**b**, **c**) Chondromyxoid fibroma-like area, H&E ×100. (**d**) Tumour with osteoid, H&E ×250. (**e**) Calcifying osteoid, H&E ×100. (**f**) Tumour permeating through bone to soft tissue, H&E ×100

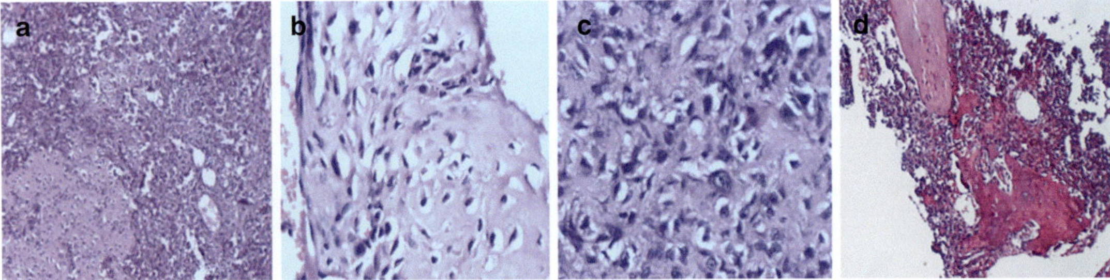

Fig. 5.35 CB-like OS in a 16-year-old boy. (**a**) Shows chondroid matrix and sheets of chondroblast-like cells, H&E ×100. (**b**) Chondroid matrix, H&E ×250. (**c**) Atypical cells and pink matrix, H&E ×400. (**d**) Destruction of bone with soft tissue extension was the helpful feature in diagnosing OS, H&E ×40

Clear Cell OS

These are osteosarcomas with predominant clear cells. They may show intracytoplasmic glycogen. Most important differential diagnosis is clear cell chondrosarcoma (Fig. 5.36). But these tumours are S100 negative compared to clear cell CS, which is S100 positive.

MFH-Like OS

This type of OS is an undifferentiated sarcoma with highly pleomorphic cells with tumour cells producing osteoid (Fig. 5.37). Numerous tumour giant cells are observed. Brisk mitosis including many atypical mitosis will be present.

5.3.8 Surface Osteosarcomas

Osteosarcoma arising on the surface of bone has a different clinical behaviour compared to intramedullary osteosarcoma. The tumour arises from the periosteal aspect of the cortex of the involved bone. The following tumours are classified as surface OS as they have unique clinical, radiographic and biological properties:

1. Parosteal OS
2. Periosteal OS
3. High-grade surface OS

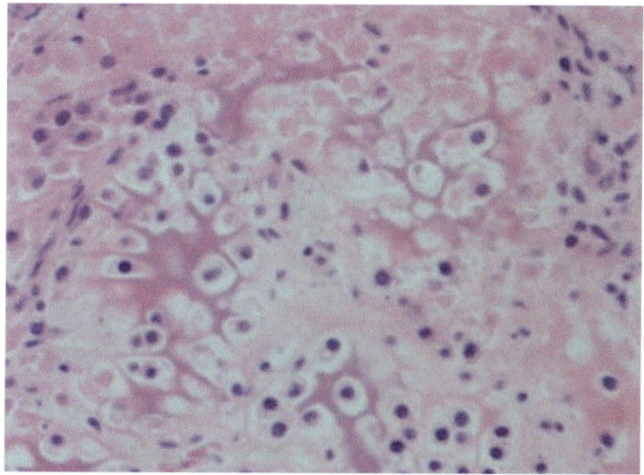

Fig. 5.36 Clear cell OS. Cells with clear cytoplasm resembling metastatic clear cell carcinoma. Lace-like osteoid can be seen, H&E ×250

5.3.8.1 Parosteal OS

Parosteal OS is a low-grade osteosarcoma (4% of all OS), in which the atypia is minimal and is difficult to diagnose on needle biopsy. Geschicter and Copeland described the conventional parosteal osteosarcoma. It is more frequent in women and occurs a decade older than conventional OS (third and fourth decades) [125]. The preferred sites are long bones of the appendicular skeleton. Around 70% of cases are seen at the posterior aspect of the distal femur. They present as a painless enlarging mass with a long history of more than 1 year.

Parosteal OS is cytogenetically characterized by ring chromosome containing amplified material from chromosome 12q13–q15. The genes involved are MDM2 and CDK4. >85% of cases show this amplification [116, 123].

Radiology

These tumours are seen as densely radio-opaque mass fixed to the cortex of the involved bone. It is centrally denser than periphery. There is little or no involvement of the medullary cavity. Both linear and circumferential growth of the tumour will be present (Fig. 5.38). Thus, on plain X-ray, they appear as very heavily ossified mass encircling bone with amorphous trabeculations. It is lobulated and less mineralized at the periphery. The tumour is attached to cortex with a broad base. MRI will confirm that there is no medullary cavity involvement.

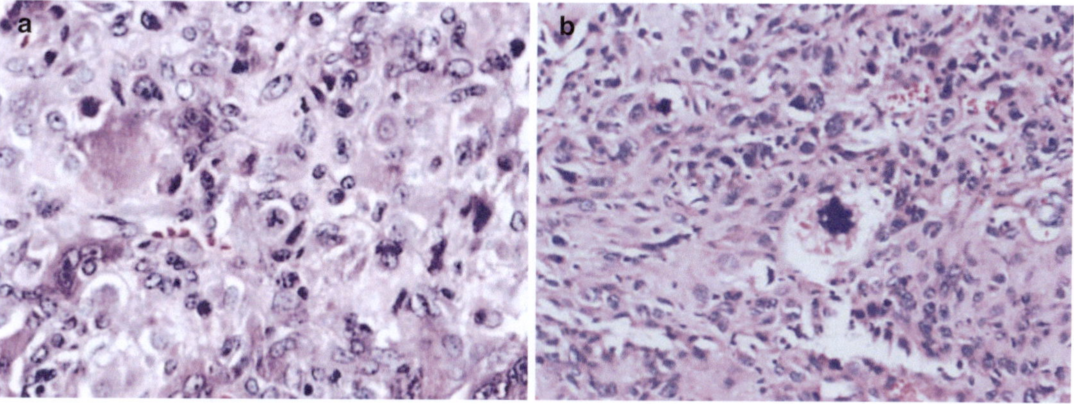

Fig. 5.37 MFH-like osteosarcoma, H&E ×250. (**a**) Tumour giant cells. (**b**) Atypical mitosis, H&E ×100

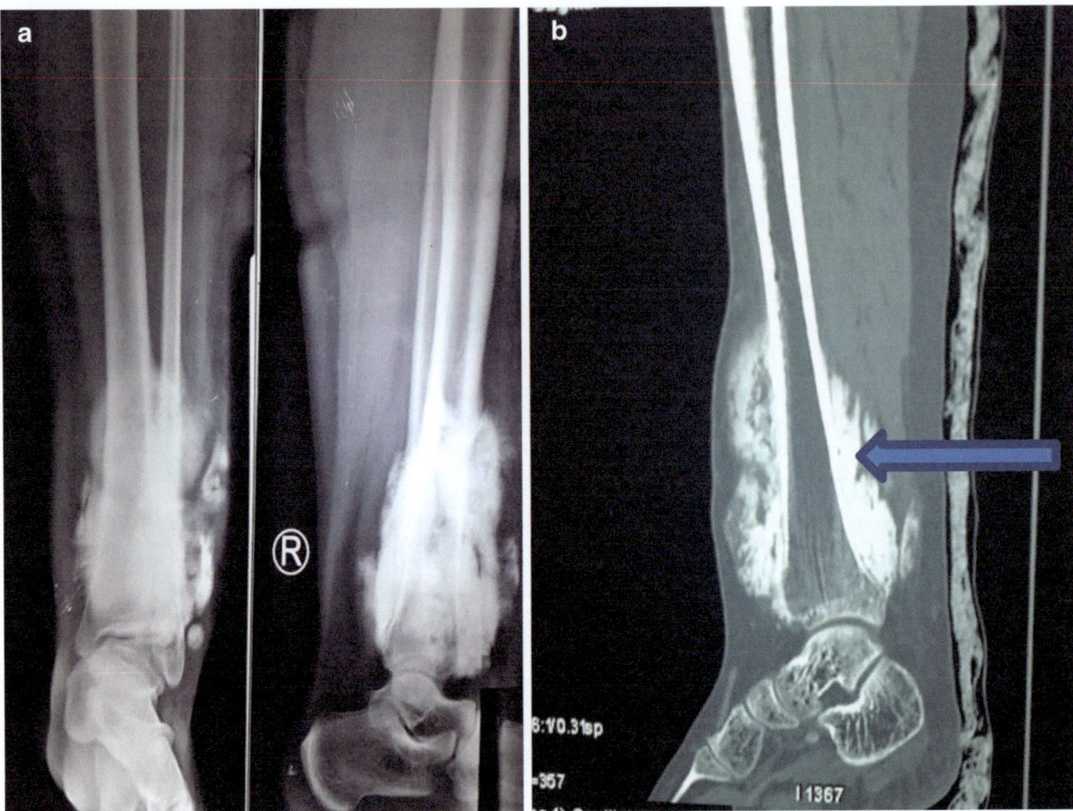

Fig. 5.38 Parosteal OS: (**a**) Plain X-ray showing a very heavily ossified mass encircling bone in the metaphysis of tibia, lobulated and less mineralized at the periphery. (**b**) MRI of parosteal OS lesion attached to cortex with a broad base and without medullary involvement

Pathology

Grossly, the tumour is well circumscribed, ivory-white and very hard due to heavy ossification. It is attached to the bone surface by a broad base. Rarely, a cartilaginous cap is seen and resembles osteochondroma. Soft and fleshy areas suggest dedifferentiation. Large tumours encircle the bone (Fig. 5.39).

Histologically, the tumour is composed of bland-looking spindle cells loosely arranged between mature trabecular bony spicules, which are part of the tumour (Fig. 5.40). The cells show only minimal atypia. Hence, it is difficult to differentiate from benign mimickers. Tumour cells may permeate into soft tissue or skeletal muscle. Bony trabeculae are with or without osteoblastic rimming. They are often parallel in arrangement. Cartilaginous areas are seen in 50% of cases. They may be in nodules or form a cap. Parosteal osteosarcomas then resemble osteochondroma (Fig. 5.41). But in OC, the marrow spaces are with marrow elements or fat in contrast to atypical spindle cells in OS. Radiology correlation will help in differentiation.

IHC

MDM2 and CDK4 are positive.

Molecular

Cytogenetics show ring chromosome (Fig. 5.58a), and FISH test for MDM2 (Fig. 5.58b) shows amplification [116, 124].

Sometimes, these tumours undergo high-grade transformation, and then they are called **dedifferentiated parosteal osteosarcoma** (Figs. 5.42 and 5.43). Hence, extensive sampling is required to rule out the possibility of dedifferentiation in these tumours. This is important for management because the dedifferentiated parosteal osteosarcomas are given adjuvant chemotherapy.

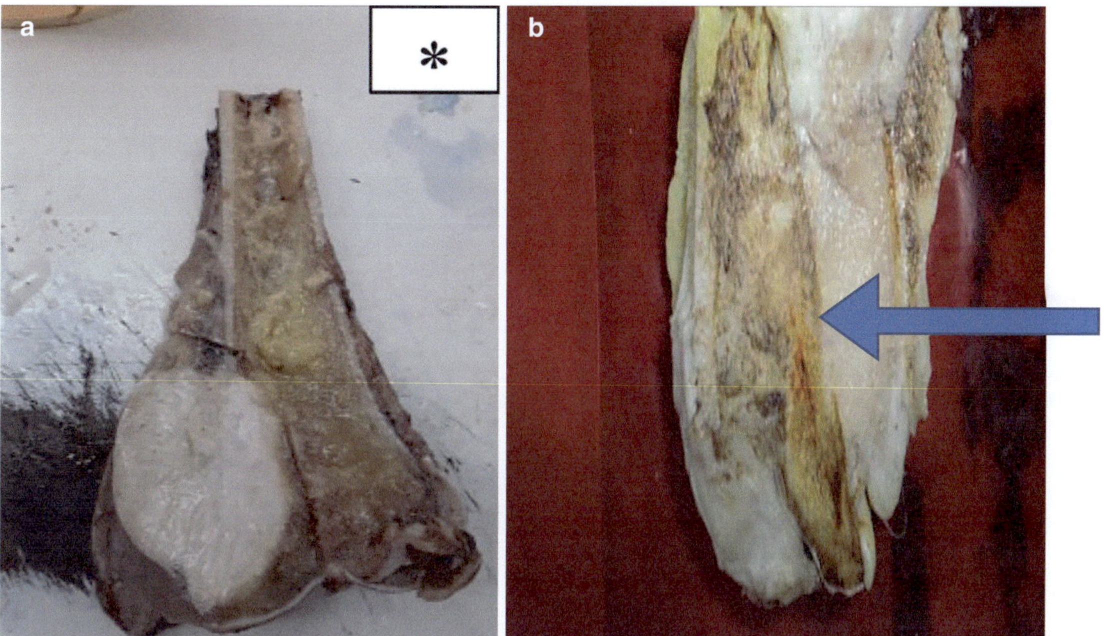

Fig. 5.39 (**a**, **b**) Gross specimen showing tumour stuck to the surface of the lower end of femur. (*gross picture: Courtesy Dr. Sanjay Gandhi, Gujarat)

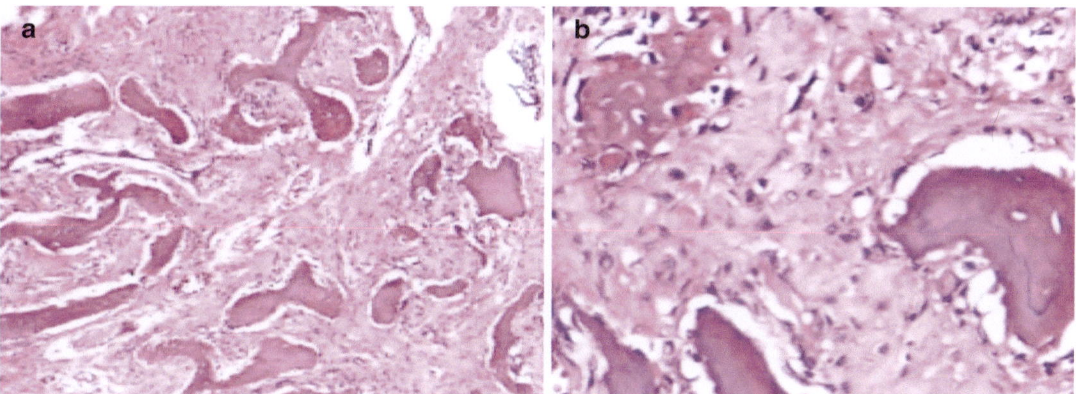

Fig. 5.40 Parosteal OS. (**a**) Low-grade spindle cell tumour with mildly atypical nuclei permeating pre-existing bony spicules, H&E ×100. (**b**) Mature bony spicules and permeating low-grade spindle cell neoplasm with woven bone, H&E ×250

Differential Diagnosis

The most important differential diagnosis is myositis ossificans (Table 5.8). A serial radiology may help to differentiate myositis ossificans. They show reduction in size as time advances. Other differentials are osteochondroma if there is a cartilaginous cap and low-grade central osteosarcoma. If radiology is not available, other low-grade osteoid-producing lesions like fibrous dysplasia, fracture callus, desmoplastic fibroma and florid reactive periostitis are important differentials. The MDM2 amplification is helpful to differentiate these benign mimics, which do not show amplification. The surrogate IHC markers are MDM2 and CDK4. FISH for MDM2 amplification is more sensitive than IHC.

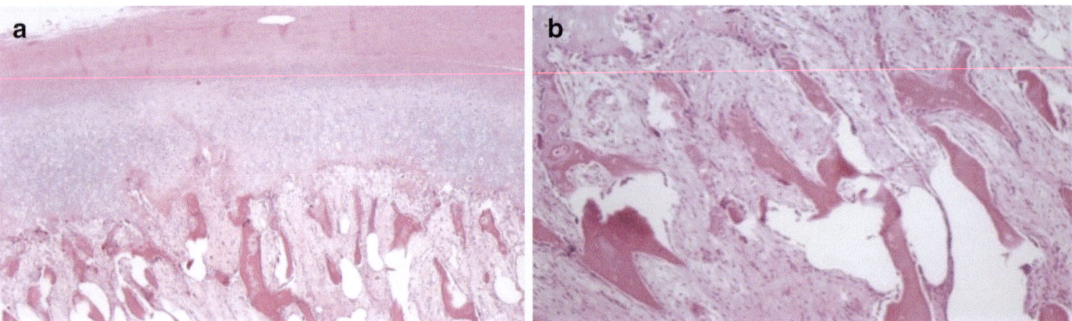

Fig. 5.41 Parosteal OS in a 31-year-old female. (**a**) Cartilaginous cap resembling osteochondroma, H&E ×100. (**b**) Beneath the cartilage, bony spicules and permeating low-grade spindle cells are seen, H&E ×100

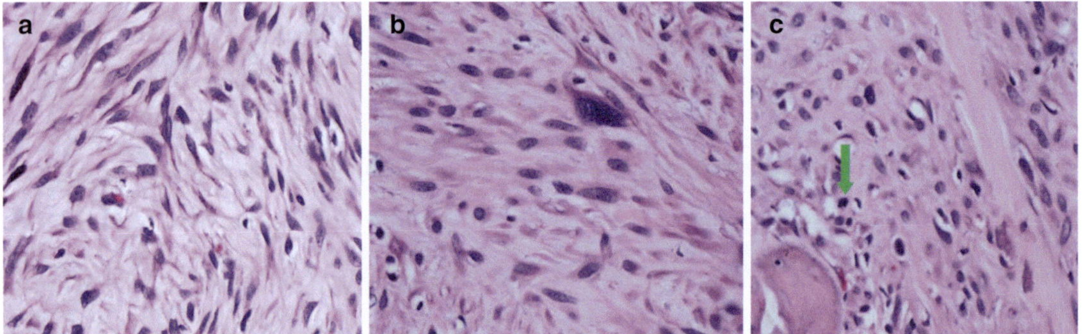

Fig. 5.42 Dedifferentiated parosteal osteosarcoma. (**a**) Cellular spindle cells, H&E ×250. (**b**) Focal high-grade areas with scattered hyperchromatic pleomorphic nuclei, H&E ×400. (**c**) Atypical mitosis (green arrow), H&E ×250

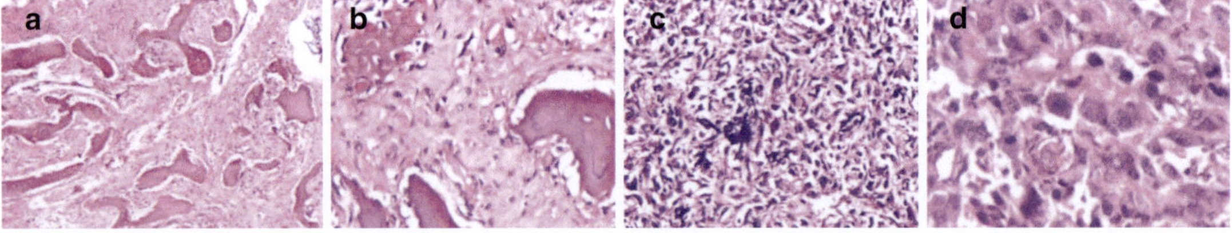

Fig. 5.43 Dedifferentiated parosteal OS. (**a**, **b**) Initial biopsy showing low-grade OS, H&E ×100. (**c**) Cellular areas with pleomorphic hyperchromatic cells, H&E ×100. (**d**) Dedifferentiated areas from resected specimen with mitotic figures, H&E ×400

Treatment

These tumours are treated with surgery alone, and the expected survival is more than 90%. Low-grade tumours rarely metastasize. But dedifferentiated parosteal OS metastasizes to lung, bones, etc. and has a poor prognosis.

5.3.8.2 Periosteal Osteosarcoma

Periosteal osteosarcoma is another surface osteosarcoma. It is considered as intermediate grade [126, 127]. Even though it morphologically resembles conventional osteosarcoma, the behaviour of these tumours is intermediate

Table 5.8 Differentiating features of parosteal OS and myositis ossificans

	Parosteal OS	Myositis ossificans
History of injury	–	+ (mass develops in 2 weeks)
Attachment to bone	Yes	No
Stroma	Hypocellular	Cellular
Mitosis	Occasional	+
Size	Increasing	Reduction in size
Histology	Reverse zoning: central osteoid/ bone and spindle cells in periphery	Zoning: central spindle cells and outer cartilage and bone
Atypical cells	+	–
IHC and molecular: MDM2 and CDK4	+	–

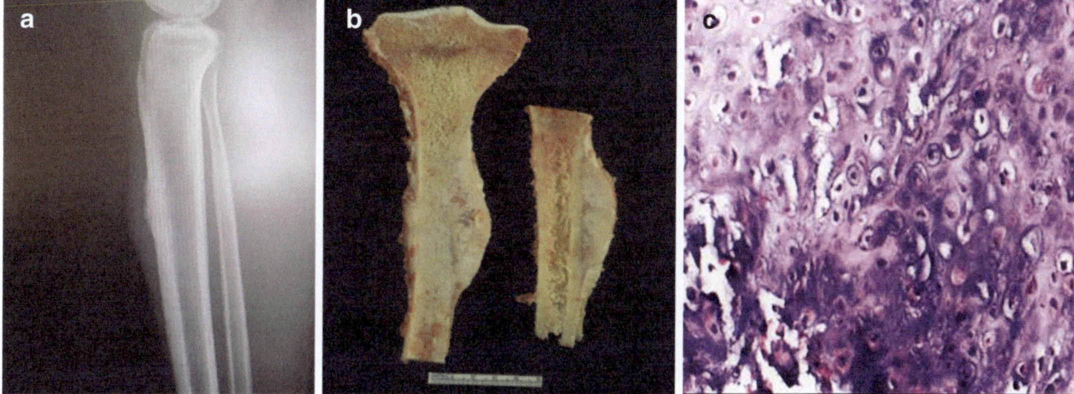

Fig. 5.44 Periosteal OS. (**a**) Plain X-ray of tibia with tumour on the surface of metadiaphyseal region. (**b**) Gross specimen with surface tumour and chondroid cut surface. (**c**) Chondroblastic OS with high-grade hyaline cartilage, H&E ×400

between low and high grade. It forms <2% of all osteosarcomas. They are mainly seen in males (1.5:1) of second and third decades and usually arise on the diaphyseal cortices of the tibia and femur.

Radiology

These tumours appear with a wide base surrounded by peripheral reactive bone. Intralesional mineralization is perpendicular to the long axis of the parent bone (hair-on-end appearance).

Pathology

Grossly, they are chondroid in appearance with glistening cut surface. Intralesional ossification can be seen. The tumour is in continuity to inner periosteum, and the outer periosteum is elevated.

Histology: Periosteal osteosarcoma is a chondroblastic variant in most of the cases (Fig. 5.44). It is composed of lobules of malignant grade III cartilage cells with peripheral spindling of cells. Heavily mineralized osseous matrix may be seen within lobule centres. Periphery of the lobules may show osteoid/chondroid matrix.

DD

1. Periosteal chondrosarcoma is the closest differential diagnosis. But CS occurs in an older age group, is metaphyseal in location and

shows chondroid type of coarse calcification in radiology. IDH mutations are seen in CS.
2. Parosteal OS is mushroom shaped, surrounds the bone, is metaphyseal in location and is fibrous and low grade on histology.
3. High-grade surface OS is similar to COS and is metadiaphyseal in location with a mixture of osteoblastic, chondroblastic and fibroblastic areas. High-grade pleomorphic malignant cells are seen.

Molecular

MDM2/CDK4 amplification is absent. IDH mutation is also absent.

Treatment and Prognosis

Surgical excision is the line of treatment. When treated with surgery alone, it has got a survival rate of 80–85%.

5.3.8.3 High-Grade Surface Osteosarcom

High-grade surface osteosarcoma is a rare lesion (<1% of all OS) that tends to affect males in the second decade. The preferred site is the femur. It can be purely lytic to sunburst-like radio-opaque. They are diaphyseal or metadiaphyseal in location [128, 131]. These tumours in later stages can have intramedullary extension [129]. Hence, a series of images may be required to demonstrate that it was a surface tumour to start with [130].

Pathology

The gross appearance is highly variable with a fleshy granular cut surface. Histologically, it is similar to COS with high-grade fibroblastic or osteoblastic osteosarcoma or a mixture of osteoblastic, chondroblastic and fibroblastic areas. Intramedullary extension as in COS can be seen in later stages. If these tumours show MDM2 amplification, it is considered as dedifferentiation in low-grade osteosarcoma [132].

Treatment and Prognosis

Treatment and prognosis of these tumours are similar to those of conventional osteosarcomas (Fig. 5.45).

Intra-cortical osteosarcoma is an extremely rare form of osteosarcoma. When an osteosarcoma is confined to the cortex, it is called intracortical osteosarcoma. Long bones are the common sites. The cases described are similar to conventional osteosarcoma grossly, histologically and biologically.

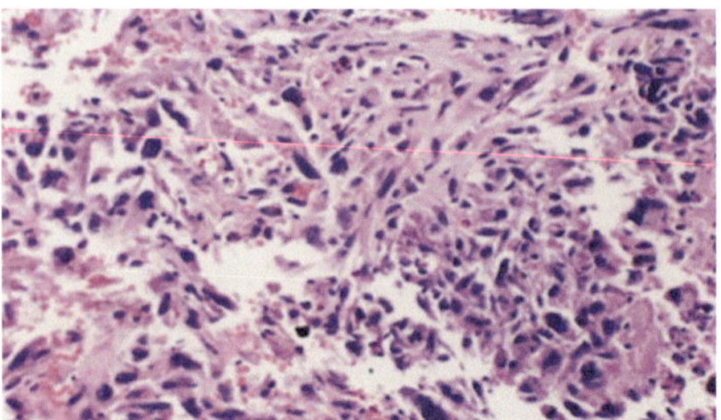

Fig. 5.45 High-grade surface OS showing features of conventional OS, H&E ×100

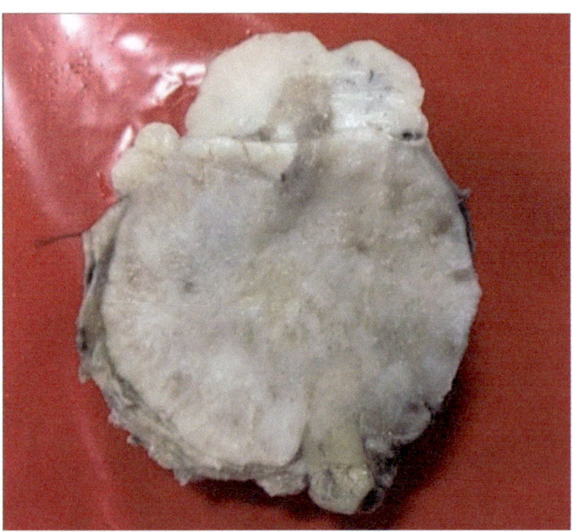

Fig. 5.46 Gross picture of OS of maxilla

5.3.9 Osteosarcoma of Jaw

The jawbone (maxilla and mandible) osteosarcomas are having a different biological property different from what is seen in conventional osteosarcoma [79, 83]. Osteosarcomas of the jaw usually occur at a decade later than conventional OS. The patients are in third and fourth decades [91, 99]. Both sexes are affected equally. It differs from conventional osteosarcomas morphologically. Majority are chondroblastic type (Fig. 5.46). Some are fibroblastic (Fig. 5.48) or osteoblastic. Another

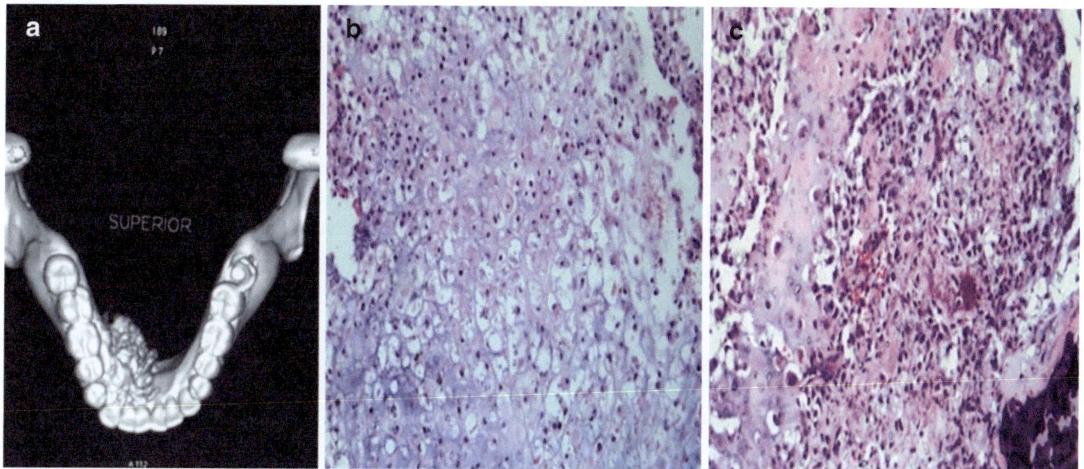

Fig. 5.47 OS mandible in a 28-year-old female. (**a**) Radiograph showing growth involving inner surface of mandible on the right side. (**b**, **c**) Histology is chondroblastic OS, H&E ×100. In jaw tumours, the morphology resembles chondromyxoid fibroma. It should not be mistaken as benign

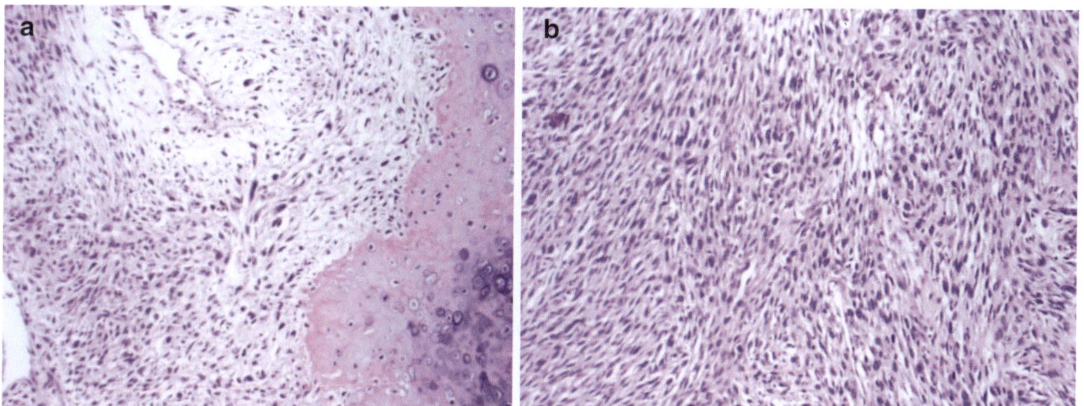

Fig. 5.48 OS mandible in a 13-year-old girl with (**a**) chondroblastic and (**b**) fibroblastic areas

peculiarity that is often observed in jaw osteosarcoma is chondromyxoid appearance (Fig. 5.47). Hence, many of them are diagnosed as benign. Systemic metastasis is very rare. They are locally aggressive tumours and are considered intermediate-grade tumours. Local relapse is common, and death due to local disease can occur in these cases [91, 99]. As cartilage tumours are rare to occur in jawbones, care should be taken not to under-diagnose these tumours as benign. Extra-gnathic osteosarcomas of skull bones are aggressive tumours [68].

5.3.10 Secondary Osteosarcoma

Osteosarcomas arising in pre-existing benign lesions or tumours and those occurring after radiation treatment for other tumours or dedifferentiation of other less aggressive bone tumours are referred to as "secondary osteosarcoma" (Fig. 5.48).

The diseases in which secondary OS arise are Paget disease of bone [133], bone infarcts, chronic osteomyelitis and implant-related OS and osteosarcomas secondary to fibrous dysplasia (Fig. 5.49). Radiation-associated osteosarcomas are also secondary osteosarcomas [134].

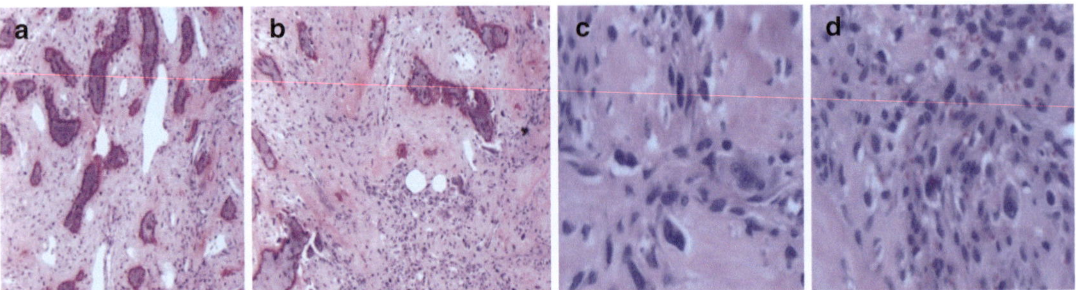

Fig. 5.49 Secondary OS occurring in fibrous dysplasia, in a 29-year-old female. (**a**, **b**) Fibrous dysplasia with woven bone in a fibrous stroma. (**c**, **d**) Osteosarcoma developed 11 years later

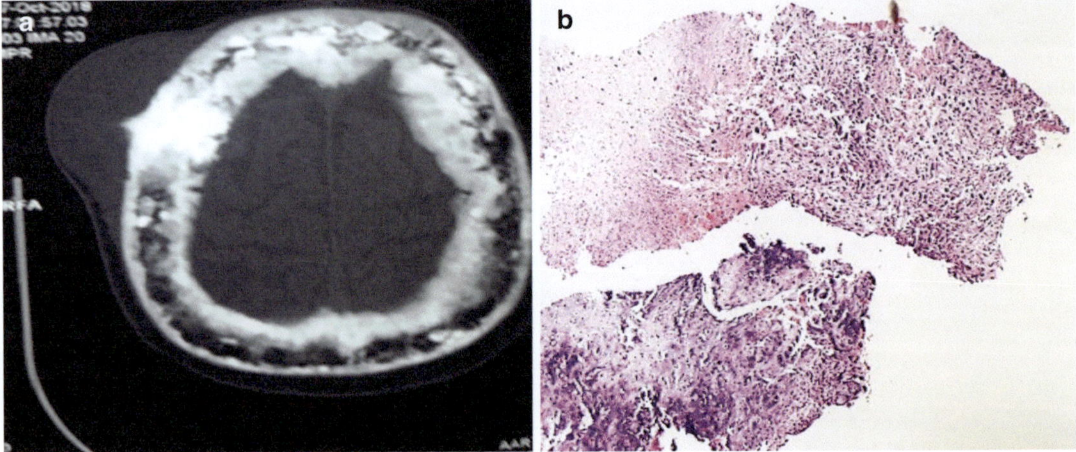

Fig. 5.50 Secondary CBOS in Paget disease. (**a**) Radiology of skull showing typical cotton wool appearance and an exophytic growth. (**b**) The exophytic growth on biopsy showed chondroblastic osteosarcoma, H&E ×40

Paget sarcoma is common in femur, humerus and pelvic bones. It is rare in spine. Radiation-induced OS occurs in bones near the radiation field. It is common in flat bones of chest wall and pelvis. They are characterized by complex karyotypes [135]. Osteosarcomas are reported to develop in osteochondromas [66].

Certain clinical syndromes are associated with osteosarcomas. The syndromes are hereditary retinoblastoma, Li-Fraumeni syndrome and Rothman-Thompson syndrome. They are also considered as secondary OS [87, 100]. Multifocal synchronous tumours can occur [57] (Fig. 5.50). In hereditary retinoblastoma, OS usually develops in lower limbs.

The secondary osteosarcomas are treated in the same way as conventional OS. They usually do not respond to chemotherapy. 30% have lung metastasis at the time of presentation. They have an aggressive clinical course, and the prognosis is worse than conventional osteosarcoma.

5.3.11 Composite Sarcoma of Bone

Rarely, osteosarcoma can be seen along with other mesenchymal sarcomas of bone. It arises from primordial mesenchymal cells with the ability to differentiate into different cell types. These

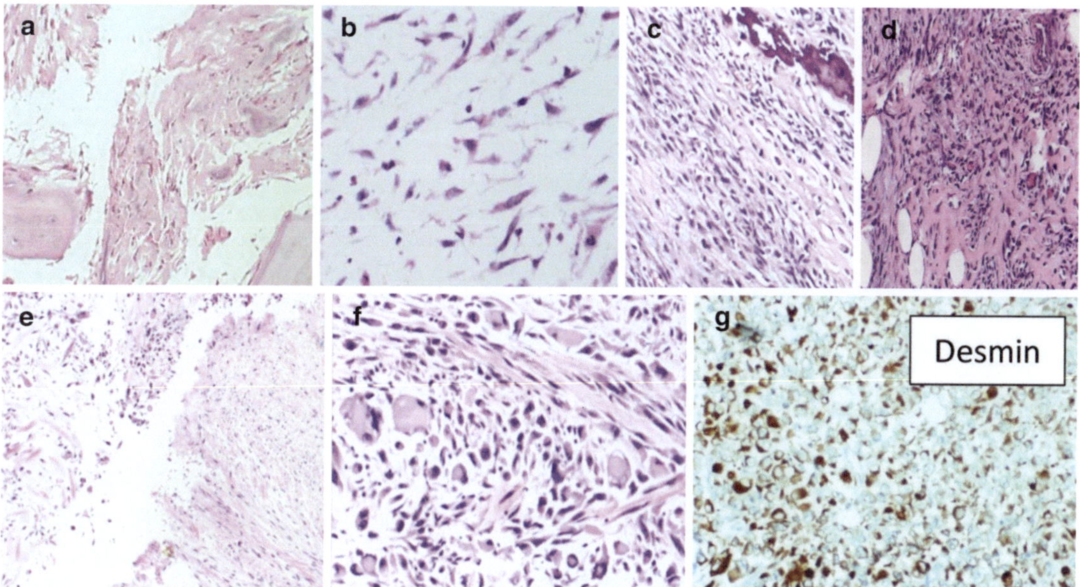

Fig. 5.51 Composite sarcoma of bone in dedifferentiated low-grade central osteosarcoma: (**a**) low-grade osteosarcoma with permeation of pre-existing bony spicules, H&E ×40. (**b**) Low-grade spindle cells, H&E ×100. (**c**, **d**) Dedifferentiation in low-grade osteosarcoma, 6 months after initial diagnosis with atypia, increased mitosis and calcifying osteoid, H&E ×100. (**e**) Rapid growth of tumour ended up in amputation of limb. Composite sarcoma: osteoblastic osteosarcoma on the right side and rhabdomyosarcoma on the left side, H&E ×40. (**f**) High power of rhabdomyosarcoma with rhabdomyoblasts, H&E ×250. (**g**) Desmin positive in rhabdomyosarcomatous areas, ×250

tumours were earlier called malignant mesenchymoma of bone [137]. First case of malignant mesenchymoma of bone was reported by Shajowicz in 1966 [140]. The recent terminology of these tumours is composite sarcomas [136]. It is usually seen in adolescents and young adults. Long tubular bones and pelvis are the common sites affected. The reported cases are seen along with conventional osteosarcomas. Liposarcoma [138, 139] or rhabdomyosarcoma [136, 141] (Fig. 5.51) is the common tumour reported along with osteosarcoma. Rarely, these tumours are seen when there is dedifferentiation in low-grade osteosarcomas.

5.3.12 Multicentric Osteosarcoma

(M-OGS) is characterized by multiple osteosarcomas arising in bone without visceral involvement [63, 74]. Lesions that arise simultaneously are referred to as synchronous (S-OGS) [57] and those that arise months to years later are referred to as metachronous (M-OGS). M-OGS has a poor prognosis (Figs. 5.52 and 5.53). Depending on the different types, they involve either long bones (type 1) or flat bones (type 2). Type 1 and 2 are synchronous and occur in children and adults, respectively. Type 3 is metachronous. Type 1 has the worst prognosis.

5.3.13 Mimickers of Osteosarcoma

The benign mimickers of osteosarcomas (Table 5.9) are myositis ossificans, exuberant callus, subungual exostosis, bizarre parosteal osteochondromatous proliferation (BPOP), sternoclavicular hyperostosis (given in Chap. 4), stress fracture, avulsion fracture (given in Chap.

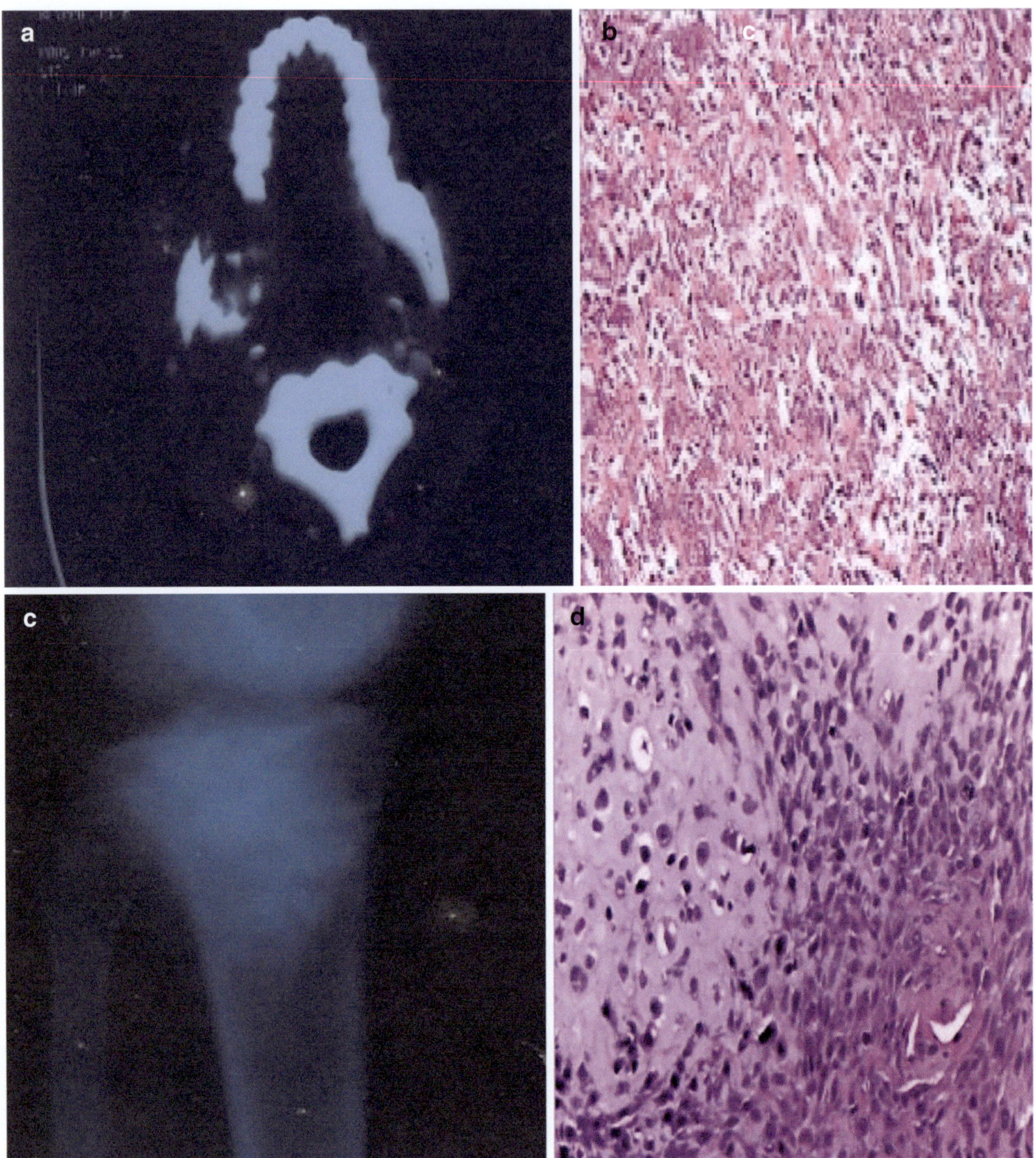

Fig. 5.52 Multifocal OS in a 19-year-old male. (**a**, **b**) Tumour mandible with osteoblastic OS. (**c**, **d**) Tibial tumour with chondroblastic OS

17) and fibro-osseous pseudotumour of digits. The differentiation from myositis is given below.

5.3.14 Osteosarcomatous Areas in Other Tumours

Table 5.10 gives a list of tumours showing osteosarcomatous areas.

5.3.15 Treatment and Prognosis of Osteosarcoma

A combination of surgery with chemotherapy is the usual treatment given [80]. The advent of chemotherapy has improved the outcome [76], and around 75% can be expected to be long-term survivors. Preoperative chemotherapy for three cycles followed by limb salvage surgery and

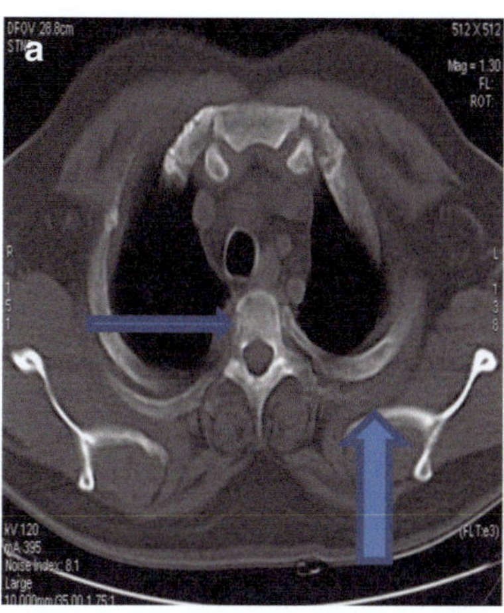

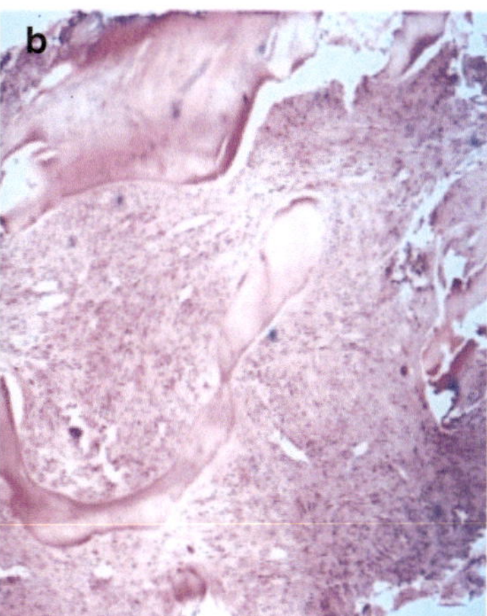

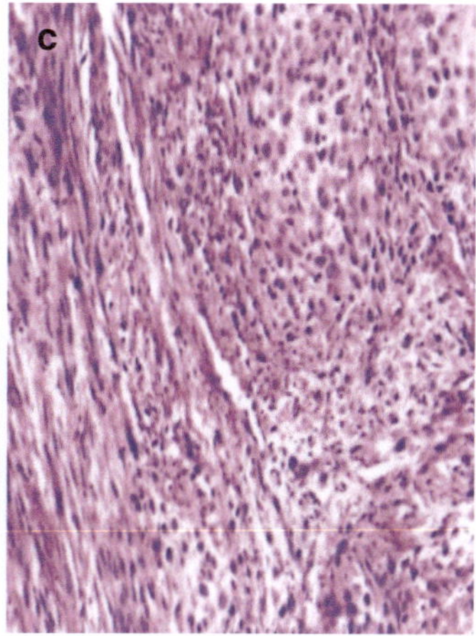

Fig. 5.53 Multifocal OS in a 40-year-old male with lytic lesions in pelvis, rib, femur, skull and vertebra. Radiological diagnosis was metastasis. Biopsy revealed conventional multifocal osteosarcoma. (**a**) Lytic lesion body of vertebra and rib (arrows). (**b**, **c**) Biopsy of femur showing osteosarcoma permeating bony trabeculae, H&E ×100

Table 5.9 Benign mimickers of osteosarcoma

Mimickers of osteosarcoma
• Myositis ossificans
• Exuberant fracture callus
• Subungual exostosis
• BPOP
• Stress fracture
• Sternoclavicular hyperostosis
• Fibro-osseous pseudotumour of digits

Table 5.10 Osteosarcomatous areas in other tumours

Other tumours with osteosarcomatous component
• Synovial sarcoma
• MPNST
• Epithelioid sarcoma
• MFH
• Other tumours: malignant phyllodes tumour Malignant mixed Mullerian tumour (MMMT)

post-operative chemotherapy is the standard line of treatment [58, 105].

Patients with OS can be categorized into two groups: (1) those that respond well to chemotherapy (at least 90% diffuse necrosis) [78] and (2) those that respond poorly (less than 90% necrosis, focal or diffuse). Most cases in which therapy failed to improve long-term survival rates fall within the latter group. Histologic necrosis after preoperative chemotherapy is usually determined by Huvos grading system. A combination of doxorubicin, high-dose methotrexate, cisplatin and ifosfamide is given preoperatively followed by limb-sparing surgery and further chemotherapy [76]. Current management protocols provide long-term survival rates of 60–80%. Even if the patient shows an excellent response to chemotherapy, continued post-operative chemotherapy is advocated. CT is also exceptionally effective in shrinking and/or circumscribing the soft tissue mass, permitting limb salvage procedures that otherwise would be impossible or extremely hazardous to perform. Radiotherapy is given for unresectable tumours [73, 101]. Surgical management can be accomplished either by limb-sparing resection or by amputation. In both procedures, adequate wide margins should be obtained. If wide margins can be obtained without sacrificing major nerves, limb salvage surgery is done so that the limb function can be preserved. Patients who have clinically apparent metastases at presentation have a poor survival (10–20%). Low-grade osteosarcomas are treated with wide excision. Chemotherapy is given to those low-grade cases with dedifferentiation.

5.3.15.1 Assessment of the Effect of Chemotherapy

Grossing of specimen after chemotherapy is given in Chap. 2. Soft tissue is removed, longitudinal cuts are done and a slice of full slab of tumour is decalcified and processed fully (Fig. 5.54).

There are many grading systems for assessing the effect of preoperative chemotherapy on the tumour. The grading systems described by Picci et al. and Huvos et al. are given in Table 5.11.

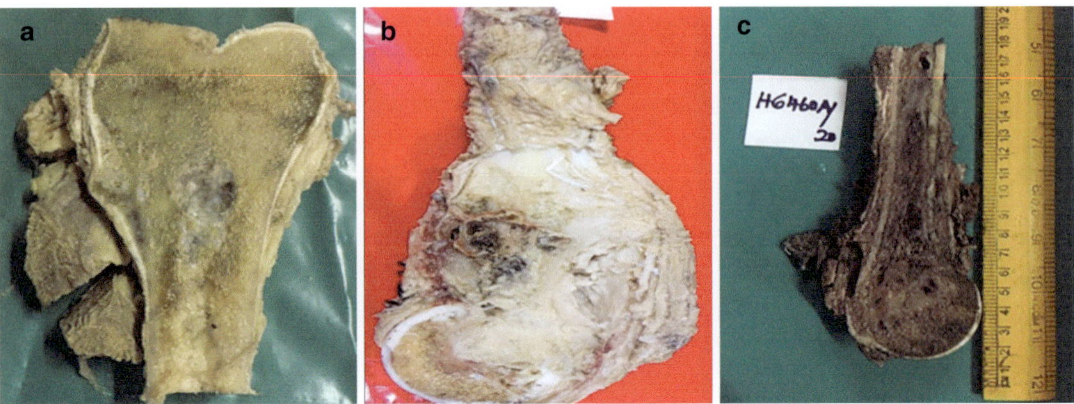

Fig. 5.54 Gross specimen of post-treatment OS. (**a**) Tibia. (**b**) Femur. (**c**) Post-chemotherapy telangiectatic OS

Table 5.11 Grading systems to assess chemotherapy effects

Picci et al.	Huvos et al.
Total response: no viable tumour	IV: No histological viable tumour
Good response: 90–99% necrosis	III: Scattered foci of viable tumour
Fair response: 60–89% necrosis	II: Areas of necrosis with viable tumour
Poor response: <60% necrosis	I: Little or no chemotherapy effect

Table 5.12 Effects of chemotherapy

Effects of chemotherapy
• Necrosis: ghost outlines of neoplasm
• Calcification/new bone formation
• Fibrosis: loosely arranged vessels and spindle cells
• Hyalinization and adipose tissue
• Granulation tissue formation
• Haemosiderin deposition
• Mucinous change and inflammation
Viable tumour cells: large atypical cells with hyperchromatic nuclei, smudged or clumped chromatin and vacuolated cytoplasm
>90% necrosis: 90% disease-free survival

The prognosis depends on good and poor responders. Those greater than 90% necrosis are considered as good responders [78]. The effects of chemotherapy include necrosis, fibrosis and replacement by fat or hyaline tissue (Table 5.12). The sum of all these changes is calculated as the percentage of necrosis. The chondroid matrix and osteoid matrix remain as such or show maturation to bone (Figs. 5.55, 5.56 and 5.57). But the nuclei in chondroid area will be necrotic with red colour (Fig. 5.55). Care should be taken not to confuse plump fibroblasts as viable tumour cells (Figs. 5.56d and 5.58). Some are of the opinion that isolated tumour cells and cartilage should be ignored when quantitating viable tumour [103].

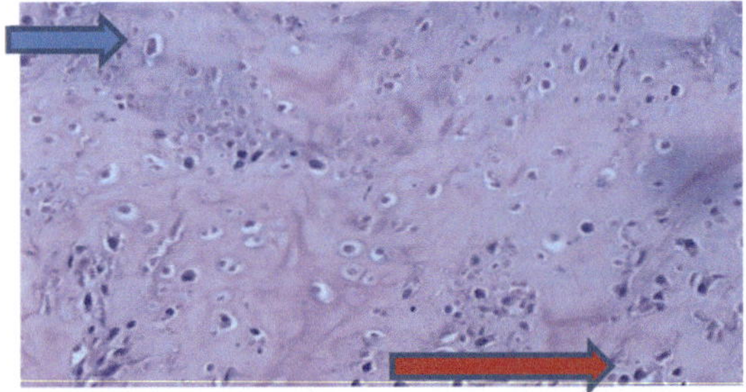

Fig. 5.55 Necrotic cartilage with pink nuclei in the upper part of the picture (blue arrow) and viable cartilage in the lower part (red arrow)

5.3.15.2 Prognosis

Several prognostic factors are associated with osteosarcoma outcomes [65]. Histological response to neoadjuvant chemotherapy [78] is currently the strongest prognostic factor in high-grade OS. Other prognostic factors are location, tumour stage and adequacy of surgical margins (Table 5.13). Proximal extremity,

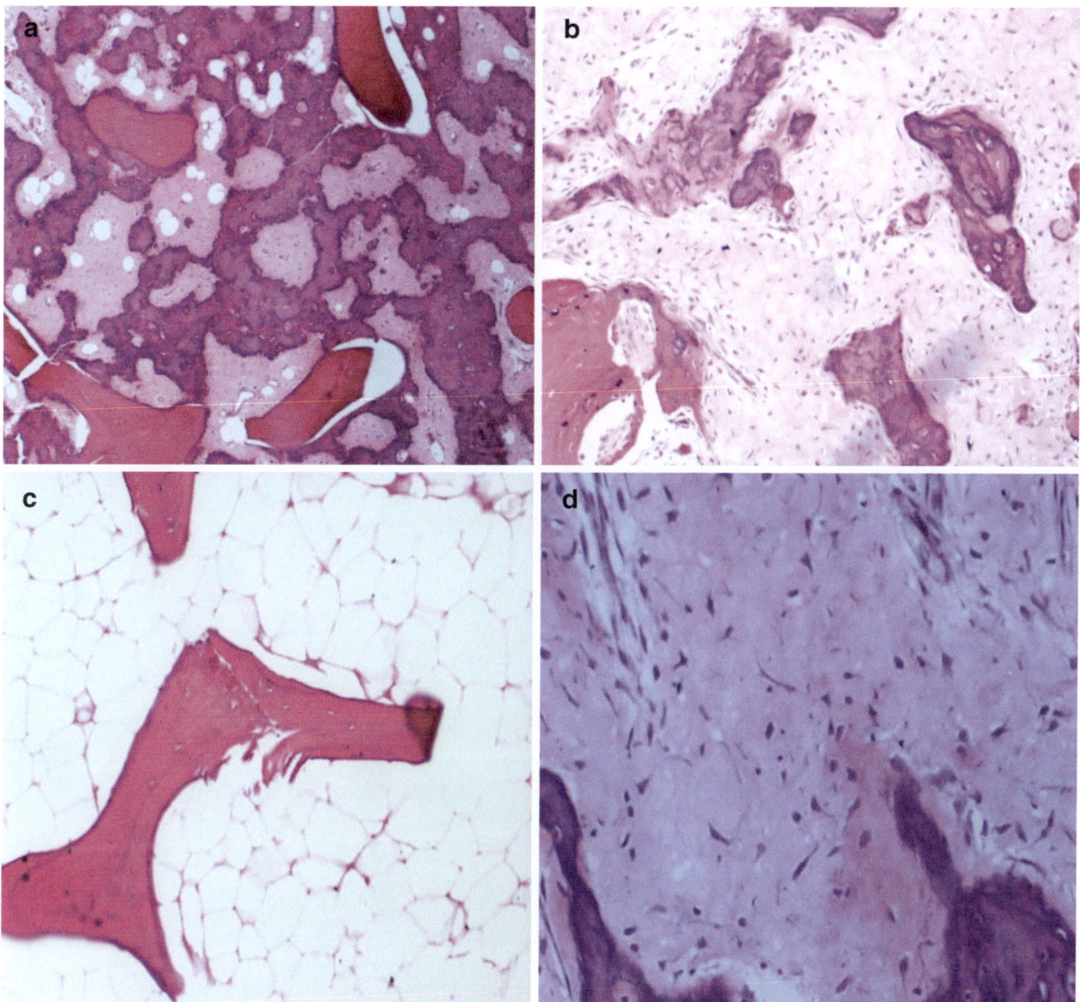

Fig. 5.56 Effects of chemotherapy in a case of OBOS. (**a**) No viable cells are seen. Maturing osteoid, calcifying osteoid, H&E ×250. (**b**) Fibroblasts with hyalinized collagen-replace tumour tissue. (**c**) Tumour replaced by fat after chemotherapy. (**d**) Plump fibroblasts and pink collagen replacing tumour, H&E ×250. It should not be mistaken for tumour cells

tumours of axial skeleton, poor response to preoperative chemotherapy, metastasis at presentation and large tumour size [94] are poor prognostic factors. In children less than 5 years, prognosis is poor [55]. Lung is the most frequent site of metastasis, followed by bone. Rarely, other malignancies are reported in treated osteosarcoma patients [104]. The cases showing Her2/neu expression and positivity for P-glycoprotein by IHC on pre-chemotherapy biopsy tissue are reported as poor responders to chemotherapy [60] (Figs. 5.60 and 5.61).

5.3.16 Cytogenetic [150] and Molecular [103, 124] findings in OS (Table 5.14)

These tests are carried out for the following:

- To differentiate from benign tumours (Fig. 5.59)
- High grade vs. low grade
- Prognosis: predictive for recurrence (Figs. 5.60 and 5.61)

  Metastatic potential

  Chemo-resistance

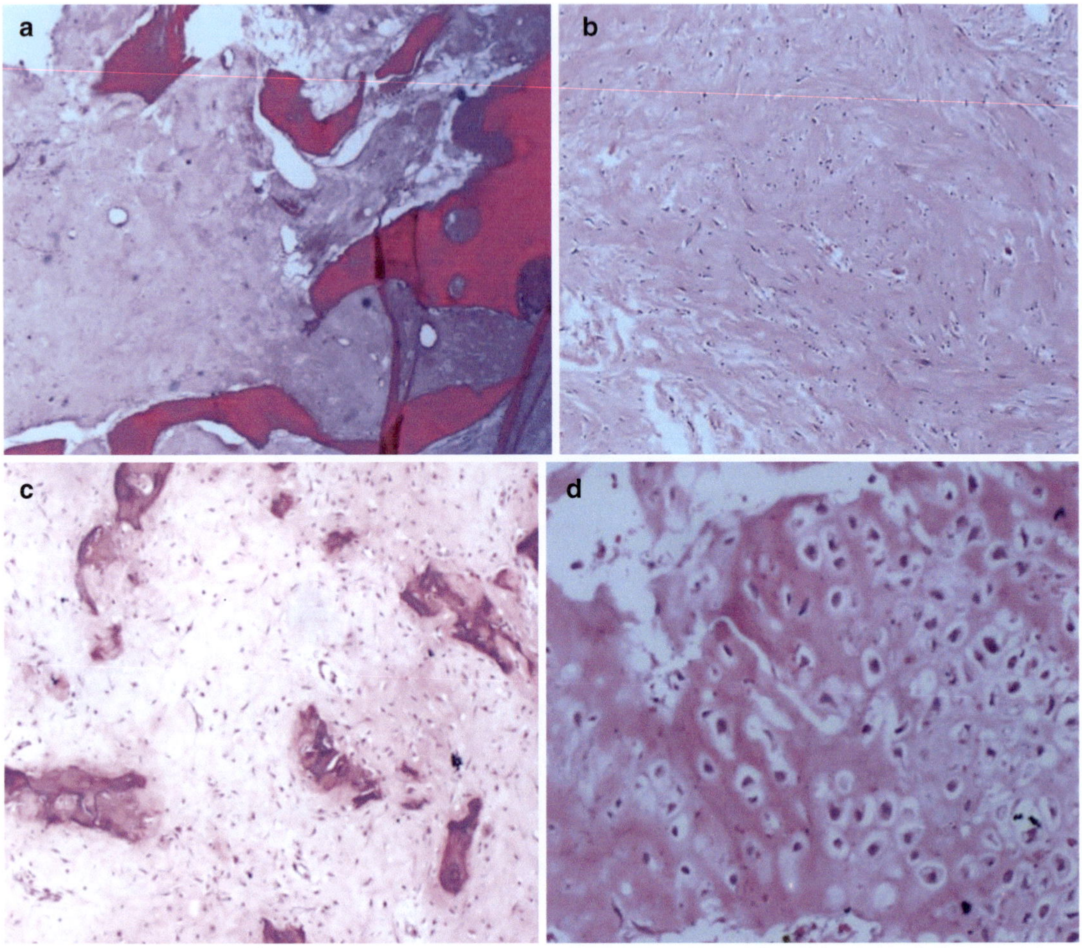

Fig. 5.57 Effects of chemotherapy in a case of CBOS. (**a**) Hyalinization, H&E ×100. (**b**) Fibroblastic proliferation, H&E ×40. (**c**) Calcifying osteoid with fibroblasts in a chondroblastic osteosarcoma with foci of viable CBOS cells, H&E ×100. (**d**) Viable residual tumour (chondroblastic OS), H&E ×250

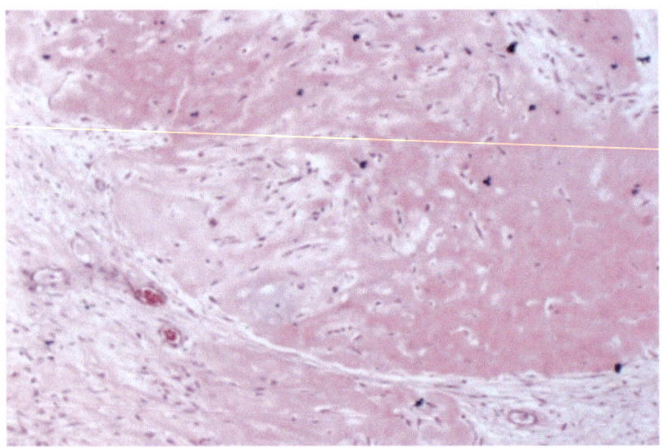

Fig. 5.58 Hyalinization with fibroblasts should not be mistaken for viable cells, H&E ×100

Table 5.13 Poor clinical and molecular prognostic factors in osteosarcoma

Poor prognostic factors	
Clinical	Molecular
• Metastasis at presentation • Tumour in axial skeleton • Size >10 cm • ↑ Alkaline phosphatase or LDH • Poor response to pre-op CT • Skip metastasis or discontinuous tumour in bone • LN involvement	**Predictive for recurrence** • Her-2/neu overexpression • Amplification of 17p11–12 • Gain of 8q21.3 • ↑ c-fos and c-Jun proto-oncogenes **Increased metastatic potential** • 13q14 LOH • DNA alteration of Rb gene • Synchronous overexpression of c-fos and c-myc

Table 5.14 Cytogenetic and molecular findings in osteosarcoma

Cytogenetics and molecular
To differentiate from benign tumours
Osteosarcoma from osteoblastoma
• OS: Rb or p53 mutations, HDM2 (MDM2) gene amplification
• Absence of these in OB (unique three-way translocation involving chromosomes 1, 2, 14)
High grade vs. low grade
• **High-grade OS**
– Complex structural and numerical chromosome alterations [59, 60, 64]
– Gain of chr 1, loss of chr 9, 10, 13, 17 and long arm of chr 6 [67, 77]
– Gain of 12p sequences: genetic pathway for aggressive OS
• **Low-grade OS**
– Ring and marker chromosome [61, 93]
– Gain of 12q 13–15 sequences → ring chromosome (MDM2, CDK4 and SAS genes)
– Amplification of MDM2 and CDK4 consistently seen in low-grade OS
Prognostic markers
Predictive for recurrence
– Her-2/neu overexpression
– Amplification of 17p11–12
– Gain of 8q21.3
– ↑ c-fos and c-Jun proto-oncogenes
Increased metastatic potential
– 13q14 LOH
– DNA alteration of Rb gene
– Synchronous overexpression of c-fos and c-myc
Chemo-resistance
– P glycoprotein-encoded MDR-1 (multidrug resistance gene) expression before chemotherapy

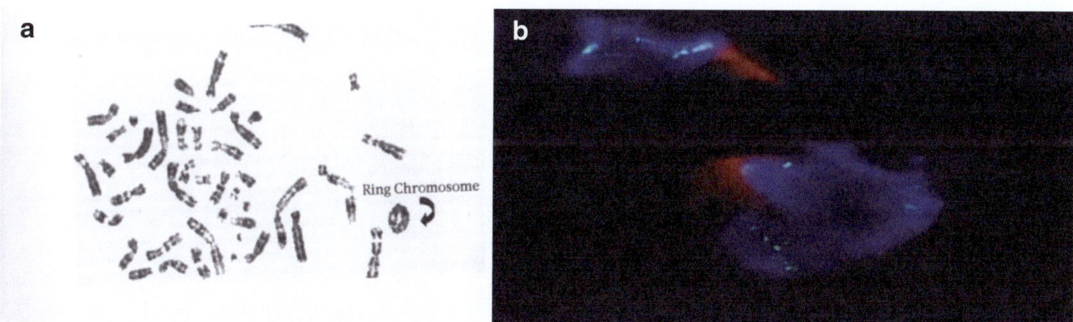

Fig. 5.59 (**a**) Conventional cytogenetics showing ring chromosome in parosteal OS (curved arrow). (**b**) MDM2 amplification by FISH

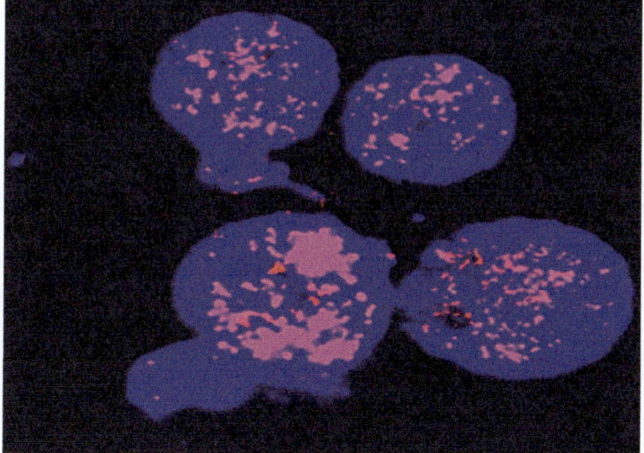

Fig. 5.60 Her2/neu amplification by FISH in OS

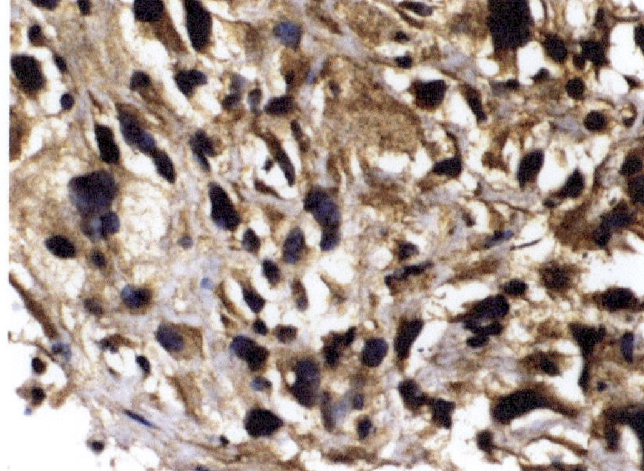

Fig. 5.61 IHC for P glycoprotein expression in initial biopsy (pre-chemotherapy biopsy) of a case of osteosarcoma. P glycoprotein, ×250. This case did not respond to neoadjuvant chemotherapy

5.4 Other Osteoid-Producing Lesions Mimicking Tumour

5.4.1 Heterotopic Ossification (Myositis Ossificans)

Myositis ossificans is a benign soft tissue neoplasm composed of spindle cells and osteoblasts, usually occurring after injury. In the early florid phase of heterotopic ossification due to increased cellular activity, there is rapid growth, and it is mistaken for sarcoma [142] (Fig. 5.62).

5.4.1.1 Clinical

The patient may or may not give a history of trauma [149]. Common locations are elbow, thigh, shoulder, buttocks, etc. Any age group can be affected, but it is more common in young males [143]. The patients present with pain and swelling.

5.4.1.2 Radiology

Radiographs show round mass with mineralization at the periphery (cloud-like pattern), 2–6 weeks after the onset of symptoms [147] (Fig. 5.63). The most important differential diagnosis is parosteal osteosarcoma [148]. In cases of difficulty, a follow-up plain X-ray shows decrease in size in case of myositis ossificans, whereas sarcoma will increase in size [145,146].

5.4.1.3 Pathology

Grossly, the lesion is well circumscribed, and the outer surface will be hard like an eggshell. Microscopically, a zonation will be evident with central fibrous tissue and outer chondroid and

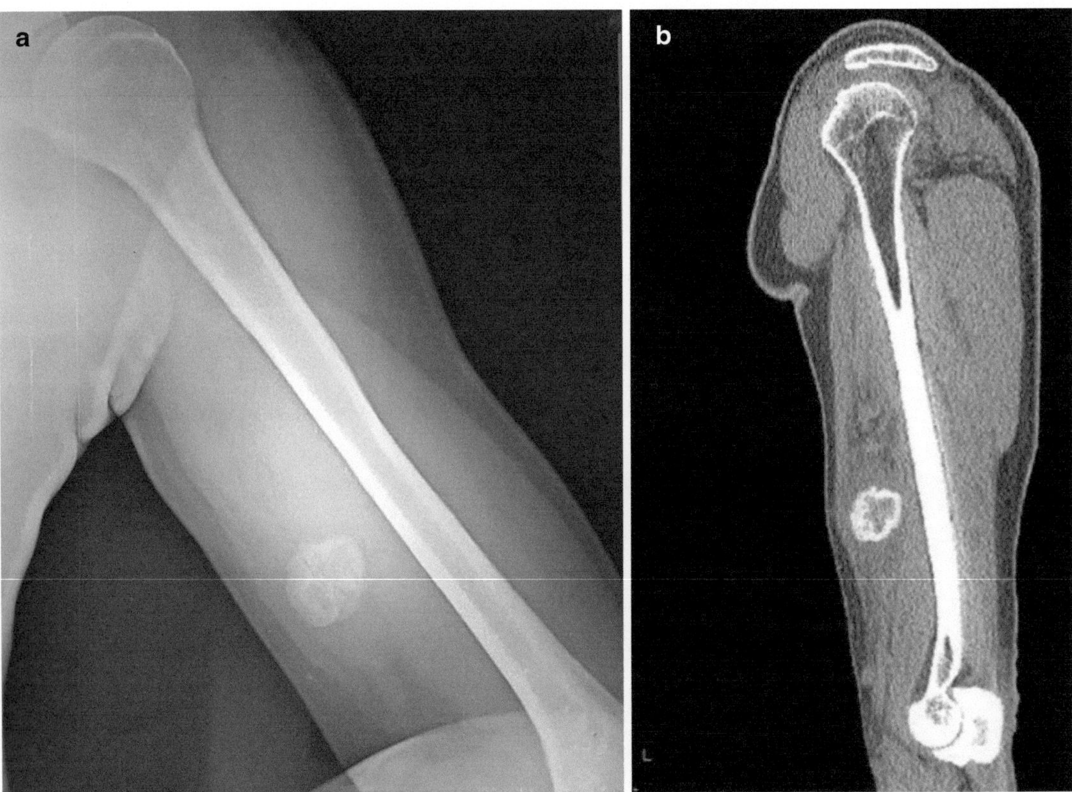

Fig. 5.62 Myositis ossificans*. (**a**) Plain X-ray showing sclerotic round mass in the soft tissue. (**b**) MRI of same case. (*Courtesy: Dr. Jayanthi, Ganga Hospital, Kovai)

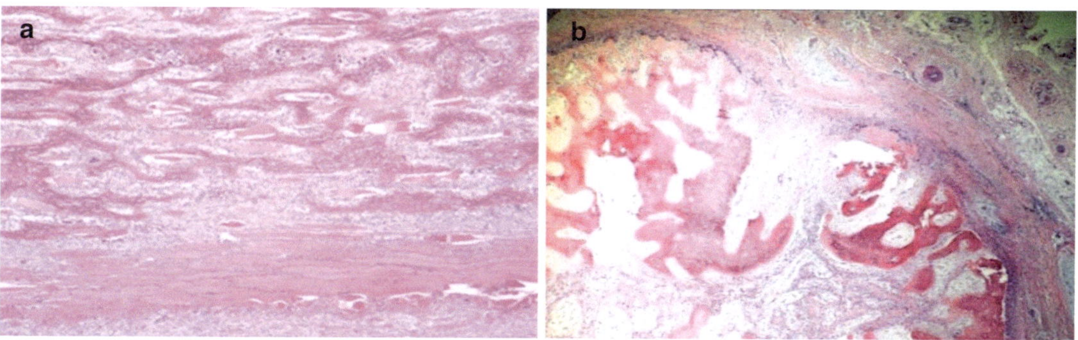

Fig. 5.63 Zoning in myositis ossificans. (**a**, **b**) Outer bone, inner cartilage and fibrous tissue, H&E ×100

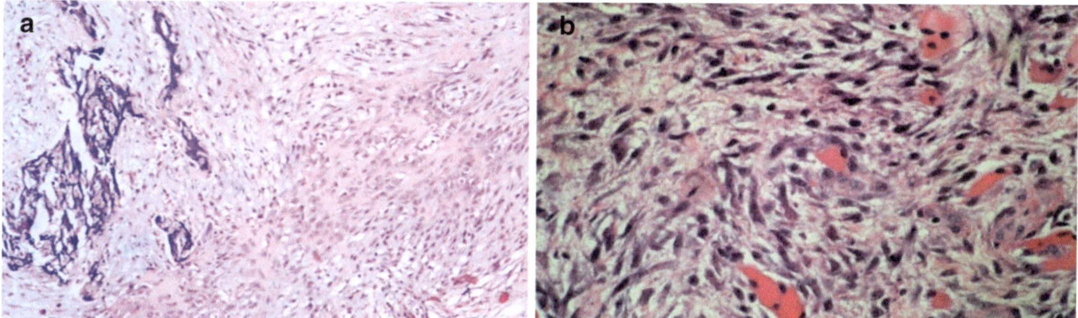

Fig. 5.64 Myositis ossificans. (**a**) Cellular fibroblastic proliferation and calcifying osteoid, H&E ×100. (**b**) Cellular area in myositis, H&E ×250

osseous tissue (Fig. 5.63). This zonation is sometimes difficult to appreciate in fragmented biopsy specimen (Fig. 5.64). The fibroblasts are bland looking, but it may show increased mitotic activity. Myositis can show atypical features [147]. Cartilage can show marked proliferation mimicking chondrosarcoma. Some of these lesions undergo cyst formation and resemble aneurysmal bone cyst. GNAS1 gene mutation has been reported in progressive heterotopic ossification [150].

The subungual exostosis, bizarre periosteal osteochondromatous proliferation (BPOP), florid reactive periostitis and fibro-osseous pseudotumour of digits are all examples of heterotopic ossification [144]. A rare lesion called as myositis ossificans progressiva occurs in young children [149] with multiple heterotopic calcification and ossification in different sites, usually hands and feet. This may be a life-threatening situation. These cases have a hereditary tendency.

5.4.1.4 Treatment and prognosis

Treatment is excision. It has got a good prognosis. Recurrence is uncommon.

5.4.2 Bone Island

Enostosis or bone islands are areas of density seen on plain X-ray. They are extremely dense with spiculated edges. It is similar to osteoma,

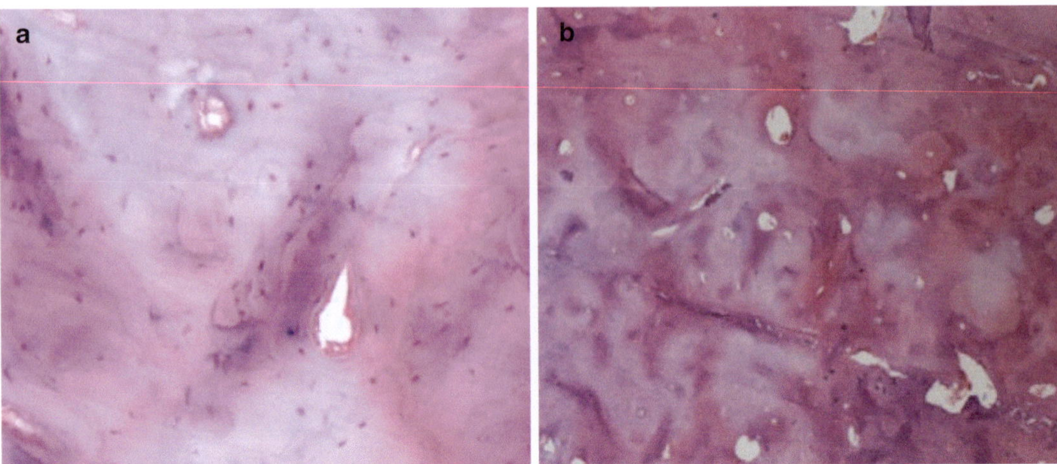

Fig. 5.65 (**a**, **b**) Bone island showing cortical bone, H&E ×400

but they are seen in medullary cavity. These benign sclerotic bone lesions are usually detected incidentally [151]. They are small, but sometimes can be of large size also.

5.4.2.1 Radiology

Enostoses can be detected on plain X-ray, CT and MRI. They are considered as one of the skeletal "do not touch" lesions. Bone islands can occur in any bone. It is more common in pelvis, long bones, spine and ribs. In long bones, it occurs in the diaphysis. The long axis of bone island and the long axis of the involved bone are parallel to each other. In the metaphysis, the bone islands are more spherical. If it is more than 2 cm, they are called giant bone islands. They can slowly increase in size over time. No uptake is seen on bone scan. This is useful to differentiate bone islands from blastic metastasis.

5.4.2.2 Pathology

PathologyCortical like bone is seen in the medullary cavity (Fig. 5.65).

5.4.2.3 DD

It should not be mistaken for blastic metastasis. Other DDs are osteoma, osteoid osteoma and osteoblastoma.

5.4.3 For stress Fracture, Insufficiency Fracture and Avulsion Injury, see Chap. 17.

Points to Remember

- The main osteoid-producing tumours are osteoid osteoma, osteoblastoma and osteosarcoma.
- Osteoid osteoma and osteoblastomas are histologically and immunohistochemically similar. The size of osteoblastoma is >2 cm.
- Osteosarcomas have many histological types, which can cause diagnostic difficulties.
- Low-grade osteosarcomas are parosteal OS and low-grade central OS
- MDM2 amplification by FISH is a useful test to differentiate low-grade OS from benign mimickers.
- Intermediate-grade osteosarcomas are periosteal OS and osteosarcomas of jawbones.
- Other osteoid-producing lesions which cause diagnostic difficulty are fracture callus and myositis ossificans.

References

Osteoma, Osteoid Osteoma, Osteoblastoma

1. Atallah N, Jay MM. Osteomas of the paranasal sinuses. J Laryngol Otol. 1981;95(3):291–304.
2. Bartlett JR. Intracranial neurological complications of frontal and ethmoidal osteomas. Br J Surg. 1971;58:607–13.
3. Bertoni F, et al. Osteosarcoma resembling osteoblastoma. Cancer. 1985;55(2):416–26.
4. Blaskiewicz DJ, Sure DR, Hedequist DJ, Emans JB, Grant F, Proctor MR. Osteoid osteomas: intraoperative bone scan-assisted resection. Clinical article. J Neurosurg Pediatr. 2009;4(3):237–44.
5. Boysen M. Osteomas of the paranasal sinuses. J Otolaryngol. 1978;7:366–70.
6. Bruneau M, Polivka M, Cornelius JF, George B. Progression of an osteoid osteoma to an osteoblastoma: case report. J Neurosurg Spine. 2005;3(3):238–41.
7. Chai JW, Hong SH, Choi JY, et al. Radiologic diagnosis of osteoid osteoma: from simple to challenging findings. Radiographics. 2010;30(3):737–49.
8. Greenspan A. Benign bone-forming lesions: osteoma, osteoid osteoma, and osteoblastoma. Clinical, imaging, pathologic, and differential considerations. Skelet Radiol. 1993;22:485–500.
9. Cheung FMF, Wu WC, Lam CK, et al. Diagnostic criteria for pseudomalignant osteoblastoma. Histopathology. 1997;31:196–200.
10. Chiou YY, Rosenthal DI, Rosenberg AE. "Beaded" osteoid osteoma: a possible transition between solitary and multicentric tumor. Skelet Radiol. 2003;32(7):412–5.
11. Cohen MD, Harrington TM, Ginsburg WW. Osteoid osteoma: 95 cases and a review of the literature. Semin Arthritis Rheum. 1983;12:265.
12. Dal Cin E, Sciot R, Samson I, et al. Osteoid osteoma and osteoblastoma with clonal chromosome changes. BrJ Cancer. 1998;78:344–8.
13. Hakim DN, Pelly T, Kulendran M, Caris JA. Benign tumours of the bone: a review. J Bone Oncol. 2015;4:37–41.
14. Lucas DR. Osteoblastoma. Arch Pathol Lab Med. 2010;134:1460–6.
15. Suster D, Mackinnon AC, Jarzembowski JA, Carrera G, Suster S, Klein MJ. Epithelioid osteoblastoma. Clinicopathologic and immunohistochemical study of 17 cases. Hum Pathol. 2022;125:68–78.
16. Davies M, Cassar-Pullicino VN, Davies AM, McCall IW, Tyrrell PN. The diagnostic accuracy of MR imaging in osteoid osteoma. Skelet Radiol. 2002;31(10):559–69.
17. de Andrea CE, Bridge JA, Schiller A. Osteoblastoma. In: Fletcher CD, Bridge JA, Hogendoorn PC, Mertens F, editors. WHO Classification of tumours of soft tissue and bone. 4th ed. Lyons: International Agency for Research on Cancer; 2013. p. 279.
18. Della Rocca C, Huvos AG. Osteoblastoma: varied histological presentations with a benign clinical course: an analysis of 55 cases. Am J Surg Pathol. 1996;20:841–50.
19. Dorfman HD, Weiss SW. Borderline osteoblastic tumors: problems in differential diagnosis of aggressive osteoblastoma and low-grade osteosarcoma. Semin Diagn Pathol. 1984;1:215–34.
20. Earhart J, Wellman D, Donaldson J, et al. Radiofrequency ablation in the treatment of osteoid osteoma: results and complications. Pediatr Radiol. 2013;43:814.
21. Feletar M, Hall S. Osteoid osteoma: a case for conservative management. Rheumatology (Oxford). 2002;41:585–6.
22. Fenichel I, Garniack A, Morag B, Palti R, Salai M. Percutaneous CT-guided curettage of osteoid osteoma with histological confirmation: a retrospective study and review of the literature. Int Orthop. 2006;30(2):139–42.
23. Frassica FJ, Waltrip RL, Sponseller PD, et al. Clinicopathologic features and treatment of osteoid osteoma and osteoblastoma in children and adolescents. Orthop Clin N Am. 1996;27:559–74.
24. Gasbarrini A, Cappuccio M, Bandiera S, et al. Osteoid osteoma of the mobile spine: surgical outcomes in 81 patients. Spine (Phila Pa 1976). 2011;36:2089.
25. Golant A, Dormans JP. Osteoblastoma: a spectrum of presentation and treatment in pediatric population. Univ Pa Orthop J. 2003;16:9–17.
26. Greco F, Tamburrelli F, Ciabattoni G. Prostaglandins in osteoid osteoma. Int Orthop. 1991;15(1):35–7.
27. Horvai A, Klein M. Osteoid osteoma. In: Fletcher CD, Bridge JA, Hogendoorn PC, Mertens F, editors. WHO Classification of tumours of soft tissue and bone. 4th ed. Lyons: International Agency for Research on Cancer; 2013. p. 277.
28. Hosalkar HS, Garg S, Moroz L, Pollack A, Dormans JP. The diagnostic accuracy of MRI versus CT imaging for osteoid osteoma in children. Clin Orthop Relat Res. 2005;433:171–7.
29. Kaplan I, Calderon S, Buchner A. Peripheral osteoma of the mandible: a study of 10 new cases and analysis of the literature. J Oral Maxillofac Surg. 1994;52:467–70.
30. Kenan S, Floman Y, Robin GC, et al. Aggressive osteoblastoma: a case report and review of the literature. Clin Orthop. 1985;195:294–8.
31. Atesok KI, Alman BA, Schemitsch EH, Peyser A, Mankin H. Osteoid osteoma and osteoblastoma. J Am Acad Orthop Surg. 2011;19(11):678–89.
32. Kneisl JS, Simon MA. Medical management compared with operative treatment for osteoid-osteoma. J Bone Jt Surg Am. 1992;74:179.
33. Angervall L, Persson S, Stenman G, Kindblom LG. Large cell, epithelioid, telangiectatic osteoblas-

toma: a unique pseudosarcomatous variant of osteoblastoma. Hum Pathol. 1999;30(10):1254–9.
34. Lucas DR, Unni KK, McLeod RA, et al. Osteoblastoma: clinicopathologic study of 306 cases. Hum Pathol. 1994;25:117–34.
35. Lucas DR. Osteoblastoma. Arch Pathol Lab Med. 2010;134(10):1460–6.
36. McHugh JB, Mukherji SK, Lucas DR. Sino-orbital osteoma: a clinicopathologic study of 45 surgically treated cases with emphasis on tumors with osteoblastoma-like features. Arch Pathol Lab Med. 2009;133(10):1587–93.
37. Mascarello JT, Krous HF, Carpenter PM. Unbalanced translocation resulting in the loss of the chromosome 17 short arm in an osteoblastoma. Cancer Genet Cytogenet. 1993;69:65–7.
38. Mirra JM, Cove K, Theros E, et al. A case of osteoblastoma associated with severe systemic toxicity. Am J Surg Pathol. 1979;3:463–71.
39. Mitchell ML, Ackerman LV. Metastatic and pseudomalignant osteoblastoma. A report of two unusual cases. Skelet Radiol. 1986;15:213–8.
40. Mungo DV, Zhang X, O'Keefe RJ, Rosier RN, Puzas JE, Schwarz EM. COX-1 and COX-2 expression in osteoid osteomas. J Orthop Res. 2002;20(1):159–62.
41. Nielsen GP, Rosenberg AE. Update on bone forming tumors of the head and neck. Head Neck Pathol. 2007;1(1):87–93. https://doi.org/10.1007/s12105-007-0023-4.
42. Pettine KA, Klassen RA. Osteoid-osteoma and osteoblastoma of the spine. J Bone Jt Surg Am. 1986;68A(3):354–61.
43. Peyser A, Applbaum Y, Khoury A, Liebergall M, Atesok K. Osteoid osteoma: CT-guided radiofrequency ablation using a water-cooled probe. Ann Surg Oncol. 2007;14(2):591–6.
44. Rosenthal DI, Hornicek FJ, Torriani M, Gebhardt MC, Mankin HJ. Osteoid osteoma: percutaneous treatment with radiofrequency energy. Radiology. 2003;229:171–5.
45. Schajowics F, Lemos C. Osteoid osteoma and osteoblastoma—closely related entities of osteoblastic derivation. Acta Orthop Scand. 1970;41(3):272.
46. Schajowics F, Lemos C. Malignant osteoblastoma. J Bone Jt Surg. 1976;58B:202–11.
47. Seki T, Fukuda H, et al. Malignant transformation of benign osteoblastoma. J Bone Jt Surg Am. 1975;57:424.
48. Sharma KV, Yarmolenko PS, Celik H, et al. Comparison of noninvasive high-intensity focused ultrasound with radiofrequency ablation of osteoid osteoma. J Pediatr. 2017;190:222.
49. Swanson KS, Guttu RL, Miller ME. Gigantic osteoma of the mandible: report of a case. J Oral Maxillofac Surg. 1992;50:635–8.
50. Tamam C, Yildirim D, Tamam M. Multicentric osteoid osteoma with a nidus located in the epiphysis. Pediatr Radiol. 2009;39(11):1238–41.
51. Unni KK, Inwards CY. Dahlin's bone tumors: general aspects and data on 10,165 cases. Philadelphia: Lippincott Williams & Wilkins; 2009.
52. Woertler K, Vestring T, Boettner F, Winkelmann W, Heindel W, Lindner N. Osteoid osteoma: CT-guided percutaneous radiofrequency ablation and follow-up in 47 patients. J Vasc Interv Radiol. 2001;12:717–22.
53. Yoshikawa S, Nakamura T, Takagi M, et al. Benign osteoblastoma as a cause of osteomalacia: a report of two cases. J Bone Jt Surg Br. 1977;59:279–86.
54. Zon Filippi R, Swee RG, Unni KK. Epithelioid multinodular osteoblastoma: a clinicopathologic analysis of 26 cases. Am J Surg Pathol. 2007;31(8):1265–8.

Osteosarcoma

55. Abate ME, Longhi A, Galletti S, Ferrari S, Bacci G. Non-metastatic osteosarcoma of the extremities in children aged 5 years or younger. Pediatr Blood Cancer. 2010;55:652–4.
56. Puri A, Jaffe N, Gelderblom H. Osteosarcoma: lessons learned and future avenues. Sarcoma. 2013;2013:641687. https://doi.org/10.1155/2013/641687.
57. Bacci G, Picci P, Ferrari S, et al. Synchronous multifocal osteosarcoma: results in 12 patients treated with neoadjuvant chemotherapy and simultaneous resection of all involved bones. Ann Oncol. 1996;7:864–6.
58. Bacci G, Bertoni F, Longhi A, et al. Neoadjuvant chemotherapy for high-grade central osteosarcoma of the extremity. Histologic response to preoperative chemotherapy correlates with histologic subtype of the tumor. Cancer. 2003;97(12):3068.
59. Bayani J, Zielenska M, Pandita A, Al-Romaih K, Karaskova J, Harrison K, Bridge JA, Sorensen P, Thorner P, Squire JA. Spectral karyotyping identifies recurrent complex rearrangements of chromosomes 8, 17, and 20 in osteosarcomas. Genes Chromosomes Cancer. 2003;36(1):7–16.
60. Baldini N, Scotlandi K, Serra M, Picci P, Bacci G, Sottili S, Campanacci M. P-glycoprotein expression in osteosarcoma: a basis for risk-adapted adjuvant chemotherapy. J Orthop Res. 1999;17(5):629–32.
61. Berner JM, Forus A, Elkahloun A, et al. Separate amplified regions encompassing CDK4 and MDM2 in human sarcomas. Genes Chromosomes Cancer. 1996;17:254–9.
62. Bertoni F, Bacchini P, Donati D, Martini A, Picci P, Campanacci M. Osteoblastoma-like osteosarcoma. The Rizzoli Institute experience. Mod Pathol. 1993;6(6):707–16.
63. Bhutani M, Pathak AK, Sengar M, et al. Multifocal osteosarcoma involving unusual sites. Cancer Invest. 2006;24:278–82.
64. Biegel JA, Zhou JY, Emanel BS. Complex karyotypes in a series of pediatric osteosarcomas. Cancer Genet Cytogenet. 1989;38:89–100.
65. Bielack SS, Kempf-Bielack B, Delling G, Exner GU, Flege S, Helmke K, Kotz R, et al. Prognostic factors in high-grade osteosarcoma of the extremities or trunk: an analysis of 1702 patients treated on

neoadjuvant cooperative osteosarcoma study group protocols. J Clin Oncol. 2002;20(3):776–90.

66. Bovée JV, Sakkers RJ, Geirnaerdt MJ, Taminiau AH, Hogendoorn PC. Intermediate grade osteosarcoma and chondrosarcoma arising in an osteochondroma. A case report of a patient with hereditary multiple exostoses. J Clin Pathol. 2002;55(3):226–9.
67. Bridge JA, Nelson M, McComb E, McGuire MH, Rosenthal H, Vergara G, Maale GE, Spanier S, Neff JR. Cytogenetic findings in 73 osteosarcoma specimens and a review of the literature. Cancer Genet Cytogenet. 1997;95(1):74–87.
68. Chen Y, Shen Q, Gokavarapu S, Lin C, Cao W, Chauhan S, Liu Z, Ji T, Tian Z. Osteosarcoma of head and neck: a retrospective study on prognostic factors from a single institute database. Oral Oncol. 2016;58:1–7.
69. Chow LT, Lin J, Yip KM, Kumta SM, Ahuja AT, King WW, Lee JC. Chondromyxoid fibroma-like osteosarcoma: a distinct variant of low-grade osteosarcoma. Histopathology. 1996;29(5):429–36.
70. Choo JY, Lee JH, Lee JY, Park YM. Cutaneous metastasis of giant cell-rich osteosarcoma. Ann Dermatol. 2016;28:247–8.
71. Chow LT. Giant cell rich osteosarcoma revisited-diagnostic criteria and histopathologic patterns, Ki67, CDK4, and MDM2 expression, changes in response to bisphosphonate and denosumab treatment. Virchows Arch. 2016;468:741–55.
72. Kerr DA, Lopez HU, Deshpande V, Hornicek FJ, Duan Z, Zhang Y, Rosenberg AE, Borger DR, Nielsen GP. Molecular distinction of chondrosarcoma from chondroblastic osteosarcoma through IDH1/2 mutations. Am J Surg Pathol. 2013;37:787–95.
73. DeLaney TF, Park L, Goldberg SI, et al. Radiotherapy for local control of osteosarcoma. Int J Radiat Oncol Biol Phys. 2005;61(2):492–8.
74. Corradi D, Wenger DE, Bertoni F, Bacchini P, Bosio S, Goldoni M, Unni KK, Sim FH, Inwards CY. Multicentric osteosarcoma: clinicopathologic and radiographic study of 56 cases. Am J Clin Pathol. 2011;136(5):799–807.
75. Martadiani ED, Asih MW, Winarti NW, Zulfariska N, Maria D, Asih KP. Reliability study of radiology interpretation in osteosarcoma. Bali Med J. 2021;10(2):915–21.
76. Ferrari S, Ruggieri P, Cefalo G, et al. Neoadjuvant chemotherapy with methotrexate cisplatin and doxorubicin with or without ifosfamide in nonmetastatic osteosarcoma of the extremity an Italian sarcoma group trial ISG/OS-1. J Clin Oncol. 2011;38:4420.
77. Fletcher JA, Gebhardt MC, Kozakewich HP. Cytogenetic aberrations in osteosarcomas. Nonrandom deletions, rings and double minute chromosomes. Cancer Genet Cytogenet. 1994;77:81–8.
78. Bacci G, Bertoni F, Longhi A, Ferrari S, Forni C, Biagini R, Bacchini P, Donati D, Manfrini M, Bernini G, Lari S. Neoadjuvant chemotherapy for high-grade central osteosarcoma of the extremity: histologic response to preoperative chemotherapy correlates with histologic subtype of the tumor. Cancer. 2003;97:3068–75.
79. Garrington GE, Scofield HH, Cornyn J, Hooker SP. Osteosarcoma of the jaws: analysis of 56 cases. Cancer. 1967;20:377–91.
80. Geller DS, Gorlick R. Osteosarcoma: a review of diagnosis, management, and treatment strategies. Clin Adv Hematol Oncol. 2010;8(10):705–18.
81. Gomez-Brouchet A, Mourcin F, Gourraud PA, et al. Galectin-1 is a powerful marker to distinguish chondroblastic osteosarcoma and conventional chondrosarcoma. Hum Pathol. 2010;41:1220–30.
82. Grimer RJ, Cannon SR, Taminiau AM, et al. Osteosarcoma over the age of 40. Eur J Cancer. 2003;39:157–63.
83. Guadagnolo BA, Zagars GK, Raymond AK, Benjamin RS, Sturgis EM. Osteosarcoma of the jaw/craniofacial region: outcomes after multimodality treatment. Cancer. 2009;115(14):3262–70.
84. Hasegawa T, Hirose T, Kudo E, et al. Immunophenotypic heterogeneity in osteosarcomas. Hum Pathol. 1991;22:583–90.
85. Hasegawa T, Shibata T, Hirose T, et al. Osteosarcoma with epithelioid features. An immunohistochemical study. Arch Pathol Lab Med. 1993;117:295–8.
86. Hmada YA, Bernieh A, Morris RW, Lewin J, Allen T. Chondroblastoma-like osteosarcoma. Arch Pathol Lab Med. 2020;144(1):15–7.
87. Hauben EI, Arends J, Vandenbroucke JP, et al. Multiple primary malignancies in osteosarcoma patients: incidence and predictive value of osteosarcoma subtype for cancer syndromes related with osteosarcoma. Eur J Hum Genet. 2003;11:611–8.
88. Hirose K, Okura M, Sato S, Murakami S, Ikeda JI, Noda Y, et al. Gnathic giant-cell-rich conventional osteosarcoma with MDM2 and CDK4 gene amplification. Histopathology. 2017;70:1171–3.
89. Hong SJ, Kim KA, Yong HS, Choi JW, Suh SI, Lee JH, Shon WY. Giant cell-rich osteosarcoma of bone. Eur J Radiol Extra. 2005;53:87–90.
90. Green JT, Mills AM. Osteogenic tumors of bone. Semin Diagn Pathol. 2014;31:21–9.
91. Junior AT, de Abreu AF, Pinto CAL, et al. Clinicopathological and immunohistochemical analysis of 25 head and neck osteosarcomas. Oral Oncol. 2003;39(5):521–30.
92. Okada K, Hasegawa T, Yokoyama R, Beppu Y, Itoi E. Osteosarcoma with cytokeratin expression: a clinicopathological study of six cases with an emphasis on differential diagnosis from metastatic cancer. J Clin Pathol. 2003;56:742–6.
93. Kanoe H, Nakayama T, Murakami H, Hosaka T, Yamamoto H, Nakashima Y, Tsuboyama T, Nakamura T, Sasaki MS, Toguchida J. Amplification of the CDK4 gene in sarcomas: tumor specificity and relationship with the RB gene mutation. Anticancer Res. 1998;18(4A):2317–21.
94. Kaste SC, Liu T, Billups CA, Daw NC, Pratt CB, Meyer WH. Tumor size as a predictor of outcome in pediatric non-metastatic osteosarcoma of the extremity. Pediatr Blood Cancer. 2004;43(7):723–8.
95. Kinra P, Valdamani S, Singh V, Dutta V. Diaphyseal giant cell-rich osteosarcoma: unusual histologi-

cal variant in an unusual site. Indian J Pathol Microbiol. 2012;55(4):600–2. https://doi.org/10.4103/0377-4929.107848.
96. Klein MJ, Siegal GP. Osteosarcoma: anatomic and histologic variants. Am J Clin Pathol. 2006;125:555–81.
97. Kramer K, Hicks DG, Palis J, et al. Epithelioid osteosarcoma of bone: immunocytochemical evidence suggesting divergent epithelial and mesenchymal differentiation in a primary osseous neoplasm. Cancer. 1993;71:2977–82.
98. Liu JJ, Liu S, Wang JG, Zhu W, Hua YQ, Sun W, Cai ZD. Telangiectatic osteosarcoma: a review of literature. Onco Targets Ther. 2013;28(6):593–602.
99. Laskar S, Basu A, Muckaden MA, D'Cruz A, Pai S, Jambhekar N, Tike P, Shrivastava SK. Osteosarcoma of the head and neck region: lessons learned from a single-institution experience of 50 patients. Head Neck. 2008;30(8):1020–6.
100. Li FP, Fraumeni JF, Mulvihill JJ, et al. A cancer family syndrome in twenty-four kindreds. Cancer Res. 1988;48:5358–62.
101. Machak GN, Tkachev SI, Solovyev YN, et al. Neoadjuvant chemotherapy and local radiotherapy for high-grade osteosarcoma of the extremities. Mayo Clinic Proc. 2003;78(2):147–55.
102. Misaghi A, Goldin A, Awad M, Kulidjian AA. Osteosarcoma: a comprehensive review. SICOT-J. 2018;4:12.
103. Pakos EE, Nearchou AD, Grimer RJ, Koumoullis HD, Abudu A, Bramer JAM, Jeys LM, et al. Prognostic factors and outcomes for osteosarcoma: an international collaboration. Eur J Cancer. 2009;45(13):2367–75.
104. Pratt CB, Meyer WH, Luo X, et al. Second malignant neoplasms occurring in survivors of osteosarcoma. Cancer. 1997;80:960–5.
105. Rosen G, Caparros B, Huvos AG, et al. Preoperative chemotherapy for osteogenic sarcoma: selection of postoperative adjuvant chemotherapy based on the response of the primary tumor to preoperative chemotherapy. Cancer. 1982;49(6):1221.
106. Salas S, de Pinieux G, Gomez-Brouchet A, et al. Ezrin immunohistochemical expression in cartilaginous tumours: a useful tool for differential diagnosis between chondroblastic osteosarcoma and chondrosarcoma. Virchows Arch. 2009;454:81–7.
107. Shinozaki T, Fukuda T, Watanabe H, Takagishi K. Giant cell rich osteosarcoma simulating giant cell tumor of bone. Kitakanto Med J. 2004;54:147–51.
108. Unni KK, Dahlin DC. Grading of bone tumors. Semin Diagn Pathol. 1984;1:165–72.
109. Unni KK, Dahlin DC. Osteosarcoma: pathology and classification. Semin Roentgenol. 1989;24:143–52.
110. Wang CS, Yin QH, Liao JS, Lou JH, Ding XY, Zhu YB. Giant cell-rich osteosarcoma in long bones: clinical, radiological and pathological features. Radiol Med. 2013;118(8):1324–34. https://doi.org/10.1007/s11547-013-0936-9.
111. Zhong J, Si L, Geng J, Xing Y, Hu Y, Jiao Q, Zhang H, Yao W. Chondromyxoid fibroma-like osteosarcoma: a case series and literature review. BMC Musculoskelet Disord. 2020;21(1):53.

Low Grade Central OS

112. Bertoni F, Bacchini P, Fabbri N, Mercuri M, Picci P, Ruggieri P, Campanacci M. Osteosarcoma. Low-grade intraosseous type osteosarcoma, histologically resembling parosteal osteosarcoma, fibrous dysplasia, and desmoplastic fibroma. Cancer. 1993;71:338–45.
113. Bonar SF. Central low-grade osteosarcoma: a diagnostic challenge. Skelet Radiol. 2012;41:365–7.
114. Endo M, Yoshida T, Yamamoto H, et al. Low-grade central osteosarcoma arising from bone infarct. Hum Pathol. 2013;44(6):1184–9.
115. Hayashi K, Tsuchiya H, Yamamoto N, Shirai T, Nishida H, Takeuchi A, Kimura H, Miwa S, Inatani H, Okamoto H, Yamada S, Ikeda H, Sawada-Kitamura S, Nojima T, Ooi A, Otsuka T. Diagnosis and treatment of low-grade osteosarcoma: experience with nine cases. Int J Clin Oncol. 2014;19(4):731–8.
116. Mariano FV, Corrêa MB, da Costa MV, de Almeida OP, Lopes MA, Dujardin F, Binh MB, Bouvier C, Gomez-Brouchet A, Larousserie F, Muret A, Louis-Brennetot C, Aurias A, Coindre JM, Guillou L, Pedeutour F, Duval H, Collin C, de Pinieux G. MDM2 and CDK4 immunohistochemistry is a valuable tool in the differential diagnosis of low-grade osteosarcomas and other primary fibro-osseous lesions of the bone. Mod Pathol. 2011;24(5):624–37.
117. Unni KK, Dahlin DC, McLeod RA, Pritchard DJ. Intraosseous well-differentiated osteosarcoma. Cancer. 1977;40:1337–47.

Small Cell Osteosarcoma

118. Ayala AG, Ro JY, Raymond AK, Jaffe N, Chawla S, Carrasco H, Link M, Jimenez J, Edeiken J, Wallace S, Murray JA, Benjamin R. Small cell osteosarcoma. A clinicopathologic study of 27 cases. Cancer. 1989;64(10):2162–73.
119. Devaney DM, Vinh TN, Sweet DE. Small cell osteosarcoma of bone: an immunohistochemical study with differential diagnostic considerations. Hum Pathol. 1993;23:1211–25.
120. Debelenko LV, McGregor LM, Shivakumar R, Dorfman D, Raimondi SC. A novel EWSR1-CREB3L1 fusion transcript in a case of small

cell osteosarcoma. Genes Chromosomes Cancer. 2011;50:1054–62.
121. Nakajima H, Sim FH, Bond JR, Unni KK. Small cell osteosarcoma of bone. Review of 72 cases. Cancer. 1997;79:2095–106.
122. Wang L, Bhargava R, Zheng T, Wexler L, Collins MH, Roulston D, Ladanyi M. EWSR1-CREB3L1 in small cell osteosarcoma. Genes Chromosomes Cancer. 2007.

Parosteal

123. Duhamel LAE, Ye H, Halai D, et al. Frequency of mouse double minute 2 (MDM2) and mouse double minute 4 (MDM4) amplification in parosteal and conventional osteosarcoma subtypes. Histopathology. 2012;60(2):357–9.
124. Gamberi G, Ragazzini P, Benassi MS, et al. Analysis of 12q13–15 genes in parosteal osteosarcoma. Clin Orthop Relat Res. 2000;377:195–204.
125. Okada K, Frassica FJ, Sim FH, Beabout JW, Bond JR, Unni KK. Parosteal osteosarcoma. A clinicopathological study. J Bone Jt Surg Am. 1994;76:366–78.

Periosteal OS

126. Robertson NJ, Newman PL. Periosteal osteosarcoma of the cranium. Ann Diagn Pathol. 2000;4(5):300–2.
127. Unni KK, Dahlin DC, Beabout JW. Periosteal osteogenic sarcoma. Cancer. 1976;37:2476–85.

High Grade Surface OS

128. Okada K, Krishnan Unni K, Swee RG, Sim FH. High grade surface osteosarcoma. Cancer. 1999;85:1044–54.
129. Staals EL, Bacchini P, Bertoni F. High-grade surface osteosarcoma: a review of 25 cases from the Rizzoli Institute. Cancer. 2008;112(7):1592–9.
130. Vanel D, Picci P, De Paolis M, Mercuri M. Radiological study of 12 high-grade surface osteosarcomas. Skelet Radiol. 2001;30:667.
131. Wold LE, Unni KK, Beabout JW, Pritchard DJ. High-grade surface osteosarcomas. Am J Surg Pathol. 1984;8:181–6.
132. Yoshida A, Ushiku T, Motoi T, Beppu Y, Fukayama M, Tsuda H, Shibata T. MDM2 and CDK4 immunohistochemical coexpression in high-grade osteosarcoma: correlation with a dedifferentiated subtype. Am J Surg Pathol. 2012;36(3):423–31.

Secondary OS

133. Hanson MF, Seton M, Merchant A. Osteosarcoma in Paget's disease of bone. J Bone Miner Res. 2006;21(suppl 2):P58–63.
134. Healey JH, Buss D. Radiation and pagetic osteogenic sarcomas. Clin Orthop Relat Res. 1991;270:128–34.
135. Mertens F, Larramedy M, Gusstavson A, et al. Radiation-associated sarcomas are characterized by complex karyotypes with frequent rearrangements of chromosome arm 3p. Cancer Genet Cytogenet. 2000;116:89–96.

Composite Sarcoma of Bone

136. Andión Catalán M, Buendía López S, Camarena Pavón N, Rubio San Simón A, Cañas Maciá T, Azorín CD. Composite sarcoma of bone with focal rhabdomyosarcoma and lymph node metastasis in an adolescent. Pediatr Blood Cancer. 2020;67(11):e28679.
137. Bertoni F, Laus M. Primary malignant mesenchymoma of bone (case report). Ital J Orthop Traumatol. 1978;4:105–8.
138. Bosman C, Boldrini R, Guzzanti V. Primary osteoliposarcoma of bone: first observation in the pediatric age group. Appl Pathol. 1988;6:56.
139. De Padua M, Bhandari TP, Pingle J. Primary osteoliposarcoma of the bone. Indian J Pathol Microbiol. 2009;52(1):80–2.
140. Schajowicz F, Cuevillas AR, Silberman FS. Primary malignant mesenchymoma of bone: a new tumor entity. Cancer. 1966;19:1423–8.
141. Van Dorpe J, Sciot R, Samson I, De Vos R, Brys P, Van Damme B. Primary osteorhabdomyosarcoma (malignant mesenchymoma) of bone: a case report and review of the literature. Mod Pathol. 1997;10:1047–53.

Myositis Ossificans

142. Cortellazzo Wiel L, Trevisan M, Murru FM, et al. Myositis ossificans mimicking sarcoma: a not so rare bioptic diagnostic pitfall. Ital J Pediatr. 2020;46:110.
143. Eckardt JJ, Ivins JC, Perry HO, Unni KK. Osteosarcoma arising in heterotopic ossification of dermatomyositis: case report and review of the literature. Cancer. 1981;48(5):1256–61.
144. Hoch B, Montag A. Reactive bone lesions mimicking neoplasms. Semin Diagn Pathol. 2011;28(1):102–12.
145. Lacout A, Jarraya M, Marcy PY, Thariat J, Carlier RY. Myositis ossificans imaging: keys to successful

diagnosis. Indian J Radiol Imaging. 2012;22(1):35–9. https://doi.org/10.4103/0971-3026.95402.
146. McCarthy EF, Sundaram M. Heterotopic ossification: a review. Skelet Radiol. 2005;34(10):609–19.
147. Nuovo MA, Norman A, Chumas J, Ackerman LV. Myositis ossificans with atypical clinical, radiographic, or pathologic findings: a review of 23 cases. Skelet Radiol. 1992;21:87–101.
148. Parikh J, Hyare H, Saifuddin A. The imaging features of post-traumatic myositis ossificans with emphasis on MRI. Clin Radiol. 2002;57:1058–66.
149. Sferopoulos NK, Kotakidou R, Petropoulos AS. Myositis ossificans in children: a review. Eur J Orthop Surg Traumatol. 2017;27:491–502.
150. Shore EM, Ahn J, Jan de Beur S, et al. Paternally inherited inactivating mutations of the GNAS1 gene in progressive osseous heteroplasia. N Engl J Med. 2002;346(2):99–106.

Bone Island

151. Pal R, Dutta P, Bhadada SK, et al. Islands of bone within bone. Postgrad Med J. 2019;95:289.
152. WHO Classification of Tumours Editorial Board. WHO Classification of tumours. In: Soft tissue and bone tumours, vol. 3. 5th ed. IARC; 2020.

6 Fibrous Tumours and Lesions of Bone

In this chapter, fibrogenic tumours, other mesenchymal tumours with predominant fibrous component and fibrohistiocytic tumours are included. The undifferentiated pleomorphic sarcoma is described as a separate entity in 2020 WHO [62]. But it is included in this chapter because it was earlier called as malignant fibrous histiocytoma.

6.1 Fibrogenic Tumours: Classification [59, 62]

- **Intermediate (locally aggressive)**
  - Desmoplastic fibroma
- **Malignant**
  - Fibrosarcoma
  - Undifferentiated pleomorphic sarcoma (old terminology—malignant fibrous histiocytoma of bone (MFH))
- **Other benign fibrous neoplasm/proliferations of bone**
  - Non-ossifying fibroma
  - Fibrous dysplasia and osteofibrous dysplasia
  - Periosteal desmoid
  - Fibrocartilaginous mesenchymoma
  - Myofibroma (congenital/infantile fibromatosis)

6.2 Desmoplastic Fibroma

This is one of the rarest neoplasms of bone (<0.1%). It is the intraosseous counterpart of fibromatosis/desmoid tumour of soft tissue. Majority of the cases are in the second or third decade. Any bone may be involved. Mandible [1, 3], pelvic bones, femur and tibia are the preferred sites. The patients present with pain and swelling.

6.2.1 Radiology

The lesions are well defined purely lytic with reactive sclerosis in the adjacent bone (Fig. 6.1a) [2]. Sometimes, there can be uneven bone destruction. The affected bone is expanded. Large lesions show cortical destruction, which is better appreciated on MRI.

6.2.2 Pathology

Grossly desmoplastic fibroma is firm and has a whorled appearance of cut surface. Microscopically, they show an infiltrative growth. They are hypocellular on low-power examination and composed of proliferating spindle cells with abundant collagen formation. Nuclei are bland

J. Kattoor et al., *Bone Tumors*, https://doi.org/10.1007/978-981-99-4738-6_6

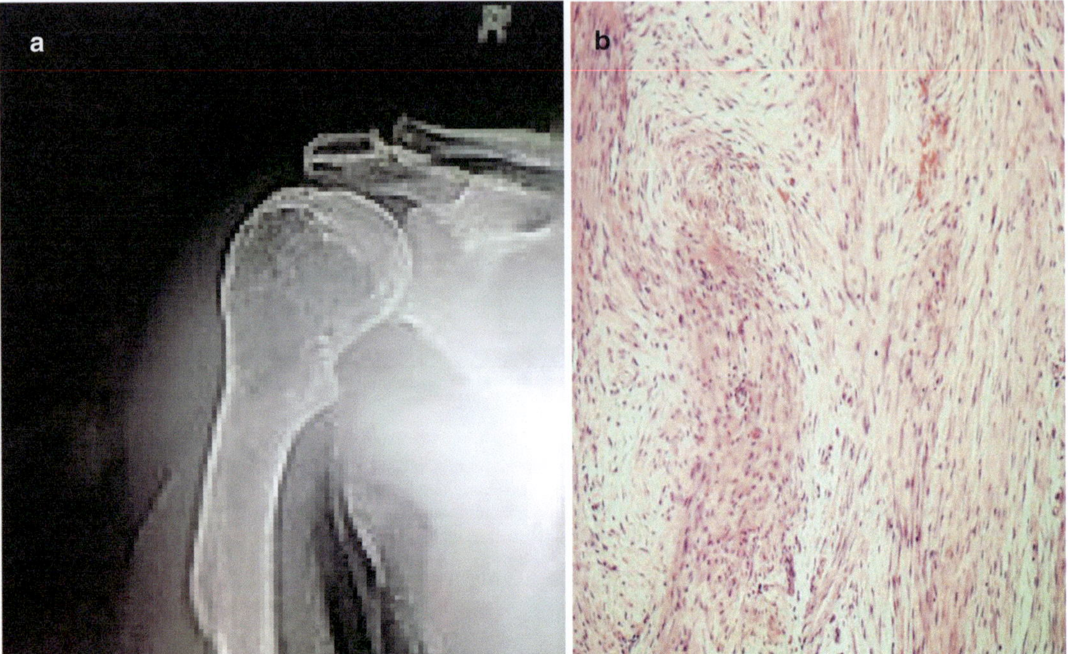

Fig. 6.1 Desmoplastic fibroma. (**a**) Lytic lesion humerus. (**b**) Loosely arranged spindle cells in fascicles with collagen, H&E ×100

without cytologic atypia. Mitotic activity is very low or absent (Fig. 6.1b). Thin-walled vessels as seen in fibromatosis can be seen in this tumour also. Differential diagnosis of this tumour is a low-grade osteosarcoma. If cellular, fibrosarcoma should be considered in the differential diagnosis. Radiology correlation is essential. Look for permeation of pre-existing bony trabeculae if there is a suspicion of malignancy. IHC shows SMA and β-catenin positivity.

6.2.3 Treatment and Prognosis

Surgical complete resection of the tumour is the treatment because this is a locally aggressive tumour. Prognosis is good if the resection is complete. In cases where curettage is done, local recurrence can occur.

6.3 Other Benign Fibrous Tumours of Bone

Non-ossifying fibroma is described in Chap. 7, under giant cell-rich lesions.

6.3.1 Fibrous Dysplasia (FD)

Fibrous dysplasia is a benign neoplasm composed of spindle cells and woven bone. This entity was considered as a tumour-like lesion. But in recent WHO (2020) [62], it is classified under the other mesenchymal tumours.

Fibrous dysplasia can cause deformity of the affected bone, and these bones are prone to deform and become fragile causing fracture [5–7]. The basic cause of fibrous dysplasia is unknown. Fibrous dysplasia can affect any bone in the body. It can be mono-ostotic or polyostotic [11]. Bones most commonly affected are craniofacial bones [17] and femur. Other bones affected are tibia, ribs and pelvic bones. The mono-ostotic form is more common.

6.3.1.1 Clinical

FD usually does not produce symptoms especially if it is mild. Symptoms develop in the second decade. In polyostotic forms, symptoms can begin early in the first decade itself. In severe forms, pain, swelling, pathological fracture, deformities and difficulty in walking are the usual symptoms. Polyostotic fibrous dysplasia [11] is associated with polyendocrinopathy and café au lait spots in McCune-Albright syndrome [4, 16, 19, 20]. In Mazabraud syndrome [18], fibrous dysplasia is associated with soft tissue myxomas [12, 17]. Complications like bone deformity due to weakening of bones can cause vision, hearing loss, arthritis and rarely malignant transformation, especially in those who receive prior radiation [63]. FD is caused by mutations in the GNAS gene [8, 10, 14, 20].

6.3.1.2 Radiology

On X-ray, fibrous dysplasia appears with a hazy ground glass appearance [27]. In long-standing lesions, pathological fracture or cyst formation can be seen (Fig. 6.2). Bone scan helps to know whether it is mono-ostotic or polyostotic.

6.3.1.3 Pathology

In FD, the normal bone is replaced by collagen-rich tissue with fibroblastic proliferation and haphazardly distributed immature woven bone (Fig. 6.3). Usually, bony fragments are not rimmed by osteoblasts. However, presence of osteoblastic rimming does not rule out the possibility of FD (Fig. 6.5d). The trabeculae of woven bone can be in different shapes resembling

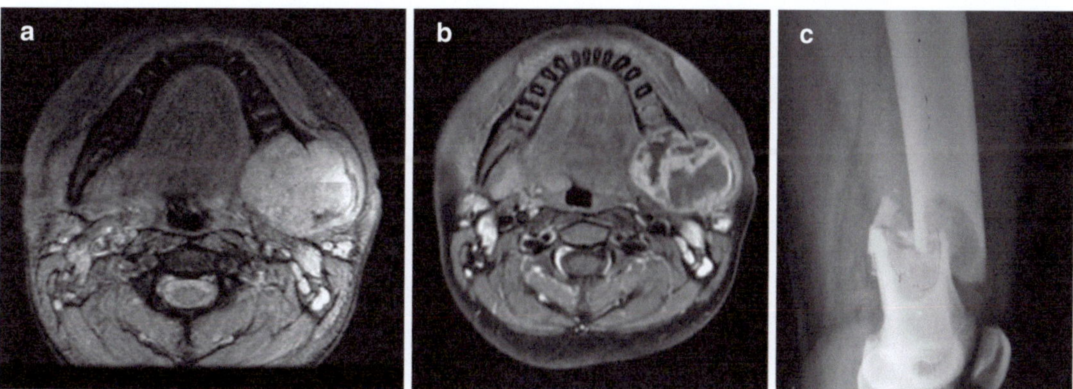

Fig. 6.2 (**a**, **b**) Fibrous dysplasia with secondary ABC in mandible in an 11-year-old girl mistaken radiologically and clinically as malignant lesion. (**c**) FD with expansile lytic appearance in the metadiaphyseal region of femur and pathological fracture

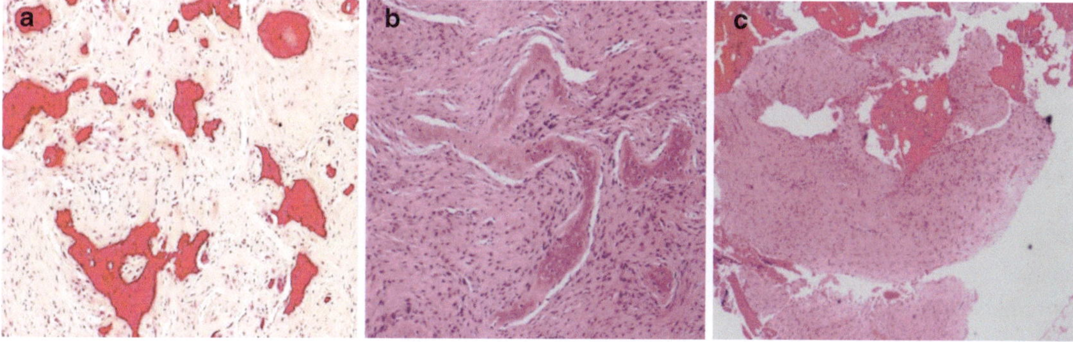

Fig. 6.3 FD: (**a**) Woven bone without osteoblastic rimming in fibrous stroma, H&E ×100. (**b**) Higher power of woven bone and cellular spindle stroma, H&E ×250. (**c**) Secondary ABC in FD, H&E ×40

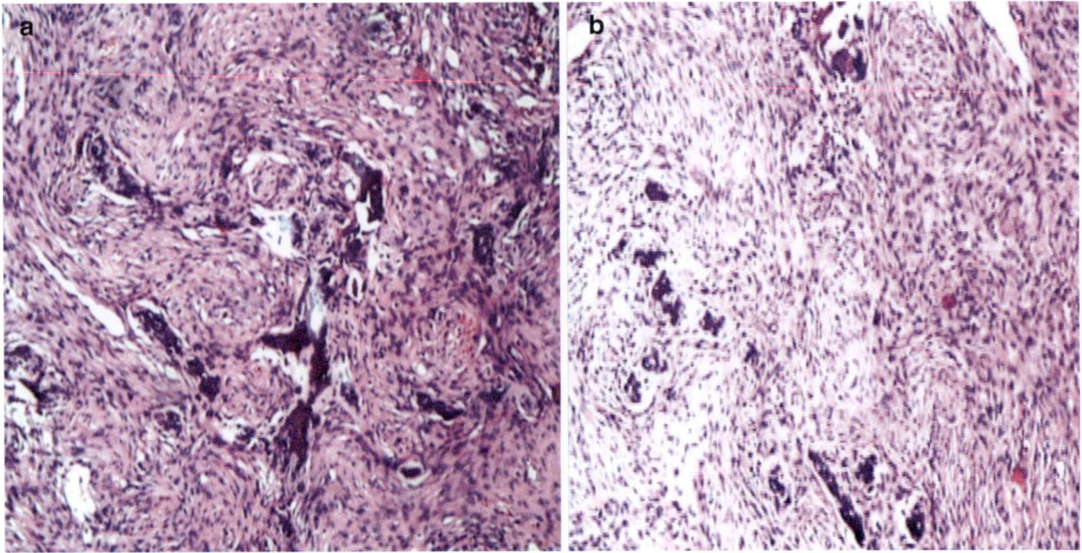

Fig. 6.4 (**a**, **b**) Spindle cell-rich FD, H&E ×100

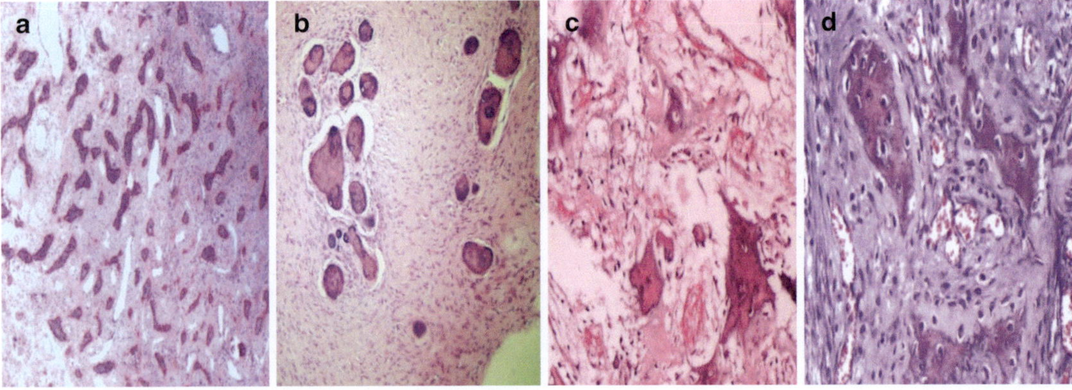

Fig. 6.5 FD: (**a**) Chinese letter pattern of woven bone, H&E ×100. (**b**) FD of maxilla-psammomatous type, H&E ×100. (**c**) Myxoid FD, H&E ×100. (**d**) Woven bone with osteoblastic rimming in FD

Chinese letters, which are curved and thin. This is described as Chinese letter pattern (Fig. 6.5a). It can form small calcified spherules that mimic psammoma bodies (Fig. 6.5b). This type is more commonly seen in jawbones and also base of skull and is usually mistaken for meningioma. In jawbones, instead of woven bone, it can be trabecular bone. Sometimes, spindle cells are seen in storiform pattern without bone production (Fig. 6.4). Fibrous dysplasia can have myxoid change in the stroma (Fig. 6.5c). Mitosis is extremely uncommon. Collection of foam cells, osteoclastic giant cells and myxoid change of stroma are present in FD. Secondary ABC formation can sometimes cause aggressive clinical and radiological appearance mimicking malignancy. Rarely, cartilage may dominate in FD, and they resemble epiphyseal plate histologically.

6.3.1.4 Differential diagnosis

This includes other fibro-osseous lesions [5–7] like ossifying fibroma [19], cemento-ossifying fibroma [15], osteoblastoma and low-grade osteosarcoma [9, 13]. Molecular test like MDM2 amplification may be helpful in differentiating low-grade OS from FD. Among all fibro-osseous lesions, the GNAS mutations are specific to fibrous dysplasia [12, 15]. The differentiation from low-grade osteosarcoma is given in Table 6.1.

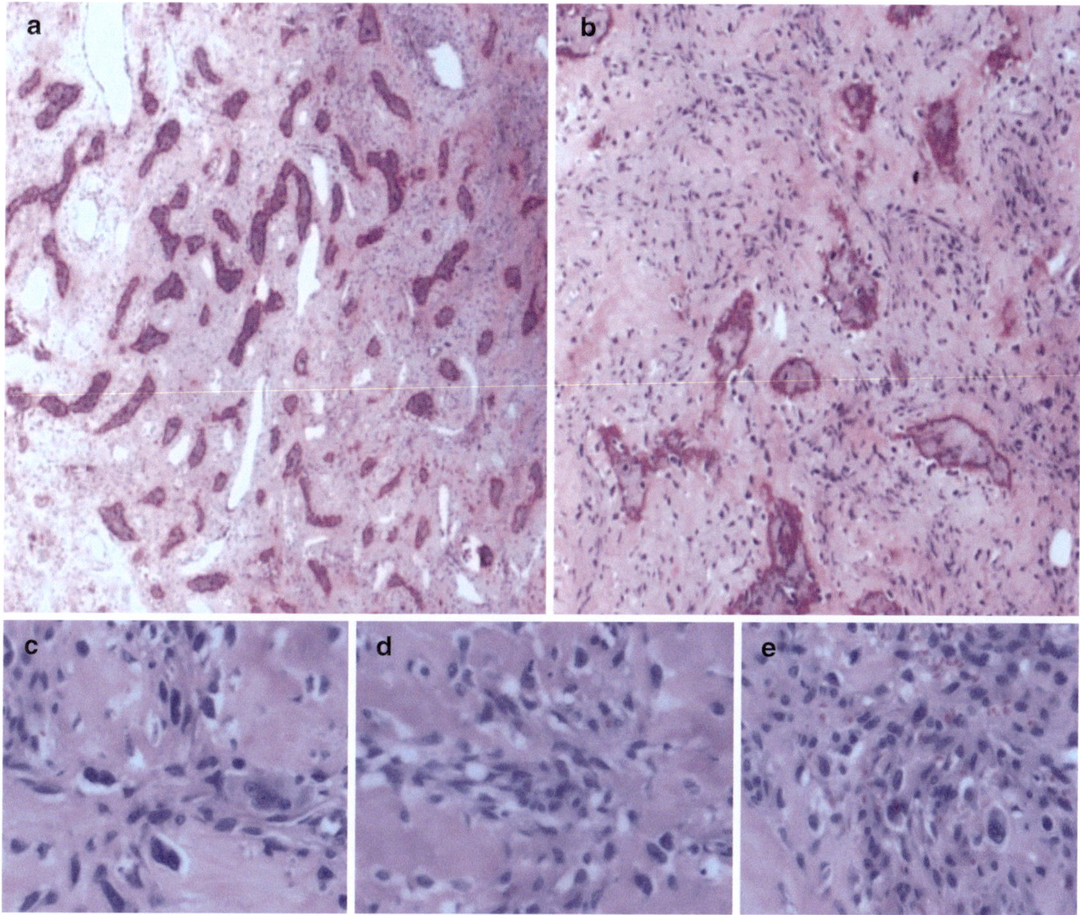

Fig. 6.6 Secondary osteosarcoma in a 29-year-old female with a diagnosis of FD 11 years back. (**a**, **b**) Fibrous dysplasia, H&E ×40. (**c**–**e**) Osteosarcoma, H&E ×250

Table 6.1 Differentiating features of fibrous dysplasia and low-grade osteosarcoma [9, 16]

	Fibrous dysplasia	Low-grade OS
Type of bone	Woven bone	Trabecular bone
Osteoblastic rimming	Usually absent	Present
Cells	Oval cells	Elongated cells
Permeation of bone	Absent	Present
Molecular	GNAS mutations	MDM2 amplification

6.3.1.5 Molecular

GNAS mutation is seen in fibrous dysplasia [20].

6.3.1.6 Treatment and Prognosis

Mono-ostotic FD with no symptoms is kept under follow-up. Symptomatic patients require either medication or surgery. Bisphosphonates are used to inhibit bone destruction. It also relieves bone pain. Bisphosphonates are given either orally or by intravenous route. Surgery is indicated when the deformity needs correction or if there is a difference in limb lengths or if there is a fracture. Surgical removal of bone lesion and replacement by bone graft can be done.

6.3.1.7 Malignancy in Fibrous Dysplasia

Rarely, malignancies can arise in fibrous dysplasia. Osteosarcoma (Fig. 6.6), fibrosarcoma and chondrosarcoma have been reported. Most of these cases had previous radiation for fibrous dysplasia. The prognosis of these cases is poor.

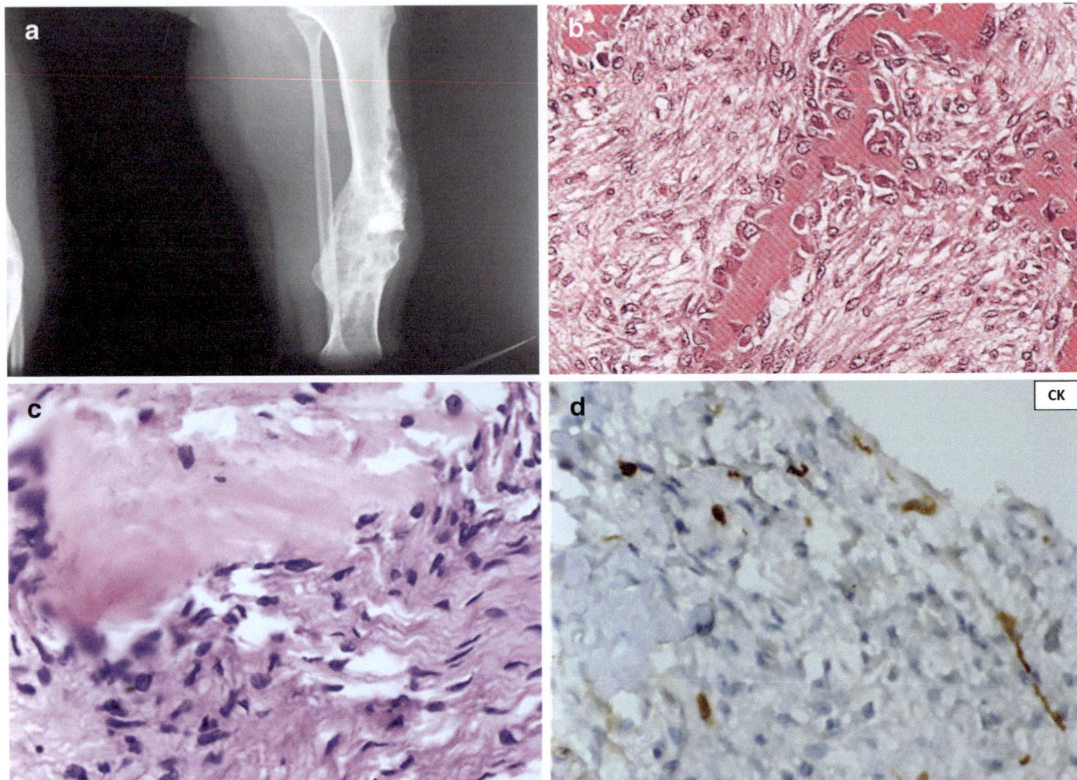

Fig. 6.7 Osteofibrous dysplasia in an 8-year-old girl. (**a**) Plain X-ray showing bowing of tibia with numerous lytic areas involving the cortex and medullary cavity. (**b**) Trabeculae of woven bone with osteoblastic rimming in a fibrous stroma, H&E ×250. (**c**) Collagenous matrix, H&E ×400. (**d**) IHC for cytokeratin showing single keratin-positive cells, CK ×250

6.3.2 Osteofibrous Dysplasia (OFD)

OFD occurs in young children below the age of 10 years [10]. It is extremely rare after 16 years [21, 22].

6.3.2.1 Clinical

Tibia and fibula are the preferred sites. 90% of cases occur at these sites. These lesions are thought to be precursors of adamantinoma occurring in adults [23, 25, 26].

6.3.2.2 Radiology

They occur as lytic mid-diaphyseal lesions with no soft tissue mass (Fig. 6.7a).

6.3.2.3 Pathology

These fibro-osseous lesions have vascularized stroma and bony trabeculae with prominent osteoblastic rimming (Fig. 6.7b, c), and they lack the characteristic Chinese letter type of woven bone seen in FD. They contain scattered cells, which are positive for cytokeratin [24] (Fig. 6.7d). But epithelial islands as seen in adamantinoma are absent.

6.3.3 Periosteal Desmoid

This is a fibrous cortical defect which occurs mainly on the posteromedial aspect of distal femur. As the cortex shows irregular destruction, it may mimic malignancy. Usually, these lesions are incidental findings. Histologically, a portion of cortex is replaced by fibrous tissue. Few benign giant cells can be seen.

6.3.4 Fibrocartilaginous Mesenchymoma

This entity was first described by Dahlin in 1984. It is one of the rarest lesions of bone. Proximal fibula is the commonest site. It can occur in other bones also. It occurs in metaphyseal area and abuts on growth plate. Cartilage, bone formation and fibroblastic proliferation can be seen. The cartilage appears as in endochondral ossification with appearance similar to epiphyseal plate. Cellular spindle cell proliferation will be seen in between. If resection is not complete, these lesions recur.

6.3.5 Myofibroma (Infantile Myofibromatosis)

Clinical: This entity usually affects infants, which can be solitary subcutaneous lesion or multiple [28]. Usually in multiple lesions, skeletal involvement is common [38]. The solitary variety involving bone is known as myofibroma, and it commonly involves craniofacial bones [34, 35, 36]. Infantile myofibroma can also occur in bone [30, 31, 32].

Radiology: These are lytic lesions with sclerotic border [33]. In the multiple variety, it affects the metaphyseal region of long bones as lucent lesions.

Pathology: Microscopically, myofibromas are composed of whorls and bundles of spindle cells with plump nuclei in a myxoid background [29]. A prominent vascular proliferation with large vascular spaces without muscular wall can be seen between the nodules. Spindle cells have a myogenic differentiation. Haemangiopericytomatous pattern is also described.

DD: These lesions should not be mistaken for low-grade sarcomas.

Treatment and Prognosis: The prognosis is good, and most of the lesions regress spontaneously [37]. Non-regressing lesions are excised. Rare forms involve visceral organs such as lung, liver or gastrointestinal tract, and these cases have a poor prognosis.

6.4 Malignant Tumours

6.4.1 Fibrosarcoma (FS)

Fibrosarcoma is a rare, malignant tumour of bone [42, 45, 47]. FS is derived from transformed spindle-shaped fibroblasts. Primary fibrosarcoma of bone may arise within the medullary canal. It can be primary or secondary. The periosteum can be a site of origin in primary fibrosarcoma [62, 63]. Secondary FS arises from pre-existing bone lesions [44, 52, 53] or bone damage induced by radiotherapy [59].

6.4.1.1 Clinical

Fibrosarcomas of bone usually occur in adults of 40 years or older. Both females and males are equally affected. Common sites are long bones [60], usually distal femur or proximal tibia or jawbones [40, 59]. FS may develop secondary to infarct, Paget disease [52] and prior radiation. Occasionally, it is multicentric [51, 54]. When multicentric, metastatic sarcomatoid carcinoma should be ruled out. Infantile congenital fibrosarcoma of bone is also described [48].

They present with persistent pain in the area of the tumour. Swelling around the bone, difficulty in moving a joint or limb and pressure symptoms caused by the tumour are the major clinical manifestations.

6.4.1.2 Radiology

It shows eccentric, osteolytic, soap bubble appearance resembling giant cell tumour. The margins can be invasive or well-defined. It is usually metaphyseal and may extend to the diaphysis or epiphysis (Fig. 6.8).

6.4.1.3 Pathology

Gross specimens have fish flesh appearance of sarcomas (Fig. 6.8c). It may destroy cortex and extend into soft tissue (Fig. 6.9). Microscopically, it is a spindle cell sarcoma with cells arranged in fascicles or herringbone pattern, resembling its soft tissue counterpart [49]. The tumour is very cellular, but pleomorphism is rare. The cells are elongated with plump vesicular nuclei. In high-

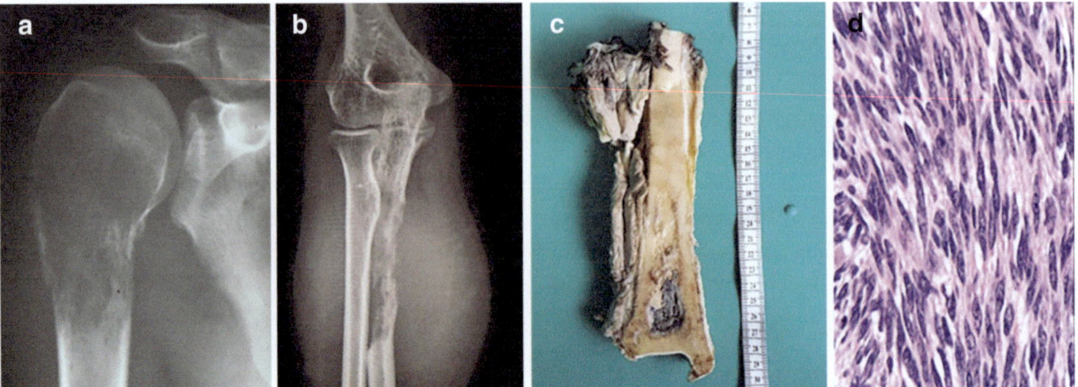

Fig. 6.8 Fibrosarcoma. (**a**) Plain X-ray of humerus with predominant lytic lesion with wide zone of transition indicating malignant nature of lesion. (**b**) Destructive lesion of ulna with involvement of diaphysis, metaphysis and epiphysis with cortical destruction and soft tissue mass. (**c**) Gross specimen showing fleshy growth in the metadiaphyseal region with areas of haemorrhage. (**d**) Spindle cell sarcoma in fascicles, H&E ×250

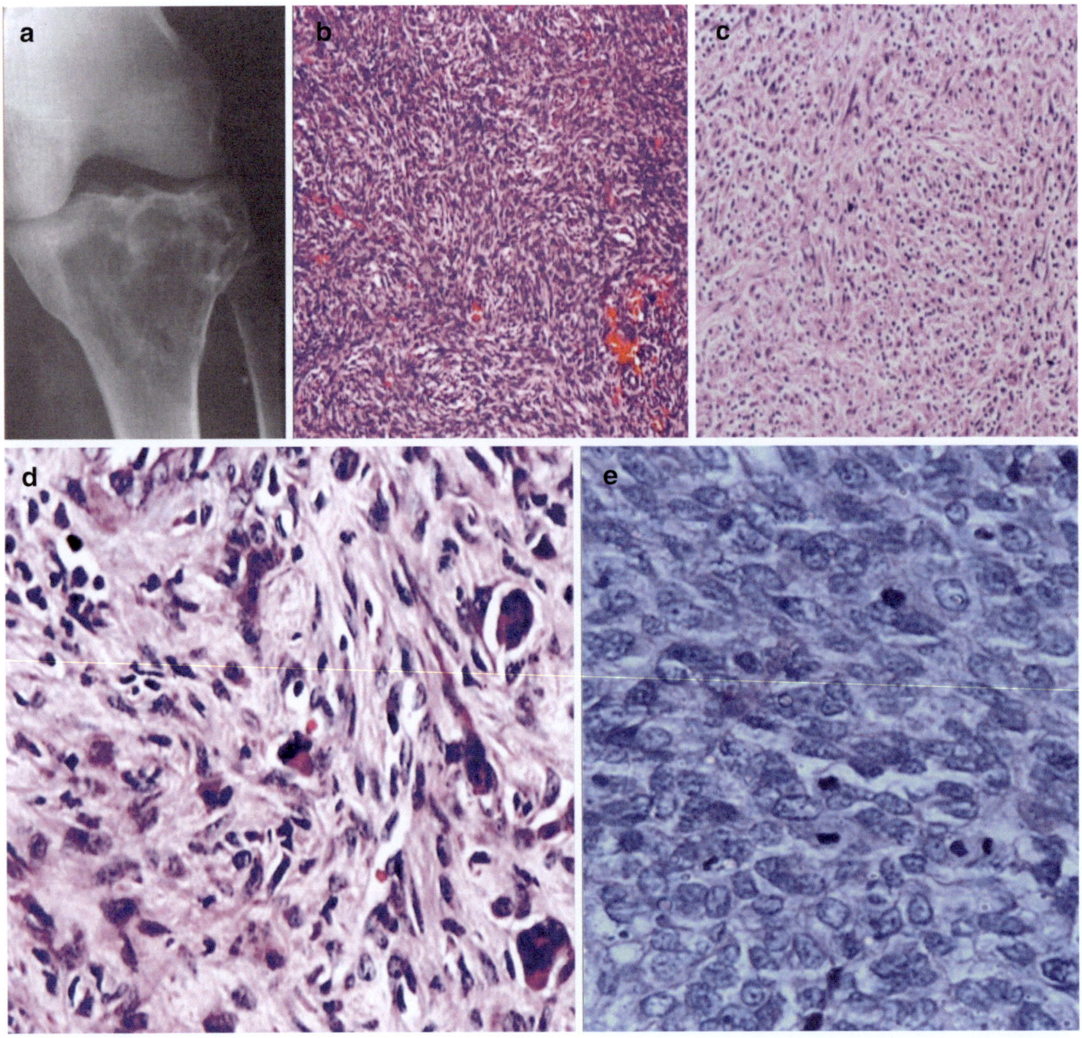

Fig. 6.9 High-grade FS of the upper end of tibia. (**a**) Plain X-ray showing lytic trabeculated lesion involving epiphysis and metaphysis resembling giant cell tumour. (**b**, **c**) Fascicles of spindle cells, H&E ×100. (**d**) High-grade areas with pleomorphism and tumour giant cells, H&E ×250. (**e**) Prominent mitotic activity, H&E ×400

grade tumours, tumour giant cells and prominent mitotic activity are seen. Areas of necrosis and haemorrhage, collagen formation and mitotic activity may be observed. No malignant osteoid will be seen. Low-grade tumours are difficult to differentiate from benign tumours like desmoplastic fibroma. The tumour will show permeation of bony trabeculae.

6.4.1.4 DD

Depending upon the grade of the tumour, DD varies. It includes desmoplastic fibroma, fibroblastic osteosarcoma, dedifferentiated chondrosarcoma [50] and metastatic sarcomatoid carcinoma. Less common are solitary fibrous tumour, leiomyosarcoma and synovial sarcoma. Some spindle cell-rich areas of giant cell tumours are mistaken for fibrosarcoma. Similarly, spindle cell adamantinoma can have fibrosarcoma-like morphology. IHC and radiology correlation will be helpful in these situations.

6.4.1.5 Treatment and Prognosis

Surgical removal is the treatment of choice [56]. Prognosis depends on the grade and stage of the tumour. High histologic grade, >50% necrosis, high mitotic activity (>20/10 HPF) and size of the tumour more than 5 cm are poor prognostic factors. Metastasis occurs to lungs and other bones [58].

6.4.2 Sclerosing Epithelioid Fibrosarcoma of Bone

Sclerosing epithelioid fibrosarcoma (SEF) is a rare and aggressive malignant neoplasm, usually occurring in soft tissue. But rarely it occurs in bone also [39].

6.4.2.1 Clinical

Usually, these tumours occur in adults (mean age 52). Long bones of the extremities are the common sites—femur, ulna and humerus [46]. Rarely is it seen in ribs and vertebrae.

6.4.2.2 Radiology

The tumours are predominantly lytic and poorly marginated.

6.4.2.3 Pathology

They are characterized by round or oval epithelioid cells arranged in linear chords or small nests in a dense collagenous matrix (Fig. 6.10). The tumour cells are small to medium sized with scanty cytoplasm and small nuclei with mild nuclear atypia. They are loosely cohesive epithelioid cells. The tumour shows permeation of pre-existing bony trabeculae [55] and can extend to soft tissue. Occasionally, it can have low-grade fibromyxoid sarcoma-like areas. Focal cartilaginous metaplasia can occur.

6.4.2.4 IHC and Molecular

MUC4 is strongly positive in these tumours [61]. They are usually negative for SATB2, which helps in differentiation from osteosarcoma (SATB2+, MUC4−). FUS and EWSR1 rearrangements by FISH are the molecular test for this entity.

6.4.2.5 Treatment and Prognosis

It is an aggressive neoplasm. Wide excision with/without radiation and/or chemotherapy is given. Some cases require amputation. Recurrences and metastasis to lung, bone and kidney are reported.

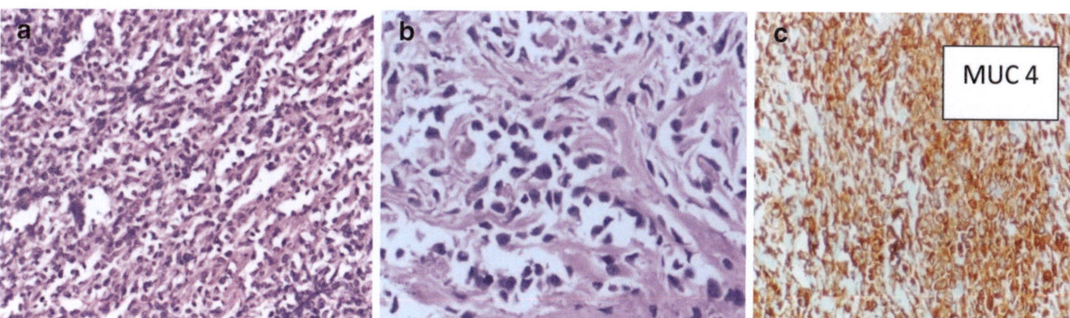

Fig. 6.10 Sclerosing fibrosarcoma. (**a**) Epithelioid cells with dense collagenous matrix, H&E ×100. (**b**) Eosinophilic matrix with epithelioid cells resembling osteoblastic osteosarcoma. (**c**) MUC4 IHC

6.5 Fibrohistiocytic Tumours

In the fifth edition of the WHO classification of soft tissue and bone tumours (2020) [62], the term "benign fibrous histiocytoma of bone" is no longer recommended. In the fourth edition of the WHO, this entity was described as a histiocytic neoplasm with morphology similar to non-ossifying fibroma. Now tumours similar to benign fibrous histiocytoma are considered as either non-ossifying fibroma or histiocytic area of giant cell tumour according to the clinical context.

6.5.1 Malignant

6.5.1.1 Undifferentiated Pleomorphic Sarcoma (UPS)

The undifferentiated pleomorphic sarcoma is a highly malignant tumour of bone without any line of differentiation [58]. This was previously known as malignant fibrous histiocytoma of bone [43]. In the recent WHO, it is a tumour under "other mesenchymal tumours".

Clinical

It occurs at any age or site. It is more common in adult males. The common sites are femur, tibia and humerus. Other rare sites are pelvis and spine. Clinically, they present with pain, swelling or both. Pathological fracture occurs in weight-bearing bones. Secondary UPS occurs in bone infarct, Paget disease or post-irradiation site. It can also occur in sites of implantation and also in diaphyseal medullary stenosis, a rare autosomal dominant disorder.

Radiology

shows lytic destructive lesion with associated soft tissue mass, in the metadiaphyseal region.

Pathology

Grossly, they are fibrous or soft. Extensive sampling to exclude osteosarcoma and dedifferentiated chondrosarcoma is indicated. Histologically, it is a high-grade pleomorphic sarcoma with spindle cells, pleomorphic tumour giant cells and sometimes histiocytes (Fig. 6.11). Brisk mitotic activity with atypical mitosis can be seen. Areas of necrosis may be present.

DD

Dedifferentiated chondrosarcoma and other pleomorphic sarcomas are the differentials of this tumour. IHC may be done to exclude other possibilities like leiomyosarcoma, rhabdomyosarcoma, osteosarcoma and sarcomatoid carcinoma. Absence of IDH1 and IDH2 mutations helps to differentiate from dedifferentiated CS.

Treatment and Prognosis

Surgical resection with chemotherapy similar to osteosarcoma is the line of treatment. Metastasis commonly occurs to lungs. Prognosis is similar to high-grade osteosarcoma or fibrosarcoma. Secondary UPS and metastatic disease carry poor prognosis.

Points to Remember

- Desmoplastic fibroma morphologically resembles fibromatosis of soft tissue.
- Fibrous dysplasia and OFD are considered as tumours and not tumour-like lesions.
- FD can be mono-ostotic or polyostotic.
- OFD is considered as a precursor of adamantinoma of bone.
- FS and undifferentiated sarcoma can resemble GCT of bone radiologically.
- The term benign fibrous histiocytoma of bone is no longer used.

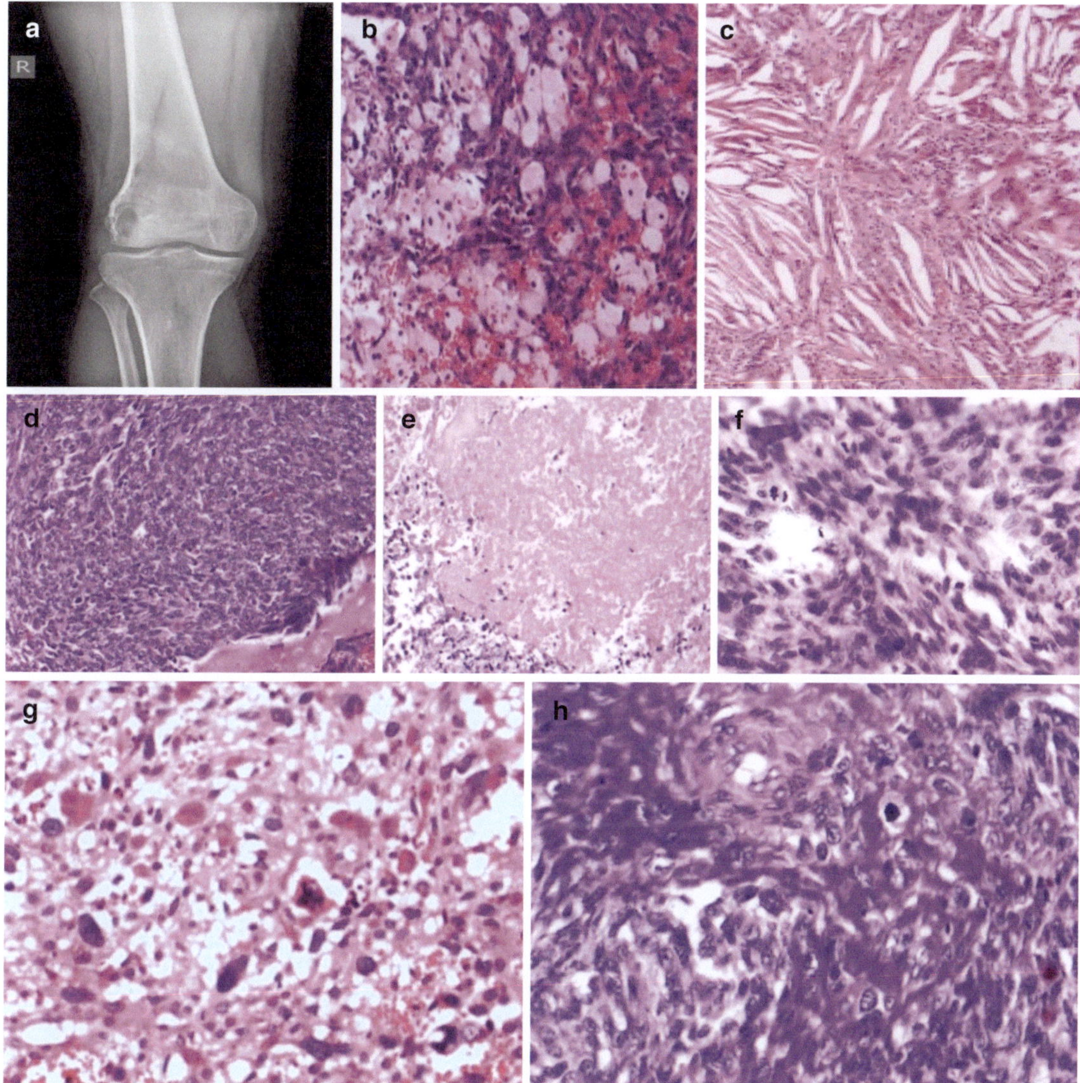

Fig. 6.11 Undifferentiated pleomorphic sarcoma in a 36-year-old male. (**a**) Plain X-ray showing lytic lesion involving epiphysis, diagnosed by radiologist as GCT. (**b**, **c**) Initial biopsy showing foamy macrophages and cholesterol clefts, H&E ×250. (**d**, **e**) Excision biopsy showing areas of necrosis, permeation, H&E ×250. (**f**) Pleomorphic cells, H&E ×250. (**g**) Tumour giant cells, H&E ×100. (**h**) Cellular area with atypical mitosis, H&E ×400. In this case, radiology and needle biopsy were misdiagnosed as giant cell tumour because of epiphyseal location and needle biopsy showing foam cells, cholesterol clefts and giant cells only

References

Desmoplastic Fibroma

1. Kahraman D, Karakoyunlu B, Karagece U, Ertas U, Gunhan O. Desmoplastic fibroma of the jaw bones: a series of twenty-two cases. J Bone Oncol. 2021;26:100333.
2. Frick MA, Sundaram M, Unni KK, Inwards CY, Fabbri N, Trentani F, Baccini P, Bertoni F. Imaging findings in desmoplastic fibroma of bone: distinctive T2 characteristics. AJR Am J Roentgenol. 2005;184(6):1762–7.
3. Talla HV, Alaparthi RK, Yelamanchili S, Naik PR. Desmoplastic fibroma of the mandible: a rare case report. J Indian Acad Oral Med Radiol. 2014;26:222–4.

Fibrous Dysplasia

4. Albright FBA, Hampton AO, Smith P. Syndrome characterized by osteitis fibrosa disseminata, areas of pigmentation and endocrine dysfunction with precocious puberty in females. N Engl J Med. 1937;216:727–46.
5. Brannon RB, Fowler CB. Benign fibro-osseous lesions: a review of current concepts. Adv Anat Pathol. 2001;8:126–43.
6. Dorfman HD. New knowledge of fibro-osseous lesions of bone. Int J Surg Pathol. 2010;18(Suppl 3):S62–5.
7. Eversole R, Su L, ElMofty S. Benign fibro-osseous lesions of the craniofacial complex. A review. Head Neck Pathol. 2008;2:177–202.
8. Tabareau-Delalande F, Collin C, Gomez-Brouchet A, Decouvelaere AV, Bouvier C, Larousserie F, Marie B, Delfour C, Aubert S, Rosset P, de Muret A, Pagès JC, de Pinieux G. Diagnostic value of investigating GNAS mutations in fibro-osseous lesions: a retrospective study of 91 cases of fibrous dysplasia and 40 other fibro-osseous lesions. Mod Pathol. 2013;26:911–21.
9. Franceschina MJ, Hankin RC, Irwin RB. Low-grade central osteosarcoma resembling fibrous dysplasia. A report of two cases. Am J Orthop. 1997;26:432–40.
10. Lee SE, Lee EH, Park H, et al. The diagnostic utility of the GNAS mutation in patients with fibrous dysplasia: meta-analysis of 168 sporadic cases. Hum Pathol. 2012;43:1234–42.
11. Lichtenstein L. Polyostotic fibrous dysplasia. Arch Surg. 1938;36:874–9.
12. Marie P. Cellular and molecular biology of fibrous dysplasia. Ann Pathol. 2001;21:489–98.
13. Muramatsu K, Hashimoto T, Seto S, et al. Low-grade central osteosarcoma mimicking fibrous dysplasia: a report of two cases. Arch Orthop Trauma Surg. 2008;128:11–5.
14. Okamoto S, Hisaoka M, Ushijima M, et al. Activating Gs(alpha) mutation in intramuscular myxomas with and without fibrous dysplasia of bone. Virchows Arch. 2000;437:133–7.
15. Patel MM, Wilkey JF, Abdelsayed R, et al. Analysis of GNAS mutations in cemento-ossifying fibromas and cemento-osseous dysplasias of the jaws. Oral Surg Oral Med Oral Pathol Oral Radiol Endod. 2010;109:739–43.
16. Schwindinger WF, Francomano CA, Levine MA. Identification of a mutation in the gene encoding the alpha subunit of the stimulatory G protein of adenylyl cyclase in McCune-Albright syndrome. Proc Natl Acad Sci U S A. 1992;89:5152–6.
17. Slootweg PJ. Maxillofacial fibro-osseous lesions: classification and differential diagnosis. Semin Diagn Pathol. 1996;13:104–12.
18. Szendroi M, Rahoty P, Antal I, et al. Fibrous dysplasia associated with intramuscular myxoma (Mazabraud's syndrome): a long-term follow-up of three cases. J Cancer Res Clin Oncol. 1998;124:401–6.
19. Toyosawa S, Yuki M, Kishino M, et al. Ossifying fibroma vs fibrous dysplasia of the jaw: molecular and immunological characterization. Mod Pathol. 2007;20:389–96.
20. Weinstein LS. G(s)alpha mutations in fibrous dysplasia and McCune-Albright syndrome. J Bone Miner Res. 2006;21(Suppl 2):S120–4.

Osteo Fibrous Dysplasia

21. Campanacci M, Laus M. Osteofibrous dysplasia of the tibia and fibula. J Bone Joint Surg Am. 1981;63:367–75.
22. Panda P, Gulia A. Osteofibrous dysplasia—an update. J Bone Soft Tissue Tumors. 2016;2(2):23–5.
23. Most MJ, Sim FH, Inwards CY. Osteofibrous dysplasia and adamantinoma. J Am Acad Orthop Surg. 2010;18:358–66.
24. Park YK, Unni KK, McLeod RA, Pritchard DJ. Osteofibrous dysplasia: clinicopathologic study of 80 cases. Hum Pathol. 1993;24(12):1339–47.
25. Gleason BC, Liegl-Atzwanger B, Kozakewich HP, Connolly S, Gebhardt MC, Fletcher JA, Perez-Atayde AR. Osteofibrous dysplasia and adamantinoma in children and adolescents: a clinicopathologic reappraisal. Am J Surg Pathol. 2008;32(3):363–76.
26. Khanna M, Delaney D, Tirabosco R, Saifuddin A. Osteofibrous dysplasia, osteofibrous dysplasia-like adamantinoma and adamantinoma: correlation of radiological imaging features with surgical histology and assessment of the use of radiology in contributing to needle biopsy diagnosis. Skeletal Radiol. 2008;37:1077–84.
27. Fitzpatrick KA, Taljanovic MS, Speer DP, Graham AR, Jacobson JA, Barnes GR, Hunter TB. Imaging findings of fibrous dysplasia with histopathologic and intraoperative correlation. AJR Am J Roentgenol. 2004;182(6):1389–98.
28. Kahn L. Adamantinoma, osteofibrous dysplasia and differentiated adamantinoma. Skeletal Radiol. 2003;32:245–58.

Myofibroma

29. Thennavan A, Narayanaswamy V, Niazi TM, Rao L, Radhakrishnan R. Infantile myofibroma eroding into the frontal bone: a case report and review of its histopathologic differential diagnosis case reports in pediatrics. Case Rep Pediatr. 2012;2012:630804. https://doi.org/10.1155/2012/630804.

30. Chung B, Enzinger FM. Infantile myofibromatosis. Cancer. 1981;48(8):1807–18.
31. Montgomery E, Speight PM, Fisher C. Myofibromas presenting in the oral cavity: a series of 9 cases. Oral Surg Oral Med Oral Pathol Oral Radiol Endod. 2000;89(3):343–8.
32. Beck JC, Devancy KO, Weatherly RA, Koopmann CF, Lesperance MM. Pediatric myofibromatosis of the head and neck. Arch Otolaryngol. 1999;125(1):39–44.
33. Koujok K, Ruiz RE, Hernandez RJ. Myofibromatosis: imaging characteristics. Pediatr Radiol. 2005;35(4):374–80.
34. Mynatt CJ, Feldman KA, Thompson LD. Orbital infantile myofibroma: a case report and clinicopathologic review of 24 cases from the literature. Head Neck Pathol. 2011;5(3):205–15.
35. Tsuji M, Inagaki T, Kasai H, Yamanouchi Y, Kawamoto K, Uemura Y. Solitary myofibromatosis of the skull: a case report and review of literature. Childs Nerv Syst. 2004;20(5):366–9.
36. Sedghizadeh PP, Allen CM, Kalmar JR, Miloro M, Suster S. Solitary central myofibroma presenting in the gnathic region. Ann Diagn Pathol. 2004;8(5):284–9.
37. Foss RD, Ellis GL. Myofibromas and myofibromatosis of the oral region: a clinicopathologic analysis of 79 cases. Oral Surg Oral Med Oral Pathol Oral Radiol Endod. 2000;89(1):57–65.
38. Kaplan SS, Ojemann JG, Grange DK, Fuller C, Park TS. Intracranial infantile myofibromatosis with intraparenchymal involvement. Pediatr Neurosurg. 2002;36(4):214–7.

Fibrosarcoma and Undifferentiated Sarcoma

39. Abdulkader I, et al. Sclerosing epithelioid fibrosarcoma primary of the bone. Int J Surg Pathol. 2002;10(3):227–30.
40. Angiero F, Rizzuti T, Crippa R, Stefani M. Fibrosarcoma of the jaws: two cases of primary tumors with intraosseous growth. Anticancer Res. 2007;27:2573–81.
41. Augsburger D, Nelson PJ, Kalinski T, Udelnow A, Knösel T, Hofstetter M, Qin JW, Wang Y, Gupta AS, Bonifatius S, Li M, Bruns CJ, Zhao Y. Current diagnostics and treatment of fibrosarcoma—perspectives for future therapeutic targets and strategies. Oncotarget. 2017;8(61):104638–53.
42. Bertoni F, et al. Primary central (medullary) fibrosarcoma of bone. Semin Diagn Pathol. 1984;1(3):185–98.
43. Bielack SS, et al. Malignant fibrous histiocytoma of bone: a retrospective EMSOS study of 125 cases. European Musculo-Skeletal Oncology Society. Acta Orthop Scand. 1999;70(4):353–60.
44. Choi JH, et al. Fibrosarcoma in bizarre parosteal osteochondromatous proliferation. Skeletal Radiol. 2001;30(1):44–7.
45. Dahlin DC, Ivins JC. Fibrosarcoma of bone. A study of 114 cases. Cancer. 1969;23(1):35–41.
46. Doyle LA, Wang WL, Dal Cin P, Lopez-Terrada D, Mertens F, Lazar AJ, Fletcher CD, Hornick JL. MUC4 is a sensitive and extremely useful marker for sclerosing epithelioid fibrosarcoma: association with FUS gene rearrangement. Am J Surg Pathol. 2012;36(10):1444–51.
47. Eyre-Brook AL, Price CH. Fibrosarcoma of bone. Review of fifty consecutive cases from the Bristol Bone Tumour Registry. J Bone Joint Surg Br. 1969;51(1):20–37.
48. Faure C, Gruner M, Boccon-Gibod L. Case report 149. Infantile congenital fibrosarcoma of humerus. Skeletal Radiol. 1981;6(3):208–11.
49. Folpe AL. Fibrosarcoma: a review and update. Histopathology. 2014;64:12–25.
50. Frassica FJ, Unni KK, Sim FH. Case report 347. Dedifferentiated chondrosarcoma: grade 4 fibrosarcoma arising in grade 1 chondrosarcoma (femur). Skeletal Radiol. 1986;15(1):77–81.
51. Gaetani S, et al. Multiple diffuse fibrosarcoma of bone. Rays. 1985;10(3):13–7.
52. Greditzer HG 3rd, et al. Bone sarcomas in Paget disease. Radiology. 1983;146(2):327–33.
53. Hinarejos P, et al. Fibrosarcoma at the site of a metallic fixation of the tibia—a case report and literature review. Acta Orthop Scand. 2000;71(3):329–32.
54. Kabukcuoglu Y, et al. Multiple diffuse fibrosarcoma of bone. Am J Orthop. 1999;28(12):715–7.
55. Kosemehmetoglu K, Ardic F, Kilpatrick SE, Aydingoz U, Sumathi VP, Michal M. Sclerosing epithelioid fibrosarcoma of bone: morphological, immunophenotypical, and molecular findings of 9 cases. Virchows Arch. 2021;478(4):767–77.
56. Nooij MA, Whelan J, Bramwell VH, Taminiau AT, Cannon S, Hogendoorn PC, Pringle J, Uscinska BM, Weeden S, Kirkpatrick A, Glabbeke M, Craft AW, European Osteosarcoma Intergroup. Doxorubicin and cisplatin chemotherapy in high-grade spindle cell sarcomas of the bone, other than osteosarcoma or malignant fibrous histiocytoma: a European Osteosarcoma Intergroup Study. Eur J Cancer. 2005;41(2):225–30.
57. Nooij MA, Whelan J, Bramwell VH, et al. Doxorubicin and cisplatin chemotherapy in high-grade spindle cell sarcomas of the bone, other than osteosarcoma or malignant fibrous histiocytoma: a European Osteosarcoma Intergroup Study. Eur J Cancer. 2005;41(2):225–30.
58. Papagelopoulos PJ, et al Primary fibrosarcoma of bone. Outcome after primary surgical treatment. Clin Orthop Relat Res. 2000;(373):88–103.

59. Pereira CM, et al. Primary intraosseous fibrosarcoma of jaw. Int J Oral Maxillofac Surg. 2005;34(5):579–81.
60. Taconis WK, van Rijssel TG. Fibrosarcoma of long bones. A study of the significance of areas of malignant fibrous histiocytoma. J Bone Joint Surg Br. 1985;67(1):111–6.
61. Wojcik JB, Bellizzi AM, Dal Cin P, Bredella MA, Fletcher CD, Hornicek FJ, Deshpande V, Hornick JL, Nielsen GP. Primary sclerosing epithelioid fibrosarcoma of bone: analysis of a series. Am J Surg Pathol. 2014;38(11):1538–44.
62. WHO Classification of Tumours. In: WHO Classification of Tumours Editorial Board, editor. Soft tissue and bone tumours. WHO classification of tumours, 5th ed. vol. 3. IARC; 2020.
63. Yabut SM Jr, et al. Malignant transformation of fibrous dysplasia. A case report and review of the literature. Clin Orthop Relat Res. 1988;(228):281–289.

7 Giant Cell-Rich Tumours

Osteoclastic giant cells (OCGCs) can be seen in a variety of lesions—both skeletal and extraskeletal. Any lytic area of bone can show OCGCs. The function of OCGC is resorption of bone. Many tumours and lesions of bone show osteoclastic giant cells. The common giant cell-rich tumours include benign and malignant tumours, reactive conditions like brown tumour of hyperparathyroidism, etc. A list of common lesions is given below.

7.1 Classification of Osteoclastic Giant Cell-Rich tumours [60]

- **Benign**
  - Aneurysmal bone cyst (ABC)
  - Non-ossifying fibroma (NOF)
- **Intermediate (locally aggressive; rarely metastasizing)**
  - Giant cell tumour of bone NOS
- **Malignant**
  - Giant cell tumour of bone, malignant
- **Other giant cell-rich lesions of bone**
  - Chondroblastoma
  - Giant cell-rich osteosarcomas
  - Giant cell reparative granuloma (GCRG)
  - Giant cell tumour of tendon sheath
  - Brown tumours of hyperparathyroidism
  - Others—osteoblastoma, clear cell chondrosarcoma, metastatic carcinoma

In this chapter, aneurysmal bone cyst, giant cell tumour of bone, malignant giant cell tumour of bone, non-ossifying fibroma and giant cell reparative granuloma are discussed.

7.2 Aneurysmal Bone Cyst (ABC)

Jaffe and Lichtenstein first described ABC as a separate entity in 1942 [7]. The aneurysmal bone cyst (ABC) was thought to be a benign tumour-like lesion. But after detection of USP6 gene arrangement in ABC, this entity is considered as a benign neoplasm.

ABC can be primary or secondary. Secondary ABC terminology is not used now. Instead, ABC-like area is preferred [60]. Here, we describe primary ABC in this chapter.

7.2.1 Clinical

Although benign in nature, they are locally destructive and may mimic malignancy clinically and radiologically. It is more common in children and young adults (first two decades of life). Females are more affected than males. Any bone can be affected. Humerus, distal femur and proximal tibia are the common sites [10]. It is also common in the posterior elements of the vertebra [14]. Pain, swelling and deformity are the common complaints. Pathologic fracture can occur. In certain sites, it can cause pressure symptoms. Rapid growth raises the suspicion of malignancy. Rarely, ABC occurs in soft tissue [11].

J. Kattoor et al., *Bone Tumors*, https://doi.org/10.1007/978-981-99-4738-6_7

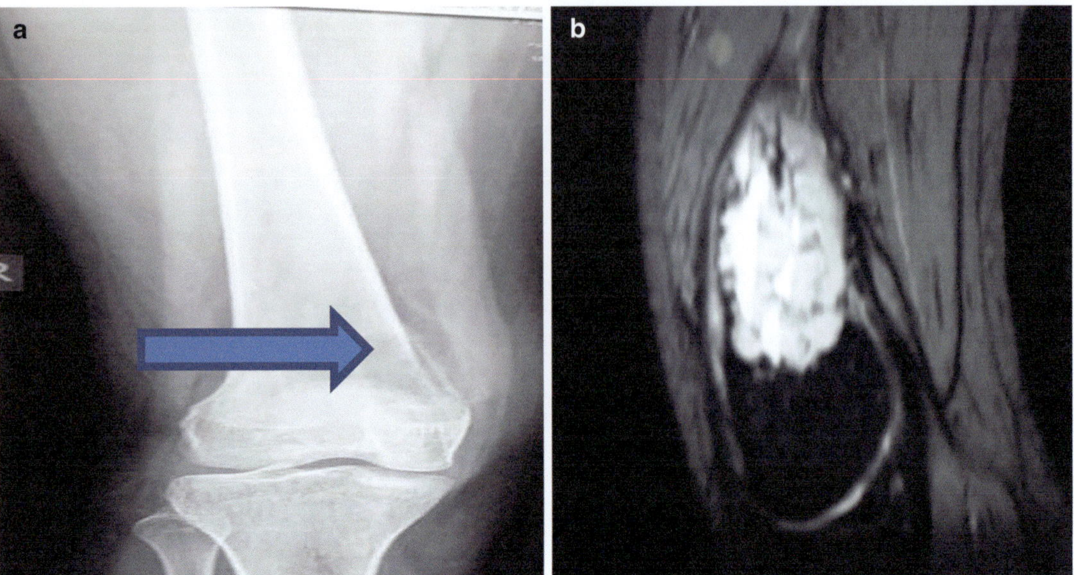

Fig. 7.1 (**a**) Plain X-ray of ABC: Eccentric lytic area metaphysis of femur. (**b**) MRI showing fluid-fluid level in ABC

7.2.2 Radiology

In long bones, it occurs in the metaphysis [15]. They are seen as eccentric and expansile cysts. The lesion may bulge into the soft tissue with a thin rim of bone at the periphery. The CT scan and MRI will show fluid-fluid levels (Fig. 7.1). Rarely, ABCs have also been known to affect an adjacent bone, especially spinal ABCs. In the flat bones, pelvis is the most common site (50%).

7.2.3 Pathology

Gross: Curetted specimen will be red and granular. If the lesion is received intact, cystic spaces separated by fibrous septa and filled with blood may be seen. Cut section will be spongy and will have a honeycomb appearance (Fig. 7.2). Sometimes, solid areas are seen. Care must be taken while grossing not to miss a solid area, which may be the primary tumour in cases of secondary ABC.

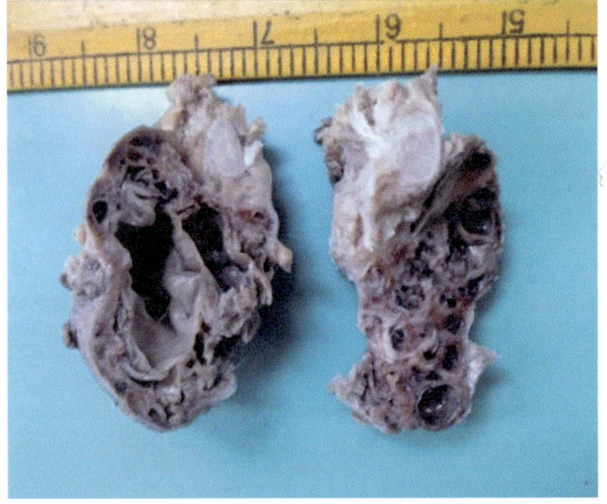

Fig. 7.2 Gross picture of ABC—multilocular cystic mass filled with blood

Microscopy shows multiple cystic spaces filled with blood. Cyst wall will show haphazardly arranged osteoclastic giant cells, fibroblastic proliferation with reactive osteoid [17] (Figs. 7.3 and 7.4) and chunky calcification [18] (Figs. 7.5, 7.6, and 7.7). The calcified material will be parallelly arranged along the cyst wall. Woven bone present shows basophilic colour and is called as blue bone. Sometimes, the mineralisation has a chondroid aura, which is seen only in ABC. Brisk mitotic activity can be seen in the spindle cells. But cytological atypia and atypical mitosis will be absent.

In **solid ABC**, cyst formation is not seen [2]. Solid proliferation of spindle elongated cells with mitosis and plenty of reactive osteoid will be present. This can be mistaken for low-grade osteosarcoma [16] (Fig. 7.8). Solid ABC seen in the small bones of hand and feet

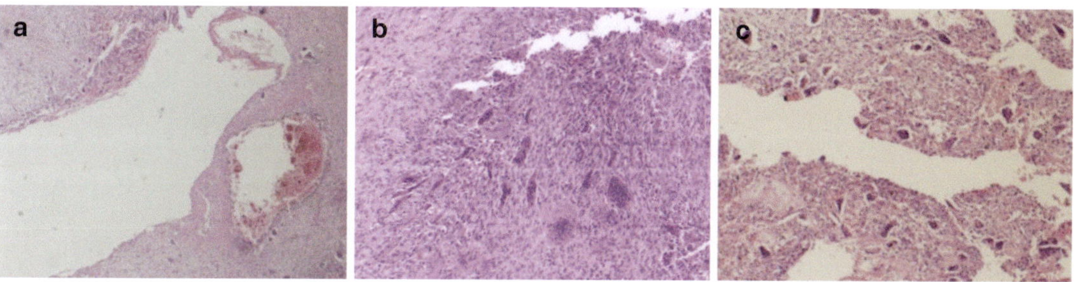

Fig. 7.3 ABC. (**a**) Cystic spaces filled with blood, H&E ×40. (**b** and **c**) Cyst wall with haphazardly arranged giant cells, elongated fibroblasts and reactive osteoid, H&E ×100

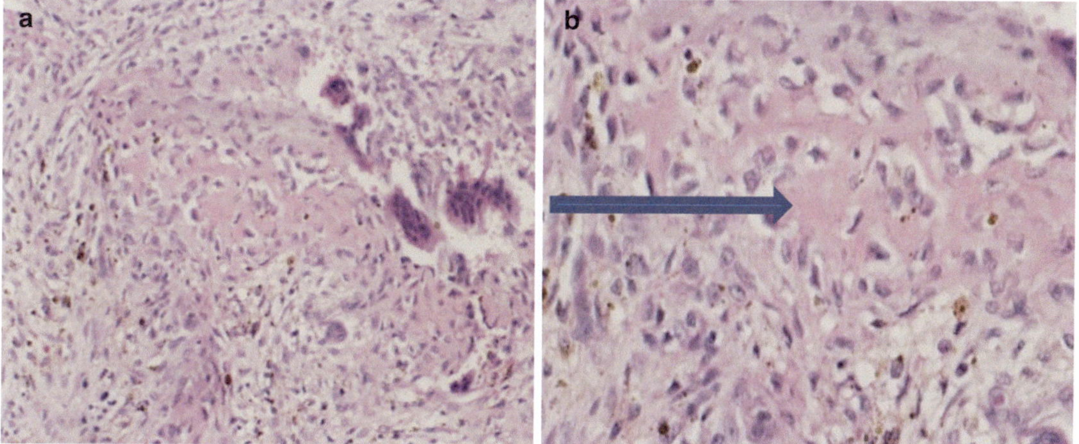

Fig. 7.4 ABC: (**a**) Reactive osteoid in the wall of ABC, H&E ×100. (**b**) Reactive osteoid, H&E ×250 (arrow)

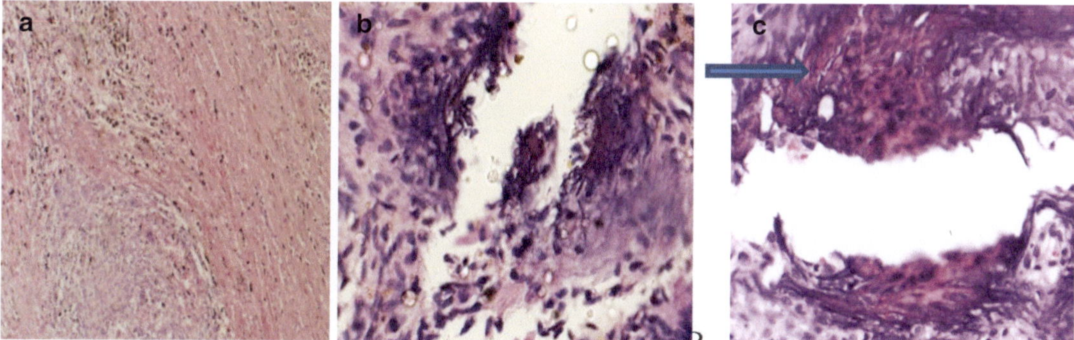

Fig. 7.5 ABC: (**a**) Haemosiderin-laden macrophages, H&E ×100. (**b** and **c**) Linear chunky calcification parallel to cyst wall (blue arrow), H&E ×400

was earlier called as giant cell reparative granuloma [6].

ABC-like areas can be seen in many tumours. These lesions were called **secondary ABC.** But this terminology is no longer used. This is much more common than primary ABC. Giant cell tumour, chondroblastoma, osteoblastoma, fibrous dysplasia, chondromyxoid fibroma and osteosarcomas are the common bone tumours, which show aneurysmal bone cyst like changes. Hence, ruling out other primary bone lesions before signing out as primary ABC is very important [3].

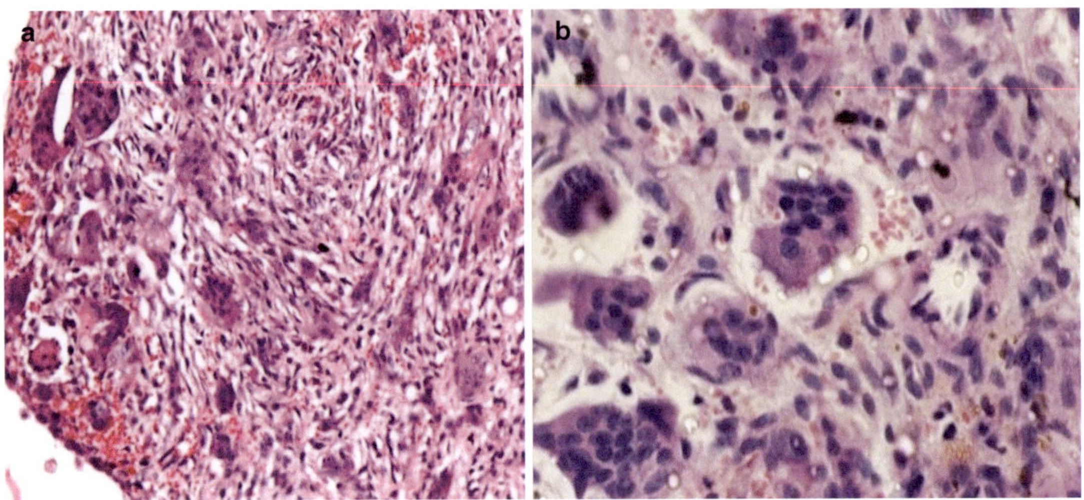

Fig. 7.6 ABC: (**a**) Osteoclastic giant cells in clusters, H&E ×100. (**b**) Cluster of giant cells, H&E ×250

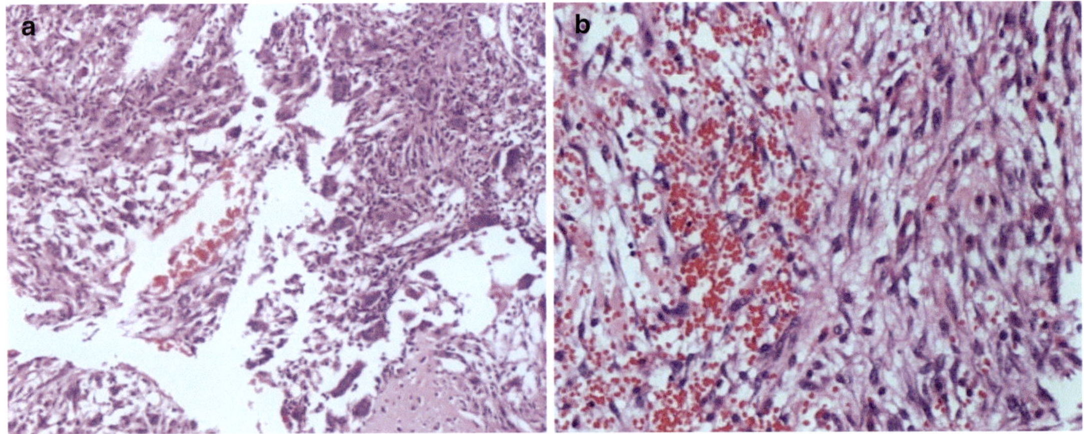

Fig. 7.7 ABC: Extravasated RBCs. (**a**) H&E ×100. (**b**) H&E ×250

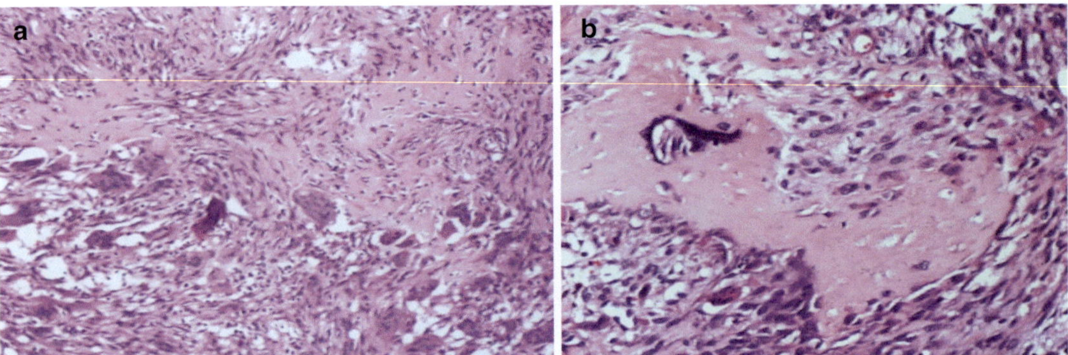

Fig. 7.8 Solid ABC: (**a**) Haphazardly arranged osteoclastic giant cells and fibroblastic stroma, H&E ×100. (**b**) Solid ABC with lots of reactive calcifying osteoid will be mistaken for osteosarcoma, H&E ×250

Table 7.1 Differentiation of ABC, GCT and telangiectatic osteosarcoma

	ABC	GCT	Telangiectatic OS
Age	<20	20–40	<20
Location in bone	Metaphysis	Epiphysis	Metaphysis
Osteoclastic giant cells (OCGCs)	Haphazard	Regular	Scattered
Stromal cells	Elongated fibroblasts	Short spindle or oval similar to nuclei in OCGC	Pleomorphic hyperchromatic
Osteoid	Reactive in between stromal cells	Reactive at the periphery	Malignant osteoid +/–
Calcification	Chunky, parallel to cyst wall	Unusual	Calcifying tumour osteoid may or may not be present
Degenerative changes	Absent	Present—cholesterol clefts, foamy macrophages	Haemorrhage and necrosis
Molecular	USP6 rearrangement	H3F3Ap.Gly34 mutations	Complex structural and numerical chromosome alterations

Abbreviations: *ABC* aneurysmal bone cyst, *GCT* giant cell tumour; OS osteosarcoma

7.2.4 Molecular studies

Molecular studies have shown a specific translocation t (16; 17) (q22; p13) in primary ABC and not in ABC-like areas of other tumours [1, 5]. The primary ABC is considered now as a neoplasm because most of the primary ABC has USP6 or CDH11 rearrangements [13].

7.2.5 DD

The differential diagnosis of ABC includes giant cell tumour, telangiectatic osteosarcoma and low-grade osteosarcoma [16]. Giant cell tumour is a disease involving epiphysis in skeletally mature individuals (usual age group of 20–40 years), with uniform arrangement of osteoclastic giant cells and stromal cells of histiocytic origin [9]. Degenerative changes are common (Table 7.1).

Telangiectatic osteosarcoma resembles ABC clinically, radiologically and morphologically. One has to look into the septa of cyst walls, which will show frank high-grade malignant cells with atypical mitosis with or without osteoid. Large cavernous and necrotic areas may mask the stromal cells. Deeper sections may reveal the malignant stromal cells. If there is clinical suspicion, a second biopsy may be helpful if sufficient solid tissue is absent in the first biopsy.

Low-grade osteosarcoma is less cellular, and one has to search for cytological atypia. In these cases, permeation of the spindle cells between bony spicules will be a helpful feature to distinguish it as osteosarcoma. IHC positivity for MDM2 or MDM2 amplification by FISH is helpful in confirming these cases as low-grade osteosarcoma.

7.2.6 Treatment and Prognosis

Aneurysmal bone cysts (ABCs) are treated surgically [4]. Small asymptomatic ABCs are kept under follow up as some of them resolve spontaneously. If the size is increasing, it has to be treated. Other treatments include selective arterial embolization and intralesional injection of methylprednisolone or calcitonin.
Recurrence usually happens within the first year after surgery. Patients are kept under regular follow up for 5 years. If any patient has received radiation, that person should be followed up for a long time as there are chances of developing post-radiation sarcoma [8].

7.3 Non-ossifying Fibroma (NOF) [63–67]

Non-ossifying fibroma is the commonest benign tumour of bone. It is also known as metaphyseal fibrous defect or fibrous cortical defect [64, 67]. It occurs due to a developmental defect [66]. The normal ossifying areas are filled with fibrous tissue.

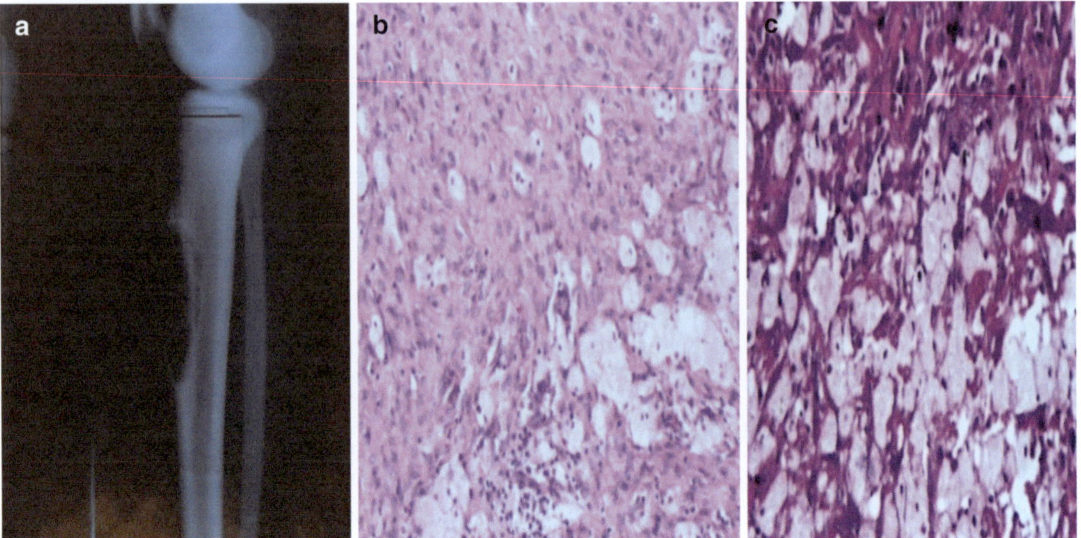

Fig. 7.9 NOF: (**a**) Plain X-ray showing eccentric metadiaphyseal lytic lesion with sclerotic border and narrow zone of transition. (**b**) Foamy macrophages and fibrous stroma, H&E ×100. (**c**) Osteoclastic giant cells and foamy macrophages, H&E ×250

Spontaneous regression of these lesions can occur. Hence, they are considered as faulty ossification.

7.3.1 Clinical

They are asymptomatic and may present with pathological fracture. Young boys are commonly affected. If a boy below 10 years present with a pathological fracture [63], most likely diagnosis is NOF.

7.3.2 Radiology

It occurs in young boys as an incidental radiographic finding. The most common site is the distal femur. Other common sites are the distal tibia, proximal tibia and fibula (Fig. 7.9a). Rarely it is reported in clavicle and ribs. Some patients have multiple lesions of same bone or polyostotic involvement. These patients should be investigated for Jaffe-Campanacci syndrome. Skin pigmentation and soft tissue haemangiomas are described in these cases.

On plain X-ray, they appear as eccentric, expansile lytic defect in the metaphyseal region. The zone of transition is narrow, and the outer margins are scalloped with a sclerotic border. On plain X-ray, the differential diagnoses are chondromyxoid fibroma, ABC and fibrous dysplasia.

7.3.3 Pathology

These lesions show loosely arranged spindle cells with storiform pattern. The cells are plump, with vesicular nuclei. Mitotic figures may or may not be present. Haemosiderin-laden macrophages, foamy histiocytes and osteoclastic giant cells in variable numbers are seen admixed with spindle cells (Fig. 7.9b, c). Giant cells are usually seen in clusters. Reactive osteoid and infarct-like necrosis may be present if there is a pathological fracture.

7.3.4 Molecular

KRAS and FGFR1 mutations are reported.

7.3.5 Differential diagnosis

The differential diagnosis [65] of non-ossifying fibroma includes the following:

- Benign fibrous histiocytoma: Clinical and radiological findings will help in the differentiation. The term BFH of bone is no longer used.
- Fibrohistiocytic area of GCT: GCT occurs in skeletally mature patients, and it extends to the articular surface of bone. Careful search will reveal areas typical of GCT with uniformly distributed giant cells.

7.3.6 Treatment

No treatment is given for small, asymptomatic non-ossifying fibromas that are discovered incidentally. Curettage and bone grafting are done in cases of pathological fracture or if >50% of diameter of bone is involved.

7.3.7 Prognosis

The prognosis for NOF is excellent. The risk of recurrence is low. Malignant transformation is not reported.

7.4 Jaffe-Campanacci Syndrome

In 1958, Jaffe described Jaffe-Campanacci syndrome [67]. It is a rare condition with multifocal non-ossifying fibromas, cafe au lait spots and axillary freckling. Other findings are mental retardation, hypogonadism or cryptorchidism, ocular abnormality and cardiovascular malformations. The two prominent features of Jaffe-Campanacci syndrome are multiple cafe au lait spots and multiple non-ossifying fibromas.

7.5 Giant Cell Reparative Granuloma (GCRG)

The term giant cell reparative granuloma is not recommended as per new WHO 2020 [60]. It is synonymous with solid ABC in the small bones of hands and feet. But some people use this terminology in gnathic bones [6, 12, 35].

GCRG was considered as a reactive process seen in the small bones of hands and feet and jawbones [41, 49]. Jaffe first described this term in 1953 [7]. It was described as a reaction to haemorrhage. In this, there is haemorrhagic cyst formation similar to aneurysmal bone cyst. It occurs in young adults in the second or third decade. The bone is expanded and lytic. The cortex may be thinned, and it can extend to the soft tissue.

7.5.1 Histology

Morphologically, GCRG consists of giant cells arranged in clusters in a spindle cell stroma. Spindle cells are fibrogenic in nature. Collagen and reactive osteoid with osteoblastic rimming can be seen (Fig. 7.10). In the jawbones, true giant cell tumours are rare except those arising in Paget disease. The differential diagnosis is brown tumour of hyperparathyroidism.

7.5.2 DD

It is difficult to differentiate GCRG from GCT [38]. In GCT, giant cells are uniformly distributed, and the stromal cells resemble nuclei of giant cells. Reactive osteoid and fibroblastic stromal cells with collagen are features in GCRG.

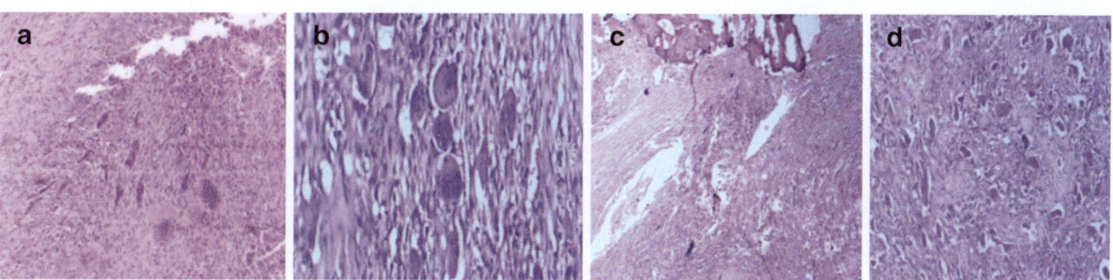

Fig. 7.10 GCRG (solid ABC): (**a**) Cluster of giant cells, H&E ×100. (**b**) H&E ×250. (**c**) Cyst formation and collagen, H&E ×100. (**d**) Reactive osteoid, H&E ×100

7.5.3 Molecular

H3.3pGly34Trp is negative in this condition, thus helping to distinguish from GCT. USP6 gene rearrangement is present in the giant cell-rich lesions of small bones of hands and feet [62] and hence they are grouped under solid ABC. But this gene rearrangement is absent in gnathic tumours and in GCT of bone.

7.5.4 Treatment

It is excision, and recurrence is rare. Complete removal results in cure.

7.6 Giant Cell Tumour of Bone (GCTB)

GCTB is a locally aggressive, rarely metastasizing intermediate-grade tumour of bone. It is composed of mononuclear stromal cells and multinucleated osteoclastic giant cells (OCGCs) [27]. The OCGCs are thought to be of histiocytic in origin. GCT accounts for 20% of benign skeletal tumours. In southern India and China, there is a high incidence of GCTB (20% of all primary bone tumours) with a slight female predominance. GCTBs mostly occur in skeletally mature individuals after closure of epiphyseal plate (80%). Peak age group is between 20 and 40 years. The common locations are at the ends of long bones [29]. Lower end of femur and upper end of tibia are the common sites involved (around 50%). The next common sites are distal end of radius, ribs and sacrum. In the vertebra, it involves the body of vertebrae. The small bones of hands and feet are rarely involved [25]. When it occurs in rare sites, other possibilities like hyperparathyroidism should be ruled out. Ilium is the most common site if pelvic bones are affected. Other rare sites are patella, sternum and hyoid bone. Giant cell-rich lesions of jawbones are usually giant cell reparative granulomas. GCTB can occur in patients with Paget disease [32].

Multicentric GCTBs are described [23, 45, 58]. This usually involves small bones of hands and feet, and they are aggressive in nature [58].

7.6.1 Clinical

Pain of variable severity and swelling are common symptoms. Rarely, patients present with pathological fracture.

7.6.2 Radiology

The lesions are lytic involving the epiphysis and extending to articular cartilage, often leaving a thin rim between tumour and cartilage [44]. There will be trabeculations giving soap bubble appearance (Fig. 7.11). Lesions can be well

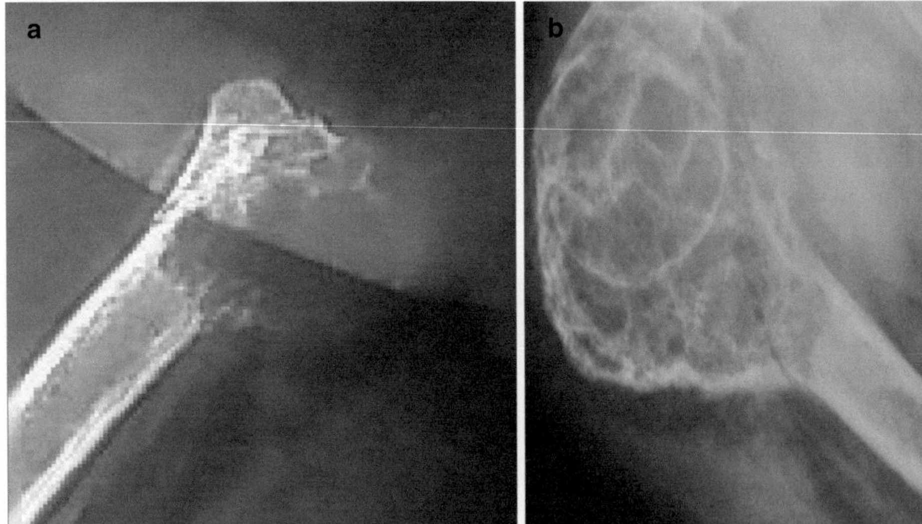

Fig. 7.11 GCT: (**a**) Plain X-ray showing epiphyseal involvement with trabeculations. (**b**) Soap bubble appearance

Table 7.2 Pathogenesis of bone resorption

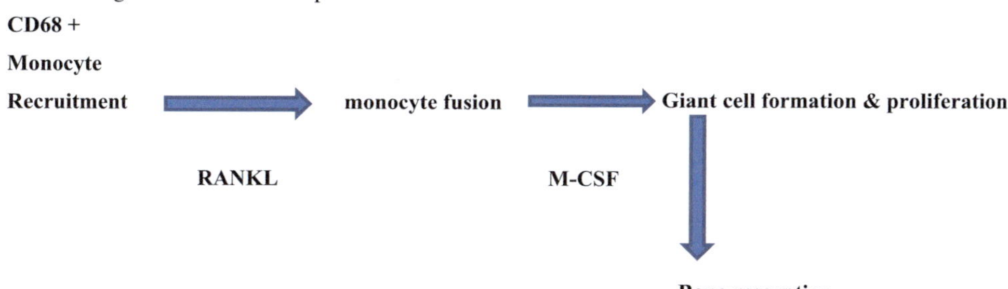

defined or poorly defined. It can extend to soft tissue by destroying the cortex. Some tumours destroy articular cartilage and extend to the joint cavity. Periosteal reaction is rare. Giant cell tumours do not produce sclerosis, but they produce a peripheral shell of ossification. Other tumours producing radiographic appearance of GCTB are fibrosarcoma, Rosai-Dorfman disease of bone, haemangioendothelioma of bone, etc. Rarely, GCTBs can occur in metaphysis, and then care should be taken to rule out more common giant cell-rich lesions in the metaphysis like aneurysmal bone cyst and osteosarcoma [39, 53]. If there are ABC like areas, CT scan can show fluid-fluid levels.

Based on radiographic appearance, Enneking and later Campanacci classified GCTBs into three stages. They are latent, active and aggressive stages, respectively.

7.6.3 Pathogenesis

Molecular studies have shown that the neoplastic mononuclear stromal cells express receptor activator of nuclear factor kappa B (RANK) ligand (RANKL). In the genesis of osteoclasts, the RANK-RANKL interaction along with the macrophage colony-stimulating factor (M-CSF) plays an important role [54]. The osteoclastic cells are recruited from blood-borne mononuclear osteoclast precursor cells (Table 7.2). Cytogenetically, telomeric associations and chromosomal end-to-end fusion are commonly seen in GCTB. In the pathogenesis of GCT, maintenance of telomere length plays an important role.

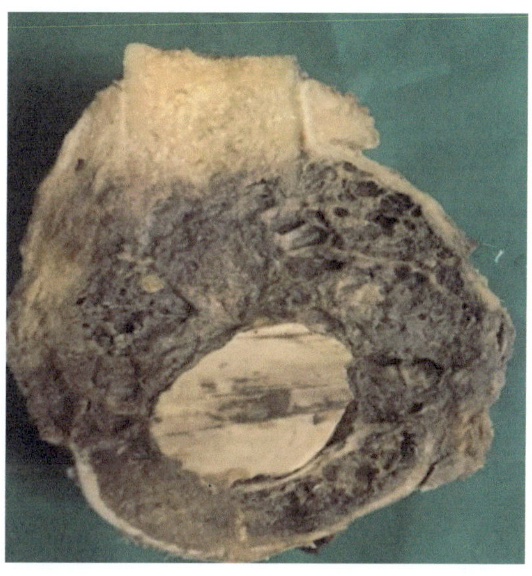

Fig. 7.12 Gross picture of giant cell tumour with ABC like changes—lower end of femur

Recently, H3F3A driver mutation has been identified in 95% of GCT of bone cases [36, 59].

7.6.4 Pathology

Gross: Specimen by curettage is soft, fleshy and brown. If a resected specimen is obtained, the tumour cut surface is chocolate brown with small cysts [20]. Sometimes, the tumour is white and fleshy simulating sarcoma. Yellow discolouration corresponding to collections of foam cells may be seen (Fig. 7.12).

Histopathology: The proliferating cells are oval to spindle with vesicular nuclei. These cells fuse to form giant cells. These osteoclastic giant

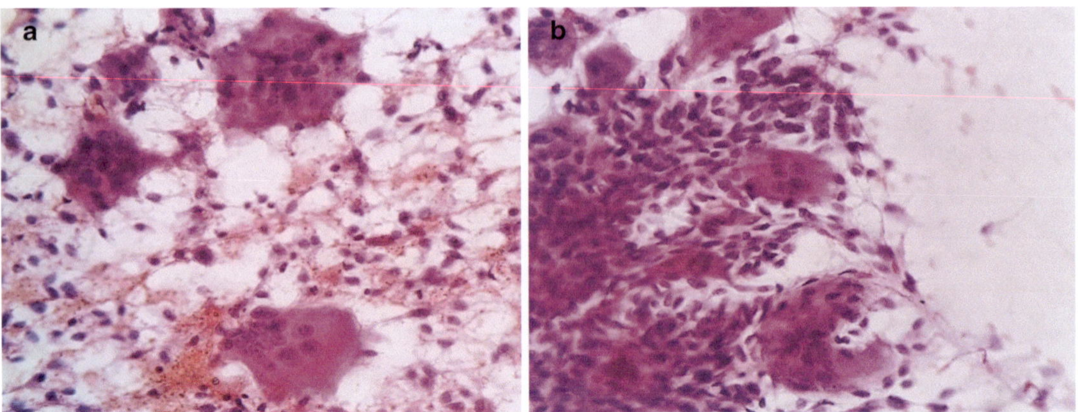

Fig. 7.13 FNAC of giant cell tumour. (**a** and **b**) Osteoclastic giant cells and stromal cells, Pap ×250

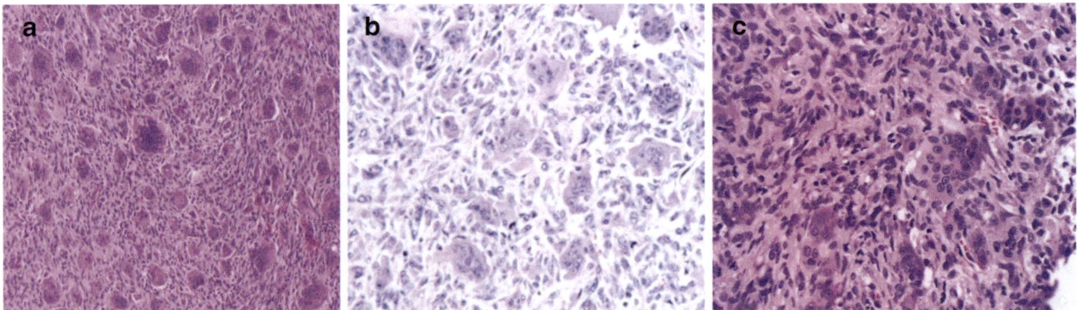

Fig. 7.14 Typical GCT: (**a**) Uniformly distributed giant cells in a spindle cell stroma, H&E ×100. (**b** and **c**) Osteoclastic giant cells with stromal cells, H&E ×250

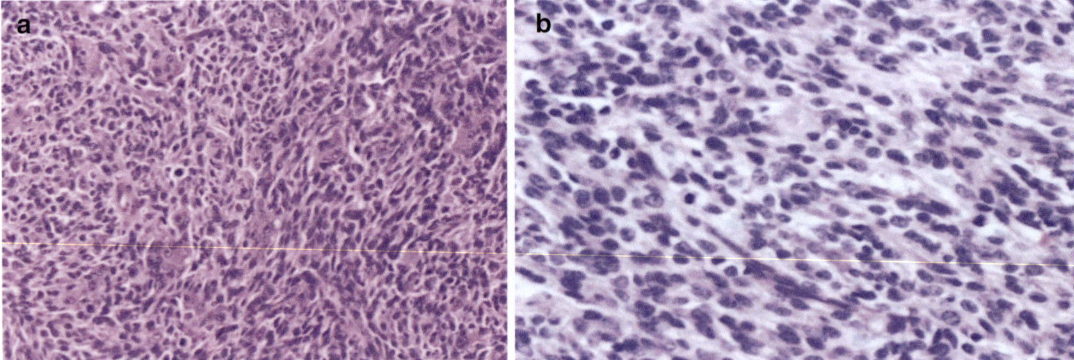

Fig. 7.15 GCT: (**a**) Giant cell-poor area resembling fibrosarcoma, H&E ×100. (**b**) H&E ×250

cells are uniformly distributed. The nuclei of giant cells and stromal cells are similar (Figs. 7.13 and 7.14). Moderate atypia may be noted in some cases. This should not be mistaken for malignancy. Brisk mitotic activity may be noted in areas. But atypical mitosis is not seen.

Many histological variations may be seen [57]. The spindle cell proliferation adjacent to this necrotic area should not be mistaken for sarcoma (Fig. 7.15). An area of necrosis/infarction without adjacent inflammatory cell reaction is frequently seen. Necrotic area usually shows

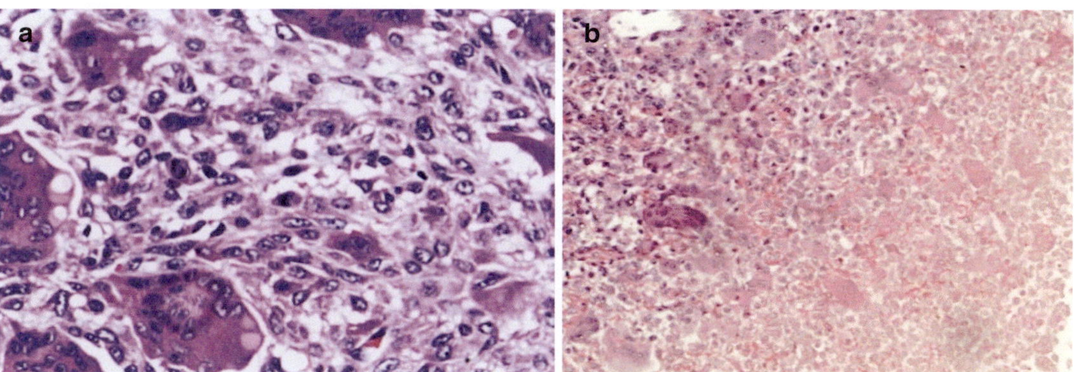

Fig. 7.16 GCT: (**a**) Nuclei of giant cells and stromal cells are similar, H&E ×250. (**b**) Infarction/necrosis: Ghost cell outlines of giant cells and stromal cells, H&E ×100

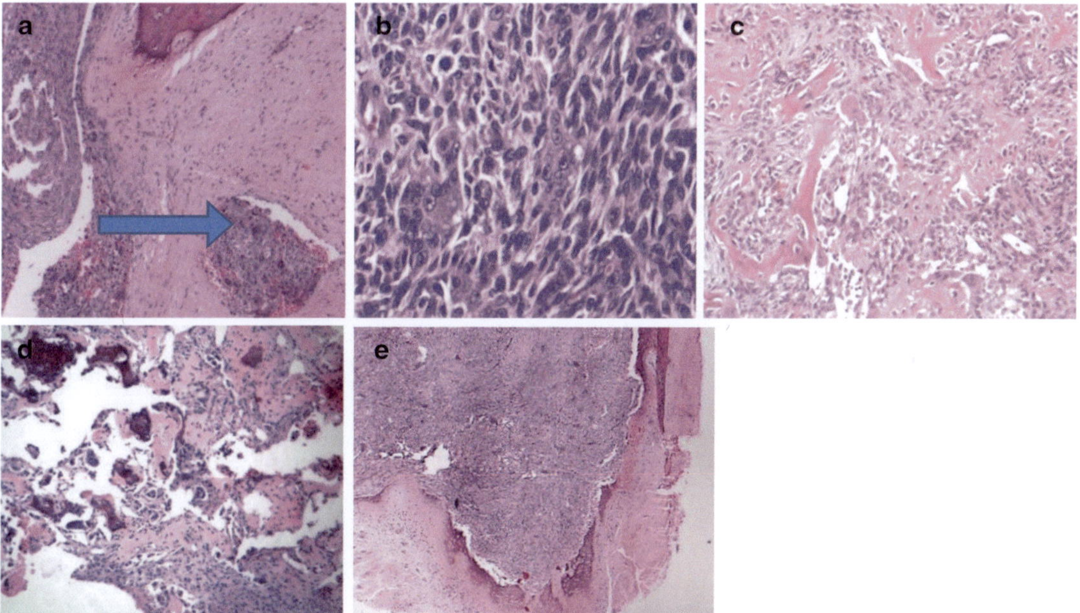

Fig. 7.17 GCT: (**a**) Vascular emboli (arrow), H&E ×100. (**b**) Mitosis, H&E ×250. (**c**) Reactive osteoid at the periphery of tumour, H&E ×100. (**d**) Calcifying osteoid, H&E ×100. (**e**) Bone at periphery, H&E ×100

cell outlines of stromal and giant cells (Fig. 7.16). Calcification is rare in giant cell tumour. Reactive osteoid formation can be seen towards periphery. Periphery of tumour may show intravascular tumour extension (Fig. 7.17). But this does not correlate with increased risk of metastasis. Degenerative changes like collection of foamy histiocytes and cholesterol clefts are common in giant cell tumour (Fig. 7.18). Areas of spindle cells in a storiform pattern resembling a fibrohistiocytic tumour may be seen. This appearance should not be mistaken for fibrous histiocytoma (Fig. 7.19). Aneurysmal bone cyst like areas are very common [20] (Fig. 7.20).

Grading of giant cell tumour has no prognostic significance. Abnormal mitosis is never seen in a typical giant cell tumour.

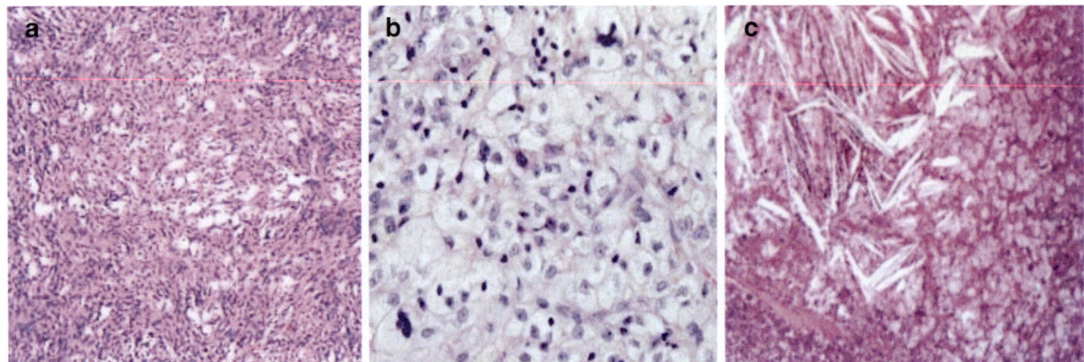

Fig. 7.18 Degenerative changes in GCT. (**a**) Foamy histiocytes, H&E ×100. (**b**) H&E ×250. (**c**) Cholesterol clefts, H&E ×250

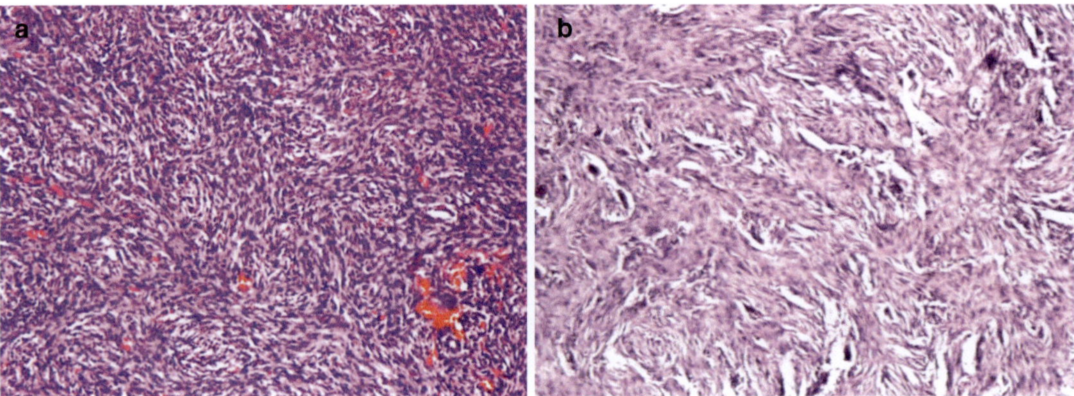

Fig. 7.19 (**a**) GCT resembling fibrosarcoma, H&E ×100. (**b**) GCT with fibrohistiocytic area and cellular spindle cell area, H&E ×100

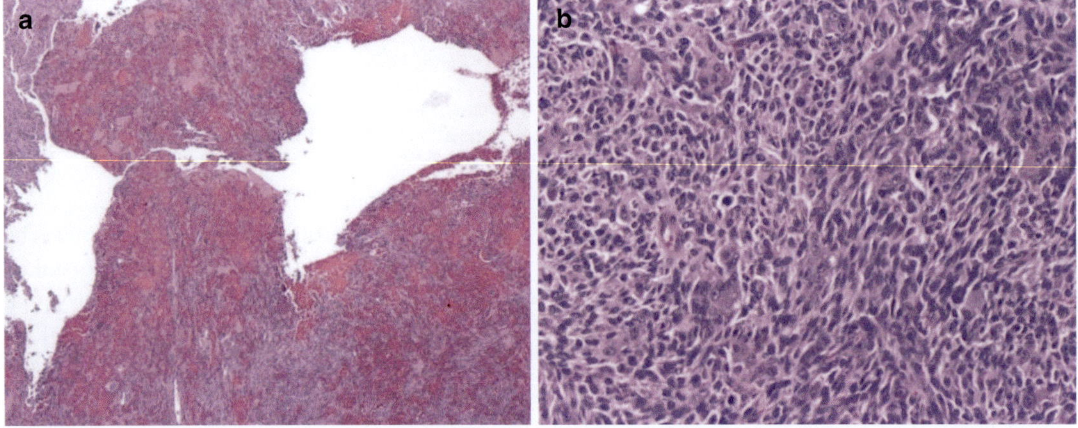

Fig. 7.20 (**a**) GCT with ABC like change, H&E ×100. (**b**) GCT with prominent mitotic activity, H&E ×100

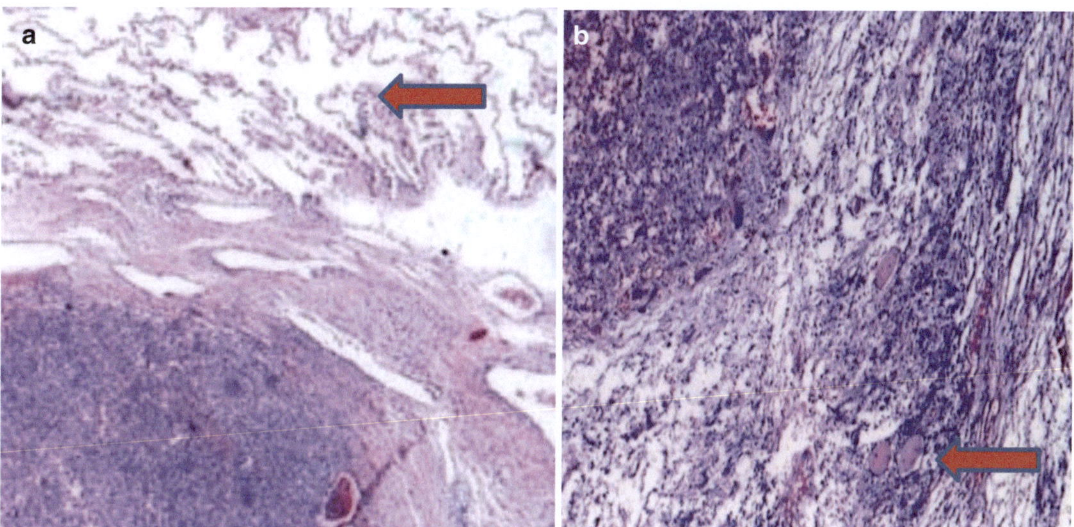

Fig. 7.21 (**a**) GCT metastasis to lung (red arrow, normal lung tissue), H&E ×100. (**b**) GCT metastasis to thyroid (red arrow, normal thyroid), H&E ×100

7.6.5 IHC

The stromal cells and OCGCs are positive for histiocytic markers CD68 and CD163 [38]. P63 shows strong and diffuse positivity in GCT [31], but it is not specific for GCT [36]. RANKL has been suggested as a good marker to differentiate GCT from other morphological mimickers. H3.3G34W is a novel marker, very specific for GCTB [19, 36, 37]. This antibody is specific and sensitive and is very useful in the diagnosis of GCT, especially in small needle core biopsies.

7.6.6 Molecular

Recently, H3F3Ap.Gly34 mutations are described in GCT [51, 52], which can be detected by IHC and molecular tests [48, 55]. A diagnosis of GCT should be made with caution if the H3F3A p. Gly34 mutation is absent (Fig. 7.21).

7.6.7 Differential Diagnosis [39, 53, 61]

1. Chondroblastoma (CB): This is also an epiphyseal tumour, formerly grouped under GCT. But chondroblastoma is a tumour of young age (<20 years), with a defined lytic lesion and a sclerotic border. The cell of origin is a chondroblast with well-defined cytoplasmic borders, abundant eosinophilic cytoplasm and cleaved/convoluted nuclei. The OCGCs are not uniformly distributed. Calcification is common and is seen around degenerated cells, giving the characteristic chicken-wire calcification. Chondroid matrix will be present. Degenerative changes are not seen.
2. Aneurysmal bone cyst (ABC): Primary ABC is usually seen in young individuals, less than 20 years. It is metaphyseal in location and is eccentrically located. Cystic spaces without lining and containing blood are the classical appearance. Cyst wall shows giant cells which are haphazardly placed. The stromal cells are elongated fibroblasts. Lots of reactive osteoid may be seen in the cyst wall. Calcification parallel to cyst wall is common. Sometimes, chicken-wire calcification can also be seen.
3. Giant cell-rich osteosarcoma: Morphologically, this is very difficult to differentiate. One has to search for atypia of the cells and atypical mitosis. Again, this is a tumour of less than 20 years' age group, metaphyseal in location with periosteal new bone formation and soft tissue extension. Marked atypia of stromal cells prompts one to search for atypical mitosis [40, 42]. Radiological correlation will help in reaching a correct diagnosis. Recently, H3F3A mutations have been described in GC-rich OS. So, they are considered as malignant GCT according to some authors [34].

Table 7.3 Differential diagnosis of giant cell tumour (GCT)

	GCT	CB	ABC	OS
Site	Epiphysis	Epiphysis	Metaphysis	Metaphysis
Age	20–40	<20	<20	<20
Stromal nuclei	Oval—similar to GC nuclei	Cleaved	Elongated	Pleomorphic
Calcification	Uncommon	Chicken wire	Amorphous	Calcifying osteoid
Others	Degeneration—foam cells, cholesterol clefts Infarction/necrosis	Chondroid matrix	Blood-filled cysts	Necrosis Atypical mitosis

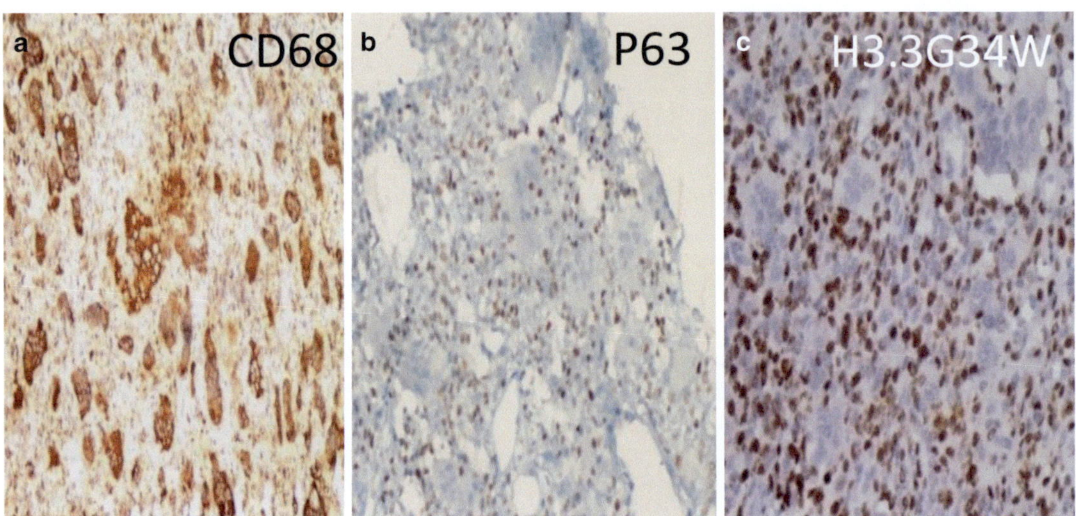

Fig. 7.22 IHC in GCT. (**a**) CD68 (both stromal cells and giant cells positive) ×250. (**b**) P63 (stromal cells diffusely strongly positive), ×100. (**c**) H3.3G34W (sensitive and specific marker for GCT, strong positivity of stromal cell nuclei), ×100

Other entities rich in giant cells will be discussed in the respective chapters [50].

Table 7.3 gives the common differential diagnosis and their features.

7.6.8 Treatment

Wide resection with adequate margins reduces local recurrence compared to intralesional curettage. The rate of local recurrence after curettage ranges between 25 and 50% [22]. Local adjuvant therapy is useful in controlling recurrence rates.

Radiotherapy is given to surgically unresectable tumours. But post-radiation sarcomatous transformation is common in these cases.

Bisphosphonates are given [56], and they act by targeting osteoclast-like giant cells by inducing apoptosis, thus limiting tumour progression. Denosumab, the monoclonal antibody developed against the RANK/RANK-L pathway, is a major invention in the treatment of GCTB [21, 26, 50]. For the treatment of GCT of bone, denosumab is the only US Food and Drug Administration (FDA)-approved drug [26]. The common site for metastasis is lung. We have encountered metastasis to lung and thyroid from a GCT of radius (Fig. 7.22). Good treatment response was reported with denosumab. Metastasis to lung is usually treated by excision (metastasectomy) [28, 46]. The clinical and molecular prognostic factors are given in Table 7.4.

7.6.9 Morphological Changes After Denosumab treatment [30, 47]

A good knowledge of morphology of treated tumours is essential. It differs significantly from the original giant cell tumour morphology and resembles other lesions like osteosarcoma (Fig. 7.23).

Woven bone is seen as a shell towards periphery in denosumab-treated GCT specimens. Bone formation can be in the form of osteoid to rounded "cement-like" structures or irregular trabeculae lined by osteoblasts. Loose fibrous tissue and thin-walled vessels can be seen between these bony trabeculae resembling osteoblastoma. The entire tumour is replaced by bone and fibrous tissue in some cases. In some other cases, a proliferation of mononuclear cells having bland, oval-to-spindle nuclei without any particular pattern is observed. In some cases, a storiform pattern may be seen. Mitoses are rare, and no atypical mitotic figures or necrosis will be seen. A marked decrease or complete absence in the number of giant cells and dense hyalinization of stroma may be mistaken for osteoblastic osteosarcoma. Denosumab-treated GCT shows minimal atypia and sparse mitosis. Pre-existing bone permeation is also absent. Some cases resemble low-grade osteosarcoma. IHC for MDM2 will help in ruling out low-grade osteosarcoma.

Table 7.4 Prognostic factors of GCT—clinical and molecular

Clinical
• Recurrence: 25–50%
• Recur in 2 years
• Metastasis <3%: benign metastasizing GCT—lung, mediastinal LN
– Rarely breast, thyroid
• 25% die with progressive disease
• 7% undergo malignant change
Prognostic molecular factors
• C-myc, c-fos overexpression: correlates with metastasis in GCT
• Urokinase plasminogen activator in tumour cells: correlates with bone destruction and local invasion
• Amplification of u-PA gene: higher biological aggressiveness
• p53 and H-ras mutation: -malignant transformation

7.6.10 Prognosis

Giant cell tumours are known to have malignant transformation even 30–40 years after treatment [24]. Hence, a long-term follow-up is mandatory [43]. Recurrences usually occur within 2 years. But late recurrences, even after 7 years, have been reported. Malignant transformation can be either as fibrosarcoma or as osteosarcoma. Metastasis usually occurs to lung, but other organs like thyroid, breast and soft tissue have been reported [22]. Giant cell tumours of radius and pelvic bone behave aggressively.

7.6.11 Multicentric GCT

Multicentric origin of GCT is rare [28]. It is usually seen in small bones of hands and feet. One

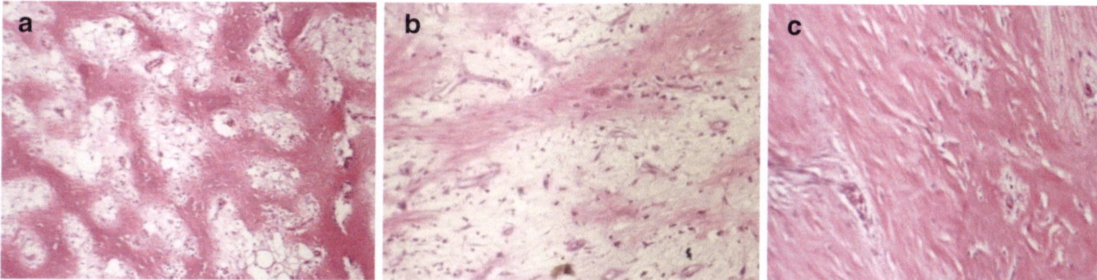

Fig. 7.23 Post-denosumab-treated GCT: (**a**) Tumour replaced by woven bone, H&E ×250. (**b**) Areas of fibroblastic proliferation, H&E ×100. (**c**) Tumour replaced by hyalinized tissue, H&E ×100

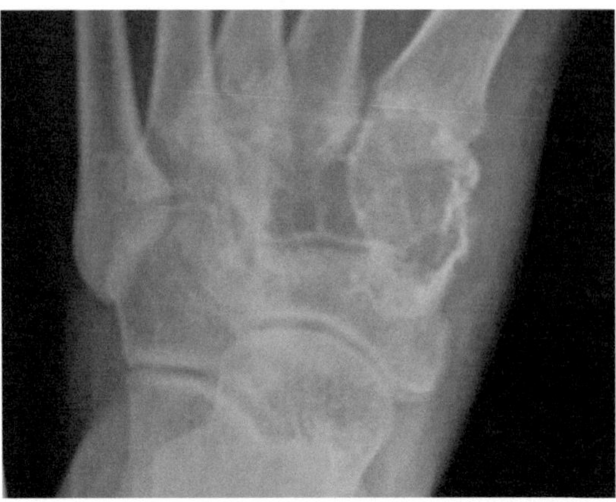

Fig. 7.24 Multicentric GCT affecting multiple metatarsal bones

Table 7.5 Differentiation of multicentric GCT and metastatic GCT

- Difficult to differentiate
- Metastatic GCT involves extraskeletal tissues—lung, lymph nodes, breast, etc
- Multicentric GCT usually affects other parts of skeleton, and it is rare
- Removal of primary tumour in metastatic GCT may result in disappearance of secondary lesions

has to rule out hyperparathyroidism in these cases (Fig. 7.24). The differentiation between multicentric and metastatic GCT is given in Table 7.5.

7.7 Giant Cell Tumour of Bone, Malignant

Rarely, GCT undergoes sarcomatous transformation [24, 57, 60]. Mostly, it is osteosarcoma. Fibrosarcoma or undifferentiated pleomorphic sarcoma is also reported. Malignant transformation can be considered as either primary or secondary malignant GCT. Secondary malignant GCT is more common than primary malignant GCT. Primary malignant GCTs are present at the time of initial diagnosis. In such cases, an area of highly pleomorphic mononuclear cells are seen in an otherwise conventional GCT. Secondary malignancy occurs at the site of previously treated GCT. In such cases, the preexisting benign GCT may not be present. Most of the malignant GCTs are secondary. They usually occur after radiotherapy. A long-term follow-up is required in GCTB because secondary malignant GCTs can occur even after 40 years.

7.7.1 Primary malignant GCT

In primary malignant giant cell tumour, areas of benign GCT will be seen. Atypical mitosis and cellular atypia may be seen in malignant areas (Fig. 7.25). These tumours may be difficult to differentiate from giant cell-rich osteosarcoma or undifferentiated pleomorphic sarcoma. But this differentiation is only of academic interest because the prognosis is the same as that of other high-grade sarcomas. The differential diagnoses are osteosarcoma, undifferentiated pleomorphic sarcoma and leiomyosarcoma. Sometimes, malignant area may be missed in a benign GCT (Fig. 7.26). Thorough sampling is essential to confirm malignancy. Grossly, the tumour may have zones of abnormal consistency, but these features are not specific. Any grossly unusual areas should be included while grossing.

7.7.2 Secondary malignant GCT

The secondary malignancy occurs usually after radiotherapy. The evidence of giant cell tumour may not be present in these cases. The malignant tumour can be fibrosarcoma, osteosarcoma or undifferentiated sarcoma (Fig. 7.27).

7.7.3 Pathogenesis

Recent studies have shown that p53 alteration and dysfunction of histone methylation (H3K27me3 loss) can lead to malignant progression of GCTB [33]. In primary, recurrent and

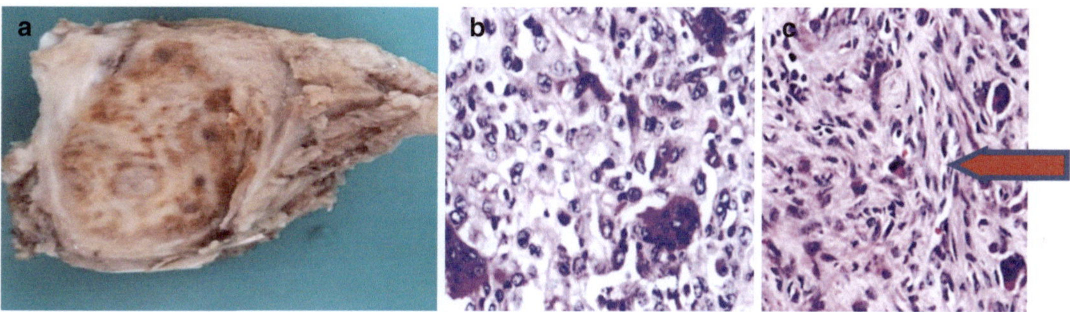

Fig. 7.25 Malignant GCT of radius. (**a**) Gross specimen with fleshy appearance. (**b**) Atypical stromal cells and osteoclastic giant cells, H&E ×400. (**c**) Malignant GCT with atypical mitosis (arrow), H&E ×250

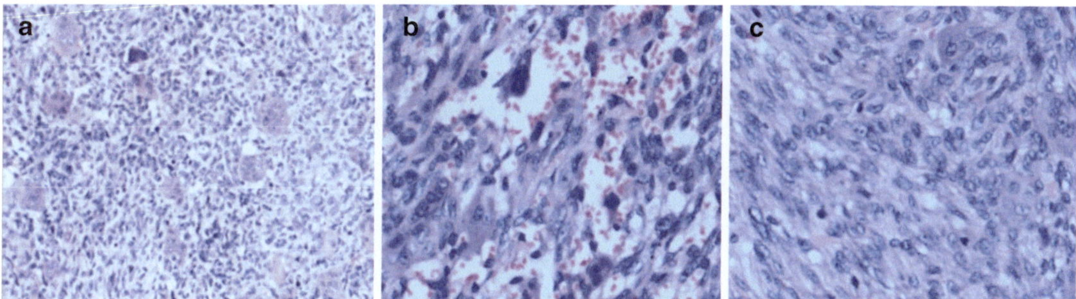

Fig. 7.26 Primary malignant GCT of skull. (**a**) Conventional GCT area, H&E ×100. (**b** and **c**) Fibrosarcoma with malignant cells in sheets without giant cells and with mitosis, H&E ×400

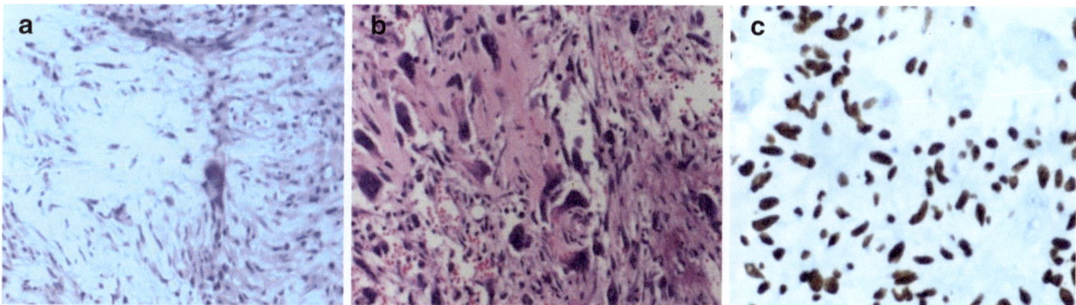

Fig. 7.27 Secondary malignant GCT with osteosarcoma. (**a**) Osteoid and malignant cells, H&E ×250. (**b**) Giant cell-rich area and osteoid, H&E ×250. (**c**) IHC for SATB2 positive in stromal cells and negative in giant cells, ×250

metastatic GCTs, allelic loss of 1p, 9q and 19q is common. TP53 and HRAS mutations are seen in secondary malignant GCT. These are also thought to play a role in malignant transformation.
Mutational testing is under evaluation as an approach to assist in the diagnosis of GCT. H3F3A mutations may help to differentiate GCT from giant cell-rich sarcomas [40, 42].

7.7.4 Treatment and Prognosis

Treatment is surgical ablation. If the sarcoma is chemo sensitive, for example osteosarcoma, adjuvant chemotherapy is given. The prognosis of primary malignant GCT is better than secondary malignancy.

Table 7.6 shows common features of some of these tumours.

Table 7.6 Other giant cell-rich lesions of bone[a]

Lesion	Cherubism	NOF	Brown tumour of HPT
Age/sex	2–7 years of age M:F ratio of 2:1	Second decade More in boys	Adults More in females
Clinical	Painless bilateral jaw swelling with upward-looking eyes	Incidental Chronic pain and/or pathologic fracture	Bones, renal stones, abdominal groans and psychic moans
Site	Jawbones	Long bones intracortical, metaphysis	Solitary or multiple Jaws, ribs, clavicles, extremities, pelvic girdle
Aetiology	A mutation in the gene SH3-binding protein 2 (SH3BP2)	Disturbance of growth or dystrophic calcification	Prolonged hyperparathyroidism
Prognosis	Stabilization or even regression after puberty	Likely to undergo spontaneous regression	Partial or complete removal of parathyroid glands followed by spontaneous tumour regression

[a] Contributed by Dr. Jayasree Geothe

Points to Remember

- Giant cell tumour of bone is an epiphyseal tumour of skeletally mature patients.
- Age of the patient is usually 20–40 years.
- Aneurysmal bone cyst and chondroblastomas are close histological mimics.
- Malignant giant cell tumour can be primary (coexisting benign and malignant areas) or secondary (at the site of previous GCT).
- Giant cell-rich osteosarcomas occur in patients less than 20 years and are metaphyseal tumours.
- To diagnose malignancy in giant cell-rich osteosarcomas, look for atypical mitoses.
- Secondary ABC terminology does not exist. Instead, it is given as ABC-like areas.
- NOF is a common metaphyseal tumour of children with OCGCs and fibrous histiocytoma-like areas.

References

Aneurysmal Bone Cyst

1. Althof PA, Ohmori K, Zhou M, et al. Cytogenetic and molecular cytogenetic findings in 43 aneurysmal bone cysts: aberrations of 17p mapped to 17p13.2 by fluorescence in situ hybridization. Mod Pathol. 2004;17(5):518–25.
2. Bertoni F, Bacchini P, Capanna R, et al. Solid variant of aneurysmal bone cyst. Cancer. 1993;71(3):729–34.
3. Bonakdarpour A, Levy WM, Aegerter E. Primary and secondary aneurysmal bone cyst: a radiological study of 75 cases. Radiology. 1978;126(1):75–83.
4. Cottalorda J, Bourelle S. Current treatments of primary aneurysmal bone cysts. J Pediatr Orthop B. 2006;15(3):155–67.
5. Dal Cin P, Kozakewich HP, Goumnerova L, Mankin HJ, Rosenberg AE, Fletcher JA. Variant translocations involving 16q22 and 17p13 in solid variant and

extraosseous forms of aneurysmal bone cyst. Genes Chromosomes Cancer. 2000;28(2):233–4.
6. Ilaslan H, Sundaram M, Unni KK. Solid variant of aneurysmal bone cysts in long tubular bones: giant cell reparative granuloma. AJR Am J Roentgenol. 2003;180(6):1681–7.
7. Jaffe HL. Aneurysmal bone cyst. Bull Hosp Joint Dis. 1950;11(1):3–13.
8. Kyriakos M, Hardy D. Malignant transformations of aneurysmal bone cyst, with an analysis of the literature. Cancer. 1991;68(8):1770–80. lesions. Cancer. 1992;70(11):2642–2649.
9. Lichtenstein L. Aneurysmal bone cyst: a pathological entity commonly mistaken for giant cell tumor and occasionally for hemangioma and osteogenic sarcoma. Cancer. 1950;3(2):279–89.
10. Martinez V, Sissons HA. Aneurysmal bone cyst: a review of 123 cases including primary lesions and those secondary to other bone pathology. Cancer. 1988;61(11):2291–304.
11. Nielsen GP, Fletcher CD, Smith MA, Rybak L, Rosenberg AE. Soft tissue aneurysmal bone cyst: a clinicopathologic study of five cases. Am J Surg Pathol. 2002;26:64–9.
12. Oda Y, Tsuneyoshi M, Shinohara N. "Solid" variant of aneurysmal bone cyst (extragnathic giant cell reparative granuloma) in the axial skeleton and long bones. A study of its morphologic spectrum and distinction from allied giant cell lesions. Cancer. 1992;70(11):2642–9.
13. Oliveira AM, Perez-Atayde AR, Inwards CY, et al. USP6 and CDH11 oncogenes identify the neoplastic cell in primary aneurysmal bone cysts and are absent in so-called secondary aneurysmal bone cysts. Am J Pathol. 2004;165(5):1773–80.
14. Rosenberg AE, Nielsen GP, Fletcher JA. Aneurysmal bone cyst. In: Fletcher CDM, Unni KK, Mertens F, editors. World Health Organization classification of tumours: pathology and genetics of tumours of soft tissue and bone. Lyon: IARC Press; 2002. p. 338–9.
15. Ruiter DJ, van Rijssel TG, van der Velde EA. Aneurysmal bone cysts: a clinicopathologic study of 105 cases. Cancer. 1977;39(5):2231–9.
16. Singh A, Majeed A, Mallick S, Khan SA, Mridha AR. Solid variant of aneurysmal bone cyst masquerading as malignancy. J Clin Diagn Res. 2017;11(7):ED35–6.
17. Vergel De Dios AM, Bond JR, Shives TC, McLeod RA, Unni KK. Aneurysmal bone cyst: a clinicopathologic study of 238 cases. Cancer. 1992;69(12):2921–31.
18. Bahk W-J, Mirra JM. Differential diagnostic value of "blue reticulated chondroid-like material" in aneurysmal bone cysts: a classic histopathologic analysis of 215 cases. Am J Clin Pathol. 2015;143:823–9.

Giant Cell Tumour

19. Amary F, Berisha F, Ye H, Gupta M, Gutteridge A, Baumhoer D, et al. H3F3A (Histone 3.3) G34W Immunohistochemistry: a reliable marker defining benign and malignant giant cell tumor of bone. Am J Surg Pathol. 2017;41:1059–68.
20. Anchan C. Giant cell tumor of bone with secondary aneurysmal bone cyst. Int J Shoulder Surg. 2008;2(3):68.
21. Balke M, Hardes J. Denosumab: a breakthrough in treatment of giant-cell tumour of bone? Lancet Oncol. 2010;11:218–9.
22. Balke M, Schremper L, Gebert C, et al. Giant cell tumor of bone: treatment and outcome of 214 cases. J Cancer Res Clin Oncol. 2008;134(9):969–78.
23. Bandyopadhyay R, Biswas S, Bandyopadhyay SK, Ray MM. Synchronous multicentric giant cell tumor. J Cancer Res Ther. 2010;6(1):106–8.
24. Bertoni F, Bacchini P, Staals EL. Malignancy in giant cell tumor of bone. Cancer. 2003;97(10):2520–9.
25. Biscaglia R, Bacchini P, Bertoni F. Giant cell tumor of the bones of the hand and foot. Cancer. 2000;88(9):2022–32.
26. Chawla S, et al. Safety and efficacy of denosumab for adults and skeletally mature adolescents with giant cell tumour of bone: interim analysis of an open-label, parallel- group, phase 2 study. Lancet Oncol. 2013;14(9):901–8.
27. Chakarun CJ, Forrester DM, Gottsegen CJ, Patel DB, White EA, Matcuk GR Jr. Giant cell tumor of bone: review, mimics, and new developments in treatment. Radiographics. 2013;33:197–211.
28. Dominkus M, Ruggieri P, Bertoni F, et al. Histologically verified lung metastases in benign giant cell tumours: 14 cases from a single institution. Int Orthop. 2006;30(6):499–504.
29. Errani C, et al. Giant cell tumor of the extremity: a review of 349 cases from a single institution. Cancer Treat Rev. 2010;36(1):1–7.
30. Hakozaki M, Tajino T, Yamada H, Hasegawa O, Tasaki K, et al. Radiological and pathological characteristics of giant cell tumor of bone treated with denosumab. Diagn Pathol. 2014;9:111.
31. Hammas N, Laila C, Youssef AL, et al. Can p63 serve as a biomarker for giant cell tumor of bone? A Moroccan experience. Diagn Pathol. 2012;7:130.
32. Hoch B, Hermann G, Klein MJ, Abdelwahab IF, Springfield D. Giant cell tumor complicating Paget disease of long bone. Skeletal Radiol. 2007;36(10):973–8.

33. Ishihara S, Yamamoto H, Iwasaki T, Toda Y, Yamamoto T, Yoshimoto M, Ito Y, Susuki Y, Kawaguchi K, Kinoshita I, Yamada Y, Kohashi K, Fujiwara T, Setsu N, Endo M, Matsumoto Y, Kakuda Y, Nakashima Y, Oda Y. Histological and immunohistochemical features and genetic alterations in the malignant progression of giant cell tumor of bone: a possible association with TP53 mutation and loss of H3K27 trimethylation. Mod Pathol. 2022;35:640–8. https://doi.org/10.1038/s41379-021-00972-x. Epub ahead of print. PMID: 34785767.
34. Ito Y, Sugita S, Segawa K, Sugawara T, Tsujiwaki M, Fujita H, et al. Giant cell-rich osteosarcoma of the vertebra with murine double minute chromosome 2- and cyclin-dependent kinase 4-positive and histone H3F3A mutant p.Gly34Trp-negative immunophenotypes. Pathol Int. 2018;68:324–6.
35. de Lange J, van den Akker HP. Clinical and radiological features of central giant-cell lesions of the jaw. Oral Surg Oral Med Oral Pathol Oral Radiol Endod. 2005;99(4):464–70.
36. Kamble A, Hui M, Rao KN, Narayanan R, Reddy BR, Uppin SG, Chandrasekhar P. Anti-Histone H3.3 G34W antibody is a sensitive and highly specific immunohistochemistry marker for the diagnosis of giant cell tumor of bone. A validation based on analysis of 198 cases from a single centre in India. Indian J Pathol Microbiol. 2022;65(3):617–29.
37. Khazaei S, et al. H3.3 G34W promotes growth and impedes differentiation of osteoblast-like mesenchymal progenitors in giant cell tumor of bone. Cancer Discov. 2020;10:1968–87.
38. Unni KK, Carrie Y. Tumors of the bones and joints. AFIP ATLAS of tumor pathology series 4. 2006.
39. Lang S. Differential diagnosis of giant cell rich lesion of bone. Pathologe. 2008;29 Suppl 2:245–9.
40. Macagno N, Caselles K, Aubert S, Audard V, Gomez-Brouchet A, Galant C, et al. Benign and malignant giant-cell rich lesions of bone: pathological diagnosis with special emphasis on recent immunohistochemistry and molecular techniques. Ann Pathol. 2018;38:92–102.
41. Mathew DG, Sreenivasan BS, Varghese SS, Sebastian CJ. Classification of giant cell lesions of the oral cavity: a fresh perspective. Oral Maxillofac Pathol J. 2016;7(2):710–6.
42. Gore MR. Giant cell rich malignancies: a meta-analysis. Ann Med Health Sci Res. 2018;8:225–32.
43. Mori Y, Tsuchiya H, Karita M, Nonomura A, Nojima T, Tomita K. Malignant transformation of a giant cell tumor 25 years after initial treatment. Clin Orthop Relat Res. 2000;381:185–91.
44. Murphey MD, Nomikos GC, Flemming DJ, Gannon FH, Temple HT, Kransdorf MJ. Imaging of giant cell tumor and giant cell reparative granuloma of bone: radiologic-pathologic correlation. Radiographics. 2001;21(5):1283–309.
45. Novais EN, Shin AY, Bishop AT, Shives TC. Multicentric giant cell tumor of the upper extremities: 16 years of ongoing disease. J Hand Surg Am. 2011;36(10):1610–3.
46. Okamoto Y, Mathew S, Daw NC, et al. Giant cell tumor of bone with pulmonary metastases. Med Pediatr Oncol. 2003;41(5):454–9.
47. Biçer OS, Tekin M. Clinical and pathological results of denosumab treatment for giant cell tumors of bone: prospective study of 14 cases. Acta Orthop Traumatol Turc. 2017;51:1–6.
48. Presneau N, Baumhoer D, Behjati S, Pillay N, Tarpey P, Campbell PJ, Jundt G, Flanagan AM. Diagnostic value of H3F3A mutations in giant cell tumour of bone compared to osteoclast-rich mimics. J Pathol Clin Res. 2015;1(2):113–23.
49. Chuong R, Kaban LB, Kozakewich H, Perez-Atayde A. Central giant cell lesions of the jaws: a clinicopathologic study. J Oral Maxillofac Surg. 1986;44(9):708–13.
50. Maharaj RC, Panigrahi S, Das BS. Effect of denosumab in giant cell tumor of bone. Oncol J India. 2017;1:34–6.
51. Righi A, Mancini I, Gambarotti M, Picci P, Gamberi G, Marraccini C, et al. Histone 3.3 mutations in giant cell tumor and giant cell-rich sarcomas of bone. Hum Pathol. 2017;68:128–35.
52. Alberto R, Irene M, Marco G, Piero P, Gabriella G, Cristina M, Paolo DTA, Lisa S, Pamela P, Alessandro F. Histone 3.3 mutations in giant cell tumor and giant cell-rich sarcomas of bone. Hum Pathol. 2017: 1–25.
53. Rosenberg AE, Nielsen GP. Giant cell containing lesion of bone and their differential diagnosis. Curr Diagn Pathol. 2001;7(4):235–6.
54. Roux S, Amazit L, Meduri G. RANK (receptor activator of nuclear factor kappa B) and RANK ligand are expressed in giant cell tumors of bone. Am J Clin Pathol. 2002;117:210–6.
55. Scotto di Carlo F, Divisato G, Iacoangeli M, Esposito T, Gianfrancesco F. The identification of H3F3A mutation in giant cell tumour of the clivus and the histological diagnostic algorithm of other clival lesions permit the differential diagnosis in this location. BMC Cancer. 2018;18:358.
56. Tse LF, Wong KC, Kumta SM, Huang L, Chow TC, Griffith JF. Bisphosphonates reduce local recurrence in extremity giant cell tumor of bone: a case–control study. Bone. 2008;42:68–73.
57. Unni KK, Inwards CY, editors. Dahalin's bone tumors: general aspects and data on 10,165 cases. 6th ed. Wolters Kluwer/Lippincott Williams and Wilkins; 2010. p. 225–247.
58. Varshney A, Rao H, Sadh R. Multicentric GCT of tarsal bones in an immature skeleton: a case report with review of literature. J Foot Ankle Surg. 2010;49(4):399.e1–4.
59. Yamamoto H, Iwasaki T, Yamada Y, Matsumoto Y, Otsuka H, Yoshimoto M, Kohashi K, Taguchi K, Yokoyama R, Nakashima Y, Oda Y. Diagnostic utility of histone H3.3 G34W, G34R, and G34V mutant-specific antibodies for giant cell tumors of bone. Hum Pathol. 2018;73:41–50.
60. WHO Classification of Tumours. In: WHO Classification of Tumours Editorial Board, editor.

Soft tissue and bone tumours. WHO classification of tumours, 5th ed., vol 3. IARC; 2020.

61. Zambo I, Pazourek L. Giant cell-rich lesions of bone and their differential diagnosis. Cesk Patol. 2017;53:61–70.
62. Agaram NP, LeLoarer FV, Zhang L, et al. USP6 gene rearrangements occur preferentially in giant cell reparative granulomas of hands and feet but not in gnathic location. Hum Pathol. 2014;45(6):1147–52.

Non-ossifying Fibroma

63. Arata MA, Peterson HA, Dahlin DC. Pathological fractures through non-ossifying fibromas. Review of the Mayo Clinic experience. J Bone Joint Surg Am. 1981;63(6):980–8.
64. Campanacci M, Laus M, Boriani S. Multiple non-ossifying fibromata with extraskeletal anomalies: a new syndrome? J Bone Joint Surg Br. 1983;65(5):627–32.
65. Dumitriu DI, Menten R, Clapuyt P. Pitfalls in the diagnosis of common benign bone tumours in children. Insights Imaging. 2014;5:645–55.
66. Jaffe HL, Lichtenstein L. Non-osteogenic fibroma of bone. Am J Pathol. 1942;18(2):205–21.
67. Mankin HJ, Trahan CA, Fondren G, Mankin CJ. Non-ossifying fibroma, fibrous cortical defect and Jaffe-Campanacci syndrome: a biologic and clinical review. Chir Organi Mov. 2009;93(1):1–7.

8 Malignant Round Cell Tumours of Bone

Malignant round cell tumours are a group of high-grade malignant tumours that are primitive in appearance. These tumours lack any particular morphologic features that would allow precise identification. They are composed of small and monotonous undifferentiated cells with scanty cytoplasm and hyperchromatic round-to-oval nuclei. They are also called small blue cell tumours because of the relatively scanty cytoplasm. These neoplasms occur in children and young adults. It involves bone and soft tissue. It comprises 20% of solid tumours in children.

The undifferentiated round cell sarcomas are considered a separate entity in the new WHO (2020) classification of soft tissue and bone [70].

8.1 Classification of Undifferentiated Small Round Cell sarcomas [70]

- Ewing sarcoma
- Round cell sarcoma with EWSR1-non ETS fusions
- CIC-rearranged sarcomas
- Sarcoma with BCOR genetic alterations
- **Other round cell tumours of bone**
  - Lymphoblastic lymphoma
  - Small cell osteosarcoma
  - Mesenchymal chondrosarcoma
  - Metastatic neuroblastoma
  - Desmoplastic small round cell tumour (DSRCT)

This chapter discusses the undifferentiated small round cell sarcomas of bone, metastatic neuroblastoma and DSRCT.

8.2 Ewing Sarcoma (ES)

The Ewing sarcoma is an aggressive childhood malignancy. Previously, it was called Ewing family of tumours (EFT), and it included classic Ewing sarcoma, Askin tumour [4] and peripheral primitive neuroectodermal tumour (PNET). But the Askin tumour and PNET terminology are not recommended now.

ES is the second most common primary malignant bone tumour. ES is common in white populations, and it is mostly seen in males. The exact origin of this tumour is unclear.

8.2.1 History

In 1921, Ewing reported a round cell sarcoma of the radius and called it "diffuse endothelioma of bone". The occurrence of Ewing sarcoma in extraskeletal sites was reported by Angervall and Enzinger. The term primitive neuroectodermal tumour (PNET) was described by Nesbitt and Vidone in 1976. Askin et al. in 1979 described a similar tumour in the thoracopulmonary region, which was called as Askin's tumour [4].

The chromosome analysis detected the t (11; 22) (q24; q12) translocation in ES cell lines in 1980.

J. Kattoor et al., *Bone Tumors*, https://doi.org/10.1007/978-981-99-4738-6_8

EWS-FLI1 chimeric gene was identified in 1992 after the cloning of translocation breakpoints [17].

8.2.2 Pathogenesis

ES was thought to be derived from primitive neuroectodermal cells. The most common translocation detected in ES is that of the EWS gene on chromosome 22 and with the FLI1 gene on chromosome 11 (>95%) [7, 9, 17, 21]. Other translocations are EWS-ERG [15] (about 5%), EWS-FEV, EWS-ETV1 [18] and EWS-ETV4 (less than 1% of cases) [6]. Structural rearrangements of FET-ETS fusion genes are common in all cases of ES [2, 10, 12]. TP53 mutations are also reported [8].

8.2.3 Clinical Features

ES is more common in males of first two decades (10–24 years). Pelvis, ribs and femur are the most common bones affected. Thirty-five percent of cases are detected with distant metastases and 5% with regional lymph node metastases at the time of diagnosis [26].

Patients with ES present with pain, swelling, venous dilation and hyperaemia. Pathological fractures occur due to bone metastasis. Spinal metastasis can progress to paralysis. Increase in the white blood cell count and erythrocyte sedimentation rate, low haemoglobin levels and increased serum levels of lactate dehydrogenase (LDH), alkaline phosphatase and C-reactive protein are also observed. Clinically and radiologically, it mimics osteomyelitis. An elevated LDH level is associated with a poor prognosis.

8.2.4 Radiological Findings

Plain radiographs show permeative and infiltrative destruction of bone. The diaphysis of the long bones is usually affected. In addition, an onion skin-like periosteal reaction is seen [11]. As the tumour grows and expands bone, it elevates the periosteum in parallel layers with deposition of new bone giving an onion peel appearance. Rarely, periosteal reaction similar to osteosarcoma with sunray appearance can be seen. This causes difficulty in differentiation from osteosarcoma. The pelvic bones are commonly affected. It is difficult to identify pelvic tumours on plain X-rays alone. Sometimes, it can expand bone and can resemble a cyst. Computed tomography (CT) is useful for identifying soft tissue involvement, destruction of the cortex and detection of pulmonary metastasis. Tumours occurring in the subperiosteal location show saucerization of cortex. MRI helps in the identification of skip lesions in the bone. The

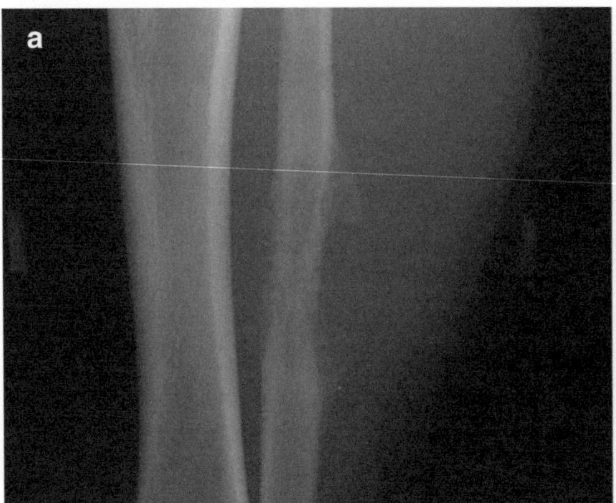

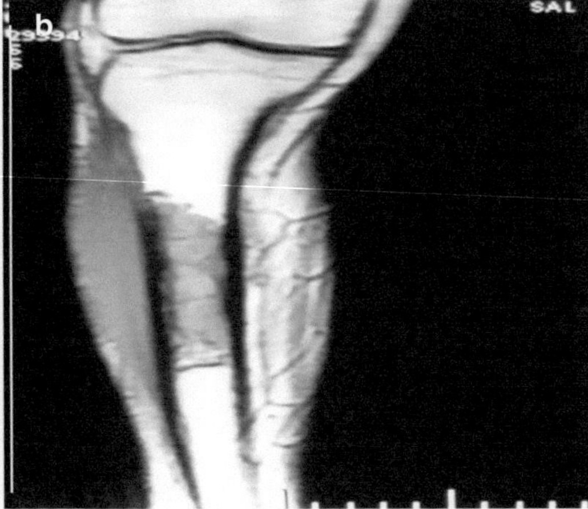

Fig. 8.1 Ewing sarcoma: (**a**) Plain X-ray showing diaphyseal destructive lesion with periosteal reaction and soft tissue extension of fibula. (**b**) MRI of ES tibia showing permeative nature and extent of lesion

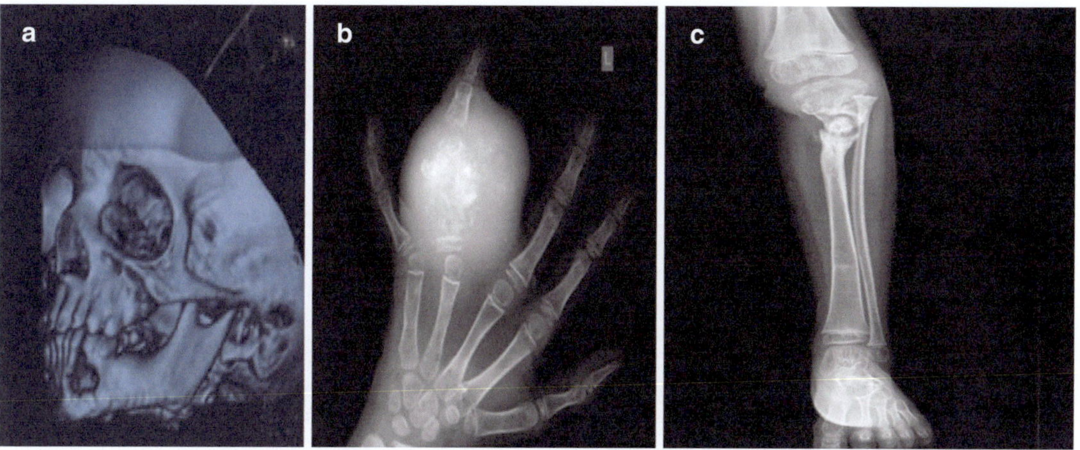

Fig. 8.2 (**a**) ES of mandible in a 2-year-old child. (**b**) ES in a 6-year-old male child involving phalanx. (**c**) ES of tibia

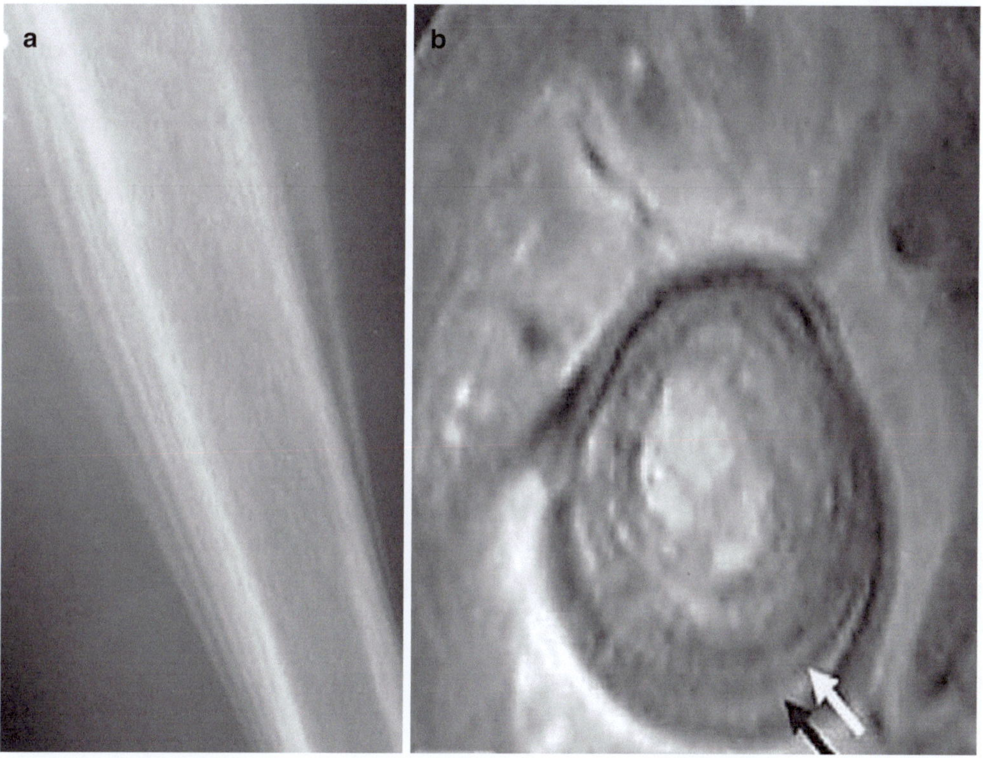

Fig. 8.3 ES of humerus showing onion peel periosteal reaction. (**a**) Plain X-ray. (**b**) MRI

radiological differential diagnoses of ES include osteomyelitis and malignant lymphoma of the bone as these are permeative lesions of bone. Other DDs are osteosarcoma, Langerhans cell histiocytosis and metastatic neuroblastoma (Figs. 8.1, 8.2, and 8.3).

8.2.5 Pathology

Grossly, the tumour involves medullary cavity with destruction of cortex and soft tissue extension. The soft tissue involvement can be extensive (Fig. 8.4). Histologically, ES is a small blue round cell tumour with round nuclei and scanty cytoplasm. Matrix formation is not seen. Small foci of eosinophilic material may be seen mimicking osteosarcoma [11]. But calcifying osteoid is absent. ES tumour cells are usually uniform round with few mitoses (Fig. 8.5a, b). They contain abundant amounts of glycogen in the cytoplasm giving a vacuolated appearance (Fig. 8.5c, d). This can be demonstrated by PAS stain. Necrosis and apoptosis can be noted, and this gives a light and dark appearance on low power (Fig. 8.6). Other patterns are alveolar (Fig. 8.7), lobular (Fig. 8.8) and filigree (Fig. 8.9) patterns. The dark blue change indicates degenerative changes. Sometimes, a prominent desmoplastic stroma separates tumour cells to lobules and can resemble desmoplastic small round cell tumour (Fig. 8.10). Papillaroid pattern (Fig. 8.11) and perivascular arrangement can be noted (Fig. 8.12). ES also demonstrates rosette formation indicating neural differentiation (Fig. 8.13). Rarely, haemangioendothelioma-like appearance (Fig. 8.14) may be noted. Some tumours can undergo crush artefact as in lymphoma of bone (Fig. 8.15).

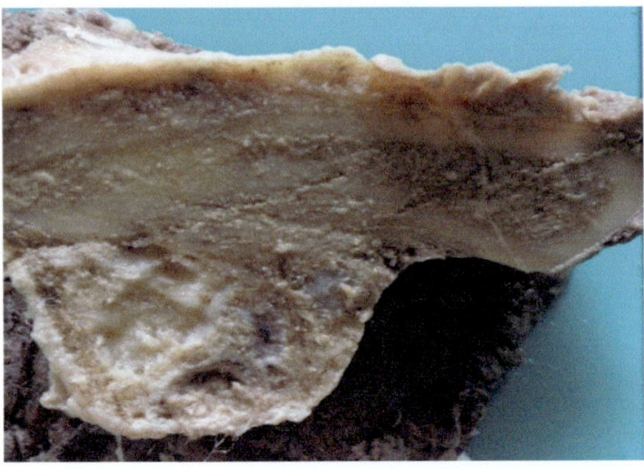

Fig. 8.4 Gross specimen of ES in a 28-year-old female. Left hemipelvectomy specimen: post-chemotherapy showing tumour with cortical involvement with necrotic and cystic change

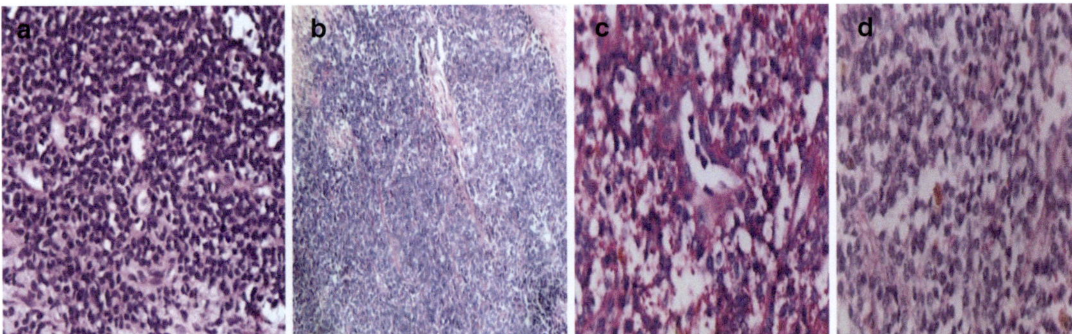

Fig. 8.5 ES. (**a** and **b**) Malignant round cell tumour, H&E ×100. (**c** and **d**) PAS with and without diastase demonstrating glycogen, PAS ×250

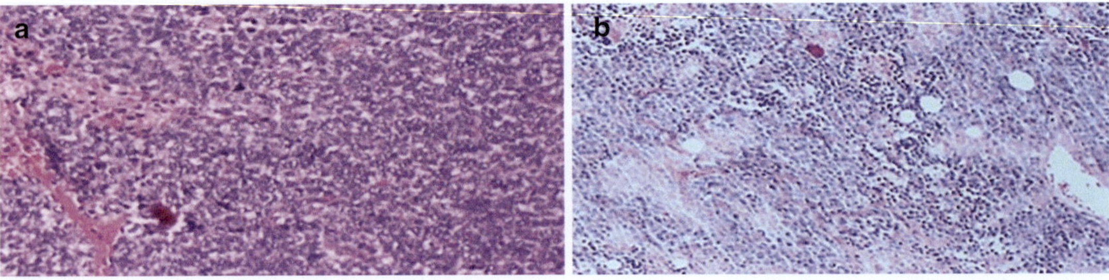

Fig. 8.6 (**a** and **b**) Classical Ewing sarcoma with primary cells (light) and secondary (dark) cells, H&E ×100

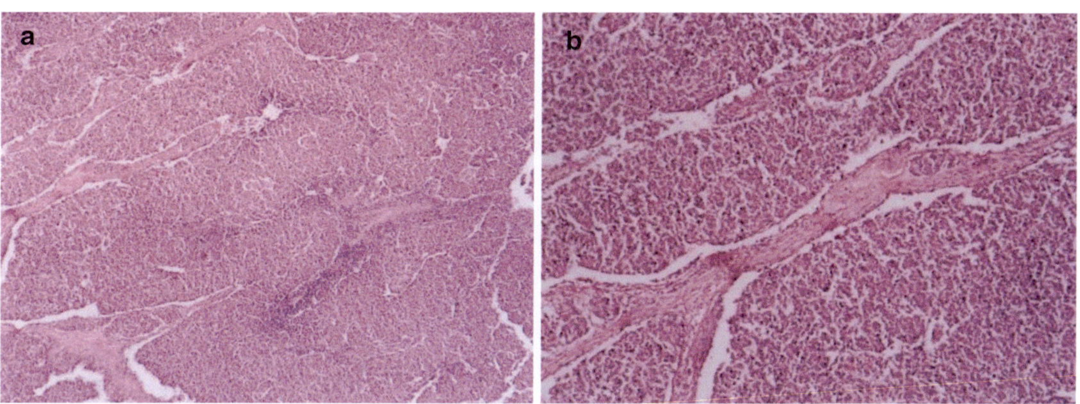

Fig. 8.7 (**a** and **b**) Classical Ewing sarcoma—alveolar pattern, H&E ×100

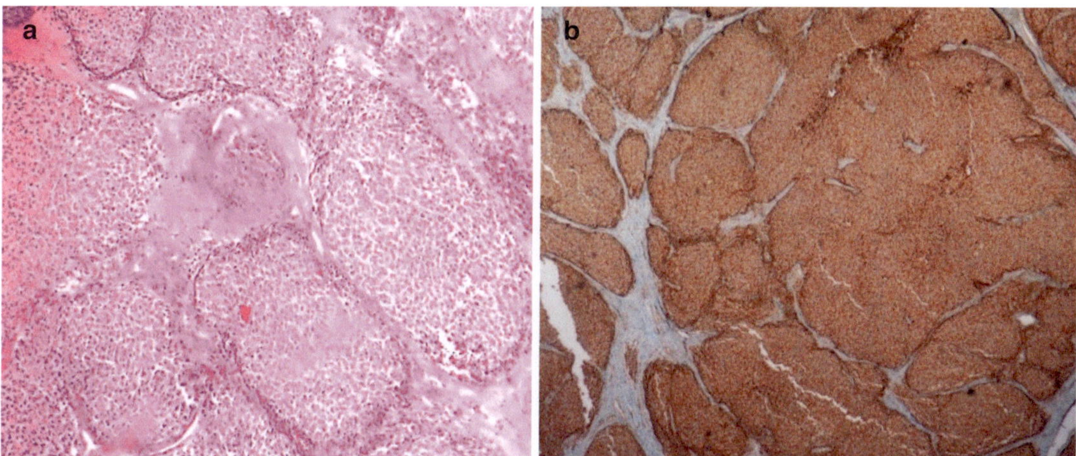

Fig. 8.8 (**a**) Classical Ewing sarcoma—lobular pattern, H&E ×100. (**b**) CD99 of same case highlighting lobular pattern, CD99 (MIC2) ×100

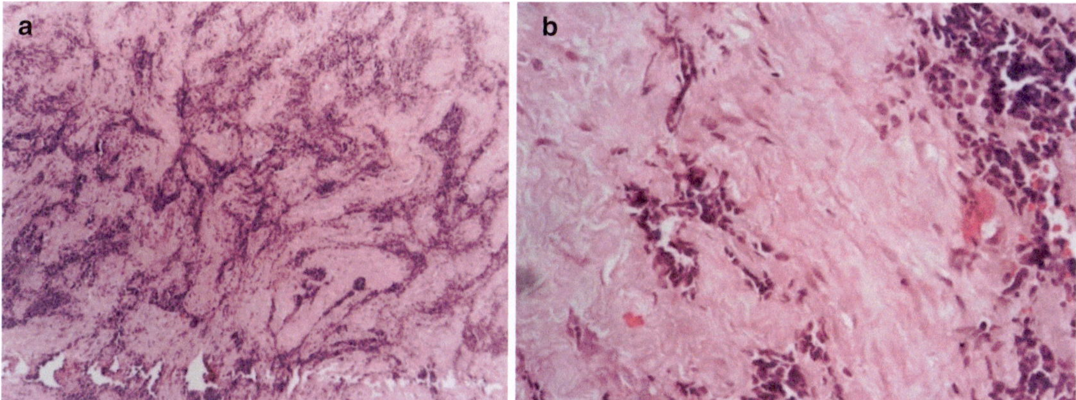

Fig. 8.9 (**a** and **b**) Ewing sarcoma with filigree pattern, H&E ×100

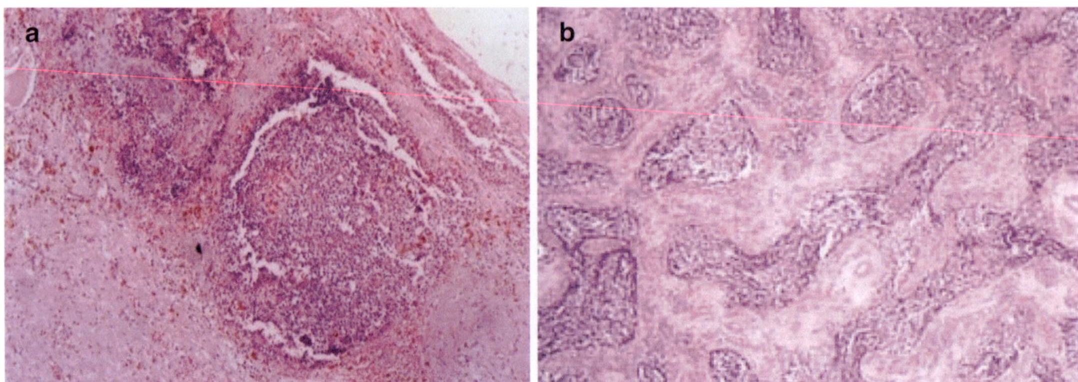

Fig. 8.10 (**a** and **b**) ES: DSRCT-like pattern—nodules of tumour set in desmoplastic stroma, H&E ×100

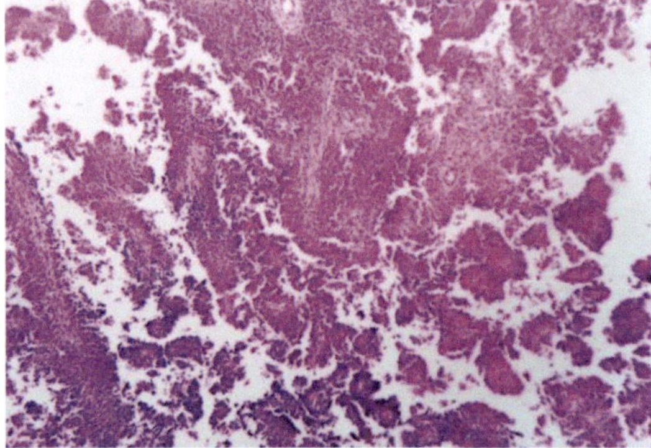

Fig. 8.11 Ewing sarcoma showing papillaroid clusters, H&E ×100

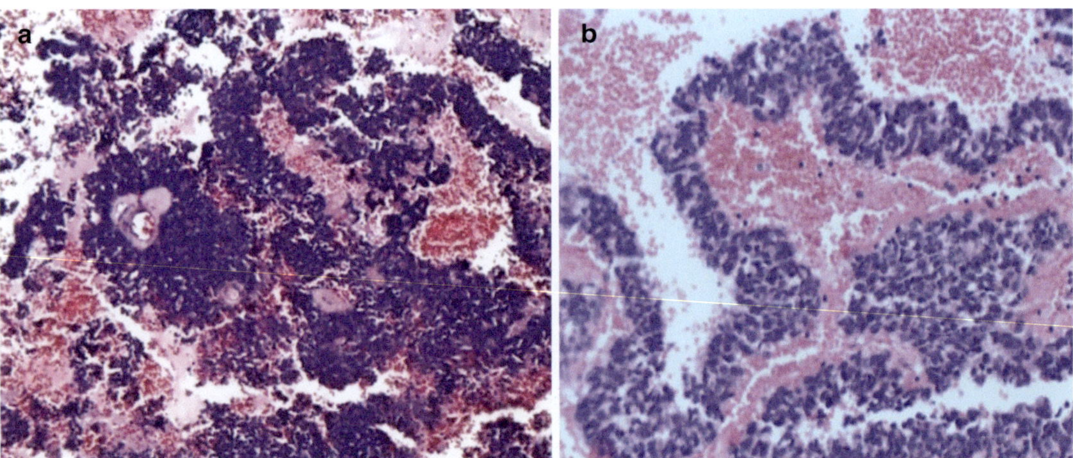

Fig. 8.12 (**a**) Ewing sarcoma with perivascular arrangement of tumour cells (perithelial pattern), H&E ×100. (**b**) H&E ×250

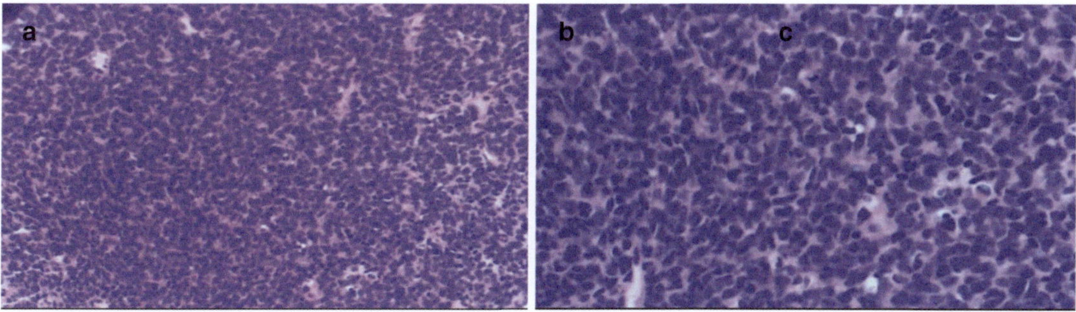

Fig. 8.13 (**a**) Ewing sarcoma with rosettes, H&E ×100. (**b**) H&E ×250

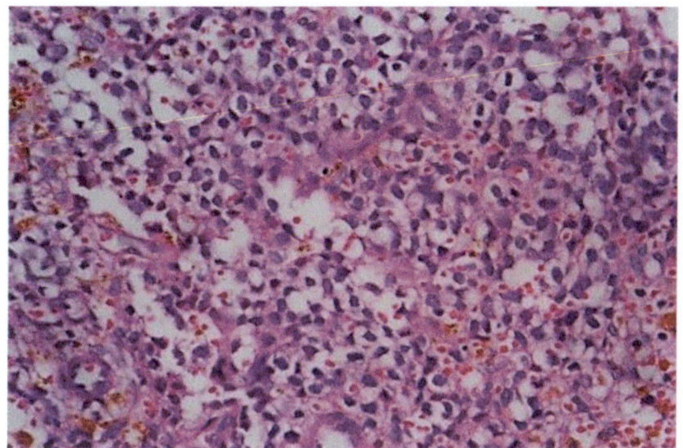

Fig. 8.14 Ewing sarcoma with haemangioendothelioma-like areas H&E ×100

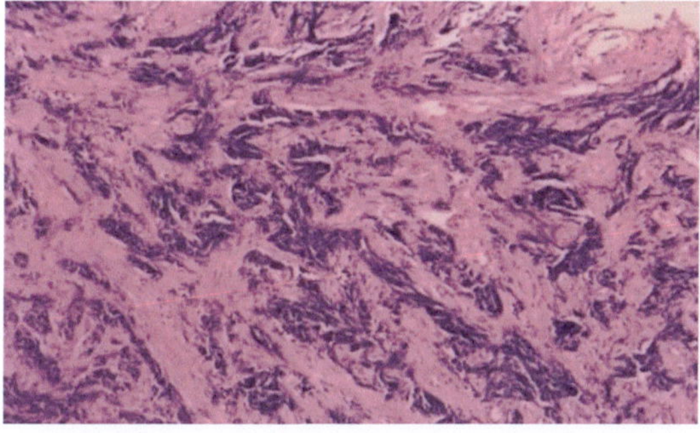

Fig. 8.15 Ewing sarcoma with crush artefact of tumour cells simulating lymphoma, H&E ×100

8.2.6 Immunohistochemistry

In over 95% of ES cases, CD99 shows crisp and strong membrane positivity [1] (Fig. 8.16). However, similar CD99 expression can be seen in other tumours like lymphoblastic leukaemia/lymphoma, rhabdomyosarcoma, round cell osteosarcoma and poorly differentiated synovial sarcoma. But these tumours may show cytoplasmic positivity also. A paranuclear dot-like positivity for CD99 can be rarely seen (Fig. 8.17), but this is considered as negative. The FLI1 antibody is now commonly used in the diagnosis of ES [14]. Its sensitivity is 63–100% and specificity 60–90% [18]. Monoclonal antibody has more specificity compared to polyclonal antibody (Fig. 8.18). The non-Ewing small round cell tumours can also express FLI1. But mesenchymal chondrosarcoma is negative for FLI1.

NKX2.2 is expressed in about 93% of ES [3] (Fig. 8.19). The staining is diffuse and strong. It is a member of NK2 family of transcription factors. Non-Ewing small round cell tumours positive for NKX2.2 are rare. Hence, it is considered as a useful marker for ES. NKX2.2 combined with crisp membrane positivity for CD99 gives 98% specificity for ES. Another tumour which gives diffuse and strong positivity for NKX2.2 is olfactory neuroblastoma [3]. Other round cell tumours like small cell carcinoma, synovial sarcoma and mesenchymal chondrosarcoma may show focal and weak staining. Cytokeratin is positive in 25% of cases of ES indicating epithelial differentiation (Fig. 8.20). Positivity for neural markers such as S-100 and neuroendocrine markers are sometimes detected in ES.

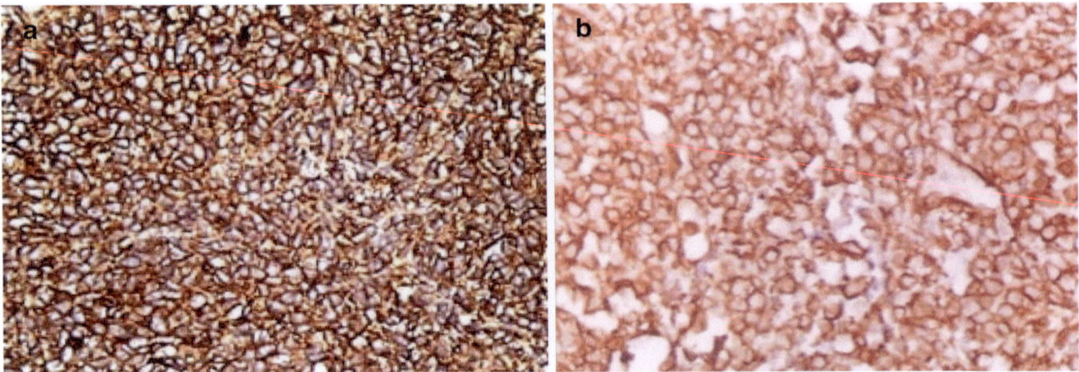

Fig. 8.16 IHC: (**a** and **b**) Crisp membrane positivity of CD99 (MIC2), ×100

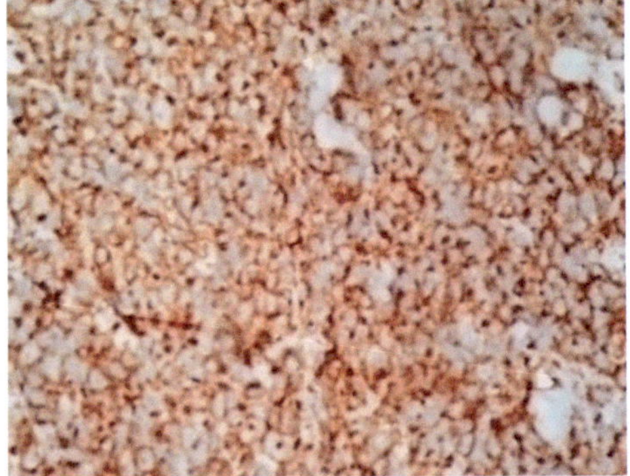

Fig. 8.17 Paranuclear dot positivity of CD99 in a case of large cell ES CD99, ×250. This finding is considered as negative for CD99. FISH confirmation mandatory in such cases

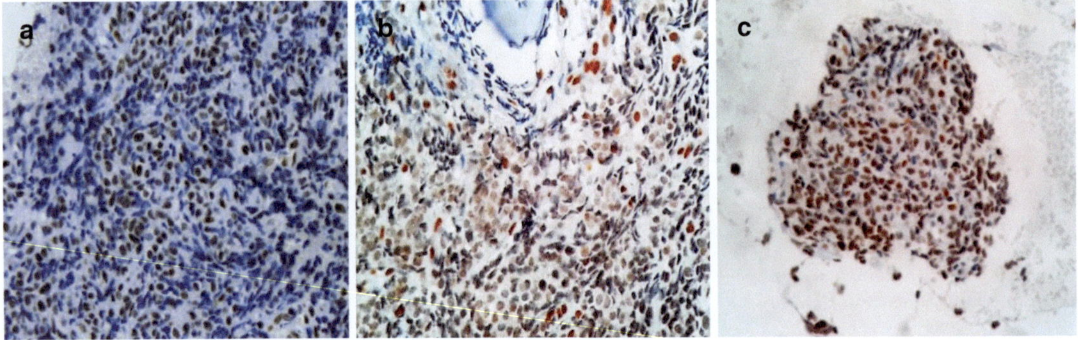

Fig. 8.18 IHC: FLI1 with strong nuclear positivity. (**a**–**c**) FLI1, ×100. FLI-1 is usually diffusely positive in the nuclei, but not a specific marker for ES. Internal control is endothelial cells

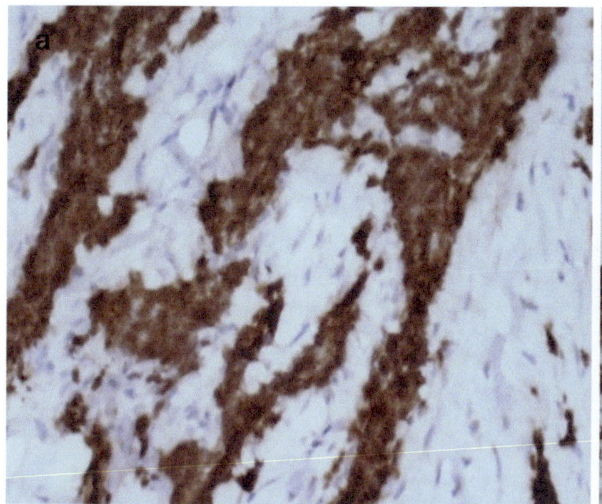

Fig. 8.19 IHC: ES in an 8-year-old girl. (**a** and **b**) NKX2.2 diffusely and strongly positive in nuclei showing extensive crush artefact NKX2.2, ×100. NKX2.2 is a very sensitive and reliable marker for ES. EWSR1 by FISH was positive in this case

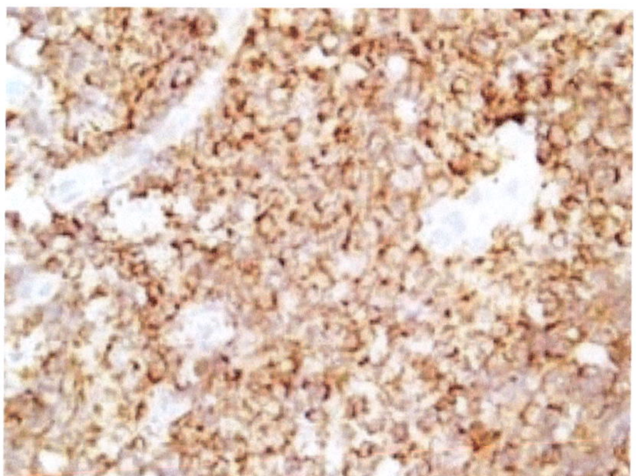

Fig. 8.20 Coexpression of cytokeratin in a case of ES in a 22-year-old female, CK ×100. This case was positive for EWSR1 FISH

8.2.7 DD

The differentiation of round cell tumours by IHC is given in Table 8.1.

8.2.8 Treatment Response

Ewing sarcoma cells may disappear completely after chemotherapy [16, 29]. Hence, there is a decrease in tumour volume after chemotherapy. This makes it difficult to assess the extent of necrosis as in osteosarcoma. There are two different methods of histologic assessment to assess the extent of necrosis. Huvos described a system similar to that of osteosarcoma samples. Necrosis is evaluated by taking full thickness of tumour as in osteosarcoma and grading the extent of necrosis relative to the percentage of residual viable tumour. The Huvos system includes four grades [24]. They involve 90–100% viability, necrosis of 50–90%, necrosis of 90–99% and 100% necrosis, respectively. Since this system is difficult in assessing necrosis in ES, Picci et al. proposed evaluating the amount of remaining viable tumour [24]. The absolute quantity of viable tumour cells is calculated. The scoring system proposed by Picci et al. includes three grades depending upon the number of low-power microscopic fields involved. This method is easy to interpret, but extensive sampling is required. The viable tumour cells are seen in the subperiosteal region, in soft tissue or in areas of haemorrhage. Recently, extracorporeal radiotherapy (ECRT) of the resected tumour during surgery and reimplantation of the same have been tried in Ewing sarcoma with good results [25].

Table 8.1 Differential diagnosis of malignant round cell tumours

Tumour type	CD99 (MIC2)	NKX2.2	Synaptophysin	Desmin	Myogenin	CK	LCA
ES	95%	100%	20%	–	–	+/–	–
NB	0%	+/–	95%	–	–	–	–
ARMS	20%	–	–	80%	90%	+/–	–
DSRCT	16%	–	5%	80%	–	90%	–
PD SS	50%	–	–	–	–	50%	–
ML	90%	–	–	–	–	–	90%

ES Ewing sarcoma, *NB* neuroblastoma, *ARMS* alveolar rhabdomyosarcoma, *DSRCT* desmoplastic small round cell tumour, *PD SS* poorly differentiated synovial sarcoma, *ML* malignant lymphoma, *CK* cytokeratin, *LCA* leucocyte common antigen

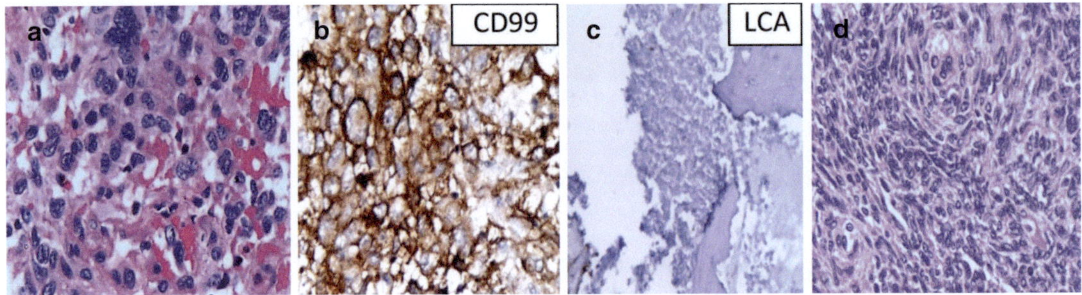

Fig. 8.21 ES after treatment. (**a**) Marked pleomorphism with convoluted nuclei resembling lymphoma, H&E ×400. (**b**) CD99 showed strong membrane positivity for CD99, ×250. (**c**) LCA was negative, LCA ×40. FISH for EWSR1 done on this case was positive. (**d**) Spindling of cells after treatment resembling spindle cell sarcoma

8.2.9 Post-treatment Morphologic Changes of Recurrent Tumours

Various post-chemotherapy changes [31] in the viable cells are nuclear membrane irregularity with pleomorphism resembling lymphoma (Fig. 8.21) or spindling of cells resembling spindle cell sarcoma-like osteosarcoma or fibrosarcoma. But all these cases showed CD99 membrane positivity with negative LCA. Confirmation by FISH for EWSR1 fusion transcript is mandatory in all cases.

8.2.10 Molecular Tests

Molecular techniques by demonstrating chromosomal translocations by reverse transcription polymerase chain reaction (RT-PCR) [17, 21] and fluorescent in situ hybridization (FISH) [28] are very useful in the confirmation of ES [43]. RT-PCR also helps in the detection of circulating tumour cells (sub-microscopic metastatic disease) in the blood or bone marrow. Probes for different translocations are available (Table 8.2). But most labs use EWSR1 break-apart probes for ES diagnosis.

Table 8.2 Types of translocations found in Ewing sarcoma

Translocation fusion gene	% of tumours exhibiting EWSR gene rearrangement
t (11;22)(q24;q12) EWSR1-FLI1	95%
t (21;22)(q22;q12) EWSR1-ERG	5%
t (7;22)(q22;q12) EWSR1-ETV1	Rare
t (17;22)(q21;q12) EWSR1-ETV4	Rare
t (2;22)(q35;q12) EWSR1-FEV	Rare

Break-apart probes are available for EWSR1 rearrangements (Fig. 8.22) [7, 25, 69]. EWSR1 rearrangements were first identified in Ewing sarcoma. Other tumours can also show EWSR1 rearrangement. They are desmoplastic small round cell tumour (DSRCT), myxoid liposarcoma (MLPS), extraskeletal myxoid chondrosarcoma (EMC), angiomatoid fibrous histiocytoma (AFH), clear cell sarcoma (CCS) and myoepithelial neoplasms. Hence, even if EWSR1 is positive, it has

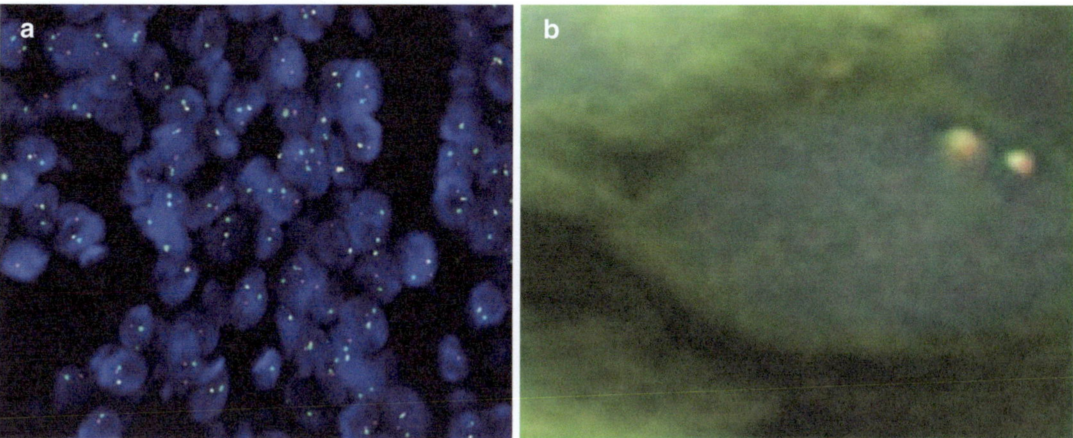

Fig. 8.22 ES: FISH for EWSR1. (**a**) EWSR1 break-apart probe—positive showing many break-apart red and green signals. (**b**) Another case—negative for EWSR1 showing fused signals

to be correlated with morphology and radiology in arriving at a diagnosis of ES.

8.2.11 ES Variants

A number of variants have been described in Ewing sarcoma [13]. All the variants should be confirmed by FISH test for EWSR1 or by RT-PCR. They are as follows:

- Atypical ES
- Adamantinoma-like ES
- Sclerosing ES
- Spindle cell sarcoma-like ES

8.2.11.1 Atypical ES [22]

The tumour cells of the atypical or large cell EFT are larger than classic EFT (20 and 24 μ). They are with vacuolated cytoplasm, irregular nuclear membranes and prominent nucleoli (Fig. 8.23). Sometimes, spindle cells can be seen.

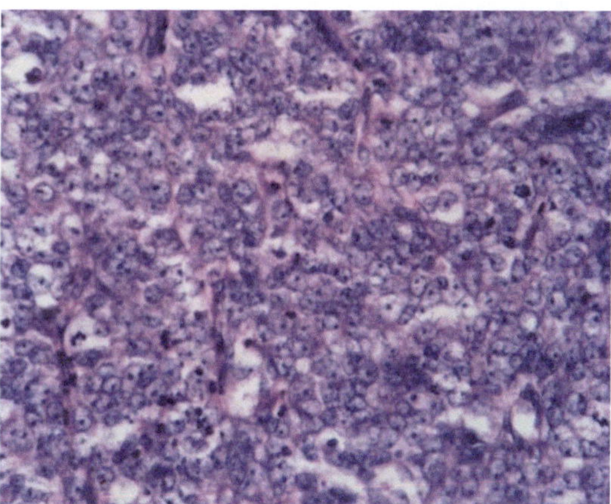

Fig. 8.23 Atypical large cell ES, H&E ×250. Cells with large vesicular nuclei with prominent nucleolus and scanty cytoplasm

The tumours are also positive for CD99 and FLI1 (Fig. 8.24) and show EWSR1 positivity by FISH. FISH test should be done in such cases for confirmation.

8.2.11.2 Adamantinoma-Like EFT

This is a rare variant usually seen in the tibia and fibula, head and neck region and also pelvis [19, 20]. They show morphological and immunohistochemical features similar to adamantinoma. The cells are seen arranged in nests with peripheral palisading. They are pleomorphic with a prominent desmoplastic stroma. Immunohistochemistry for cytokeratins and squamous markers is positive.

8.2.11.3 Sclerosing EFT

This tumour has hyalinized eosinophilic matrix and resembles sclerosing epithelioid fibrosarcoma or sclerosing rhabdomyosarcoma. Adequate sampling is required to demonstrate typical features of classical ES (Fig. 8.25).

8.2.11.4 Spindle Cell Sarcoma-Like EFT

Tumour cells are spindle shaped and resemble synovial sarcoma (Fig. 8.26).

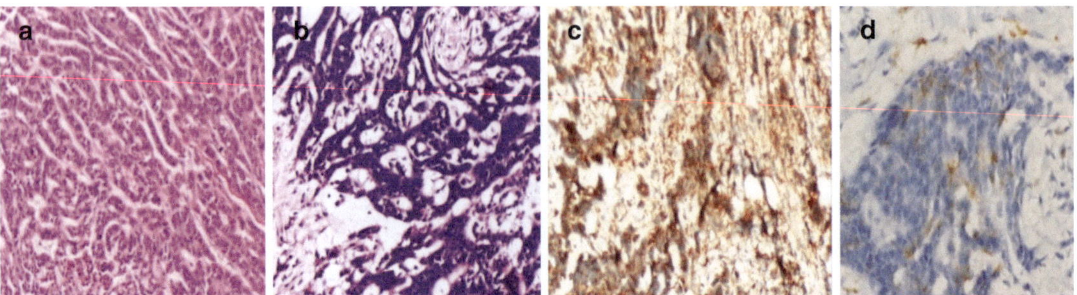

Fig. 8.24 ES—adamantinoma-like. (**a** and **b**) Cords and nests of cells, H&E ×100. (**c**) CD99 ×100. (**d**) Synaptophysin ×100. These cases should be confirmed by FISH

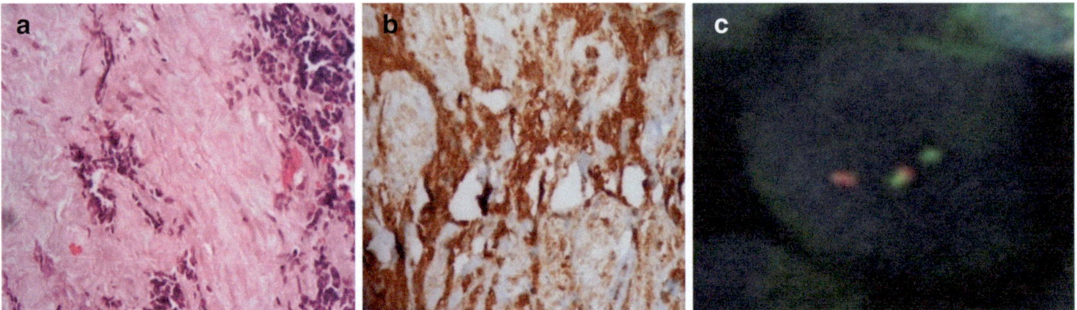

Fig. 8.25 (**a**) ES—sclerosing variant, H&E ×40. (**b**) CD99 ×100. (**c**) EWSR1-positive break-apart signals

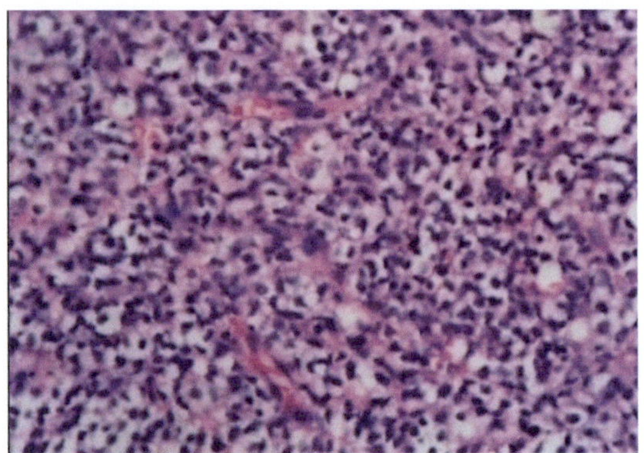

Fig. 8.26 ES showing spindling of cells resembling synovial sarcoma, H&E ×100

8.2.12 Treatment and Prognosis

Thirty-five percent of ES patients present with metastasis at the time of diagnosis [5, 23]. Patients with lung metastasis alone have a better prognosis. Other metastatic sites are bone or bone marrow. Survival has increased with new chemotherapeutic agents. But late relapses, even 10 years after treatment, have been reported. Size ≥8 cm and presence of metastatic disease are regarded as poor prognostic factors. Cases with p53 or p16/p14ARF genetic alterations have more aggressive behaviour. Their response to chemotherapy is poor. The occurrence of relapse can be predicted by the histologic response to initial chemotherapy.

8.3 Round Cell Sarcomas with EWSR1-Non-ETS Fusion

This entity is composed of round and spindle cells. EWSR1-NFATC2, FUS-NFATC2 and EWSR1-PATZ1 sarcomas come under this group. These sarcomas are rare [32, 33, 65, 66].

EWSR1-NFATC2 is seen predominantly in bone. Femur, humerus, radius and tibia are the common sites involved. It can also occur in soft tissue of extremities, head and neck and chest wall.

FUS-NFATC2 occurs exclusively in bones. But **EWSR1-PATZ1** sarcomas [66, 68] are more common in the deep soft tissue. Chest and abdomen are the common sites involved. They are also seen in head and neck, extremities and CNS.

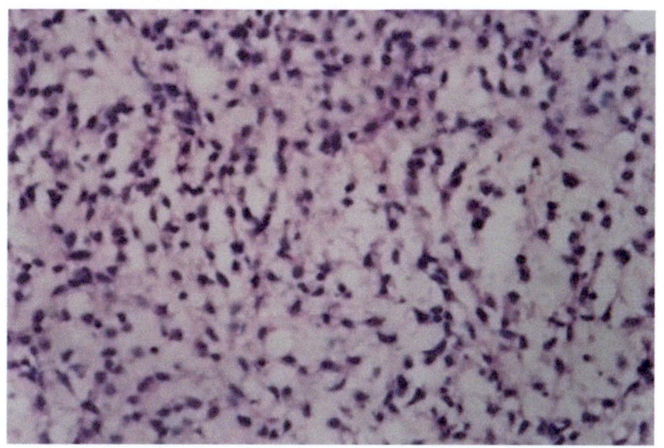

Fig. 8.27 Spindling of tumour cells in a myxoid background, H&E ×100

EWSR1-NFATC2 and FUS-NFATC2 sarcomas [32, 33] occur in children and adolescents, whereas EWSR1-PATZ1 occurs mainly in adults. EWSR1-NFATC2 and FUS-NFATC2 sarcomas show a male preponderance (M:F = 5:1).

8.3.1 Pathology

Grossly, these tumours are solid with firm or fleshy cut surface. EWSR1-PATZ1 sarcomas are solid and cystic.

Microscopy: The sarcomas with NFATC2 fusion are with round or spindle-shaped cells (Fig. 8.27) having clear-to-pale eosinophilic cytoplasm and monomorphic or markedly pleomorphic nuclei. Background shows myxomatous stroma. Tumour cells are arranged in cords, nests, trabecular or acinar pattern. Sometimes, sheets of cells without matrix may also be seen. Mitotic activity is variable. Areas of necrosis can be seen.

8.3.2 IHC

In 50% of cases, CD99 is strongly positive. NKX2.2 and PAX-7 can be positive. Dot-like staining of cytokeratin and focal positivity for CD138 may be present.

8.3.3 DD

Includes myoepithelial tumour, plasmacytoma and lymphomas.

8.3.4 EWSR1-PATZ1

EWSR1-PATZ1 sarcomas have small round and spindle cells in a fibrous stroma. Mitosis is sparse, and necrosis may be absent. IHC shows coexpression of desmin, myogenin and myo-D1 and neurogenic markers like S100, SOX10 and GFAP. CD99 is usually negative. CD34 can be positive.

8.3.5 Molecular Pathology

EWSR1-NFATC2 fusion genes arise from a derivative 22-ring chromosome and show amplification, whereas FUS-NFACT2 fusion gene does not show amplification. Hence, they are different from other undifferentiated round cell sarcomas like Ewing sarcomas, EWSR1-PATZ1 sarcomas and CIC rearranged and sarcomas with BCOR genetic alteration. PATZ1 gene is very close to EWSR1 focus, and interpretation of break-apart signal by FISH is difficult [67]. Fusion transcripts can be detected by next-generation sequencing (NGS).

8.3.6 Prognosis

Metastasis to lungs, bones and skin has been reported. Recurrences are common. Response to conventional chemotherapy is poor. EWSR1-PATZ1 sarcomas are found to be aggressive.

8.4 CIC-Rearranged Sarcoma

CIC-rearranged sarcomas are aggressive tumours arising in soft tissues of children and young adults. CIC-DUX4 Ewing-like sarcoma is an infrequent bone tumour (<5% of CIC-arranged sarcoma occurs in bone) [30, 34–36]. Since this tumour has morphological similarities for Ewing sarcoma, it is described here. CIC rearrangement is the most common genetic abnormality detected in EWSR1-negative small blue round cell tumours. They have a distinct pathogenesis. They show morphological overlap and variable CD99 positivity similar to ES.

8.4.1 Clinical

CIC-DUX4 sarcomas occur in the soft tissues of extremities and trunk, followed by viscera. Gastrointestinal and genitourinary regions are the main sites of visceral involvement. They are rare in the bone. Young males (25–35 years) are mainly affected. Ewing sarcoma mainly occurs in children (<15 years).

8.4.2 Pathology

Grossly, these are well-circumscribed tumours with a fleshy cut surface. Large areas of haemorrhage and necrosis can be seen. A mixture of round, spindle and epithelioid cells is seen in a lobulated pattern separated by fibrous stroma [38, 42]. The tumour cells are larger than ES cells and show more pleomorphism. Prominent nucleoli can be seen. The cytoplasm is abundant. The stroma shows myxoid change, which is a prominent feature of these tumours. This finding is absent in Ewing sarcoma. Necrosis and brisk mitotic activity are common.

8.4.3 IHC

CD99 expression is variable with some of them showing diffuse positivity and some being totally negative. In ES, it is diffuse and strong membranous reactivity with CD99. Nuclear WT1 positivity is seen in CIC-rearranged sarcomas, and this is a consistent finding. ETV4 will be positive in 95% of tumours. NKX2.2 is negative. CD31 and ERG positivity may be present [37].

8.4.4 Molecular

CIC-DUX4 gene fusion (t (4; 19) or t (10; 19) translocation) by FISH is the confirmatory test and is present in 95%.

8.4.5 Prognosis

CIC-rearranged tumours are aggressive tumours. They have a high metastatic rate, mainly to the lung. They do not respond to chemotherapy regimen given for ES. The 5-year survival rate is only 40–45%.

8.5 Sarcomas with BCOR Genetic Alterations (BCOR-CCNB3 Sarcoma)

Pierron et al. first described BCOR genetic alterations. Recurrent gene fusions of BCOR (encoding Bcl-6 interacting co-repressor) and CCNB3 (cyclin B3) were identified in a group of undifferentiated round cell sarcomas in adolescents and young adults [27, 39, 44, 45].

8.5.1 Clinical

This tumour predominantly occurs in males and is common in the second decade [43]. It usually arises in bone and frequently shows soft tissue extension. They may attain large size (median in one series 10 cm). The common sites of involvement are pelvis, lower limbs and paraspinal region. It is rarely seen in head and neck, lungs and kidney.

8.5.2 Radiology

These tumours are large with cortical destruction and soft tissue extension.

8.5.3 Pathology

They have a soft and fleshy cut surface. Microscopically, these tumours are cellular and composed of small round-to-plump cells with scanty pale-to-eosinophilic cytoplasm [41]. Nuclei are angulated and hyperchromatic with fine chromatin. Nucleoli are usually absent. Prominent mitotic activity and numerous apoptotic bodies will be seen (Fig. 8.28). Small areas of tumour cell necrosis can be seen. Cells may be short spindly in some cases. Prominent gaping vessels with intravascular thrombi are described. Some tumours show solid areas of plump spindle cells resembling synovial sarcoma. Recurrent sarcoma may show higher degree of pleomorphism with large, highly atypical spindle cells

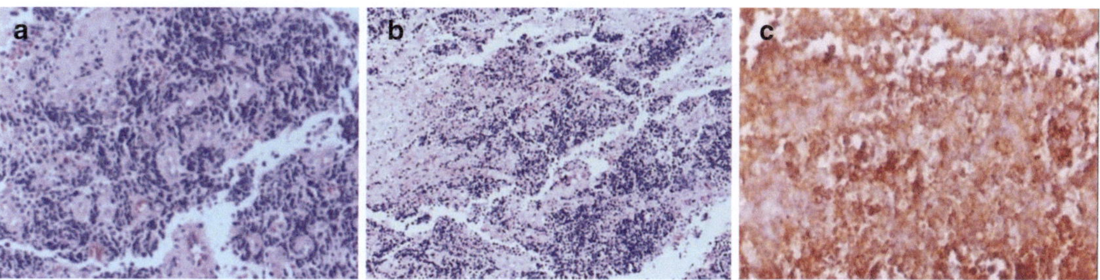

Fig. 8.28 (**a** and **b**) Round cells in fibrous stroma, H&E ×100. (**c**) CD99 with cytoplasmic positivity, ×100

Table 8.3 Undifferentiated small round cell sarcomas [42, 43, 45]

	ES	EWSR1-non-ETS-FUS-NFATC2	EWSR1-non-ETS EWSR1-PATZ1	CIC rearranged	Sarcoma with BCOR
Clinical	Bone and ST 88% bone, 12% ST	**Exclusively bone**	**ST** Chest wall, abdomen	**Deep ST** Bone <5%	Bone/ST 1.5:1 **Children: -males**
Cells	Uniform small round	**Round and spindle cells** in **myxohyaline background**	**Small round and/ or spindled** + fibrous stroma	Undifferentiated round cells. Rarely spindle/epithelioid	Small round cells, rich capillary network. Short spindle as in SS
CD99	95% membranous	50%	Not consistent	Patchy 80%; membranous in 20%	50%
CK	25%	Focal dot-like	–		–
NKX2.2	++	+/–	–	**Negative**	–
Other IHC	FLI1, ERG	CD138	**Myogenic and neurogenic**	**WT1** **ETV4** **NUT in CIC-NUTM1** CK, S100 Myogenic markers,Calretinin, ERG rarely	**SATB2** TLE1 Cyclin D1 **Cyclin B3**
Molecular	EWSR1-FLI1 (85%)	FUS-NFATC2	EWSR1-PATZ1	CIC-DUX4	BCOR-CCNB3 BCOR-ITD (infants)
Survival	65–70%	Better survival	Aggressive	Highly aggressive	72–80%

and osteoid deposition. Metastatic focus may also show similar morphology.

8.5.4 IHC

Immunohistochemical staining for BCOR and CCNB3 shows strong and diffuse positivity [40, 46]. Cyclin B3 is positive in BCOR-CCNB3 sarcomas. This is helpful to differentiate from other BCOR-positive tumours. SATB2, TLE1 and cyclin D1 are the other IHC markers positive in these tumours. CD99 shows weak positivity or may be completely absent [47].

8.5.5 Molecular

BCOR gene rearrangements and BCOR-ITD can be seen.

8.5.6 DD

Other undifferentiated round cell sarcomas like classic Ewing sarcoma, alveolar rhabdomyosarcoma and poorly differentiated synovial sarcomas are the main differentials. But all these tumours are negative for BCOR-CCNB3 fusion transcripts. See Table 8.3 for differentiating features of undifferentiated small round cell sarcomas of bone and soft tissue.

8.5.7 Treatment and Prognosis

Treatment is same as that of ES, and these tumours respond to Ewing sarcoma chemotherapy. Prognosis is also similar to ES. Some patients present with metastasis at the time of presentation. Metastasis occurs mainly to lung. Bone, viscera and soft tissue are other sites of metastasis.

8.6 Other Round Cell Tumours of Bone

Lymphomas (see chapter on haematological malignancies of bone), mesenchymal chondrosarcoma (see chapter on chondrosarcoma), small cell osteosarcomas (see chapter on osteosarcoma) and metastatic neuroblastomas are other round cell tumours of bone (see chapter on metastatic tumours of bone). Rhabdomyosarcomas, retinoblastoma (Fig. 8.30) and desmoplastic small round cell tumour (DSRCT) are primary soft tissue tumours, which rarely metastasize or directly involve bone. Langerhans cell histiocytosis can be a differential diagnosis of round cell tumours of bone (see chapter on histiocytic lesions).

8.7 Metastatic Neuroblastoma

Neuroblastoma (NB) is a primitive neoplasm of neuroectodermal origin [56]. It is the third most common malignant tumour in the childhood, following lymphoma/leukaemia and brain tumours. The peak incidence is 0–4 years (40% in less than 1 year) [55]. It is rarely diagnosed prenatally during the third trimester, on ultra sonogram. It occurs anywhere in the sympatho-adrenal neuroendocrine system. Bone and bone marrow are preferred sites of metastasis [49, 50, 54, 57]. All patients with metastatic (stage 4) disease are in the high-risk category [51, 53], especially those diagnosed after 18 months of age. At the time of diagnosis, the high-risk category includes age more than 1 year, metastases, amplification of the *MYCN* oncogene and unfavourable histology.

Histologically, malignant round cells with or without rosettes and neurofibrillary material are seen. If there are no rosettes or neurofibrillary material, IHC is mandatory. In children more than 5 years, the most important differential diagnoses are Ewing sarcoma, lymphoma/leukaemia and rarely small cell osteosarcoma. A panel of antibodies consisting of synaptophysin, chromogranin [48], NB84 [58], CD99, LCA and Tdt is mandatory. Cells of a neuroblastoma are diffusely positive for synaptophysin and chromogranin, while negative for CD99, LCA and Tdt (Figs. 8.29 and 8.30).

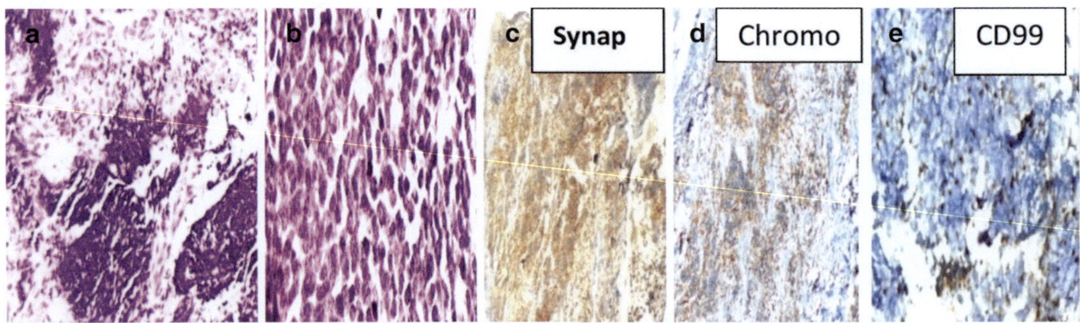

Fig. 8.29 (**a**) Metastatic neuroblastoma to mandible in a 2-year-old girl. H&E ×40. US abdomen revealed adrenal NB. (**b**) H&E ×250. (**c–e**) IHC: Synaptophysin and chromogranin are diffusely positive, and CD99 is negative, ×100

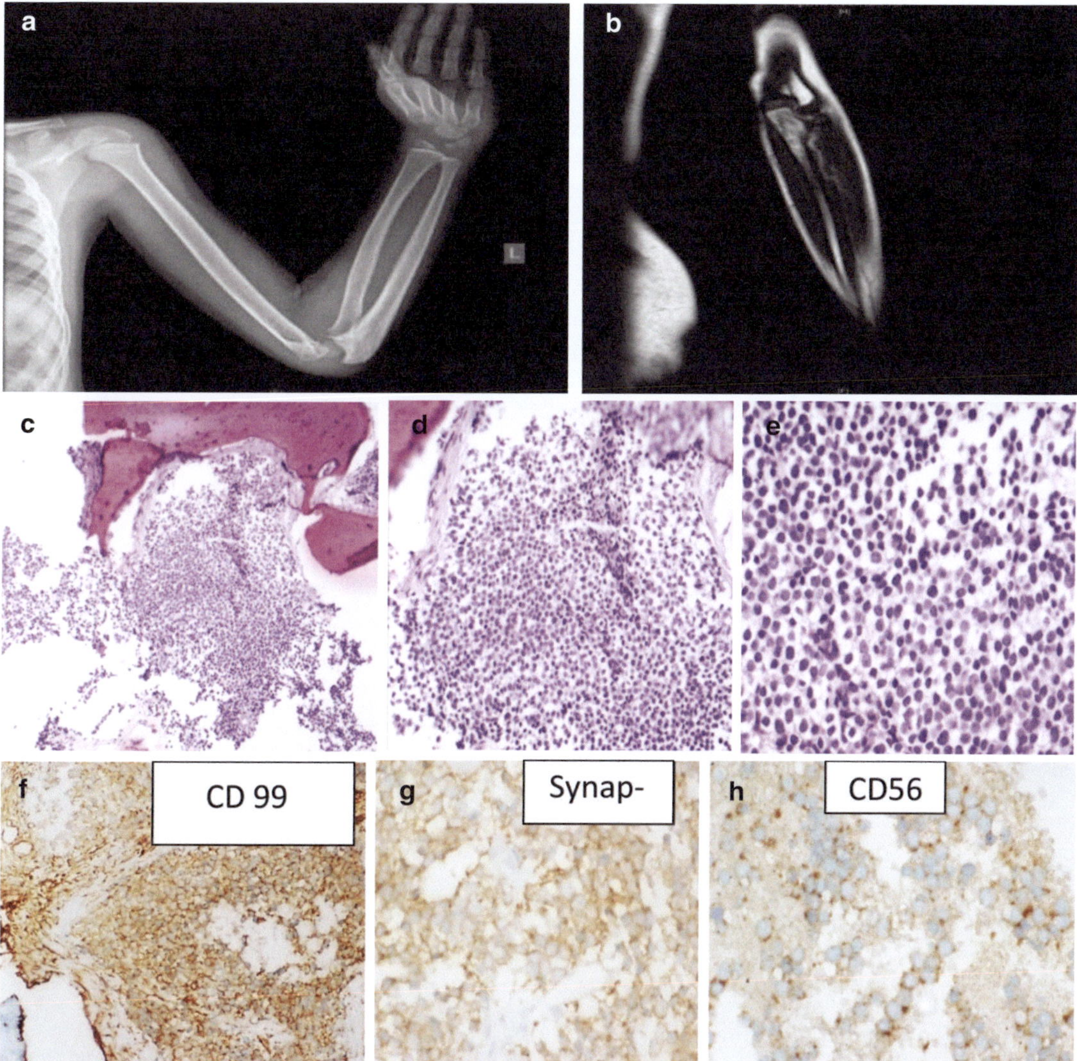

Fig. 8.30 Metastatic retinoblastoma to ulna in a 7-year-old child. Retinoblastoma was diagnosed when the child was 1 year old. (**a** and **b**) Plain X-ray and MRI of hand. (**c**) Bone with round cell neoplasm, H&E ×40. (**d**) H&E ×100. (**e**) Malignant round cells in sheets, H&E ×250. (**f**–**h**) IHC: Synaptophysin and CD56 were positive, and CD99 showed cytoplasmic positivity, ×100. As the clinical diagnosis was ES, FISH test for EWSR1 was done and was negative

PHOX2 is a useful marker in the diagnosis of peripheral neuroblastic tumours [52]. There is an unequivocal role of genetics in the diagnosis and prognosis of neuroblastomas, including N-myc amplification of the *MYCN* oncogene, and histologic findings.

8.8 Desmoplastic Small Round Cell Tumour of Bone (DSRCT)

Desmoplastic small round cell tumour (DSRCT) is an extremely rare malignant tumour occurring in the abdomen that usually affects adolescents and young males [59]. DSRCT may rarely metastasize to bone, but primary occurrence in bone is extremely rare. There are a few case reports of primary DSRCT of bone.

8.8.1 Clinical

DSRCT of bone has been reported in ilium, femur, skull, maxilla [63] and tibia. It occurs in children and young adults [62].

8.8.2 Radiology

No pathognomonic findings are described. Combination of PET/CT and MRI is done for the diagnosis of primary DSRCT of bone [64]. Tumour causes a wide area of destruction. The overlying cortex is thickened. PET/CT is commonly taken as part of workup.

8.8.3 Pathology

The tumour shows diffuse growth replacing marrow space. Cortical destruction is seen. Tumor cells are round with small amount of pale-to-clear cytoplasm. Nuclei are with fine chromatin and inconspicuous nucleoli. Desmoplastic stroma may be evident in resected tumours (Fig. 8.31).

8.8.4 IHC

Immunohistochemical staining shows multi-lineage potential with cells staining positive for CK, desmin, CD99, WT1 [60] and NSE

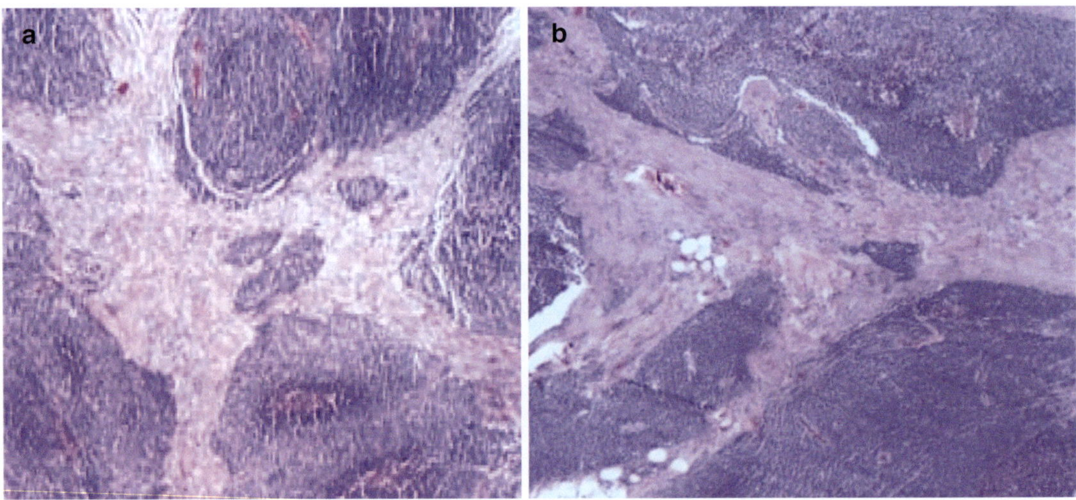

Fig. 8.31 DSRCT: (**a**) Small round cells in a desmoplastic stroma dividing the tumour into lobules, H&E ×100. (**b**) H&E ×250

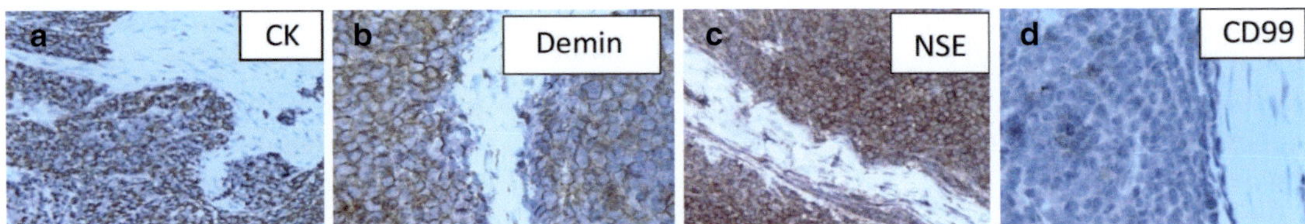

Fig. 8.32 DSRCT IHC: Multi-lineage of the tumour evident by positivity for (**a**) cytokeratin, (**b**) desmin, (**c**) NSE and (**d**) CD99. Unlike Ewing sarcoma, CD99 is weak and patchy, ×250

(Fig. 8.32). Desmin usually shows paranuclear dot positivity.

8.8.5 Molecular

FISH/RT-PCR is done for confirming EWS-WT1 gene rearrangement [61] [t (11; 22) (p13: q12)].

8.8.6 DD

Other malignant round cell tumours of bone like Ewing sarcoma, small cell osteosarcoma and malignant lymphoma. IHC and molecular tests help in diagnosis.

8.8.7 Treatment and Prognosis

Chemotherapy is the line of management as in other malignant round cell tumours. Prognosis is poor. Only 15–30% have 5-year overall survival.

Points to Remember

- Malignant round cell tumours are a heterogeneous group of tumours.
- Ancillary testing is essential for proper categorization.
- NKX2.2 is a reliable marker for Ewing sarcoma.
- CIC-rearranged sarcoma is more common in soft tissue. They do not respond to chemotherapy and is an aggressive tumour.
- Sarcoma with BCOR genetic alteration has a better prognosis and responds to chemotherapy.
- Metastatic neuroblastoma is the commonest round cell tumour in children below 5 years, and they are usually negative for CD99.
- In desmoplastic small round cell tumour, multiple IHC markers are positive.

References

Ewing Sarcoma

1. Ambros IM, Ambros PF, Strehl S, Kovar H, Gadner H, Salzer-Kuntschik M. MIC2 is a specific marker for Ewing's sarcoma and peripheral primitive neuroectodermal tumors. Evidence for a common histogenesis of Ewing's sarcoma and peripheral primitive neuroectodermal tumors from MIC2 expression and specific chromosome aberration. Cancer. 1991;67(7):1886–93.
2. Arvand A, Denny CT. Biology of EWS/ETS fusions in Ewing's family tumors. Oncogene. 2001;20:5747–54.
3. Yoshida A, Sekine S, Tsuta K, Fukayama M, Furuta K, Tsuda H. NKX2.2 is a useful immunohistochemical marker for Ewing sarcoma. Am J Surg Pathol. 2012;36:993–9.
4. Askin FB, Rosai J, Sibley RK, Dehner LP, McAlister WH. Malignant small cell tumor of the thoracopulmonary region in childhood: a distinctive clinicopathologic entity of uncertain histogenesis. Cancer. 1979;43(6):2438–51.
5. Bacci G, Ferrari S, Bertoni F, Rimondini S, Longhi A, Bacchini P, Forni C, Manfrini M, Donati D, Picci P. Prognostic factors in nonmetastatic Ewing's sarcoma of bone treated with adjuvant chemotherapy: analysis of 359 patients at the Instituto Ortopedico Rizzoli. J Clin Oncol. 2000;18:4–11.
6. Barr FG, Womer RB. Molecular diagnosis of Ewing family tumors: too many fusions? J Mol Diagn. 2007;9(4):437–40. https://doi.org/10.2353/jmoldx.2007.070080.
7. Baldauf MC, Orth MF, Dallmayer M, et al. Robust diagnosis of Ewing sarcoma by immunohistochemical detection of super-enhancer-driven EWSR1-ETS targets. Oncotarget. 2018;9:1587–601.
8. Kelleher C, Thomas DM. Molecular pathogenesis and targeted therapeutics in Ewing sarcoma/primitive neuroectodermal tumours. Clin Sarcoma Res. 2012;2(1):6.
9. Siligan C, Ban J, Bachmaier R, et al. EWS-FLI1 target genes recovered from Ewing's sarcoma chromatin. Oncogene. 2005;24(15):2512–24.
10. Sharrocks D. The ETS-domain transcription factor family. Nat Rev Mol Cell Biol. 2001;2(11):827–37.
11. de Alava E, Lessnick SL, Sorensen PH. Ewing sarcoma. In: Fletcher CDM, Bridge JA, Hogendoorn PCW, Mertens F, editors. WHO classification of tumours of soft tissue and bone. Lyon: WHO Press; 2013. p. 305–9.

12. Delattre O, Zucman J, Plougastel B, Desmaze C, Melot T, Peter M, Kovar H, Joubert I, de Jong P, Rouleau G, Aurias A, Thomas G. Gene fusion with an ETS DNA-binding domain caused by chromosome translocation in human tumours. Nature. 1992;359(6391):162–5.
13. Folpe AL, Goldblum JR, Rubin BP, Shehata BM, Liu W, Dei Tos AP, Weiss SW. Morphologic and immunophenotypic diversity in Ewing family tumors: a study of 66 genetically confirmed cases. Am J Surg Pathol. 2005;29(8):1025–33.
14. Folpe AL, Hill CE, Parham DM, O'Shea PA, Weiss SW. Immunohistochemical detection of FLI-1 protein expression: a study of 132 round cell tumours with emphasis of CD99-positive mimics of Ewings's sarcoma/primitive neuroectodermal tumour. Am J Surg Pathol. 2004;24:1657–62.
15. Maire G, Brown CW, Bayani J, et al. Complex rearrangement of chromosomes 19, 21, and 22 in Ewing sarcoma involving a novel reciprocal inversion-insertion mechanism of EWS-ERG fusion gene formation: a case analysis and literature review. Cancer Genet Cytogenet. 2008;181(2):81–92.
16. García-Castellano JM, Yordi A, Nagib H, John H. Histopathologic and radiologic assessment of chemotherapeutic response in Ewing's sarcoma: a review. Sarcoma. 2012;2012:357424, 8 pages. https://doi.org/10.1155/2012/357424.
17. Downing JR, Head DR, Parham DM, et al. Detection of the (11;22)(q24;q12) translocation of Ewing's sarcoma and peripheral neuroectodermal tumor by reverse transcription polymerase chain reaction. Am J Pathol. 1993;143(5):1294–300.
18. Jeon IS, Davis JN, Braun BS, Sublett JE, Roussel MF, Denny CT, Shapiro DN. A variant Ewing's sarcoma translocation (7; 22) fuses the EWS gene to the ETS gene ETV1. Oncogene. 1995;10(6):1229–34.
19. Bishop JA, Alaggio R, Zhang L, Seethala RR, Antonescu CR. Adamantinoma-like Ewing family tumors of the head and neck: a pitfall in the differential diagnosis of basaloid and myoepithelial carcinomas. Am J Surg Pathol. 2015;39(9):1267–74.
20. Mahadevan P, Ramkumar S, Gangadharan VP. Adamantinoma-like Ewing's family tumor of the Sino nasal region: a case report and a brief review of literature. Case Rep Pathol. 2019;2019:5158182, 6 pages. https://doi.org/10.1155/2019/51581822019.
21. Mangham DC, Williams A, McMullan DJ, McClure J, Sumathi VP, Grimer RJ, Davies AM. Ewing's sarcoma of bone: the detection of specific transcripts in a large, consecutive series of formalin-fixed, decalcified, paraffin-embedded tissue samples using the reverse transcriptase-polymerase chain reaction. Histopathology. 2006;48:363–76.
22. Nascimento AG, Unii KK, Pritchard DJ, Cooper KL, Dahlin DC. A clinicopathologic study of 20 cases of large-cell (atypical) Ewing's sarcoma of bone. Am J Surg Pathol. 1980;4(1):29–36.
23. Ozaki T. Diagnosis and treatment of Ewing sarcoma of the bone: a review article. J Orthop Sci. 2015;20(2):250–63.
24. Picci P, Rougraff BT, Bacci G, Neff JR, Sangiorgi L, Cazzola A, Baldini N, Ferrari S, Mercuri M, Ruggieri P. Prognostic significance of histopathologic response to chemotherapy in nonmetastatic Ewing's sarcoma of the extremities. J Clin Oncol. 1993;11:1763–9.
25. Puri A, Gulia A, Agarwal MG, Jambhekar NA, Laskar S. Extracorporeal irradiated tumor bone: a reconstruction option in diaphyseal Ewing's sarcomas. Indian J Orthop [serial online]. 2010 [cited 2012 Nov 13];44:390–396.
26. Rekhi B, Mridha A, Kattoor J. Small round cell lesions of the bone: diagnostic approach, differential diagnoses and impact on treatment. Indian J Pathol Microbiol. 2019;62(2):199–205.
27. Rekhi B, Kembhavi P, Mishra SN, Shetty O, Bajpai J, Puri A. Clinicopathologic features of undifferentiated round cell sarcomas of bone & soft tissues: an attempt to unravel the *BCOR-CCNB3- & CIC-DUX4*-positive sarcomas. Indian J Med Res. 2019;150(6):557–74.
28. Rekhi B, Vogel U, Basak R, Desai SB, Jambhekar NA. Clinicopathological and molecular spectrum of Ewing sarcomas/PNETs, including validation of EWSR1 rearrangement by conventional and array FISH technique in certain cases. Pathol Oncol Res. 2014;20(3):503–16.
29. Rosen G, Juergens H, Caparros B, Nirenberg A, Huvos AG, Marcove RC. Combination chemotherapy (T-6) in the multidisciplinary treatment of Ewing sarcoma. Natl Cancer Inst Monogr. 1981;56:289–99.
30. Siegele B, Roberts J, Black JO, Rudzinski E, Vargas SO, Galambos C. DUX4 immunohistochemistry is a highly sensitive and specific marker for CIC-DUX4 fusion-positive round cell tumor. Am J Surg Pathol. 2017;41(3):423–9.
31. Van der Woude HJ, Bloem JL, Taminiau AHM, Nooy MA, Hogendoorn PC. Classification of histopathologic changes following chemotherapy in Ewing's sarcoma of bone. Skeletal Radiol. 1994;23:501–7.
32. Wang GY, Thomas DG, Davis JL, Ng T, Patel RM, Harms PW, Betz BL, Schuetze SM, McHugh JB, Horvai AE, Cho SJ, Lucas DR. EWSR1-NFATC2 translocation-associated sarcoma clinicopathologic findings in a rare aggressive primary bone or soft tissue tumor. Am J Surg Pathol. 2019;43(8):1112–22.
33. Yoshida A, Hashimoto T, Ryo E, Yoshida KI, Motoi T, Yatabe Y, Mori T. Confirmation of NKX3-1 expression in EWSR1-NFATC2 sarcoma and mesenchymal chondrosarcoma using monoclonal antibody immunohistochemistry, RT-PCR, and RNA in situ hybridization. Am J Surg Pathol. 2021;45(4):578–82.

CIC-Rearranged Sarcoma

34. Antonescu CR, Owosho AA, Zhang L, et al. Sarcomas with CIC-rearrangements are a distinct pathologic entity with aggressive outcome: a clinicopathologic and molecular study of 115 cases. Am J Surg Pathol. 2017;41(7):941–9.

35. Italiano A, Sung YS, Zhang L, et al. High prevalence of *CIC* fusion with double-homeobox (DUX4) transcription factors in *EWSR1*-negative undifferentiated small blue round cell sarcomas. Genes Chromosomes Cancer. 2012;51:207–18.
36. Brcic I, Brodowicz T, Cerroni L, Kashofer K, Serbanescu GL, Kasseroler MT, Amann G, Scheipl S, Szkandera J, Leithner A, Liegl-Atzwanger B. Undifferentiated round cell sarcomas with CIC-DUX4 gene fusion: expanding the clinical spectrum. Pathology. 2020;52(2):236–42.
37. Kojima N, Arai Y, Satomi K, et al. Co-expression of ERG and CD31 in a subset of CIC-rearranged sarcoma: a potential diagnostic pitfall. Mod Pathol. 2022;35:1439–48.
38. Yamada Y, Kuda M, Kohashi K, et al. Histological and immunohistochemical characteristics of undifferentiated small round cell sarcomas associated with CIC-DUX4 and BCORCCNB3 fusion genes. Virchows Arch. 2017;470:373–80.

BCOR-CCNB3 Sarcoma

39. Alfaro-Cervello C, Andrade-Gamarra V, Nieto G, et al. Congenital undifferentiated sarcoma associated to BCORCCNB3 gene fusion. Pathol Res Pract. 2017;213:1435–9.
40. Kao YC, Sung YS, Zhang L, et al. BCOR overexpression is a highly sensitive marker in round cell sarcomas with BCOR genetic abnormalities. Am J Surg Pathol. 2016;40:1670–8.
41. Li WS, Liao IC, Wen MC, et al. BCOR-CCNB3-positive soft tissue sarcoma with round-cell and spindle-cell histology: a series of four cases highlighting the pitfall of mimicking poorly differentiated synovial sarcoma. Histopathology. 2016;69: 792–801.
42. Matsuyama A, Shiba E, Umekita Y, et al. Clinicopathologic diversity of undifferentiated sarcoma with *BCOR-CCNB3* fusion: analysis of 11 cases with a reappraisal of the utility of immunohistochemistry for BCOR and CCNB3. Am J Surg Pathol. 2017;41:1713–21.
43. Peters TL, Kumar V, Polikepahad S, et al. BCOR-CCNB3 fusions are frequent in undifferentiated sarcomas of male children. Mod Pathol. 2015;28:575–86.
44. Pierron G, Tirode F, Lucchesi C, et al. A new subtype of bone sarcoma defined by BCOR-CCNB3 gene fusion. Nat Genet. 2012;44:461–6.
45. Puls F, Niblett A, Marland G, Gaston CL, Douis H, Mangham DC, Sumathi VP, Kindblom LG. BCOR-CCNB3 (Ewing-like) sarcoma: a clinicopathologic analysis of 10 cases, in comparison with conventional Ewing sarcoma. Am J Surg Pathol. 2014;38(10):1307–18.
46. Shibayama T, Okamoto T, Nakashima Y, et al. Screening of BCOR-CCNB3 sarcoma using immunohistochemistry for CCNB3: a clinicopathological report of three pediatric cases. Pathol Int. 2015;65:410–4.
47. Sumathi VP, Kindblom L-G. BCOR-CCNB3 (Ewing-like) sarcoma—a clinicopathologic analysis of 10 cases, in comparison with conventional Ewing sarcoma. Am J Surg Pathol. 2014;38:1307–18.

Neuroblastoma

48. Carlei F, Polak JM, Ceccamea A, Marangos PJ, Dahl D, Cocchia D, Michetti F, Lezoche E, Speranza V. Neuronal and glial markers in tumours of neuroblastic origin. Virchows Arch A Pathol Anat Histopathol. 1984;404(3):313–24.
49. Botía González CM, Sirvent Cerdá SI, Azorín D. Bone metastasis of primitive occult neuroblastoma. https://doi.org/10.1594/EURORAD/CASE.
50. Brignole C, Pastorino F, Perri P, Amoroso L, Bensa V, Calarco E, Ponzoni M, Corrias MV. Bone marrow environment in metastatic neuroblastoma. Cancers. 2021;13:2467.
51. DuBois SG, Kalika Y, Lukens JN, et al. Metastatic sites in stage IV and IVS neuroblastoma correlate with age, tumor biology, and survival. J Pediatr Hematol Oncol. 1999;21:181–9.
52. Bielle F, Fréneaux P, Jeanne-Pasquier C, Maran-Gonzalez A, Rousseau A, Lamant L, Paris R, Pierron G, Nicolas AV, Sastre-Garau X, Delattre O, Bourdeaut F, Peuchmaur M. PHOX2B immunolabeling—a novel tool for the diagnosis of undifferentiated neuroblastomas among childhood small round blue-cell tumors. Am J Surg Pathol. 2012;36:1141–9.
53. Huang C, Jiang S, Liao X, Li Y, Li S, Yang J. Bone and bone marrow involvement in neuroblastoma. Medicine (Baltimore). 2020;99(2):e22505. https://doi.org/10.1097/MD.0000000000022505.
54. Granchi D, Corrias MV, Garaventa A, Baglìo SR, Cangemi G, Carlini B, Paolucci P, Giunti A, Baldini N. Neuroblastoma and bone metastases: clinical significance and prognostic value of Dickkopf 1 plasma levels. Bone. 2011;48(1):152–9.
55. Hubbard AK, Spector LG, Fortuna G, et al. Trends in international incidence of pediatric cancers in children under 5 year of age: 1988-2012. JNCI Cancer Spectr. 2019;3:pkz007.
56. Shohet J, Foster J. A review and update on neuroblasoma. BMJ. 2017;357:j1863.
57. Kuroda T, Morikawa N, Matsuoka K, Fujino A, Honna T, Nakagawa A, Kumagai M, Masaki H, Saeki M. Prognostic significance of circulating tumor cells and bone marrow micrometastasis in advanced neuroblastoma. J Pediatr Surg. 2008;43(12):2182–5.
58. Miettinen M, Chatten J, Paetau A, Stevenson A. Monoclonal antibody NB84a in the differential diagnosis of neuroblastoma and other small round cell tumors. Am J Surg Pathol. 1998;22:327–32.

DSRCT

59. Gerald WL, Miller HK, Battifora H, Miettinen M, Silva EG, Rosai J. Intra-abdominal desmoplastic small round-cell tumor. Report of 19 cases of a distinctive type of high-grade polyphenotypic malignancy affecting young individuals. Am J Surg Pathol. 1991;15(6):499–513.
60. Hill DA, Pfeifer JD, Marley EF, Dehner LP, Humphrey PA, Zhu X, Swanson PE. WT1 staining reliably differentiates desmosplastic small round cell tumour from Ewing sarcoma/primitive neuroectodermal tumour. Am J Clin Pathol. 2000;114:345–53.
61. Ladanyi M, Gerald WL. Specificity of the EWS/WT1 gene fusion for desmoplastic small round cell tumour. J Pathol. 1996;180(4):462.
62. Murphy A, Stallings RL, Howard J, O'Sullivan M, Hayes R, Breatnach F, McDermotta MB. Primary desmoplastic small round cell tumour of bone: report of a case with cytogenetic confirmation. Cancer Genet Cytogenet. 2005;156:167–71.
63. Rekhi B, Basak R, Desai SB, Jambhekar NA. t (11; 22) (p13; q12) EWS-WT 1 positive desmoplastic small round cell tumor of the maxilla: an unusual case indicating the role of molecular diagnosis in round cell sarcomas. J Postgrad Med. 2010;56(3): 201–5.
64. Tateishi U, Hasegawa T, Kusumoto M, Oyama T, Ishikawa H, Moriyama N. Desmoplastic small round cell tumor: imaging findings associated with clinicopathologic features. J Comput Assist Tomogr. 2002;26:579–83.

EWSR1-Non-ETS Sarcoma

65. Bode-Lesniewska B, Fritz C, Exner GU, Wagner U, Fuchs B. EWSR1-NFATC2 and FUS-NFATC2 gene fusion-associated mesenchymal tumors: clinicopathologic correlation and literature review. Sarcoma. 2019;2019:9386390. https://doi.org/10.1155/2019/9386390.
66. Chougule A, Taylor MS, Nardi V, et al. Spindle and round cell sarcoma with EWSR1-PATZ1 gene fusion: a sarcoma with polyphenotypic differentiation. Am J Surg Pathol. 2019;43(2):220–8.
67. Flucke U, van Noesel MM, Siozopoulou V, Creytens D, Tops BBJ, van Gorp JM, Hiemcke-Jiwa LS. EWSR1—the most common rearranged gene in soft tissue lesions, which also occurs in different bone lesions: an updated review. Diagnostics (Basel). 2021;11:1093.
68. Michal M, Rubin BP, Agaimy A, et al. EWSR1-PATZ1-rearranged sarcoma: a report of nine cases of spindle and round cell neoplasms with predilection for thoracoabdominal soft tissues and frequent expression of neural and skeletal muscle markers. Mod Pathol. 2021;34:770–85.
69. Tsuda Y, Zhang L, Meyers P, Tap WD, Healey JH, Antonescu CR. The clinical heterogeneity of round cell sarcomas with EWSR1/FUS gene fusions: impact of gene fusion type on clinical features and outcome. Genes Chromosomes Cancer. 2020;59(9):525–34.
70. WHO Classification of Tumours. In: WHO Classification of Tumours Editorial Board, editor. Soft tissue and bone tumours. WHO classification of tumours, 5th ed., vol. 3. IARC; 2020.

9 Haematological Neoplasms of Bone

9.1 Plasma Cell Myeloma

Myeloma is a haematological malignancy, and it is the most common primary neoplasm of bone. Multiple myeloma (MM) is a plasma cell dyscrasia. Monoclonal plasma cells in the bone marrow undergo malignant transformation, resulting in increased production of monoclonal immunoglobulins. This in turn causes end-organ damage like lytic lesions of bone, renal failure, anaemia and hypercalcaemia. This is called CRAB criteria—hypercalcaemia, renal failure, anaemia and lytic bone lesions. Classification of plasma cell neoplasm is given in Table 9.1.

Bone disease is a prominent criterion to diagnose MM [1, 10]. 80% of the patients present with osteolytic lesions at diagnosis. Pathological fracture is common in myeloma patients (60%).

Myeloma bone disease (MBD) consists of a single lytic lesion in any part of skeleton with osteopenia. The bones commonly affected are that of skull, vertebrae and long bones. The prognosis is poor if the number of lesions is more.

Table 9.1 Classification of plasma cell neoplasms

Classification of plasma cell neoplasm (WHO 2017—Revised 4th edition) [19]
Non-IgM monoclonal gammopathy of undetermined significance
Plasma cell myeloma
Plasmacytoma
Monoclonal immunoglobulin deposition diseases
Plasma cell neoplasms with associated paraneoplastic syndrome

9.1.1 Pathophysiology of Myeloma Bone Disease

The main mechanism of MBD is increased osteoclastogenesis with decreased osteoblastic activity [5, 6]. There are certain factors involved in this mechanism. During progression to plasma cell myeloma, osteolysis releases growth factors embedded in bone matrix resulting in increased osteoclastic activity. Receptor activator of nuclear factor kappa-B ligand (RANKL) [9, 14] and osteoprotegerin (OPG) system have an important role in the pathogenesis [2, 3].

The coupling mechanism by osteoclasts and osteoblasts that is involved in bone remodelling is lost in MM. Increased osteoclastic activity and reduced bone formation result in extensive bone loss. In metastasis from breast and prostate, the osteoclastic as well as osteoblastic activity is increased.

9.1.2 Clinical Features

Most of the myeloma patients present with haematologic problems. Myeloma is a disease of adults above 40 years of age [8]. It is more common in males. The bones containing haematopoietic marrow are mostly affected. Pain, neurologic

J. Kattoor et al., *Bone Tumors*, https://doi.org/10.1007/978-981-99-4738-6_9

symptoms and pathological fracture are the common presenting symptoms. Osteosclerotic myeloma is associated with peripheral neuropathy. Usually, diagnosis is made by laboratory findings and bone marrow examination.

9.2 Solitary plasmacytoma of bone (SPB)

involves single site of abnormal growth of plasma cells. It can be within bone or extraskeletal in location. Risk of developing multiple myeloma is high in these patients. Solitary plasmacytoma of bone is an intraosseous neoplasm without involvement of other bones, with proliferation of clonal plasma cells. There will be no evidence of plasma cell myeloma (PCM) elsewhere.
More than 50% of tumours are seen in axial skeleton. Vertebra followed by pelvis, long bones, ribs, skull and clavicle are the common sites. It rarely affects small bones of hands and feet. Most cases progress to plasma cell myeloma. Patients have serum or urinary M component. When plasmacytoma is diagnosed, a workup for plasma cell myeloma should be done. Laboratory diagnosis of myeloma is as per ASCO guidelines [11].

9.2.1 Pathogenesis

Immunoglobulin heavy- and light-chain genes show clonal rearrangement with mutations in the variable region of heavy-chain gene.

9.2.2 Laboratory findings

ASCO guidelines are followed [11] for the diagnosis of myeloma:

- Serum calcium level [40]: higher than the upper limit of normal (>1 mg/dL higher than upper limit of normal or >11 mg/dL).
- Alkaline phosphatase: lower or normal. Alkaline phosphatase values especially the bone-specific alkaline phosphatase are useful in differentiating metastatic tumours and other bone lesions [12].
- Renal insufficiency (creatinine >2 mg/dL or creatinine clearance <40 mL/min).
- Anaemia (haemoglobin <10 g/dL).

Serum-free light chain (SFLC) testing is useful in diagnosing and monitoring plasma cell disorders (dyscrasias). Light chains are proteins produced by plasma cells.

9.2.3 Radiology

Punched-out areas of bone destruction (moth-eaten appearance) are the classical finding. This is seen mainly in ribs, pelvic bones, sternum, skull and vertebrae. Associated osteoporosis is common. Ballooned-out expansion of bone can be seen. Metastatic carcinomas, lymphomas and hyperparathyroidism can have similar radiological findings as in myeloma. But myelomas are not positive on bone scan, whereas metastasis and lymphomas are positive. As there is no bone formation in response to bone destruction, bone scan is normal in myeloma. Solitary plasmacytomas are usually lytic and expansile. Sclerotic myelomas have a rim of sclerosis around a lytic area or are completely sclerotic as in blastic metastasis. Combined morphological and functional MRI provides optimal bone marrow assessment for staging [19].

9.2.4 Pathology

Gross appearance of myeloma is fleshy dark red or brown mass [28]. They are soft and friable. Sometimes, they can be white fish-flesh appearance as in lymphoma. Soft tissue extension is evident in some cases. Rarely, extensive amyloid with grey, waxy appearance may be present.

Microscopy: Microscopic examination will show sheets of mature and immature plasma cells with or without amyloid [10, 16]. Amyloid shows positivity for Congo red, and under polarizer, it shows apple green birefringence (Figs. 9.1, 9.2, 9.3, and 9.4). Sometimes, increased number of plasmablasts with nucleoli can be seen. Rarely, undifferentiated highly pleomorphic cells indistinguishable from lymphoma may be observed. Some myelomas can have prominent thick-walled capillaries with

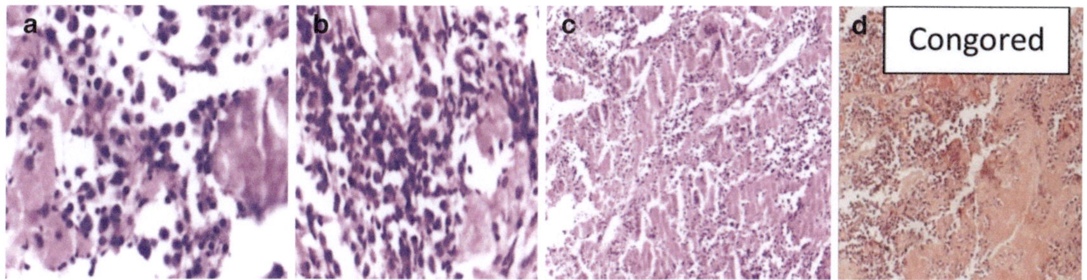

Fig. 9.1 Plasmacytoma ilium with amyloid deposition. (**a**, **b**) Sheets of plasma cells, H&E ×250. (**c**) Extensive pink amyloid, H&E ×100. (**d**) Congo red stain shows salmon pink appearance, ×100

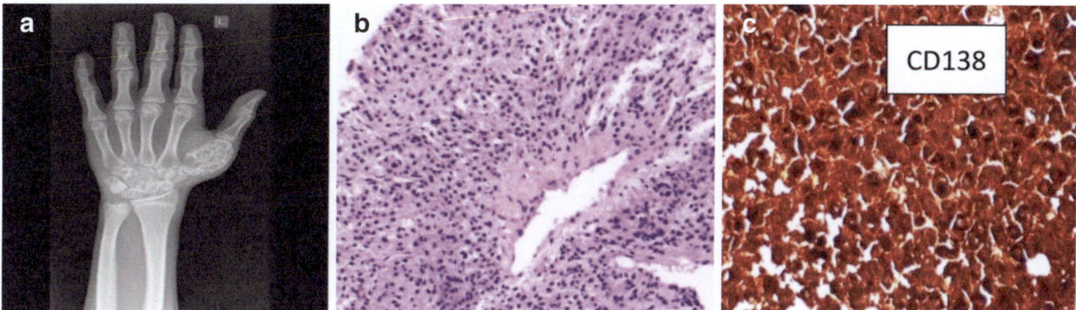

Fig. 9.2 A rare case of plasmacytoma metacarpal bone in a 16-year-old boy. (**a**) Plain X-ray shows soap bubble appearance of the first metacarpal bone. (**b**) Sheets of plasma cells, H&E ×100. (**c**) CD138 strongly positive, ×250

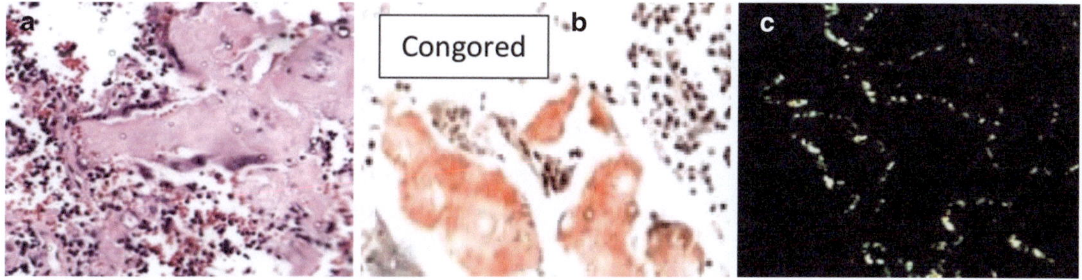

Fig. 9.3 Plasmacytoma with extensive amyloid. (**a**) Sheets of plasma cells with extensive amyloid deposits, H&E ×100. (**b**) Congo red showing positivity, ×100. (**c**) Apple green birefringence under polarizer, ×100

amyloid deposition and resemble neuroendocrine tumours. Stag horn type of vessels resembling haemangiopericytoma may also be seen. Mitotic figures are usually sparse in typical myeloma. Amyloid deposition can be so extensive so as to mask the tumour cells. In such cases, myeloma workup should be done before labelling it as primary amyloidosis. The main cause of the presence of amyloid in bone is myeloma. Rare exception is haemodialysis-induced amyloidosis.

The criteria given by the NCCN and the International Myeloma Working Group [17] for the diagnosis and staging of plasma cell myeloma are given in Tables 9.2 and 9.3.

9.2.5 IHC

Immunohistochemical stains for plasma cells are CD138 (Fig. 9.2) and CD38. CD20 and LCA are weak in myeloma. CD56 is positive. CD56 is

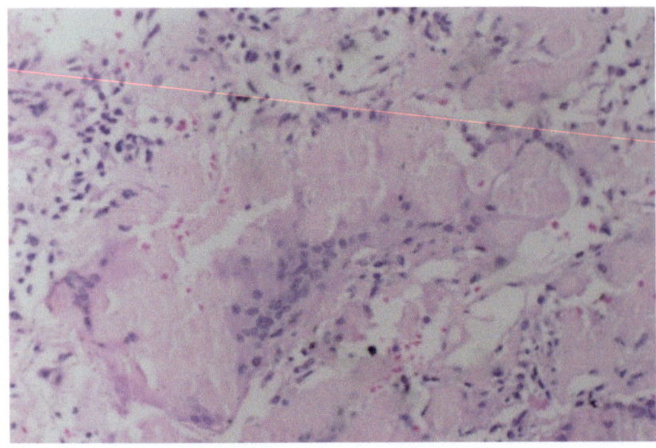

Fig. 9.4 Plasmacytoma with predominant amyloid and giant cells, H&E ×100

Table 9.2 Criteria for the diagnosis of plasma cell myeloma

Criteria for plasma cell myeloma diagnosis (International Myeloma Working Group) [33]
Clonal bone marrow plasma cells ≥10% or bony or extramedullary plasmacytoma (confirmed by biopsy)
One or more myeloma-defining events
• Serum calcium level >0.25 mmol/L (>1 mg/dL) higher than the upper limit of normal or >2.75 mmol/L (>11 mg/dL)
• Renal insufficiency (creatinine >2 mg/dL [>177 µmol/L] or creatinine clearance <40 mL/min)
• Anaemia (haemoglobin <10 g/dL or haemoglobin >2 g/dL below the lower limit of normal)
• One or more osteolytic bone lesions on skeletal **radiography, CT or FDG PET-CT**
More than one of the biomarkers of malignancy
• Clonal bone marrow plasma cells ≥60%
• Abnormal serum-free light chain (FLC) ratio ≥100 (involved kappa) or <0.01 (involved lambda)
• One or more focal ≥5 mm lesions on MRI scans
• Bone marrow plasma cells (BMPCs) ≥60%
• Involved/uninvolved serum-free light chain ratio ≥100

also useful for detecting residual disease. It also serves as a potential response criterion. Plasmacytoma is monoclonal and shows kappa or lambda light-chain restriction (Fig. 9.5). 60–70% has both free light chains and a serum monoclonal (M) protein.

Table 9.3 Staging of myeloma

Stage I criteria are as follows:
• Beta-2 microglobulin ≤3.5 g/dL and albumin ≥3.5 g/dL
• Standard risk for CA
• Normal LDH
Stage II comprises patients who do not meet the criteria for stage I or stage III
Stage III consists of the following:
• Beta-2 microglobulin of 5.5 g/dL or more
and either
• High risk for CA *or* high LDH

9.2.6 DD

Differential diagnosis includes osteomyelitis, reactive plasmacytosis, lymphomas, metastatic carcinomas and melanomas or epithelioid vascular tumours. Cytokeratin, CD31, CD138, LCA, CD20 and kappa and lambda can be used as a panel of markers to differentiate these tumours. Solitary plasmacytoma should be differentiated from osteomyelitis, plasmablastic lymphoma and lymphoplasmacytic lymphoma.

9.2.7 Treatment

Myeloma is treated with chemotherapy. High-dose chemotherapy and stem cell transplant are required in some cases. Solitary plasmacytoma is treated with surgery followed by radiotherapy. Radiotherapy is also given when there is severe pain especially for vertebral tumours. Bisphosphonates [18] and RANKL inhibitors [14, 15] are used in treatment.

9.2.8 Prognosis

The poor prognostic factors are anaemia, involvement of spinal cord and renal failure [7]. Hypercalcaemia is an adverse prognostic factor in a case of myeloma [21]. Fifty percent of solitary plasmacytoma cases develop myeloma in 2–3 years.

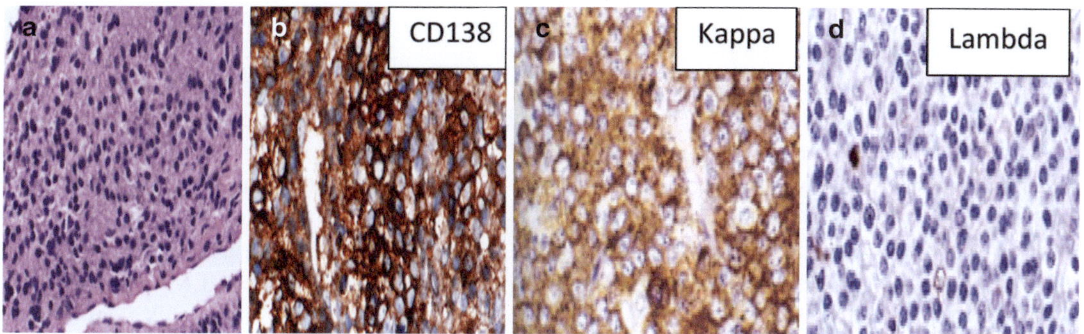

Fig. 9.5 (**a**) Tumour from vertebra in an elderly male, H&E ×250 Plasmacytoma/ Metastatic carcinoma. (**b**) CD138 positive, ×400. CK was negative. (**c**) Kappa ×250. (**d**) Lambda ×250. Plasmacytoma with kappa light-chain restriction

9.3 Malignant Lymphoma (ML) of Bone

In 1939, Jackson and Parker described primary lymphoma of bone. Bone lymphomas account for 3–7% of extra-nodal lymphomas, and lymphomas constitute about 7% of all bone malignancies. The terminology bone lymphoma is restricted to those cases primarily involving bone (single bone or multiple bones) with or without regional lymph node involvement. There should not be visceral or generalized lymph node involvement [23].

9.3.1 Clinical

he disease occurs in older adults (>40 years) and predominantly in males [22, 23]. Multiple bone involvement is common [27, 28]. Femur, pelvis, vertebra and humerus are the most common sites. In the long bones, the metadiaphyseal region is affected [33, 35]. Involvement of the small bones of the hands and feet is very rare. Soft tissue extension can be seen. In spite of extensive involvement, patient can be without many symptoms.

9.3.2 Lab findings

Some of the laboratory findings are useful in suspecting malignant lymphoma. Elevated serum LDH is a useful parameter. Anaemia, increased alkaline phosphatase (ALP), increased erythrocyte sedimentation rates (ESRs), low platelet counts and increased calcium levels are other findings described in primary non-Hodgkin lymphoma (NHL) of bone.

9.3.3 Radiology

A permeative growth pattern is seen. On plain X-rays, they are lytic with moth-eaten appearance. Sclerotic areas may also be seen. Cortical erosion and destruction with soft tissue extension may be present. Periosteal reaction similar to Ewing sarcoma or extensive involvement of long bones, sometimes involving the entire bone, may be seen [32]. Sometimes, bilateral symmetrical involvement is also noted. Multiple bones can be involved [40, 41]. The findings are non-specific, and there is overlap with other round cell tumours like Ewing sarcoma. Sometimes, the lesion is not evident on plain X-ray which may look normal. But MRI shows signal abnormalities with extensive involvement of the marrow (Fig. 9.6) [25, 26]. When you see abnormal marrow signal on MRI or increased uptake on bone scan, with inconspicuous plain radiograph, lymphoma has to be ruled out.

9.3.4 Pathology

Gross appearance: Bone lymphomas on cut section are fleshy grey-white or haemorrhagic [29, 33]. Depending on the host bone response, the tumour can be very sclerotic, and biopsy specimens may require decalcification [24].

Needle biopsy will show extensive crush artefact [39], and morphology of cells is difficult to make out. One may have to search for areas where cells can be visualized better. The dictum is that "When **you see extensive crush artefact on a bone biopsy, rule out lymphoma".**

Some of the lymphomas elicit fibrotic stromal reaction and appear spindly mimicking a sarcoma. This is especially seen in anaplastic large cell lymphoma (ALCL) [30]. Diffuse large B-cell lymphoma (DLBCL) is the commonest histological subtype [28, 35] (Figs. 9.7 and 9.8) followed by lymphoblastic lymphoma (Fig. 9.9), Burkitt lymphoma and ALCL (Figs. 9.10 and 9.11). Further subtyping of lymphoma is done by immunohistochemistry alone or in combination with flow cytometry [25]. Rosette forming lymphomas are described which can cause diagnostic difficulty [34].

T cell lymphomas are unusual in bone. Adult T-cell leukaemia/lymphoma (ATLL), especially acute variant, can present as lytic bone lesions, and these cases are associated with hypercalcaemia [38]. Hodgkin lymphoma infiltration of bone is usually secondary to nodal involvement (Fig. 9.12). The infiltrate can be polymorphic resembling osteomyelitis, which is also a differential diagnosis on radiology. Usually, follicular

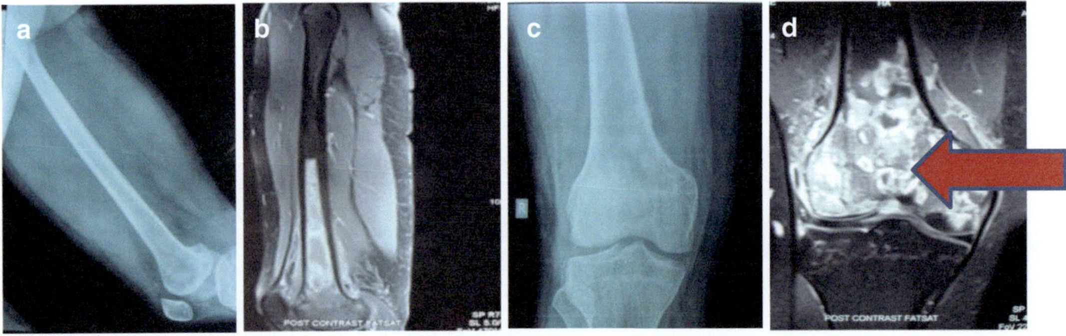

Fig. 9.6 ML—radiology of two cases. (**a** and **c**) Plain X-ray looks normal. (**b** and **d**) MRI with abnormal marrow signal. The extent of disease is also evident on MRI

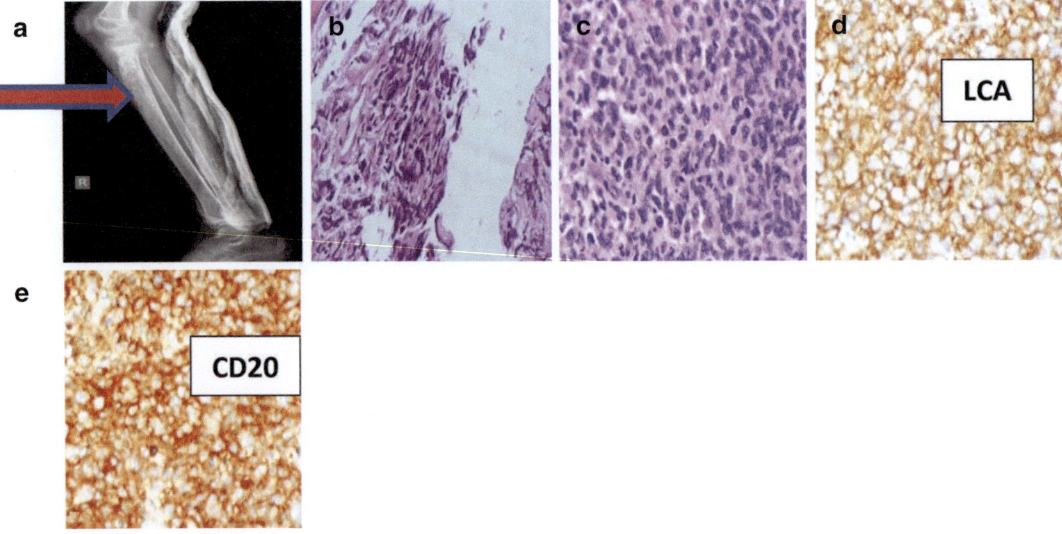

Fig. 9.7 ML—DLBCL of the upper tibia. (**a**) Plain X-ray showing destructive permeative lesion in the upper tibia. (**b**) Scanner view with tumour cells showing crush artefact, H&E ×40. (**c**) Higher power showing large monotonous looking cells, H&E ×400. (**d**) IHC-LCA-diffuse strong membranous positivity, ×250. (**e**) CD20 (B-cell marker) showing diffuse strong membrane positivity, ×250

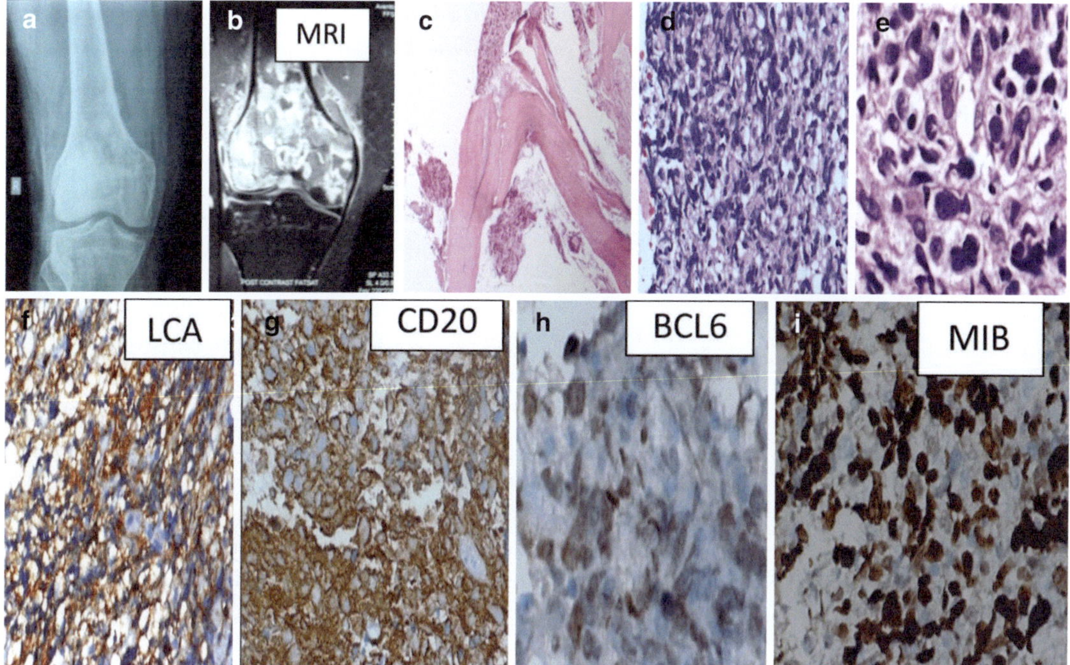

Fig. 9.8 DLBCL in a 24-year-old male presented with pain in leg. (**a**) Plain X-ray showed non-specific findings. Initial biopsy reported as inflammatory lesion. (**b**) Subsequently, MRI was taken and showed abnormal signals. (**c**) Cells with extensive crush artefact. (**d**) Large cells and crushed cells, H&E ×250. (**e**) Discrete large pleomorphic malignant cells, H&E ×400. (**f**) LCA ×100. (**g**) CD20 with strong membrane positivity, ×250. (**h**) BCL6 showing nuclear positivity, ×250. BCL2 was negative. (**i**) MIB1 labelling index 80%, ×250

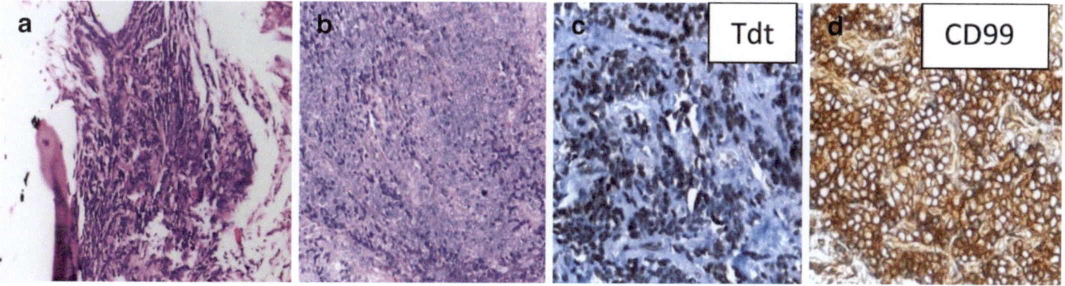

Fig. 9.9 Lymphoblastic lymphoma bone in a 13-year-old boy. (**a**) Scanner view showing extensive crush artefact. (**b**) Higher power showing immature lymphoid cells in sheets. (**c**) Tdt showed diffuse positivity. LCA was negative. (**d**) CD99 showing strong membrane positivity as in Ewing sarcoma. A panel of IHC markers are essential for proper diagnosis of round cell neoplasm of bone

lymphomas and chronic lymphocytic lymphoma/leukaemia will not present as primary lymphomas of bone [23, 29, 33]. They show secondary involvement of bone (Fig. 9.13). Rosette forming lymphoma is described which will cause diagnostic difficulty [34].

9.3.5 IHC

Minimum IHC in a suspected case should include LCA, CD3, CD20, CD30 and Tdt. CD99 can show strong membrane positivity, especially in lymphoblastic lymphomas [23,

37]. A panel of antibodies like desmin, synaptophysin and NKX2.2 might be required in selected cases to rule out other malignant round cell tumours [28]. Additional studies such as flow cytometry and other ancillary tests will help in proper typing of tumours.

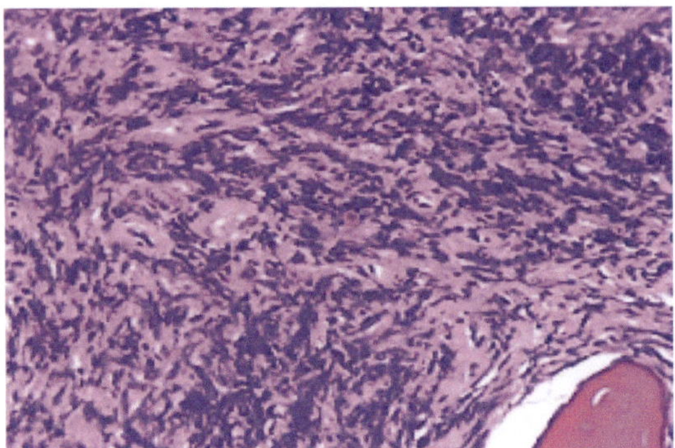

Fig. 9.10 Spindling of cells in ALCL mimicking sarcoma, H&E ×100

9.3.6 DD

Other round cell sarcomas of bone [35], myeloma and osteomyelitis are the differential diagnosis.

9.3.7 Treatment and Prognosis

Depending on the stage of the disease and the grade and type of the lymphoma, chemotherapy and radiotherapy are given [31]. Primary DLBCLs have a good prognosis [28, 35]. Age more than 60 years is thought to be an adverse factor for survival [36]. In general, prognosis of primary bone lymphoma is said to be better

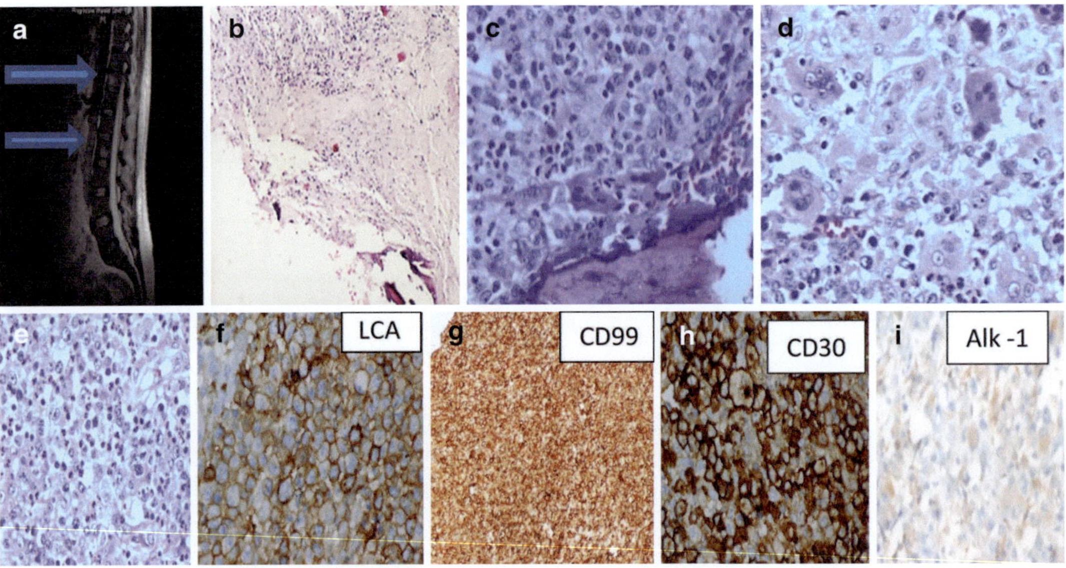

Fig. 9.11 Alk-negative ALCL vertebra in a 37-year-old lady who presented with paraplegia. PET scan revealed lesions in humerus and femur also. (**a**) MRI showing multiple thoracic and lumbar vertebrae involved with destructive lesions. (**b**) Bone with sheets of neoplastic cells, H&E ×40. (**c** and **d**) Large pleomorphic cells with tumour giant cells, H&E ×400. (**e**) Mixture of pleomorphic malignant cells and inflammatory cells, H&E ×250. (**f**) LCA ×250. (**g**) CD99 with strong membrane positivity, ×100. (**h**) CD30 showing diffuse strong positivity, ×250. (**i**) Alk1 was negative, ×100

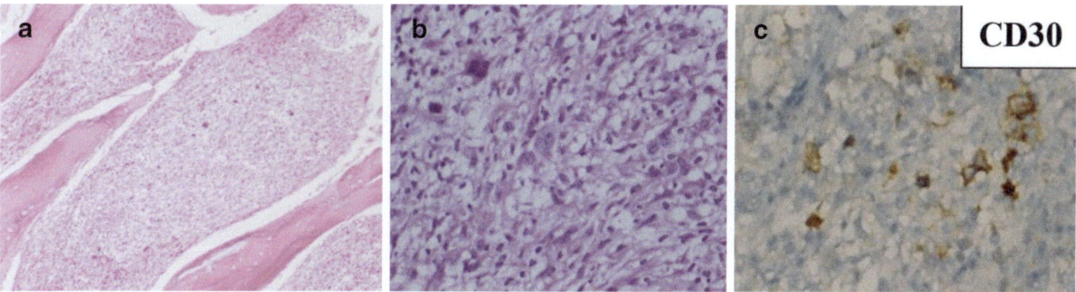

Fig. 9.12 Secondary involvement of bone from a nodal Hodgkin lymphoma. (**a**) Bone with diffuse infiltration of neoplasm, H&E ×100. (**b**) High power showing a mixture of cells including RS cells, H&E ×250. (**c**) CD30 positive in RS cells, ×250

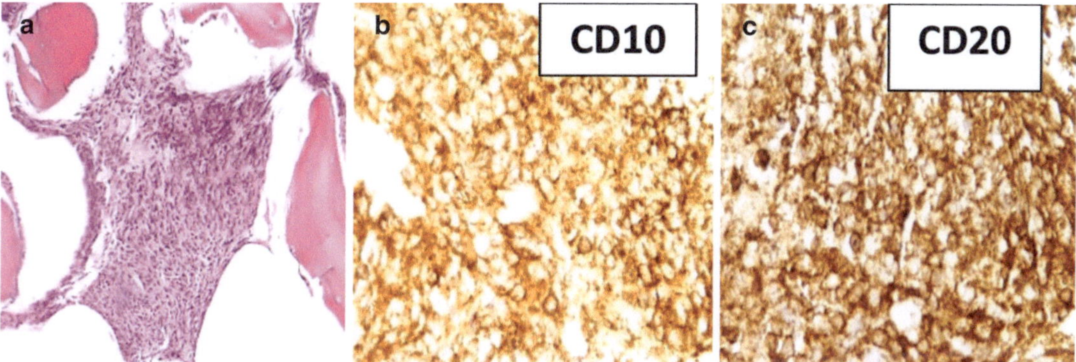

Fig. 9.13 Follicular lymphoma secondary involvement of bone. (**a**) Bone with cells showing crush artefact, H&E ×40. (**b**) CD10 positive, ×100. (**c**) CD20 diffusely positive, ×100

than nodal and non-osseous extra-nodal diffuse large B-cell lymphoma (DLBCL). Other poor prognostic factors are multifocality and soft tissue extension. Soft tissue extension and multifocality are poor prognostic factors [28, 29, 40].

Points to Remember

- Myeloma is the commonest malignant primary bone tumour.
- Criteria for plasma cell myeloma diagnosis are that of the International Myeloma Working Group.
- In plasmacytoma, the entire biopsy may show amyloid. Myeloma workup should be done in such cases.
- The main cause of the presence of amyloid in bone is myeloma.
- When multiple bones are involved in an adult, rule out myeloma and metastasis. Lymphoma is the third possibility.
- In malignant lymphoma of bone, plain X-ray can be normal, but MRI shows abnormal signals.
- When a bone biopsy shows extensive crush artefact of tumour cells, rule out lymphoma.
- DLBCL is the commonest lymphoma subtype in bone.
- Bone involvement in follicular lymphoma and Hodgkin lymphoma is usually secondary.

References

Myeloma/Plasmacytoma

1. Hameed A, Brady JJ, Dowling P, Clynes M, O'Gorman P. Bone disease in multiple myeloma: pathophysiology and management. Cancer Growth Metastasis. 2014;7:33–43.
2. Bataille R, Chappard D, Marcelli C, et al. Mechanisms of bone destruction in multiple myeloma: the importance of an unbalanced process in determining the severity of lytic bone disease. J Clin Oncol. 1989;7(12):1909–14.
3. Bataille R, Chappard D, Marcelli C, et al. Recruitment of new osteoblasts and osteoclasts is the earliest critical event in the pathogenesis of human multiple myeloma. J Clin Invest. 1991;88:62–6. https://doi.org/10.1172/JCI115305.
4. Caers J, Paiva B, Zamagni E, et al. Diagnosis, treatment, and response assessment in solitary plasmacytoma: updated recommendations from a European Expert Panel. J Hematol Oncol. 2018;11:10.
5. Terpos E, Ntanasis-Stathopoulos I, Gavriatopoulou M, Dimopoulos MA. Pathogenesis of bone disease in multiple myeloma: from bench to bedside blood. Cancer J. 2018;8:7.
6. Roodman GD. Pathogenesis of myeloma bone disease. Leukemia. 2009;23:435–41. https://doi.org/10.1038/leu.2008.336.
7. Kyle RA, Rajkumar SV. Criteria for diagnosis, staging, risk stratification and response assessment of multiple myeloma. Leukemia. 2009;23(1):3–9.
8. Kyle RA. Multiple myeloma: review of 869 cases. Mayo Clin Proc. 1975;50:29–40.
9. Lai FP, Cole-Sinclair M, Cheng WJ, et al. Myeloma cells can directly contribute to the pool of RANKL in bone bypassing the classic stromal and osteoblast pathway of osteoclast stimulation. Br J Haematol. 2004;126:192–201. https://doi.org/10.1111/j.1365-2141.2004.05018.
10. Børset M, Sundan A, Waage A, Standal T. Why do myeloma patients have bone disease? A historical perspective. Blood Rev. 2020;41:100646.
11. Mikhael J, Ismaila N, Cheung MC, Costello C, Dhodapkar MV, Kumar S, Lacy M, Lipe B, Little RF, Nikonova A, Omel J, Peswani N, Prica A, Raje N, Seth R, Vesole DH, Walker I, Whitley A, Wildes TM, Wong SW, Martin T. Treatment of multiple myeloma: ASCO and CCO joint clinical practice guideline. J Clin Oncol. 2019;37(14):1228–63.
12. Russano F, Pisani O, Venditti F, Pantano A, Rago A, Siniscalchi E, Cerchiara L, Franceschini L, De Rosa L, Mariani M, Andriani S, Cudillo L, Garcia M, Cantonetti M, Mohamed S, Anaclerico B, Caravita T, Stocchi F, Cimino G, Gumenyuk S, Vozella F, Avvisati G. Alkaline phosphatase (alp) levels in multiple myeloma and solid cancers with bone lesions: is there any difference? J Bone Oncol. 2021;26:100338.
13. Ohana N, Rouvio O, Nalbandyan K, Sheinis D, Benharroch D. Classification of solitary plasmacytoma, is it more intricate than presently suggested? A commentary. J Cancer. 2018;9(21):3894–7.
14. Parrondo RD, Sher T. Prevention of skeletal related events in multiple myeloma: focus on the RANK-L pathway in the treatment of multiple myeloma. Onco Targets Ther. 2019;12:8467–78.
15. Ring ES, Lawson MA, Snowden JA, Jolley I, Chantry AD. New agents in the treatment of myeloma bone disease. Calcif Tissue Int. 2018;102:196–209. https://doi.org/10.1007/s00223-017-0351-7.
16. Vincent Rajkumar S. Multiple myeloma: 2020 update on diagnosis, risk-stratification and management. Am J Haematol. 2023;95(11):1444.
17. Terpos E, et al. International Myeloma Working Group recommendations for the treatment of multiple myeloma-related bone disease. J Clin Oncol. 2013;31:2347–57.
18. Terpos E, Roodman GD, Dimopoulos MA. Optimal use of bisphosphonates in patients with multiple myeloma. Blood. 2014;121:3325–8.
19. Walker R, Barlogie B, Haessler J, et al. Magnetic resonance imaging in multiple myeloma: diagnostic and clinical implications. J Clin Oncol. 2007;25(9):1121–8.
20. Swerdlow SH, Campo E, Harris NL, Jaffe ES, Pileri SA, Stein H, Thiele J, editor. WHO classification of tumours of haematopoietic and lymphoid tissues, Revised 4th ed., vol. 2; 2017.
21. Zagouri F, Kastritis E, Zomas A, et al. Hypercalcemia remains an adverse prognostic factor for newly diagnosed multiple myeloma patients in the era of novel antimyeloma therapies. Eur J Haematol. 2017;99:409–14. https://doi.org/10.1111/ejh.12923.

Malignant Lymphoma

22. Muller A, Dreyling M, Roeder F, Baur-Melnyk A, Knosel T, Klein A, Birkenmaier C, Jansson V, Durr HR. Primary bone lymphoma: clinical presentation and therapeutic considerations. J Bone Oncol. 2020;25:1–6.
23. Bindal P, Desai A, Delasos L, Mulay S, Vredenburgh J. Primary bone lymphoma: a case series and review of literature. Case Rep Hematol. 2020;10:4254803, 6 pages.
24. Cleven AHG, Ferry JA. In: WHO classification of soft tissue and bone tumours, WHO classification of tumours, 5th ed., vol. 3. 2020. pp. 489–491.
25. Hermann G, Klein MJ, Abdelwahab IF, Kenan S. MRI appearance of primary non-Hodgkins lymphoma of bone. Skeletal Radiol. 1997;26:629–32.
26. Heyning FH, Kroon HM, Hogendoorn PC, Taminiau AH, van der Woude HJ. MR imaging characteristics in primary lymphoma of bone with emphasis on non-aggressive appearance. Skeletal Radiol. 2007;36:937–44.

27. Wu H, Zhang L, Shao H, et al. Prognostic significance of soft tissue extension, international prognostic index, and multifocality in primary bone lymphoma: a single institutional experience. Br J Haematol. 2014;166:60–8.
28. Wu H, Bui MM, Leston DG, et al. Clinical characteristics and prognostic factors of bone lymphomas: focus on the clinical significance of multifocal bone involvement by primary bone large B-cell lymphomas. BMC Cancer. 2014;14:900.
29. Demircay E, Hornicek FJ Jr, Mankin HJ, Degroot H 3rd. Malignant lymphoma of bone: a review of 119 patients. Clin Orthop Relat Res. 2013;471:2684–90.
30. Lones MA, Sanger W, Perkins SL, Medeiros LJ. Anaplastic large cell lymphoma arising in bone: report of a case of the monomorphic variant with the t(2;5)(p23;q35) translocation. Arch Pathol Lab Med. 2000;124:1339–43.
31. Müller A, Dreyling M, Roeder F, et al. Primary bone lymphoma: clinical presentation and therapeutic considerations. J Bone Oncol. 2020;25:100326.
32. O'Neill J, Finlay K, Jurriaans E, Friedman L. Radiological manifestations of skeletal lymphoma. Curr Probl Diagn Radiol. 2009;38:228–36.
33. Ramadan KM, Shenkier T, Sehn LH, Gascoyne RD, Connors JM. A clinicopathological retrospective study of 131 patients with primary bone lymphoma: a population-based study of successively treated cohorts from the British Columbia Cancer Agency. Ann Oncol. 2007;18:129–35.
34. Rekhi B, Gulia A. "Rosette forming" primary high-grade B-cell lymphoma, presenting as a scapular mass, masquerading Ewing sarcoma: a rare case with diagnostic implications. Indian J Pathol Microbiol. 2021;64(3):617–9.
35. Govi S, Christie D, Messina C, et al. The clinical features, management and prognostic effects of pathological fractures in a multicenter series of 373 patients with diffuse large B-cell lymphoma of the bone. Ann Oncol. 2014;25:176–81.
36. Sharma A, Ahmed R, Agrawal N, Kapoor J, Sharma A, Khushoo V, Agrawal P, Bhurani D, Mirgh SP. Primary bone lymphoma: a 13 year retrospective institutional analysis in the chemo-immunotherapy era. Indian J Hematol Blood Transfus. 2021;37(2):240–8.
37. Sung CO, Ko YH, Park S, et al. Immunoreactivity of CD99 in non-Hodgkin's lymphoma: unexpected frequent expression in ALK-positive anaplastic large cell lymphoma. J Korean Med Sci. 2005;20:952–6.
38. Takahashi T, Tsukuda H, Itoh H, Kimura H, Yoshimoto M, Tsujisaki M. Primary and isolated adult T-cell leukemia/lymphoma of the bone marrow. Intern Med. 2011;50:2393–6.
39. Unni KK, Inwards CY. Dahlin's bone tumors: general aspects and data on 10,165 cases. United Kingdom: Wollters Kluwer Health/Lippincott Williams & Wilkins; 2010.
40. WHO Classification of Tumours. In: WHO Classification of Tumours Editorial Board, editor. Soft tissue and bone tumours. WHO classification of tumours, 5th ed., vol. 3. IARC; 2020.
41. Zhang X, Zhu J, Song Y, Ping L, Zheng W. Clinical characterization and outcome of primary bone lymphoma: a retrospective study of 61 Chinese patients. Sci Rep. 2016;6:28834.

10 Histiocytic Lesions of Bone

Histiocytic disorders are a group of diseases derived from macrophages and dendritic cells. Histiocytic neoplasm of bone comes under the haematopoietic neoplasms of bone in the WHO 2020 classification [32]. The LCH-NOS and disseminated, ECD and RDD are included in the WHO classification. The histiocytic disorders are grouped as dendritic cell disorders, macrophage related and malignant histiocytosis [18]. They occur mainly in children but can also occur in adults.

Langerhans cell histiocytosis (LCH) is the most common dendritic cell disorder. Erdheim-Chester disease (ECD) and juvenile xanthogranuloma (JXG) are also derived from dendritic cells (Table 10.1). Sinus histiocytosis with massive lymphadenopathy (Rosai-Dorfman disease (RDD) and haemophagocytic lymphohistiocytosis (HLH) are macrophage-related tumours.

Table 10.1 Histiocytic lesions of bone

Histiocytic lesions of bone
Langerhans cell histiocytosis (LCH)
LCH-NOS (not otherwise specified)
LCH, Disseminated
Erdheim-Chester disease (ECD)
Rosai-Dorfman disease (RDD)
Xanthoma of bone

10.1 Langerhans Cell Histiocytosis (LCH)

LCH belongs to a group of disorders having cells resembling dendritic cells of skin along with a mixture of marrow cells like eosinophils, T lymphocytes and multinucleated giant cells [4, 5]. Paul Langerhans first described the dendritic cells in 1892, and thus the name Langerhans cell histiocytosis was given for this group of tumours. When the Langerhans cell accumulates in the skin, bone and lung, they form clusters and become tumours. They are also called eosinophilic granulomas. The Langerhans cells show racquet-shaped Birbeck granules in the cytoplasm, which is seen only by electron microscopy.

The unifocal disease is called as eosinophilic granuloma. Multiple systems are involved in Hand-Schüller-Christian disease and Letterer-Siwe disease. A common name for this group of diseases was given by Lichtenstein, called as histiocytosis X. The X indicates that the cell of origin is uncertain. Later, histiocytosis X was renamed as Langerhans cell histiocytosis because the cell of origin was thought to be dysfunctional epidermal Langerhans cells. Recently, abnormal cells in LCH have been thought to be derived

J. Kattoor et al., *Bone Tumors*, https://doi.org/10.1007/978-981-99-4738-6_10

from myeloid dendritic cells. They share the same antigens (CD1a, S100 and CD207) and possess the Birbeck granules of Langerhans cells of epidermis.

Based on the number of lesions and systems involved, LCH is divided into three groups.

Unifocal localized form (70%): Usually, a single bone or a few bones are involved in this form. But rarely can it involve lung also. The typical example is eosinophilic granuloma. Patients usually present between 5 and 15 years of age. This type should be distinguished from lung LCH, which is mostly seen in adults who are smokers.

Multifocal unisystem (chronic recurring) form (20%): This involves multiple bones or multiple lesions in the same bone. The liver, spleen, lymph nodes and skin are also involved. They present at a younger age than localized form, with lytic lesions of bone, rashes and eruptions on the skin of scalp and ear. In 50% of cases, pituitary stalk is involved causing diabetes insipidus. Hand-Schüller-Christian disease is an example of this (triad of diabetes insipidus, exophthalmos and lytic bone lesions).

Multifocal multisystem (fulminant) form (10%): This is a rapidly progressing form with multisystem involvement. They are usually fatal. It is a disease occurring below the age of 2 years. They present with anaemia, thrombocytopenia and involvement of the reticuloendothelial system. Typical example is Letterer-Siwe disease. Even with treatment, prognosis is very poor.

10.1.1 Bone Lesions

LCH can involve any bone. The most common bones involved are skull, femur, ribs, vertebrae, mandible and pelvis. The lytic lesions are well defined and have a "punched-out" appearance, especially in the skull bones. This is due to asymmetric destruction of the inner and outer cortices. Mastoid bone is a preferred site. Skull bone disease lacks periosteal reaction. Skull lesions can cause a map-like appearance referred to as a geographic skull. In the vertebra, body of the vertebra is commonly involved. Long bone involvement is more common in children than in adults (Fig. 10.1).

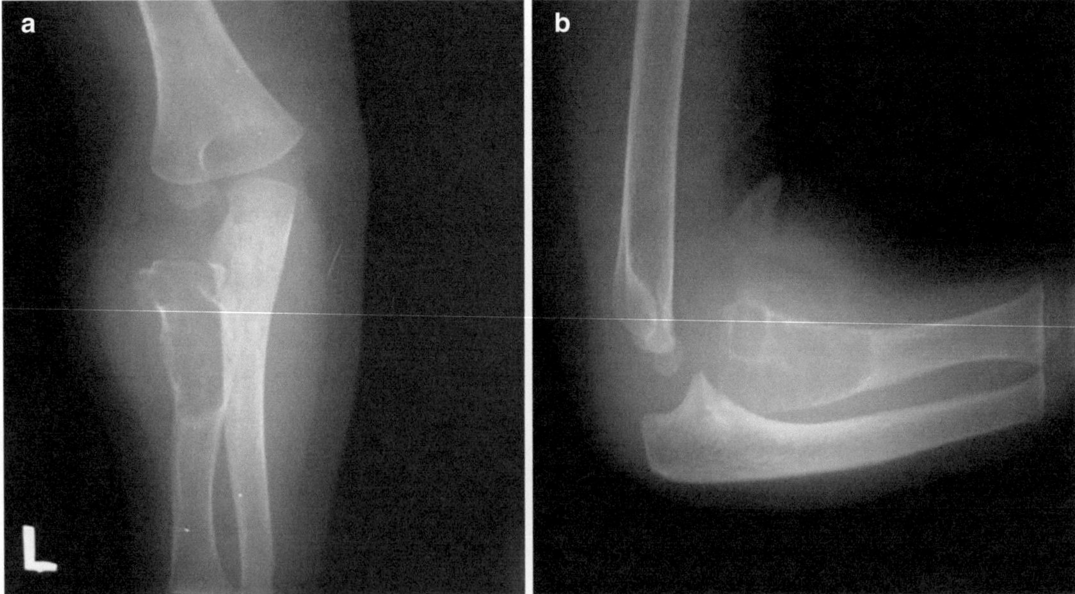

Fig. 10.1 LCH: Plain X-ray. (**a**) Lytic lesion in the upper radius in a 1-year-old child with well-defined borders. (**b**) Lesion in the upper ulna in an 8-year-old child

10.1.2 Clinical

Patients may be asymptomatic or may present with focal pain, swelling or pathologic fractures. The bones commonly involved are the femur, humerus and tibia.

10.1.3 Radiology

They involve the diaphysis or metaphysis. Initially, the lesions are lytic, expansile and aggressive (Fig. 10.2). In the chronic lesions, they appear sclerotic with periosteal new bone formation. Sometimes, it can have a sharply defined sclerotic margin.

10.1.4 Pathology

The lesions of LCH are composed of cells with abundant eosinophilic cytoplasm. The nuclei of LCH cells resemble epidermal dendritic cells with cleaved nuclei having nuclear grooves. Eosinophils are common. Other inflammatory cells like lymphocytes, plasma cells and neutrophils are often present in variable numbers. Multinucleated giant cells can be seen (Fig. 10.3). Large areas of necrosis may be seen in LCH of bone. Cells are seen as clusters. If cells are in sheets, lymphoma has to be ruled out. In the lymph node, cells are seen in the sinusoids.

10.1.5 IHC

The positives antibodies are CD1a (Fig. 10.4), S100 protein and langerin (CD207) [6]. CD207 is a type II transmembrane C-type lectin.

10.1.6 Differential Diagnosis

Other histiocytic/dendritic lesions, lymphoma and Langerhans cell sarcoma are the usual differentials. In Rosai-Dorfman disease (RDD), the histiocytes are negative for CD1a or langerin. The classical emperipolesis seen in RDD is absent in LCH. Erdheim-Chester disease is seen in older age group. The histiocytes seen in ECD are foamy in

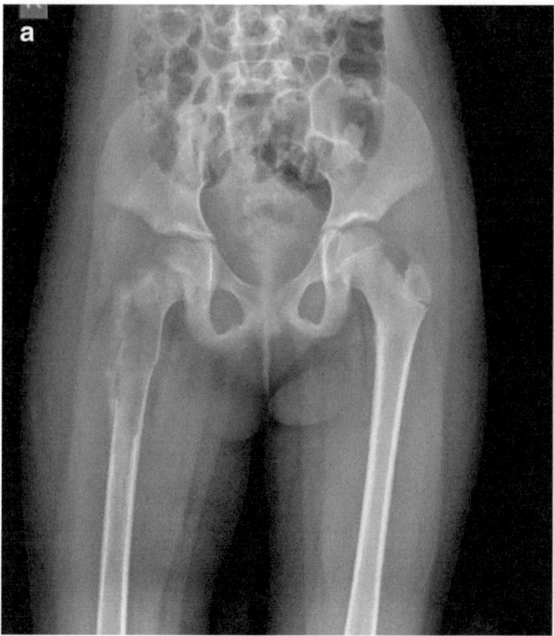

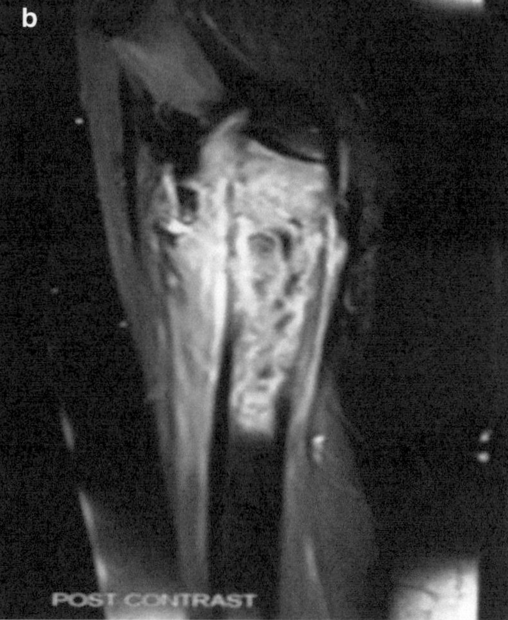

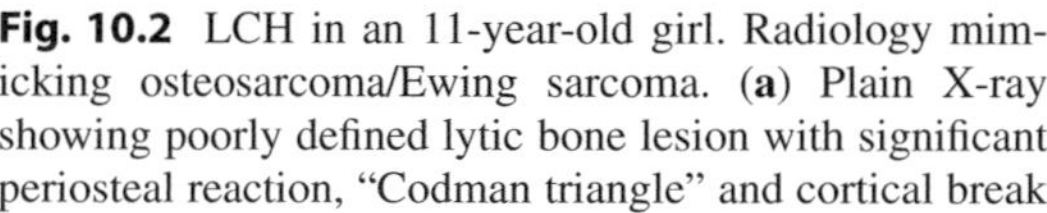

Fig. 10.2 LCH in an 11-year-old girl. Radiology mimicking osteosarcoma/Ewing sarcoma. (**a**) Plain X-ray showing poorly defined lytic bone lesion with significant periosteal reaction, "Codman triangle" and cortical break in the upper femur. (**b**) MRI showing heterogeneously enhancing lesion of right femur with marrow involvement, cortical break and significant soft tissue component

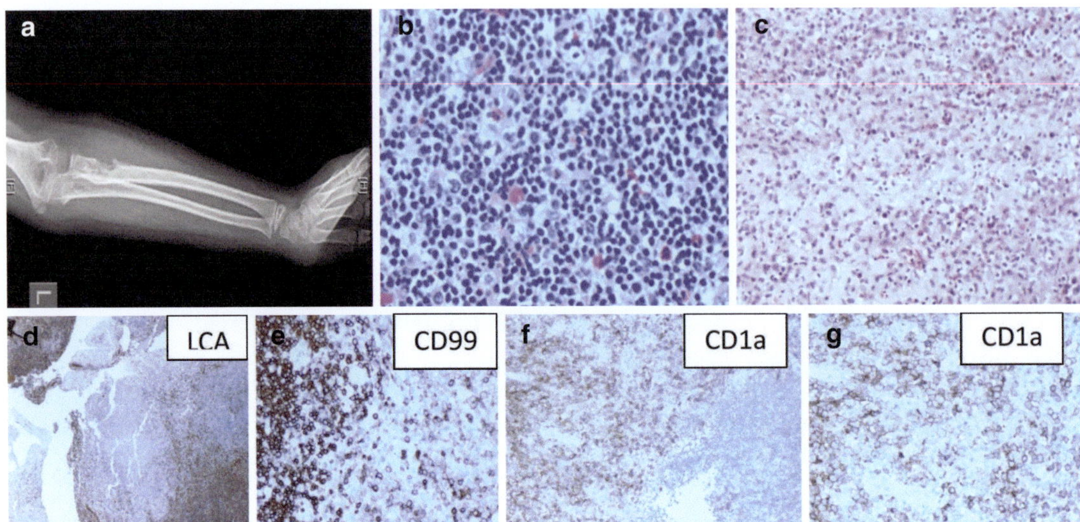

Fig. 10.3 LCH in an 8-year-old girl. (**a**) Plain X-ray with lytic lesion in the upper radius-metadiaphyseal region with periosteal reaction. Radiology diagnosis was Ewing sarcoma. (**b**) Microscopy showed pale and dark areas. Dark area with polymorphous population of lymphoid cells, H&E ×250. (**c**) Pale area showing histiocytes admixed with eosinophils, H&E ×100. (**d**) LCA highlighting lymphocytes in dark area, LCA ×100. (**e**) CD99 positive in lymphoid cells, ×250. (**f**) CD1a-positive cells in sheets in pale area, ×100. (**g**) CD1a ×250

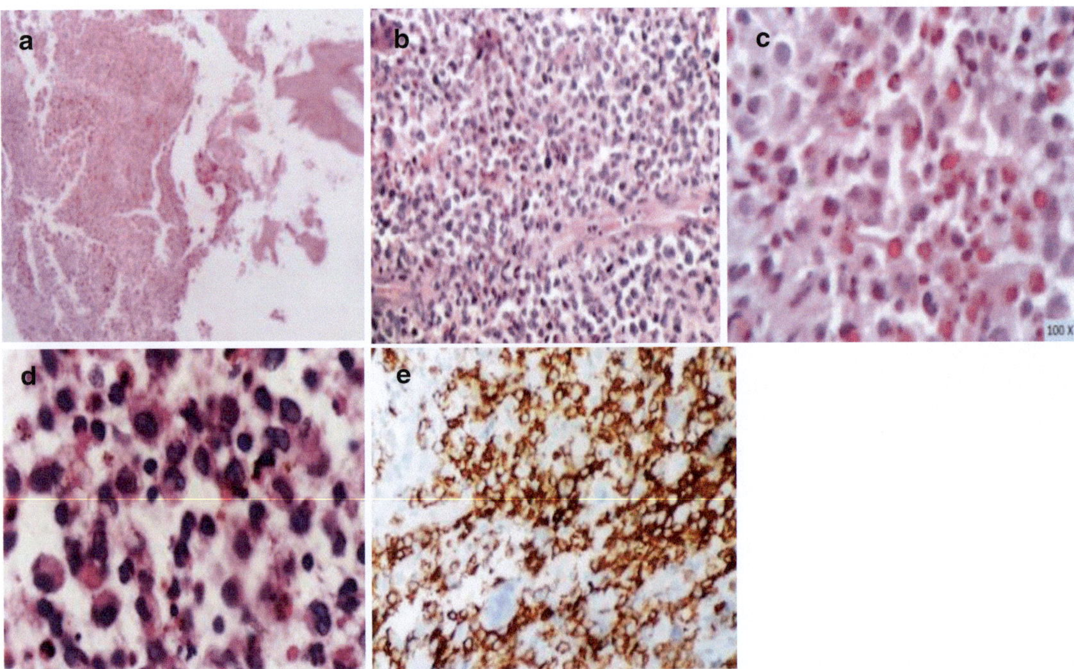

Fig. 10.4 LCH: (**a**) H&E ×40. (**b**) Mixture of histiocytes and eosinophils, H&E ×100. (**c**) Histiocytic cells (Langerhans cells) are with well-defined cell borders, moderate cytoplasm and cleaved/convoluted nuclei mixed with eosinophils, H&E ×250. (**d**) H&E ×400. (**e**) Cells are diffusely positive for CD1a, ×100

nature, and CD1a and langerin will be negative. Juvenile xanthogranuloma shows foamy histiocytes and Touton giant cells. Lymphomas show markedly atypical cells. Blastomycosis infection can have similar type of histiocytes. Rarely, osteomyelitis comes in the differential.

10.1.7 Molecular

BRAF or MAP2K1 mutations are seen [1–3].

10.1.8 Treatment

Unifocal bone lesions are usually treated by curettage. No adjuvant treatment is required. The lesion may also regress spontaneously. Some patients are treated with radiotherapy. Systemic chemotherapy is required for cases with multisystem involvement. Inhibitors of BRAF and MEK are being tried for cases that are positive for BRAF and MEK mutation.

10.1.9 Prognosis

More than 99% of unifocal disease has good prognosis. The involvement of bone marrow, liver or lung is considered as poor prognostic factors. Young age at diagnosis, hepatosplenomegaly, thrombocytopenia and involvement of more than three bones are poor prognostic indicators.

10.2 Erdheim-Chester Disease (ECD)

ECD is first described by Chester in 1930. It is a disease of unknown aetiology involving bone, lung and pituitary [14].

10.2.1 Clinical Features

This disease occurs mainly in adult males. The usual age group is 45–55 years. Clinically, they may be asymptomatic or may have systemic symptoms like weight loss [7]. They may also have bone pain. Some patients will have progressive disease with multisystem involvement [14]. They may present with diabetes insipidus because of involvement of pituitary [8] or it may affect lung (pulmonary fibrosis), heart (cardiac failure) or brain (cerebral symptoms) [13].

10.2.2 Radiology

The characteristic feature of ECD is bilateral symmetric sclerotic bony lesions [10], usually affecting metadiaphyseal regions of long bones (Fig. 10.5). Flat bones are not usually affected.

10.2.3 Pathology

There will be accumulation of foamy histiocytes, lymphocytes and variable degrees of fibrosis in the affected tissues [12]. In bone, the bony trabeculae are thickened giving a pagetoid appearance. Multinucleated giant cells may be present. Immunohistochemically, the histiocytes are CD1a negative (Fig. 10.6), but other histiocytic markers like S100, CD68 and CD163 will be positive [9].

10.2.4 Molecular

BRAF mutations are seen in EDD also [11].

10.2.5 Differential diagnosis

This includes other histiocytic lesions like LCH, xanthogranuloma, Rosai-Dorfman disease, histiocyte-rich lesions of bone like non-ossifying fibroma giant cell tumour and also metastatic renal cell carcinoma. Radiological findings and immunohistochemistry help in proper diagnosis.

10.2.6 Treatment and Prognosis

There is no specific treatment. Chemotherapy and steroids have been tried. The prognosis is good if only bone lesions are present. Systemic involvement carries a poor prognosis [15]. Some

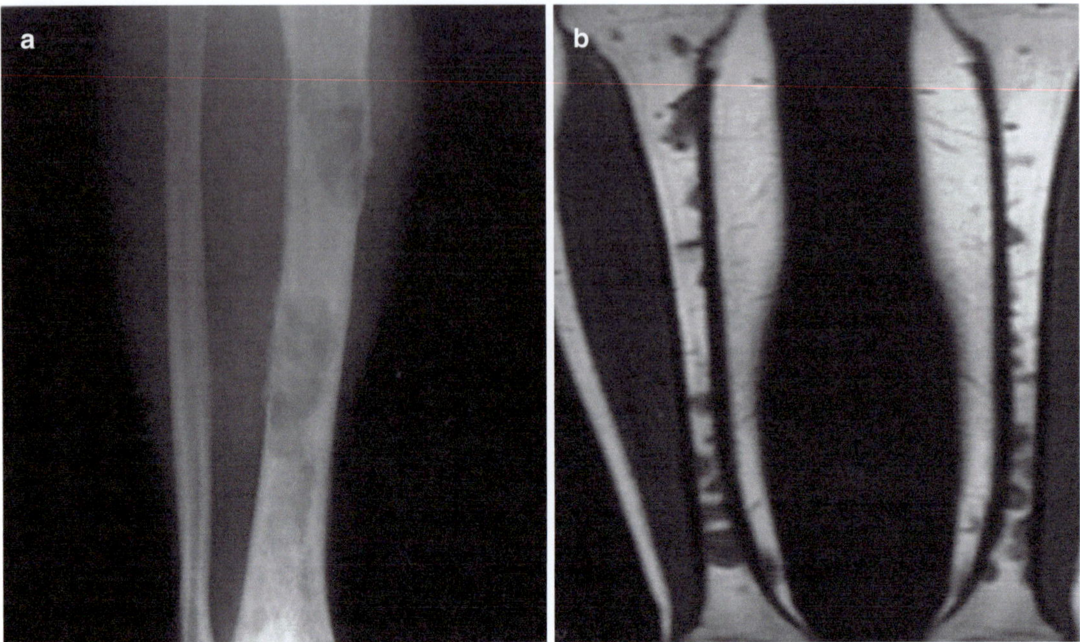

Fig. 10.5 ECD: (**a** and **b**) Bilateral symmetrical involvement of tibia in a 62-year-old lady. Multiple lytic and sclerotic lesions are seen. She presented with weight loss, polydipsia and pain in both legs

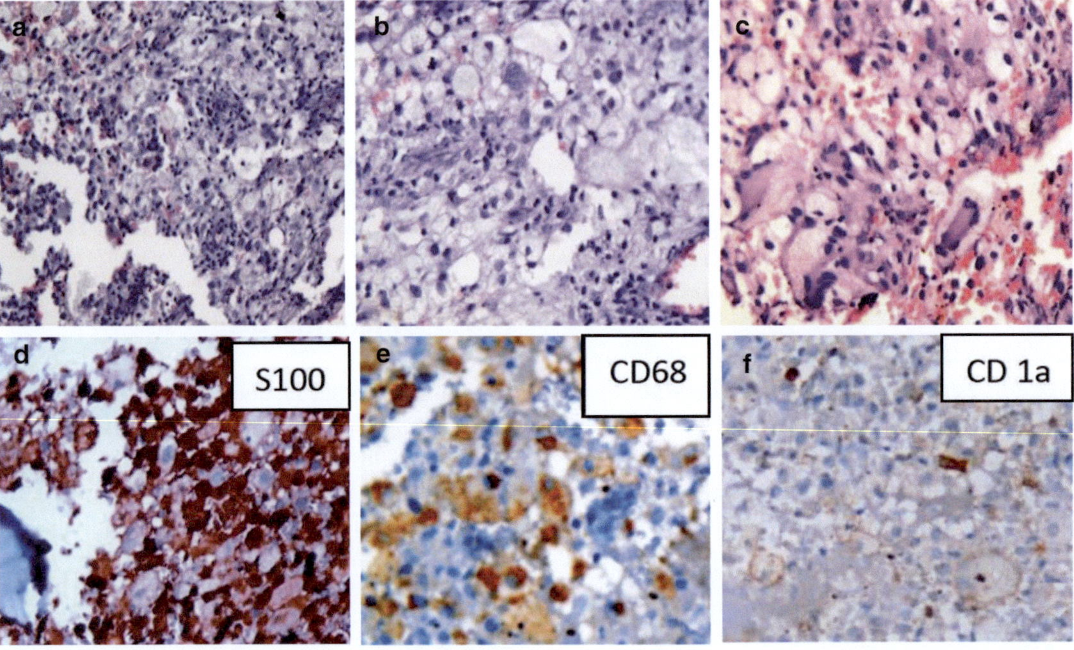

Fig. 10.6 ECD in a 62-year-old female: (**a**) Collection of foamy histiocytes admixed with lymphocytes and multinucleated giant cells, H&E ×100. (**b**) Sheets of foamy histiocytes, H&E ×250. (**c**) Giant cells (Touton type and foreign body type), H&E ×250. (**d**) S100 ×250. (**e**) CD68 ×250. (**f**) CD1a, ×250 (negative)

patients will have progressive disease with diabetes insipidus because of the involvement of pituitary or it may affect lung (pulmonary fibrosis), heart (cardiac failure) or brain (cerebral symptoms).

10.3 Rosai-Dorfman Disease (RDD)

RDD is also known as sinus histiocytosis with massive lymphadenopathy (SHML). It is a rare disorder, first described by Rosai and Dorfman in 1969 [19, 25]. The aetiology is unknown. The patients usually present with massive lymphadenopathy of neck with fever, increased ESR and leukocytosis. There is involvement of extra-nodal sites in some cases [17]. Rarely the extra-nodal sites alone are involved without involvement of lymph nodes. The extra-nodal sites are the orbit, eyelid, upper respiratory tract, salivary gland, skin, bone and testes.

RDD rarely has bone involvement (only in 28% of cases) [26]. Primary bone RDDs occur in less than 10% of cases. Since osseous RDD is rare and because of the dense inflammatory component, it is confused with other lesions, such as lymphoma, Langerhans cell histiocytosis (LCH), osteomyelitis, storage diseases and sarcoma.

10.3.1 Clinical

All age groups are involved, but it usually occurs in first and second decades. The patients may be asymptomatic and present as incidental findings [22]. Pain and swelling are the main symptoms. Depending on the site of involvement, pressure symptoms can be present. It can involve any bone [21, 23]. Long bones, skull, vertebrae and small bones are mainly involved. Sometimes, multiple bones are involved.

10.3.2 Radiology

The lesions are lytic or mixed lytic and sclerotic and involve metaphysis (Fig. 10.7). The margins are ill defined. The differential diagnosis includes metastatic disease, osteomyelitis, eosinophilic granuloma, giant cell tumour, etc.

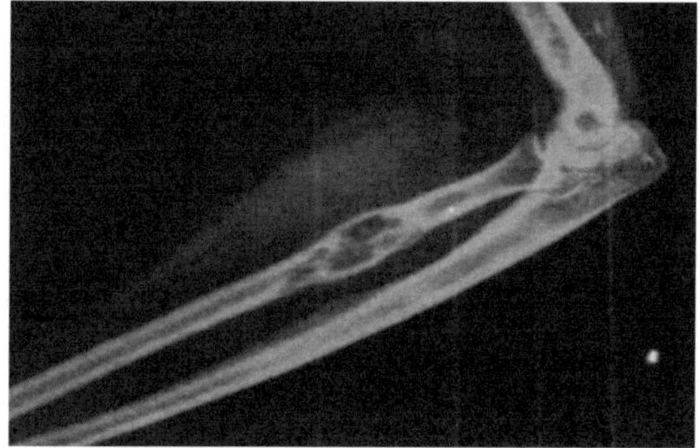

Fig. 10.7 SHML of radius with mixed lytic and sclerotic lesion involving metadiaphyseal area

- **Courtesy: Dr. Jayasree Geothe**

10.3.3 Pathology

Mixed inflammatory cells including lymphocytes, plasma cells, scattered eosinophils, neutrophils and collection of histiocytes are seen in the marrow spaces. A pale and dark area is observed. The histiocytes are seen in groups or sheets, and they appear pale at low-power examination. Darker areas are mainly lymphocytes and plasma cells. The histiocytes are with abundant pale, eosinophilic to vacuolated cytoplasm with phagocytosis of lymphocytes and plasma cells. This is known as "emperipolesis". This finding is absent in other histiocytic diseases like LCH and EDD. The bony trabeculae are not seen in this area, or they may be sparse. Reactive bone formation and areas of fibrosis can be seen in the adjacent area. Sometimes RDD and ECD can occur in same patient [24].

10.3.4 IHC

Histiocytes are positive for S-100 protein, CD68 and CD163 (histiocytic markers). They are negative for CD1a and langerin (CD207) (Fig. 10.8). Recently, OCT2 has been found to be positive in RDD [16]. Differential diagnosis includes other histiocyte-rich lesions like LCH, ECD, GCT and fracture site. The distinguishing feature is emperipolesis of histiocytes.

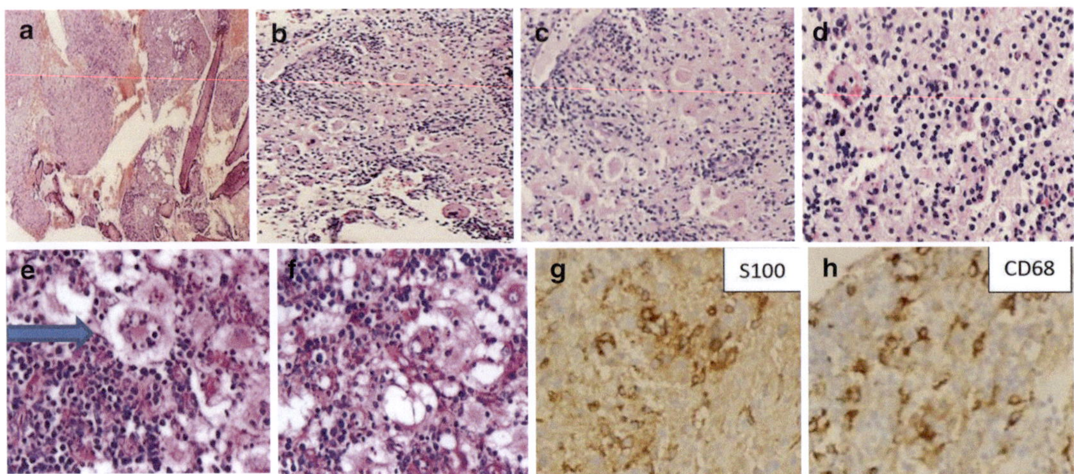

Fig. 10.8 SHML. (**a**) Low power showing cells in sheets, H&E ×40. (**b** and **c**) Pale and dark areas, H&E ×100. (**d**) Low power of pale area showing clusters of histiocytes, H&E ×100. (**e**, **f**) Histiocytes with emperipolesis. Cytoplasm shows ingested lymphocytes, H&E ×400. (**g**) S100 ×100. (**h**) CD68 ×250 (both histiocytic markers). These histiocytes are negative for CD1a and langerin

10.3.5 Molecular

Activation of RAS/MPK pathway has been implicated in the pathogenesis of RDD. KRAS and MAP2K1 mutations are described in this disease [20].

10.3.6 Treatment and Prognosis

Lesions may resolve spontaneously. If symptomatic, surgical removal is the treatment of choice. In most patients, treatment consists of curettage. The outcome of primary intraosseous RDD is good. In recurrent cases, lesions may develop at new sites like other bone, lymph nodes or soft tissue.

10.4 Xanthoma of Bone

Xanthoma of bone is a very rare benign primary bone tumour [28]. Histologically, it is characterized by sheets of foamy histiocytes and multinucleated giant cells.

10.4.1 Clinical

Patients are usually males, more than 20 years. It occurs commonly in flat bones [30]. Pelvis, ribs and skull are preferred sites. Other bones involved are mandible [27], calcaneum [29], femur [31], etc. They may be detected as incidental finding. The lesions are usually solitary. Some patients present with pain.

10.4.2 Radiology

An expansile lytic lesion with a sclerotic margin is seen.

10.4.3 Pathology

Gross appearance: These are bright yellow well-circumscribed lesions.

Microscopy shows sheets of foam cells, cholesterol crystals and giant cells. Xanthoma of bone is a diagnosis of exclusion. Many bone lesions are rich in foamy histiocytes like ECD,

RDD, fibrous dysplasia, giant cell tumour (GCT) and non-ossifying fibroma (NOF). Underlying diseases have to be excluded before giving a diagnosis of xanthoma. Radiology and clinical features will help in excluding other entities. Metastatic clear cell carcinoma, especially from kidney, is the most important differential diagnosis.

10.4.4 IHC

Xanthoma cells are CD68 positive and cytokeratin (CK) negative. CD10 and CK will be positive in clear cell RCC. CD1a is negative. Other histiocytic markers are positive (Fig. 10.9).

10.4.5 Treatment

Xanthoma of bone is a benign lesion. They are treated with curettage. Prognosis is excellent.

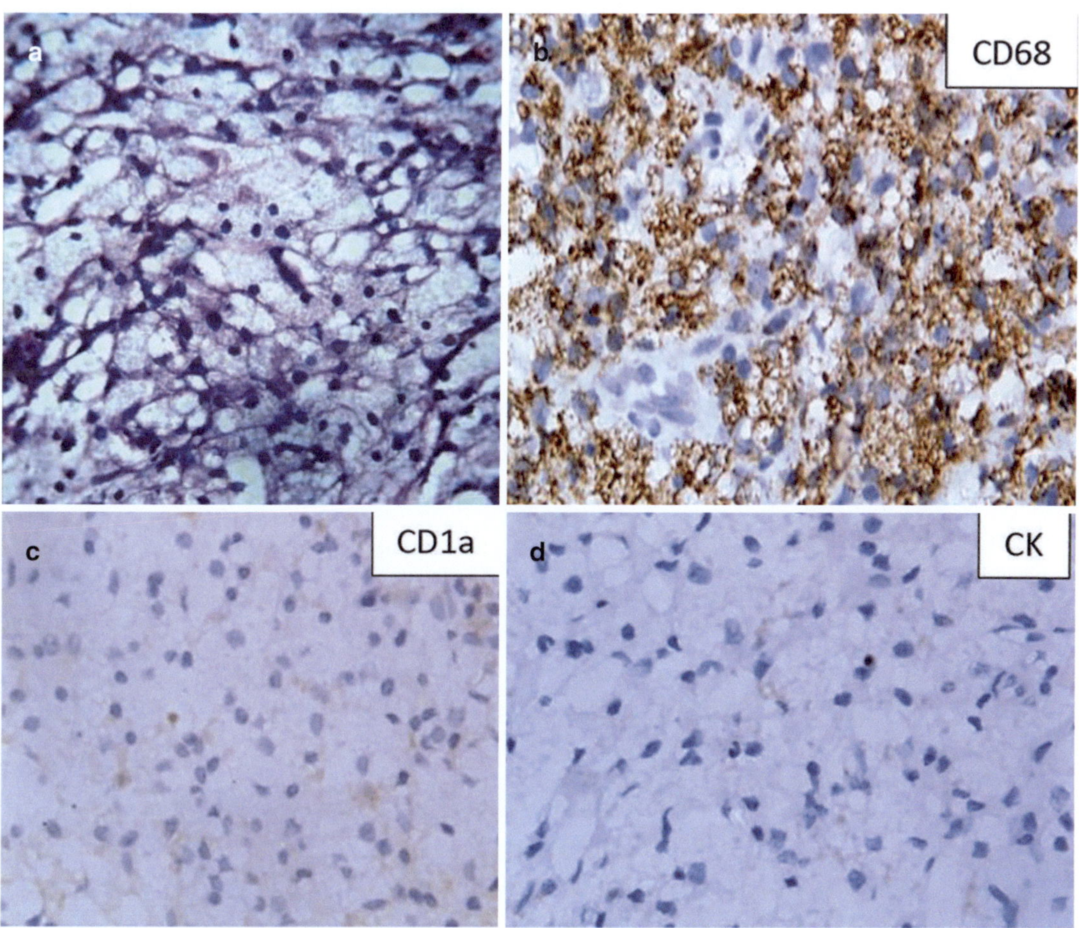

Fig. 10.9 Xanthoma of bone: (**a**) Foamy histiocytes mimicking metastatic carcinoma, H&E ×250. (**b**) CD68, ×100. (**c**) CD1a, ×100. (**d**) CK, ×100 (both CD1a and CK are negative)

Points to Remember

- **LCH** is divided into LCH, NOS and LCH, disseminated.
  Unifocal (localized) form (70%), e.g. eosinophilic granuloma.
  Multifocal unisystem (20%), e.g. Hand-Schüller-Christian disease.
  Multifocal multisystem, e.g. Letterer-Siwe disease.
  Langerhans cell with grooved nuclei, CD1a and langerin positive. Birbeck granules in EM.

Admixed eosinophils.

- **ECD**: Bilateral symmetric lytic lesions of long bones; flat bones not affected. Associated diabetes insipidus, cardiac failure and pulmonary fibrosis may be present. Histiocytic markers positive, CD1a negative.
- **RDD**: Rare in bones. Pale and dark areas. Pale areas with sheets of histiocytes with emperipolesis. S100 positive, CD1a and langerin negative.

References

Langerhans Cell Histiocytosis

1. Badalian-Very G, Vergilio JA, Degar BA, MacConaill LE, Brandner B. Recurrent BRAF mutations in Langerhans cell histiocytosis. Blood. 2010;116:1919–23.
2. Go H, Jeon YK, Huh J, Choi SJ, Choi YD, et al. Frequent detection of BRAF(V600E) mutations in histiocytic and dendritic cell neoplasms. Histopathology. 2014;65:261–72.
3. Hervier B, Haroche J, Arnaud L, Charlotte F, Donadieu J, et al. Association of both Langerhans cell histiocytosis and Erdheim-Chester disease linked to *BRAF* V600E mutation. Blood. 2014;124:1119–26.
4. Nakamine H, Yamakawa M, Yoshino T, Fukumoto T, Enomoto Y, Matsumura I. Langerhans cell histiocytosis and Langerhans cell sarcoma: current understanding and differential diagnosis. J Clin Exp Hematop. 2016;56(2):109–18.
5. Kilpatrick SE, Wenger DE, Gilchchrist GS, Shives TC, Wollan PC, Unni KK. Langerhans' cell histiocytosis of bone: a clinicopathologic analysis of 263 paediatric and adult cases. Cancer. 1995;76:2471–84.
6. Pileri SA, Grogan TM, Harris NL, Banks P, Campo E, Chan JK, Favera RD, Delsol G, De Wolf-Peeters C, Falini B, Gascoyne RD, Gaulard P, Gatter KC, Isaacson PG, Jaffe ES, Kluin P, Knowles DM, Mason DY, Mori S, Müller-Hermelink HK, Piris MA, Ralfkiaer E, Stein H, Su IJ, Warnke RA, Weiss LM. Tumours of histiocytes and accessory dendritic cells: an immunohistochemical approach to classification from the International Lymphoma Study Group based on 61 cases. Histopathology. 2002;41(1):1–29.

Erdheim Chester Disease

7. Chasset F, Barete S, Charlotte F, et al. Cutaneous manifestations of Erdheim-Chester disease (ECD): clinical, pathological, and molecular features in a monocentric series of 40 patients. J Am Acad Dermatol. 2016;74(3):513–20.
8. Courtillot C, Laugier Robiolle S, Cohen Aubart F, et al. Endocrine manifestations in a monocentric cohort of 64 patients with Erdheim-Chester disease. J Clin Endocrinol Metab. 2016;101(1):305–13.
9. Diamond EL, Dagna L, Hyman DM, et al. Consensus guidelines for the diagnosis and clinical management of Erdheim-Chester disease. Blood. 2014;124(4):483–92.
10. Egan AJ, Boardman LA, Tazelaar HD, Swensen SJ, Jett JR, Yousem SA, et al. Erdheim-Chester disease: clinical, radiologic, and histopathologic findings in five patients with interstitial lung disease. Am J Surg Pathol. 1999;23:17–26.
11. Maloku E, Loo EY. Erdheim-Chester disease—a review of molecular genetic and clinical features. Adv Mol Pathol. 2020;3:57–64.
12. Haroche J, Cohen Aubart F, Amoura Z. Erdheim-Chester disease. Blood. 2020;135(16):1311–8.
13. Lachenal F, Cotton F, Desmurs-Clavel H, Haroche J, Taillia H, Magy N, et al. Neurological manifestations and neuroradiological presentation of Erdheim-Chester disease: report of 6 cases and systematic review of the literature. J Neurol. 2006;253:1267–77.
14. Alotaibi S, Alhafi O, Nasr H, Eltayeb K, Elyamany G. Erdheim-Chester disease: case report with aggressive multisystem manifestations and review of the literature. Case Rep Oncol. 2017;10:501–7.
15. Toya T, Ogura M, Toyama K, Yoshimi A, Shinozaki-Ushiku A, Honda A, Honda K, Hosoya N, Murakami Y, Kawashima H, Nannya Y, Arai S, Nakamura F, Shinoda Y, Nangaku M, Miyagawa K, Fukayama M, Moriya-Saito A, Katayama I, Ogura T, Kurokawa M. Prognostic factors of Erdheim–Chester disease: a nationwide survey in Japan. Haematologica. 2018;103(11):1815–24.

Rosai-Dorfman Disease

16. Ravindran A, Goyal G, Go RS. Rosai-Dorfman disease displays a unique monocyte-macrophage pheno-

type characterized by expression of OCT2. Am J Surg Pathol. 2021;45:35–44.
17. Al-Saad K, Thorner P, Ngan BY, et al. Extranodal Rosai-Dorfman disease with multifocal bone and epidural involvement causing recurrent spinal cord compression. Pediatr Dev Pathol. 2005;8:593–8.
18. Demicco EG, Rosenberg AE, Björnsson J, Emile JF, Abla O, Fraitag S, et al. Revised classification of histiocytoses and neoplasms of the macrophage-dendritic cell lineages. Blood. 2016;127:2672–81.
19. Foucar E, Rosai J, Dorfman R. Sinus histiocytosis with massive lymphadenopathy (Rosai-Dorfman disease): review of the entity. Semin Diagn Pathol. 1990;7:19–73.
20. Garces S, Medeiros LJ, Patel KP, et al. Mutually exclusive recurrent KRAS and MAP2K1 mutations in Rosai-Dorfman disease. Mod Pathol. 2017;30:1367–77.
21. Goyal G, Ravindran A, Young JR, et al. Clinicopathological features, treatment approaches, and outcomes in Rosai-Dorfman disease. Haematologica. 2019;105:348–57.
22. Rybak LD, Krishnan Unni K, Petur Nielsen G. Primary Rosai-Dorfman disease of bone: a clinicopathologic study of 15 cases. Am J Surg Pathol. 2010;34:1324–33.
23. Mosheimer BA, Oppl B, Zandieh S, et al. Bone involvement in Rosai-Dorfman disease (RDD): a case report and systematic literature review. Curr Rheumatol Rep. 2017;19:29.
24. Razanamahery J, Diamond EL, Cohen-Aubart F, et al. Erdheim-Chester disease with concomitant Rosai-Dorfman like lesions: a distinct entity mainly driven by MAP2K1. Haematologica. 2020;105:e5–8.
25. Rosai J, Dorfman RF. Sinus histiocytosis with massive lymphadenopathy. A newly recognized benign clinicopathological entity. Arch Pathol. 1969;87:63–70.
26. Sundaram C, Uppin Shantveer G, Chandrashekar P, et al. Multifocal osseous involvement as the sole manifestation of Rosai-Dorfman disease. Skeletal Radiol. 2005;34:658–64.

Xanthoma of Bone

27. Morel D, Kelsch RD, Nolan PJ. Primary xanthoma of the mandible: report of a rare case. Head Neck Pathol. 2016;10:245–51.
28. Bertoni F, Krishnan Unni K, McLeod RA, Sim FH. Xanthoma of bone. Am J Clin Pathol. 1988;90(4):377–84.
29. Ahmed G, Al Dosari M, El-Mahi M, Abolfotouh SM. Primary xanthoma of calcaneus bone: case report. Int J Surg Case Rep. 2014;5:699–702.
30. Alhaneedi G, Salameh M, AbuHejleh H. Xanthoma of bone: a mini review. Arch Surg Oncol. 2018;4:2471–671.
31. Hossain MI, Khan AKMS. Primary xanthoma of femur: a case report. Bangladesh J Med Sci. 2015;14(4):396–8.
32. WHO Classification of Tumours. In: WHO Classification of Tumours Editorial Board, editor. Soft tissue and bone tumours. WHO classification of tumours, 5th ed., vol. 3. IARC; 2020.

11 Notochordal Tumours

Notochordal derived lesions are a spectrum of lesions which include notochordal rest or notochordal remnant and chordoma, a malignant tumour. Mirra and Brien described "giant notochordal hamartoma" in 2001. The present terminology by the WHO for this lesion is "benign notochord cell tumour (BNT)." Recently, Carter et al. have described a new entity atypical notochordal cell tumour (ANCT).

11.1 WHO Classification of Notochordal Tumours (WHO 2020) [60]

- **Benign**
  - Benign notochordal tumour
- **Malignant**
  - Chordoma NOS
    Chondroid chordoma
  - Poorly differentiated chordoma
  - Dedifferentiated chordoma

11.2 Benign

11.2.1 Benign Notochordal Tumour (BNT)

The giant notochordal rest and notochordal hamartoma are benign notochordal cell tumours (BNTs). These should not be mistaken for chordoma [1]. This lesion is thought to be a precursor of chordoma [3, 8]. But they rarely transform to chordoma. Similar to chordomas, these lesions also have a predilection for sacrococcygeal [5] and spheno-occipital regions. Most tumours are small [2] and asymptomatic. They are usually detected at autopsy. Sometimes, it becomes large and can be detected on imaging. Usually, they are tiny or small, less than 5 mm. Multifocal BNTs are described [5].

11.2.1.1 Radiology

BNTs are occult on radiographs and often discovered incidentally on magnetic resonance imaging (MRI). No contrast enhancement will be seen on CT and MRI [57]. There is no destruction of bone, and lesions may appear sclerotic and lack soft tissue extension. They show intralesional fat, a feature helpful to distinguish from chordoma [33].

11.2.1.2 Pathology

Histologically, they are seen in marrow spaces and may be mistaken for permeation [6, 7]. Cells are small pink or with vacuolated cytoplasm resembling adipocytes (Fig. 11.1a). They lack lobulation and myxoid matrix as seen in chordomas. There will be no cytologic atypia. Cytokeratin, EMA and brachyury are positive as in chordomas (Fig. 11.1b).

11.2.1.3 Treatment

Asymptomatic patients with BNT, can be followed up with serial imaging. The symptomatic

J. Kattoor et al., *Bone Tumors*, https://doi.org/10.1007/978-981-99-4738-6_11

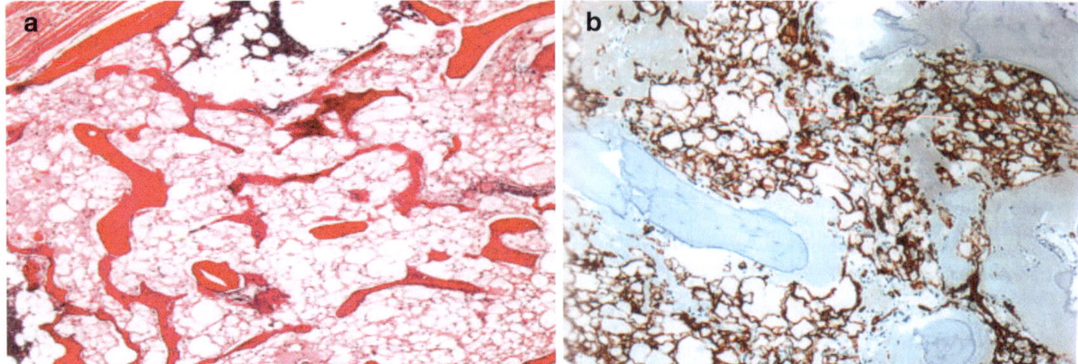

Fig. 11.1 (**a**) Cells resembling adipocytes in between bony trabeculae, H&E ×40. (**b**) Cells are positive for cytokeratin, CK ×100

BNTs are treated conservatively by excision [4]. Chordoma arising in BNT is extremely rare [56].

11.3 Chordoma NOS

Chordomas are malignant notochordal tumours with locally aggressive behaviour and potential for metastasis [55, 59]. They are very rare tumours. It represents up to 4% of primary malignant bone tumours [11, 27]. Depending on their location, chordomas are predominantly subdivided into clival [17, 26] (38%) and sacrococcygeal [35, 36] (45%). The rest are cervical, thoracic and lumbar [37]. Multifocal chordomas can occur [47].

11.3.1 Pathogenesis

In 1858, Muller hypothesized that these tumours are of notochordal origin. In 1894, Ribbert first introduced the term "ecchordosis physaliphora" [39]. The most important evidence of notochordal origin is the finding of gene duplication in the transcription factor T gene (brachyury) in familial chordoma [45]. Brachyury is encoded by TBXT, a transcription factor essential for notochordal development. It is seen in familial chordomas. Recently, the role of tyrosine kinase receptor expression and activation of downstream signalling are implicated in tumour growth and progression [14, 40]. The germline duplication of brachyury, which occurs in familial chordomas, plays an important role in notochord differentiation.

11.3.2 Clinical

Chordomas occur in adults above 40 years of age [15]. It is uncommon below 30 years. It is rare in children and adolescents (5%). But there are case reports of chordomas occurring in children [41]. The youngest case in our experience is 4 years. Males are more affected than females. In the cranial chordomas, both males and females are equally affected. Extra-axial chordomas are also reported. This mainly occurs in wrist and feet. The most common symptoms are pain and constipation for sacral chordomas. Spheno-occipital chordomas have symptoms referable to pressure on cranial nerves, and commonly nerves to the eye are affected [34]. It can also present as dysfunction of pituitary gland by destroying the gland or it can present as a swelling in the cerebello-pontine angle.

11.3.3 Radiology

Chordomas are destructive lytic tumours in the midline [50, 53]. In sacral chordomas, there will be destruction of bone with soft tissue mass anteriorly [22], better appreciated in lateral view of plain X-ray (Fig. 11.2). Chordomas are usually missed due to overlying gas shadows in the antero-posterior view. Hence, delay in diagnosis can occur. The tumour is better appreciated on MRI and is seen as lobulated mass (Fig. 11.3). Displacement of rectum may be seen. Residual bone or calcification within the tumour will be seen as densities. In cranial chordomas, destruction of clivus is the common finding.

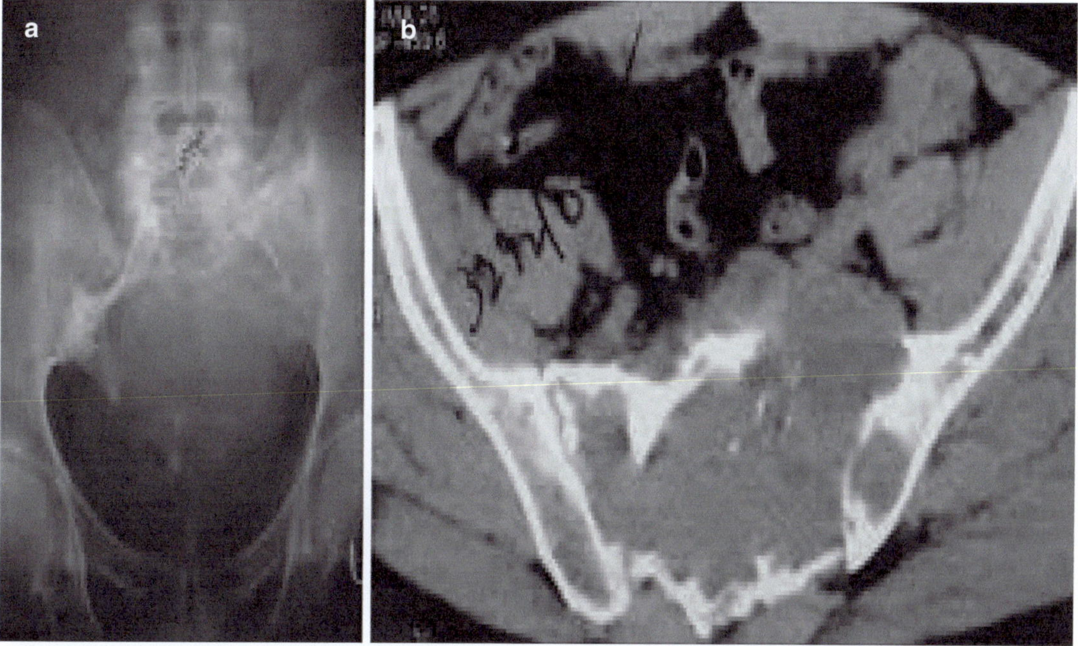

Fig. 11.2 Chordoma sacrum. (**a**) Plain X-ray showing large destructive lesion sacrum. (**b**) MRI of the same lesion

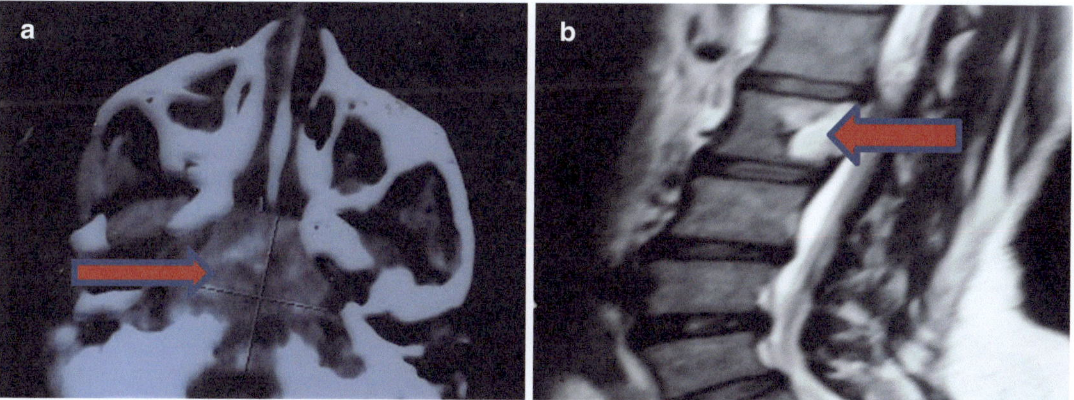

Fig. 11.3 (**a**) Chondroid chordoma clivus. (**b**) Chordoma of vertebra (red arrows)

Cranial, thoracic and lumbar chordomas produce destruction of body with or without sclerosis [32].

11.3.4 Pathology

Grossly, chordomas are lobulated with fibrous septa and gelatinous glistening cut surface (Fig. 11.4). It may resemble chondrosarcoma or mucinous adenocarcinoma.

In 1857, Virchow first described the physaliferous cells (bubble appearing) in this tumour [18]. Physaliferous cells are the large cells seen in classical chordomas. These cells are seen in groups or lobules separated by fibrous septa, and they are seen surrounded by a basophilic extracellular matrix rich in mucin and glycogen (Figs. 11.5 and 11.6). The cytoplasm of physaliferous cells is rich in glycogen. It can be demonstrated by periodic acid-Schiff (PAS) technique [49] and is diastase labile, but remains after treatment with hyaluronidase. The cells appear in cords in the myxoid matrix. Individual cells are small pink to large vacuolated. Cytoplasm is vacuolated with single or multiple vacuoles. Cells with single vacuole may resemble signet ring cells. Multivacuolated cells are the "physaliferous cells." Sometimes, spindle or epithelioid cells can predominate [16] (Fig. 11.7). But cytological atypia will be minimal in these cells. Large cells with smudged nuclei giving pseudosarcomatous appearance can be seen. These findings are not considered as dedifferentiation. Rarely, giant cell-rich chordomas can occur.

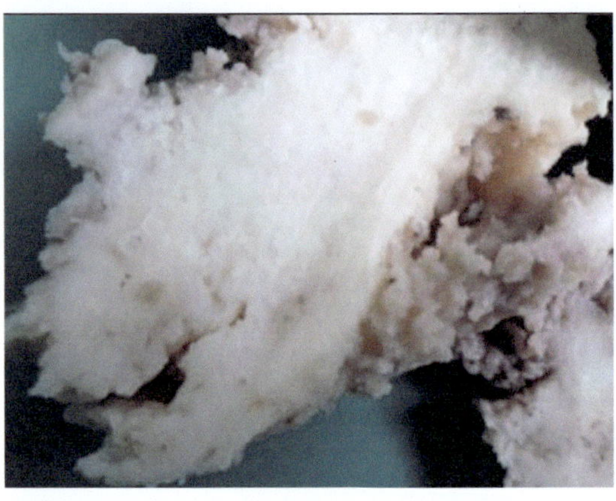

Fig. 11.4 Gross picture of a sacral chordoma with a whitish gelatinous cut surface

11.3.5 IHC

Chordomas are positive for cytokeratin and EMA and show variable positivity for S100. The diagnostic sensitive and specific marker is brachyury [10, 30].

11.3.6 Chondroid Chordoma

Is a variant of chordoma, typically occurring at the spheno-occipital region [56]. They resemble chondrosarcomas (Fig. 11.8). Typical areas of chordoma may be present. Sometimes, it is very difficult to differentiate it from chondrosarcoma. IHC for cytokeratin and brachyury positivity confirms chordoma diagnosis. Podoplanin and S100 are positive in chondrosarcomas. But CK and brachyury together have 98% sensitivity and 100% specificity in the diagnosis of chordoma [32]. If the location is midline with low-grade chondrosarcoma appearance, a diagnosis of

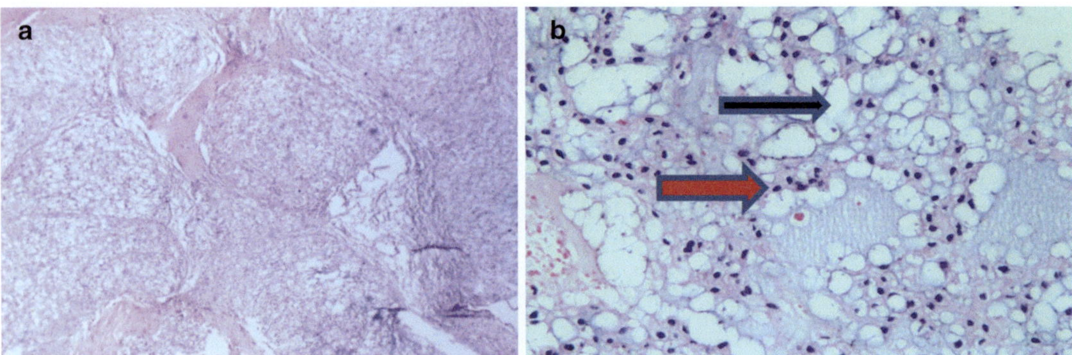

Fig. 11.5 Chordoma. (**a**) Tumour cells in lobules, H&E ×100. (**b**) Small pink cells in cords (black arrow) admixed with large physaliferous cells (red arrow) with multivacuolated cytoplasm in a myxoid stroma, H&E ×250

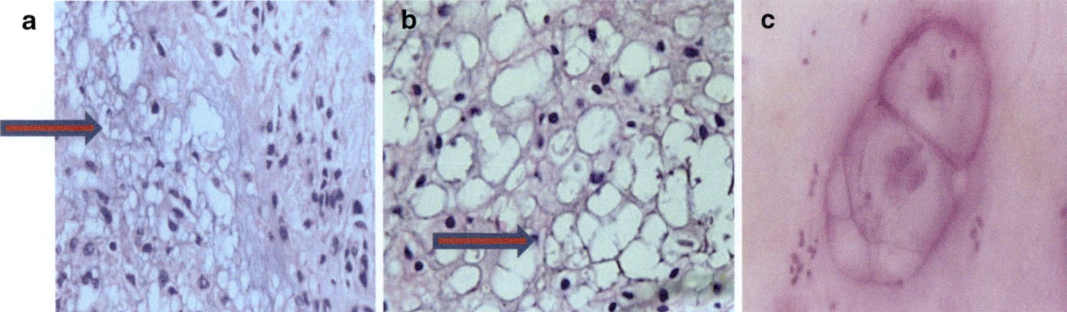

Fig. 11.6 Physaliferous cells. (**a**) Multivacuolated large cells with bubbly cytoplasm (red arrow), H&E ×100. (**b**) H&E ×250. (**c**) Cytology of physaliferous cells, Pap ×1000

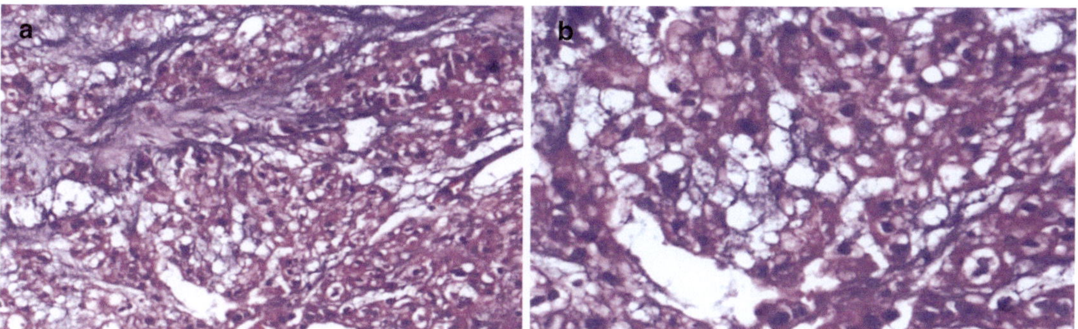

Fig. 11.7 Chordoma. (**a**) Epithelioid type of cells may predominate, H&E ×100. (**b**) Epithelioid cells and myxoid stroma. Typical physaliferous cells may be absent, making diagnosis difficult especially in a needle biopsy. IHC will help in arriving at a diagnosis

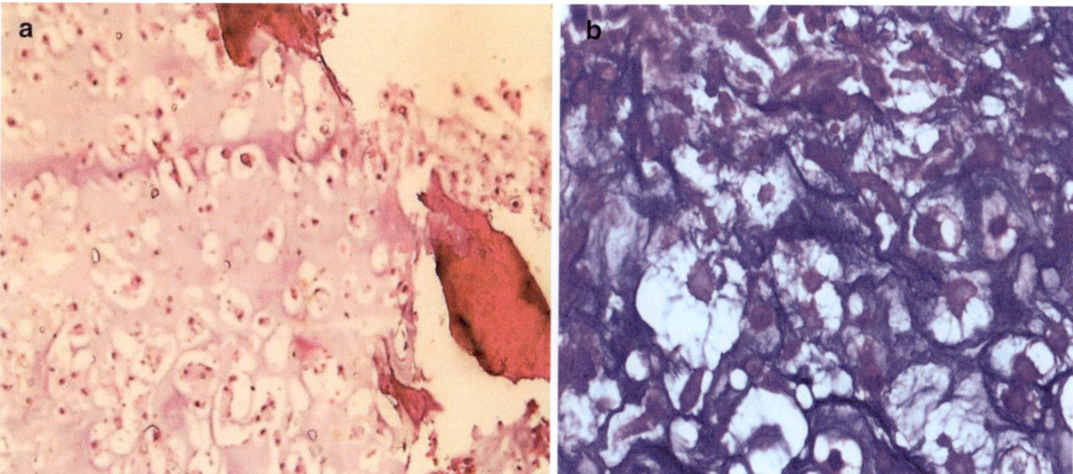

Fig. 11.8 Chondroid chordoma of clivus. (**a**) Cells have a chondroid appearance with a more myxoid stroma, H&E ×100. (**b**) H&E ×400. These cases are difficult to differentiate from chondrosarcoma. Brachyury stain will be positive in these cases

chondroid chordoma is justified. Management of chondroid chordomas and low-grade chondrosarcoma is same [29]. Rosenberg et al. reported excellent prognosis for skull base chondrosarcomas when compared to chordomas [42, 43]. Hence, an attempt should be made to separate them from chordomas at this site.

Table 11.1 Differential diagnosis of chordoma

- Metastatic Ca: lacks lobulation, more cytological atypia, CK+, brachyury−
- Myxopapillary ependymoma: GFAP+, brachyury−
- Myxoid CS (chordoid sarcoma): CK−, brachyury−, S100+
- Chordoid meningioma: location, CK−, brachyury−, S100+, EMA+

11.3.7 Differential diagnosis

The diagnosis of chordoma is straightforward. The differential diagnosis of sacral chordoma includes metastatic carcinoma and myxopapillary ependymoma (Table 11.1). Metastatic carcinoma will have more cytological atypia, and they are not lobulated. In some cases, intracytoplasmic mucin can be demonstrated by mucicarmine or periodic acid-Schiff (PAS). This is absent in chordoma. Myxopapillary ependymomas can be differentiated by IHC stains (brachyury negative,

GFAP positive). Myoepitheliomas and chondrosarcomas are brachyury negative [51]. Brachyury shows nuclear strong positivity in >95% of chordomas [24]. Brachyury can be positive in some other tumours [31]. Extraskeletal myxoid chondrosarcoma mimics chordoma morphologically. Hence, it is also called chordoid sarcoma. But these tumours are negative for CK and brachyury. Chordoid meningioma is a differential in skull base chordomas. These tumours are CK and brachyury negative and S100 and EMA positive.

11.3.8 Treatment and prognosis

Radical resection is the treatment of choice. In many cases, excision will not be complete [13]. Radiotherapy is required in these cases. Proton beam radiotherapy is found to have good results in skull base tumours [31]. Tyrosine kinase inhibitors like imatinib and sunitinib have been tried in chordomas [14, 44, 52].

Incompletely excised tumours recur [19]. Metastasis is rare, but can occur to lung, soft tissue and bones [54]. Most metastasis occurs between 3 and 7 years [12]. Metastasis to distal bone is rapid to develop and has the worst prognosis. Metastasis is common in young patients and is a poor prognosticator [19, 23]. Metastasis is rare in skull-based lesions.

11.4 Poorly Differentiated Chordoma

Poorly differentiated chordoma is a neoplasm with notochordal differentiation characterized by SMARCB1 expression [58]. This is a rare tumour. The main differences from conventional and dedifferentiated chordoma are given in Table 11.2.

11.4.1 Clinical

It is commonly seen in axial skeleton. The most common site is skull base (clivus), followed by cervical vertebra and sacrum. This type of chordoma is common in children and young adults. Females are commonly affected (M:F = 1:2). Patients present with weight loss and other nonspecific symptoms like headache and cranial nerve symptoms.

Table 11.2 Features of conventional, poorly differentiated and dedifferentiated chordomas

	Chordoma	PD chordoma	Dedifferentiated chordoma
Morphology	Lobules of epithelioid cells + physaliferous cells	Sheets of epithelioid cells	Low-grade areas + high-grade sarcoma—fibrosarcoma or osteosarcoma or rhabdomyosarcoma
Physaliferous cells	Present	Absent	Present in low-grade area
IHC	CK, EMA S100 variable Brachyury	CK Brachyury INI 1 loss	CK Brachyury in classical area
Molecular	Brachyury encoded by TBXT HER1 (EGFR)	SMARC B1 deletion Co-deletion of EWSR1	Same as chordoma

Abbreviations: *PD* poorly differentiated, *CK* cytokeratin, *EMA* epithelial membrane antigen

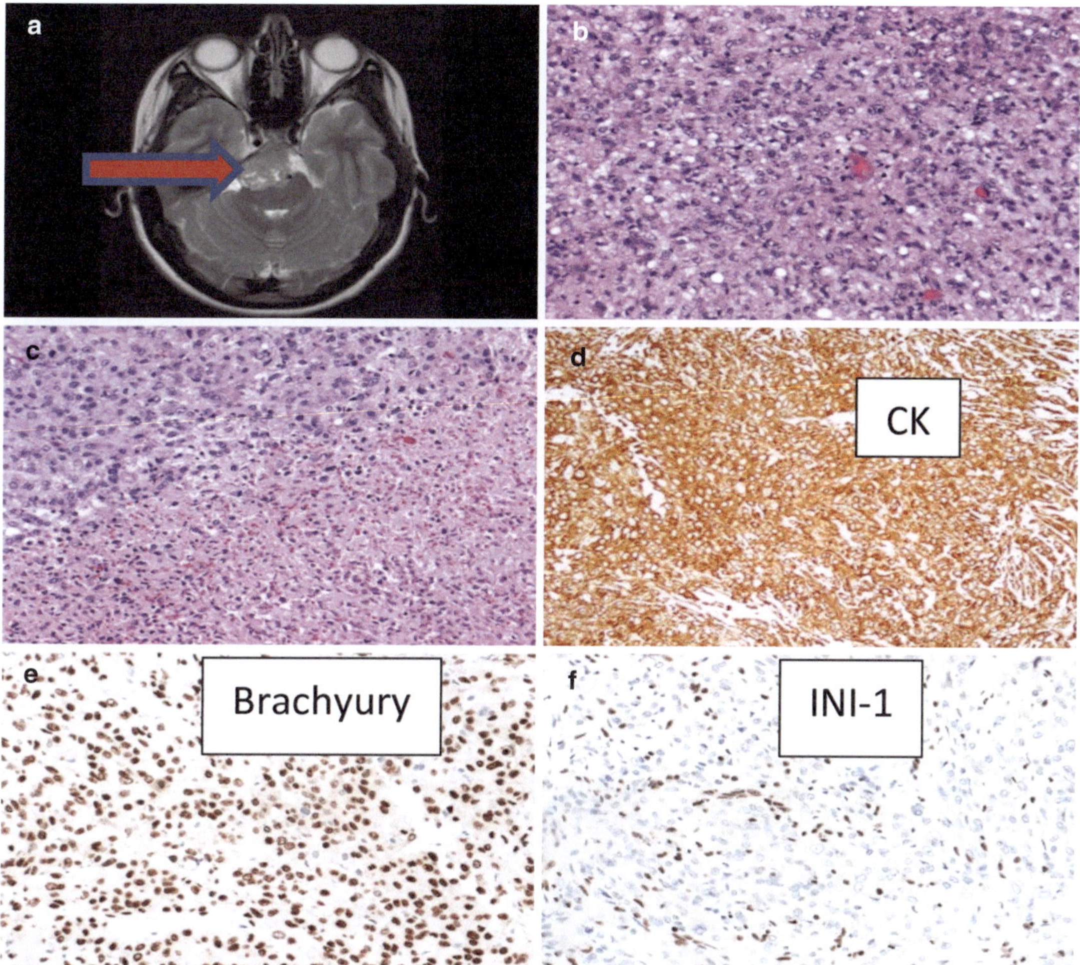

Fig. 11.9 Poorly differentiated chordoma in a child. (**a**) MRI showing an intracranial midline mass (red arrow). (**b** and **c**) Sheets of rhabdoid/epithelioid cells are seen, H&E ×100. No physaliferous cells. (**d**) Cytokeratin ×100. (**e**) Brachyury ×100 (nuclear positivity). (**f**) Tumour also shows INI-1 loss of expression ×100 (internal control endothelial cells positive)

11.4.2 Pathology

Size of the tumour varies between 2 and 10 cm, most of them around 5 cm. Microscopy shows sheets and nests of epithelioid cells, many showing rhabdoid morphology. Cells are with abundant cytoplasm, with cytoplasmic vacuoles and moderately pleomorphic vesicular nuclei. Mitotic activity is often increased. Typical physaliferous cells are absent. Extracellular myxoid stroma will also be seen focally. Geographical necrosis is seen in many cases. Cells are positive for CK and brachyury and show loss of staining with SMARCB1 (INI 1 loss) (Fig. 11.9). FISH for SMARCB1 deletions with co-deletion of EWSR1 is the confirmatory test.

11.4.3 DD

Rhabdoid tumour and rhabdoid meningioma are the close differential diagnosis.

11.4.4 Treatment and prognosis

These tumours are treated with a combination of surgery, radiotherapy and chemotherapy. Prognosis is poor.

11.5 Dedifferentiated Chordomas

These are very rare type of chordomas showing areas of typical chordoma with abrupt transition to high-grade spindle cell sarcoma [46]. This usually occurs after radiation.

11.5.1 Clinical

Commonly occur in sacrococcygeal sites with rapidly enlarging mass. It presents de novo or secondary to conventional chordoma.

11.5.2 Radiology

This is similar to conventional chordoma, but on MRI can show a bimorphic appearance.

11.5.3 Pathology

Grossly, the high-grade component has solid fleshy appearance with adjacent lobulated gelatinous cut surface of conventional chordoma. The sarcomatous area can be fibrosarcoma or osteosarcoma or rhabdomyosarcoma (Fig. 11.10). The dedifferentiated component is negative for brachyury but can show focal cytokeratin positivity.

11.5.4 DD

Dedifferentiated chondrosarcoma is a close differential.

11.5.5 Treatment and prognosis

Surgical removal is the only treatment option. Radiation and chemotherapy have no beneficial effects. Prognosis is very poor with early metastasis and high mortality.

11.6 Extra-Axial Chordoma

Chordomas are rare malignant tumours considered to arise from notochordal remnants that persist in the axial location. When they arise from extra-axial notochord remnants, they are referred to as extra-axial chordomas [9, 21]. They are extremely rare. Few cases are reported in other bones and rare cases in soft tissue. The bone cases can be intramedullary or intra-cortical. Specific marker like brachyury is required for correct diagnosis.

11.6.1 Pathogenesis

Regression of notochord occurs in different stages during the maturity of embryo. In areas where the notochord has not regressed are the

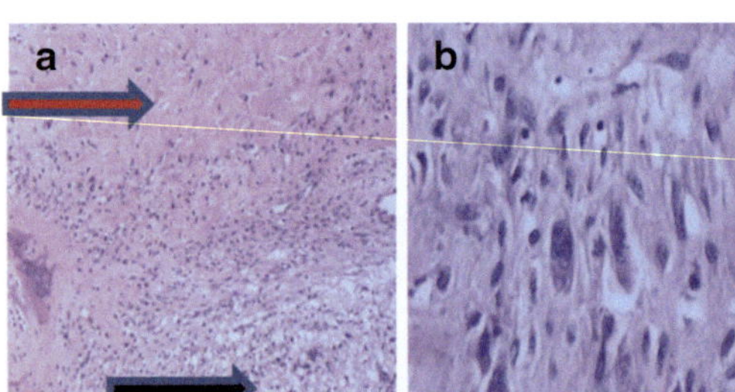

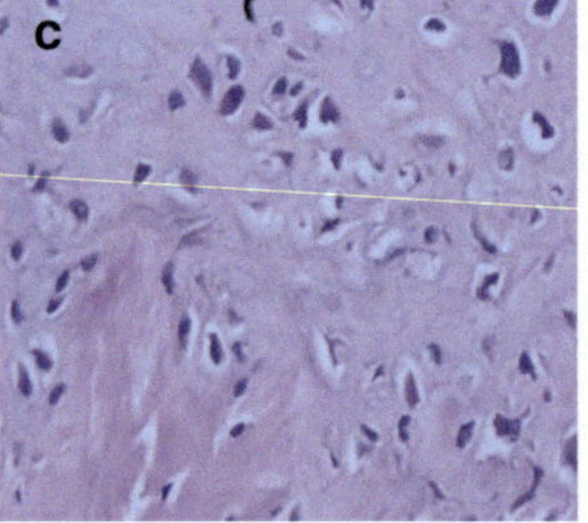

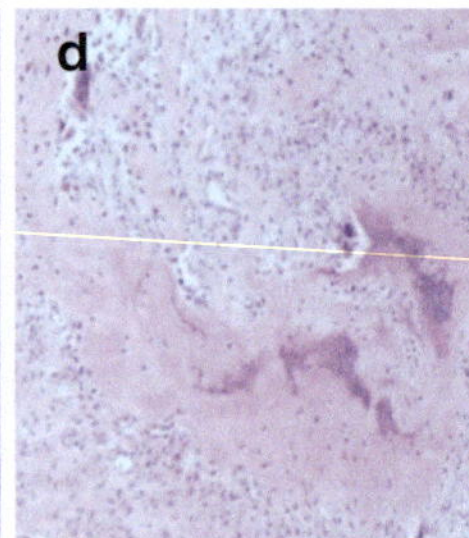

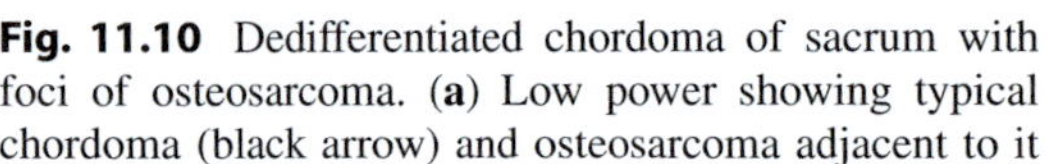

Fig. 11.10 Dedifferentiated chordoma of sacrum with foci of osteosarcoma. (**a**) Low power showing typical chordoma (black arrow) and osteosarcoma adjacent to it (red arrow), H&E ×40. (**b** and **c**) Pleomorphic malignant cells producing osteoid, H&E ×250. (**d**) Osteosarcoma with calcifying osteoid, H&E ×100

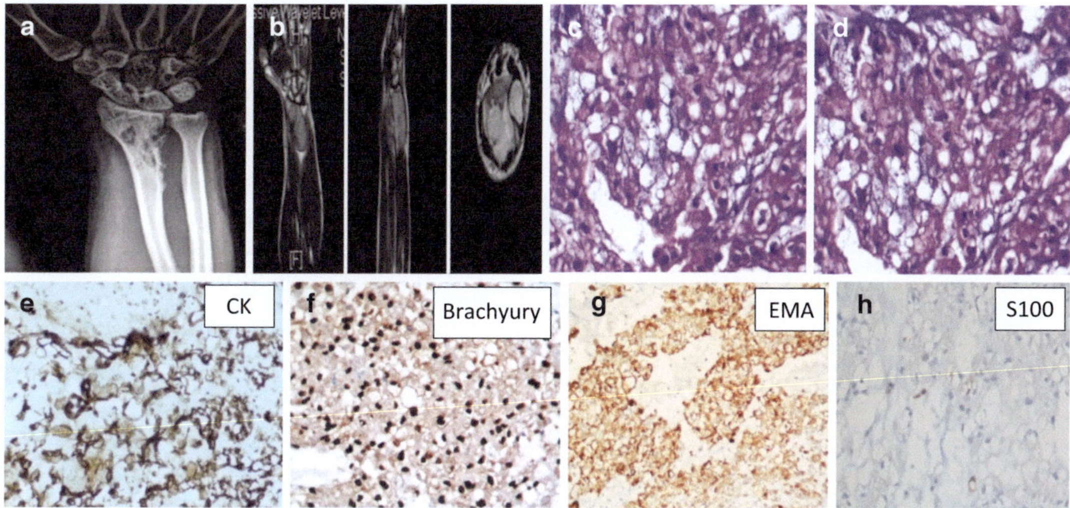

Fig. 11.11 Extra-axial chordoma of radius in a 38-year-old male. Extensive search for midline primary was negative. (**a** and **b**) Plain X-ray and MRI showing destructive lesion at the lower end of the radius. (**c** and **d**) Chordoma with typical histology, H&E ×250. (**e**) Cytokeratin ×250. (**f**) Brachyury with strong nuclear positivity ×100. (**g**) EMA ×100. (**h**) S100 ×100 (negative). (IHC Courtesy: Dr. Bharat Rekhi, Tata Memorial Hospital, for doing brachyury for our case and sharing the picture)

sites of extra-axial chordomas. The common locations are sacrococcygeal, cranial, spheno-occipital, nasopharyngeal and vertebral regions.

11.6.2 Clinical

The extra-axial bone chordomas have been reported in various sites like tibia [38], rib, metatarsals, ulna, femur, pubis and radius [21, 48]. Two soft tissue brachyury-positive tumours were reported in juxta-articular location involving the thumb and the wrist [25]. One case was reported in lung parenchyma also.

11.6.3 Pathology

The morphology of the tumour is exactly similar to conventional chordoma (Fig. 11.11). IHC for S100 (80%), CK and brachyury (100%) confirms the diagnosis [20]. Metastasis from conventional sites should be excluded before calling this tumour as extra-axial [25].

11.6.4 Treatment and Prognosis

Radical resection with a wide margin is the treatment of choice. It is extremely rare. Late recurrence is reported, even after 12 years. Metastasis is less frequent.

11.7 Atypical Notochordal Cell Tumour (ANCT)

This is a recently described entity from Mayo Clinic, USA [28]. These cases were atypical by radiology and histology from BNT to some extent, but insufficient to qualify as chordoma. They showed minimal destruction of bone and soft tissue extension unlike BNT. Histologically also, these cases had myxoid matrix, which is usually absent in BNT. But long-term follow-up of these cases showed behaviour same as BNT. Hence, they can be treated conservatively with follow-up radiology.

Points to Remember

- Chordomas are notochordal cell tumours.
- Chords of cells in basophilic matrix.
- Characteristic cell is physaliferous cells (bubble like).
- Brachyury is the specific marker. Other positive IHC markers are CK, EMA and S100.
- Poorly differentiated chordomas are recently described and included in 2020 WHO classification.
- Physaliferous cells are absent in PD chordomas. Brachyury positive, INI 1 loss and SMARC B1 deletion on molecular study.
- Dedifferentiated and extra-axial chordomas are rare.

References

Benign Notochordal Tumour (BNCT)

1. Chauvel A, Taillat F, Gille O, et al. Giant vertebral notochordal rest: a new entity distinct from chordoma. Histopathology. 2005;47:643–52.
2. Corsi A, De Maio F, Mancini F, et al. Notochordal inclusions in the vertebral bone marrow. J Bone Miner Res. 2008;23:572–5.
3. Deshpande V, Nielsen GP, Rosenthal DI, Rosenberg AE. Intraosseous benign notochord cell tumors (BNCT): further evidence supporting a relationship to chordoma. Am J Surg Pathol. 2007;31: 1573–7.
4. Amer HZM, Hameed M. Intraosseous benign notochordal cell tumor. Arch Pathol Lab Med. 2010;134:283–8.
5. Iorgulescu JB, Laufer I, Hameed M, et al. Benign notochordal cell tumors of the spine: natural history of 8 patients with histologically confirmed lesions. Neurosurgery. 2013;73:411–6.
6. Kreshak J, Larousserie F, Picci P, et al. Difficulty distinguishing benign notochordal cell tumor from chordoma further suggests a link between them. Cancer Imaging. 2014;14:4.
7. Yamaguchi T, Suzuki S, Ishiiwa H, et al. Benign notochordal cell tumors: a comparative histological study of benign notochordal cell tumors, classic chordomas, and notochordal vestiges of fetal intervertebral discs. Am J Surg Pathol. 2004;28:756–61.
8. Yamaguchi T, Suzuki S, Ishiiwa H, Ueda Y. Intraosseous benign notochordal cell tumors: overlooked precursors of classic chordomas? Histopathology. 2004;44:597–602.

Chordoma

9. Cesinaro AM, Maiorana A, Collina G, Fano RA. Extraaxial chordoma. Report of a case with immunohistochemical study. Pathologica. 1993;85(1100):755–60.
10. Abenoza P, Sibley RK. Chordoma: an immunohistologic study. Hum Pathol. 1986;17:744–7.
11. Walcott BP, Nahed BV, Mohyeldin A, Coumans J-V, Kahle KT, Ferreira MJ. Chordoma: current concepts, management, and future directions. Lancet Oncol. 2012;13:e69–76.
12. Catton C, O'Sullivan B, Bell R, et al. Chordoma: long-term follow-up after radical photon irradiation. Radiother Oncol. 1996;41:67–72.
13. Gill CM, Fowkes M, Shrivastava RK. Emerging therapeutic targets in chordomas: a review of the literature in the genomic era. Neurosurgery. 2020;6(2):E118–23.
14. Tamborini E, Miselli F, Negri T, et al. Molecular and biochemical analyses of platelet-derived growth factor receptor (PDGFR) B, PDGFRA, and KIT receptors in chordomas. Clin Cancer Res. 2006;12:6920–8.
15. Eriksson B, Gunterberg B, Kindblom LG. Chordoma. A clinicopathologic and prognostic study of a Swedish national series. Acta Orthop Scand. 1981;52:49–58.
16. Fan F, Templeton K, Damjanov I. Epithelioid cellular chordoma of the sacrum: a potential diagnostic problem. Ann Diagn Pathol. 2005;9(3):139–42.
17. Fernandez-Miranda JC, Gardner PA, Snyderman CH, et al. Clival chordomas: a pathological, surgical, and radiotherapeutic review. Head Neck. 2014;36:892.
18. Fletcher CD, Bridge JA, Hogendoorn PCW, et al. WHO classification of tumours of soft tissue and bone. Lyon: IARC; 2013. p. 328–9.
19. Frezza AM, Botta L, Trama A, et al. Chordoma: update on disease, epidemiology, biology and medical therapies. Curr Opin Oncol. 2019;31:114.
20. Oakley GJ, Fuhrer K, Seethala RR. Brachyury, SOX-9, and podoplanin, new markers in the skull base chordoma vs chondrosarcoma differential: a tissue microarray-based comparative analysis. Mod Pathol. 2008;21(12):1461–9.
21. Suzuki H, Yamashiro K, Takeda H, Nojima T, Usui M. Extra-axial soft tissue chordoma of wrist. Pathol Res Pract. 2011;207(5):327–31.
22. Hsieh PC, Xu R, Sciubba DM, et al. Long-term clinical outcomes following en bloc resections for sacral chordomas and chondrosarcomas: a series of twenty consecutive patients. Spine (Phila Pa1976). 2009;34:2233–9.
23. Lee J, Bhatia NN, Hoang BH, Ziogas A, Zell JA. Analysis of prognostic factors for patients with

chordoma with use of the California Cancer Registry. J Bone Joint Surg. 2012;94:356–63.
24. Jambhekar NA, Rekhi B, Thorat K, Dikshit R, Agrawal M, Puri A. Revisiting chordoma with brachyury, a "new age" marker: analysis of a validation study on 51 cases. Arch Pathol Lab Med. 2010;134:1181–7.
25. Abraham J, Clemens MW, Oates S. Aggressive metastatic chordoma in the wrist. Plast Reconstr Surg Glob Open. 2014;2:e245. https://doi.org/10.1097/GOX.0000000000000218.
26. Deruaz J-P, Uske A, de Tribolet N. Skull base chordomas: presentation of six cases and review of the literature. J Clin Neurosci. 1994;1:7–18.
27. Chen JW. A historical recount of chordoma. J Neurosurg Spine. 2018;28:422–8. https://doi.org/10.3171/2017.7.SPINE17668.
28. Carter JM, Wenger DE, Rose PS, Inwards CY. Atypical notochordal cell tumors. a series of notochordal-derived tumors that defy current classification schemes. Am J Surg Pathol. 2017;41:39–48.
29. Fernandez-Miranda JC, Gardner PA, Snyderman CH, Devaney KO, Mendenhall WM, Suárez C, Rinaldo A, Ferlito A. Clival chordomas: a pathological, surgical, and radiotherapeutic review. Head Neck. 2014;36:892–906.
30. Meis J, Giraldo AA. Chordoma: an immunohistochemical study of 20 cases. Arch Pathol Lab Med. 1988;102:553–6.
31. Miettinen M, Wang Z, Lasota J. nuclear brachyury expression is consistent in chordoma, common in germ cell tumors and small cell carcinomas, and rare in other carcinomas and sarcomas: an immunohistochemical study of 5229 cases. Am J Surg Pathol. 2015;39(10):1305–12.
32. Mitchell A, Scheithauer BW, Unni KK, Forsyth PJ, Wold LE, McGivney DJ. Chordoma and chondroid neoplasms of the spheno-occiput. An immunohistochemical study of 41 cases with prognostic and nosologic implications. Cancer. 1993;72:2943–9.
33. Nishiguchi T, Mochizuki K, Ohsawa M, et al. Differentiating benign notochordal cell tumors from chordomas: radiographic features on MRI, CT, and tomography. Am J Roentgenol. 2011;196:644–50.
34. Noël G, Habrand JL, Jauffret E, et al. Radiation therapy for chordoma and chondrosarcoma of the skull base and the cervical spine. Prognostic factors and patterns of failure. Strahlenther Onkol. 2003;179:241–8.
35. van Wulfften Palthe ODR, Ferreira A, et al. Sacral chordoma: a clinical review of 101 cases with 30-year experience in a single institution. Spine J. 2019;19:869–79.
36. Dijkstra PDS, Peul WC, Vleggeert-Lankamp CLA. Chordoma: a systematic review of the epidemiology and clinical prognostic factors predicting progression-free and overall survival. Eur Spine J. 2018;27:3043–58.
37. Papagelopoulos PJ, Mavrogenis AF, Galanis EC, et al. Chordoma of the spine: clinicopathological features, diagnosis,and treatment. Orthopedics. 2004;27(12):1256–63.
38. O'Donnell P, Tirabosco R, Vujovic S, et al. Diagnosing an extra-axial chordoma of the proximal tibia with the help of Brachyury, amolecule required for notochordal differentiation. Skeletal Radiol. 2007;36(1):59–65.
39. Park HH, Lee KS, Ahn SJ, et al. Ecchordosis physaliphora: typical and atypical radiologic features. Neurosurg Rev. 2017;40:87.
40. Presneau N, Shalaby A, Idowu B, et al. Potential therapeutic targets for chordoma: PI3K/AKT/TSC1/TSC2/mTOR pathway. Br J Cancer. 2009;100(9):1406–14.
41. Ridenour RV, Ahrens WA, Folpe AL, Miller DV. Clinical and histopathologic features of chordomas in children and young adults. Pediatr Dev Pathol. 2010;13(1):9–17.
42. Rosenberg AE, Brown GA, Bhan AK, Lee JM. Chondroid chordoma–a variant of chordoma. A morphologic and immunohistochemical study. Am J Clin Pathol. 1994;101:36–41.
43. Rosenberg AE, Nielsen GP, Keel SB, Renard LG, Fitzek MM, Munzenrider JE, Liebsch NJ. Chondrosarcoma of the base of skull-A Clinicopathologic study of 200 cases with emphasis on its distinction from Chordoma. Am J Surg Pathol. 1999;23:1370–8.
44. Stacchiotti S, Marrari A, Tamborini E, et al. Response to imatinib plus sirolimus in advanced chordoma. Ann Oncol. 2009;20(11):1886–94.
45. Vujovic S, Henderson S, Presneau N, et al. Brachyury, a crucial regulator of notochordal development, is a novel biomarker for chordomas. J Pathol. 2006;209(2):157–65.
46. Saito T, Hasegawa TS, et al. Dedifferentiated chordoma: a case report. Jpn J Clin Oncol. 1998;28(12):766–71.
47. Smith DS, French G, Miller M. Multifocal benign notochordal cell tumours. Histopathology. 2007;51:412–4.
48. Sugath S, Jayashree SMB. Unusual presentation of Chordoma in distal radius. J Bone Soft Tissue Tumors. 2018;4(2):33–5.
49. Crawford T. The staining reactions of chordoma. J Clin Pathol. 1958;11:110.
50. Kaiser TE, Pritchard DJ, Unni KK. Clinicopathologic study of sacrococcygeal chordoma. Cancer. 1984;53(11):2574–8.
51. Tirabosco R, Mangham DC, Rosenberg AE, Vujovic S, Bousdras K, Pizzolitto S, De Maglio G, den Bakker MA, Di Francesco L, Kalil RK, Athanasou NA, O'Donnell P, McCarthy EF, Flanagan AM. Brachyury expression in extra-axial skeletal and soft tissue chordomas: a marker that distinguishes chordoma from mixed tumor/myoepithelioma/parachordoma in soft tissue. Am J Surg Pathol. 2008;32(4):572–80.
52. Meng T, Jin J, Jiang C, Huang R, Yin H, Song D, Cheng L. Molecular targeted therapy in the treatment of chordoma: a systematic review. Front Oncol. 2019;9:1–16.
53. Unni KK. Dahlin's bone tumors: general aspects and data on 10165 cases. 6th ed. Wolters Kluwer/Lippincott Williams & Wilkins; 2010. p. 248–61.

54. Young VA, Curtis KM, Temple HT, Eismont FJ, DeLaney TF, Hornicek FJ. Characteristics and patterns of metastatic disease from chordoma. Sarcoma. 2015;2015:517657.
55. Yamaguchi T, Imada H, Iida S, Szuhai K. Notochordal tumors: an update on molecular pathology with therapeutic implications. Surg Pathol Clin. 2017; 10:637.
56. Yamaguchi T, Yamato M, Saotome K. First histologically confirmed case of a classic chordoma arising in a precursor benign notochordal lesion: differential diagnosis of benign and malignant notochordal lesions. Skeletal Radiol. 2002;31:413–8.
57. Yamaguchi T, Iwata J, Sugihara S, et al. Distinguishing benign notochordal cell tumors from vertebral chordoma. Skeletal Radiol. 2008;37(4):291–9. https://doi.org/10.1007/s00256-007-0435-y.
58. Yeter HG, Kosemehmetoglu K, Soylemezoglu F. Poorly differentiated chordoma: review of 53 cases. APMIS. 2019;127(9):607–15.
59. Ulici V, Hart J. Chordoma-A review and differential diagnosis. Arch Pathol Lab Med. 2022;146(3):386–95. https://doi.org/10.5858/arpa.2020-0258-RA).
60. WHO Classification of Tumours. Soft tissue and bone tumours, vol. 3. Edited by the WHO Classification of Tumours Editorial Board. 5th ed. IARC; 2020.

12 Vascular Tumours of Bone

Vascular tumours of bone are classified as benign, borderline and malignant vascular tumours.

12.1 WHO Classification of Vascular Tumours of Bone [47]

- **Benign**
  - Haemangioma
  - Angiomatosis
- **Intermediate (locally aggressive or borderline)**
  - Epithelioid haemangioma
- **Malignant**
  - Epithelioid haemangioendothelioma NOS
  - Angiosarcoma

12.2 Benign

12.2.1 Haemangioma

Haemangiomas are the most common diagnoses among connective tissue tumours. However, haemangiomas of bone are of minor importance when surgical procedures for diagnoses and therapy are concerned. Most of these lesions are asymptomatic and are detected accidentally while taking images for other reasons [1]. Gorham disease or disappearing or phantom bone disease also called as massive osteolysis is a form of bone haemangioma. This is a rare disorder affecting children or young adults with partial or complete disappearance of one or more bones [7, 12]. Haemangiomas of bone can be solitary or may affect two or more bones of a single extremity. Sometimes, they may involve soft tissue and cause deformities.

12.2.1.1 Clinical

Haemangioma can be capillary or cavernous type. 70% of cases are in the third to sixth decades. It is rare in infants. Females are more affected. Cranium (50%) and vertebrae (20%) are the common sites involved. They are usually solitary. Multifocal involvement is seen especially in vertebral column. In the extremities, one or more lesions of the same bone or two or three bones of the same limb may be seen [34]. Patients are asymptomatic. Pain and swelling may be a feature in some cases. Fractures including compression fracture may occur. During surgery, severe haemorrhage can occur, especially in jaw bones.

12.2.1.2 Radiology

Haemangioma is characterized by lytic area with coarse striations especially in long bones. In flat bones, the bone is expanded and lytic with radially oriented striations. Destruction of cortex can be present, but complete cortical destruction with soft tissue involvement may not be present. In the vertebral body, haemangioma shows vertical striations or multiple lytic foci. These patterns are commonly known as corduroy cloth pattern and honeycomb pattern respectively. The changes produced thus are known as polka-dot appearance

J. Kattoor et al., *Bone Tumors*, https://doi.org/10.1007/978-981-99-4738-6_12

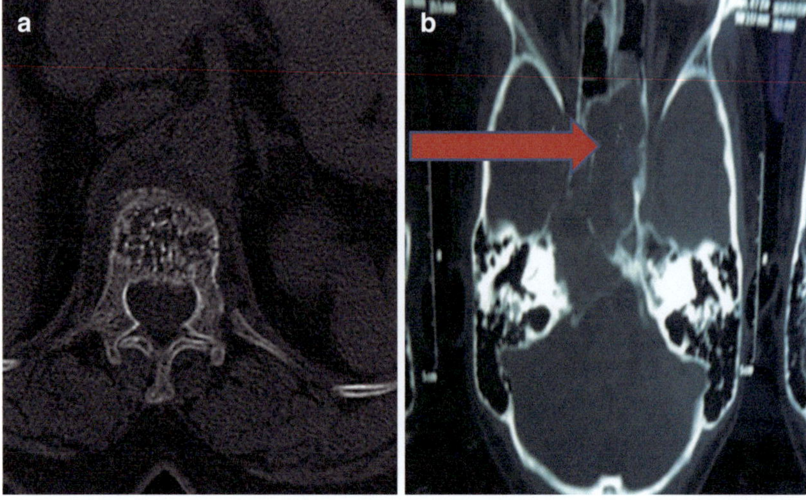

Fig. 12.1 (**a**) Haemangioma of vertebra showing polka-dot appearance. (**b**) MRI of skull showing large destructive lesion (red arrow). Courtesy Fig. 12.1a: Dr. Jayanthi

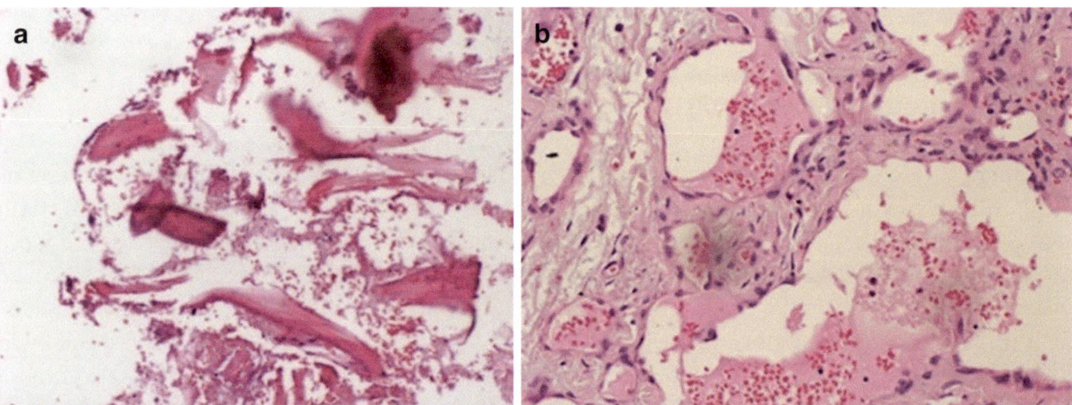

Fig. 12.2 Cavernous haemangioma bone. (**a**) Multiple blood-filled spaces in between bony trabeculae, H&E ×40. (**b**) Large dilated spaces lined by flattened endothelial cells filled with blood, H&E ×250

(Fig. 12.1). In skull bones, it produces thickened trabeculae arranged in a spoke-wheel pattern, which is described as sunburst appearance. In long bones, the findings are non-specific. Fine trabeculations and end of bone involvement may resemble giant cell tumour. Massive involvement of soft tissue is associated with phleboliths.

12.2.1.3 Pathology

Grossly, haemangiomas are blue with honeycomb appearance. A firm fleshy appearance is seen in cellular tumours. Most haemangiomas are cavernous; occasionally, a capillary component may also be seen (Figs. 12.2 and 12.3). Reactive new bone rimmed by osteoblasts can also occur, simulating osteoblastoma.

12.2.1.4 Treatment and Prognosis

Haemangiomas are treated conservatively. In inaccessible sites, radiation may be required. Massive haemangiomas with soft tissue extension may require amputation.

12.2.2 Angiomatosis

Diffuse skeletal haemangiomatosis is a rare disorder affecting spine, pelvis, skull, ribs and shoulder [48, 49]. These lesions may affect visceral organs also. Prognosis is poor in such cases. In the bone, angiomatosis presents as multiple cystic lesions with or without soft tissue involvement. Soft tissue involvement is more

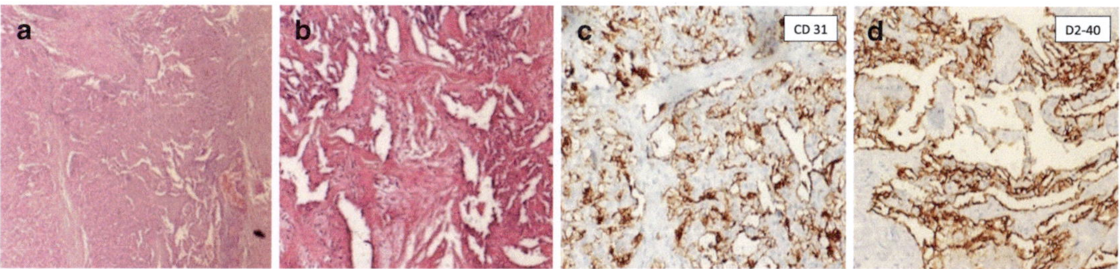

Fig. 12.3 Capillary haemangioma of skull. (**a** and **b**) Thin-walled vascular channels, H&E ×100. (**c**) Endothelial cells are positive for CD31 ×250. (**d**) D2–40 also positive ×250

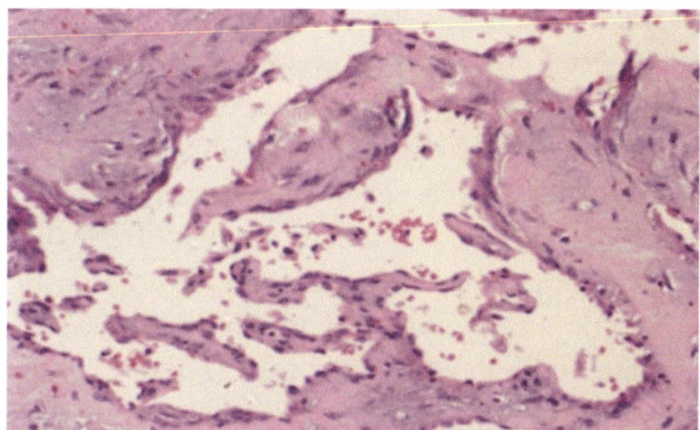

Fig. 12.4 Angiomatosis: Cystic vascular channels lined by flattened endothelial cells, H&E ×250

common (60–70%). The spleen is affected in many cases.

12.2.2.1 Clinical

The presenting complaints are pain, swelling or pathological fracture. Depending upon the clinical behaviour, they are divided into aggressive or nonaggressive. The bones affected can be regional or disseminated. In the regional involvement, there is destruction of one or more bones of same anatomic region. The trunk bones are typically affected in the disseminated form.

12.2.2.2 Pathology

Microscopy shows multiple vascular spaces lined by normal endothelial cells filled with erythrocytes (Fig. 12.4). Recently, WT1 immunomarker has been found to be useful in differentiating angiomatosis from haemangiomas [20].

12.2.3 Gorham Disease or Massive Osteolysis (Phantom Bone Disease)

Gorham disease is an aggressive form of angiomatosis [50]. It is also known as massive osteolysis. Malignant transformation to angiosarcoma is very rare. The syndromes associated with this disease are Von Hippel-Lindau syndrome, Maffucci syndrome, Klippel-Trenaunay syndrome, Kasabach-Merritt syndrome, Parkes Weber syndrome and Osler-Weber-Rendu disease.

12.2.3.1 Clinical

The patients present with pain and disability. Radiologically, there is progressive dissolution of one or more bones. The lesion may start in bone or soft tissue.

12.2.3.2 Radiology

In bone, it starts as a lytic lesion. If in soft tissue, bone rarefaction is seen on the surface with thinning and tapering producing sucked candy appearance.

12.2.3.3 Pathology

There is increased vascularity in the bone extending to soft tissues. Histologic changes may be non-specific. Sometimes, the histology resembles lymphangioma. Few cases are associated with lymphangioma of mediastinum. Treatment consists of reconstructive surgery and radiation.

12.2.4 Glomus Tumour of Bone

Primary glomus tumours of bone are extremely rare. Glomus tumour may erode bone or arise within it. Distal phalanx of a finger is usually involved. Histologically, there is proliferation of small round cells around capillaries.

12.3 Intermediate (Locally Aggressive) Tumours

12.3.1 Epithelioid Haemangioma (EH)

In 1979, Rosai described this entity as "histiocytoid haemangioma" and later called it as epithelioid haemangioma. This is a locally aggressive vascular neoplasm [3]. In this tumour, endothelial cells are epithelioid with abundant eosinophilic cytoplasm. These plump endothelial cells bulge from the vessel wall into the lumen, sometimes obscuring the lumen and forming sheet of cells.

12.3.1.1 Clinical

Epithelioid haemangiomas present as solitary lesions. Long tubular bones and short tubular bones of lower extremities are mainly involved followed by flat bones, vertebrae and small bones of hands.

12.3.1.2 Radiology

These tumours are predominantly lytic with sharply defined or sclerotic margins. Sometimes, the margins are lobulated. Rarely, they destroy the cortex and extend to soft tissue.

12.3.1.3 Pathology

The tumour can be very small (5–7 mm) or large (up to 15 cm). Cut surface is well defined with soft solid red and haemorrhagic. The cells of EH are epithelioid with abundant cytoplasm, and the nuclei are lobated with few of them showing grooves [23, 24]. The chromatin is fine, and small nucleoli are present. The cells may be arranged in lobules. Spaces are lined by plump epithelioid cells giving a tombstone appearance (Fig. 12.5). Large, clear intracytoplasmic vacuoles containing RBCs are usually present. Well-formed vessels in lobules will be present in the periphery. Sheets and cords of cells can be seen focally. Mitotic figures are rare. An inflammatory infiltrate composed of eosinophils and plasma cells is seen admixed with these tumour cells. These tumours are considered as low-grade malignant tumours because they can rarely recur (11%) or metastasize (2.7%). Small foci of necrosis can be seen.

Haemorrhagic epithelioid and spindle cell haemangioma is a variant of EH of bone [9, 18]. They are multifocal and affect the distal extremities. In this tumour, a mixture of epithelioid and spindle cell in lobules with extravasated red blood cells is seen.

12.3.1.4 IHC

CD31, CD34, FLI1 [14, 32] and ERG are the usual endothelial markers positive in EH. CK and EMA are also positive. Some cases show positivity for FOS or FOSB.

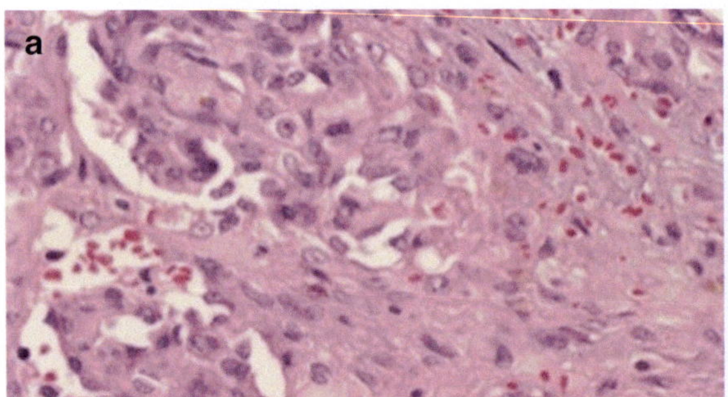

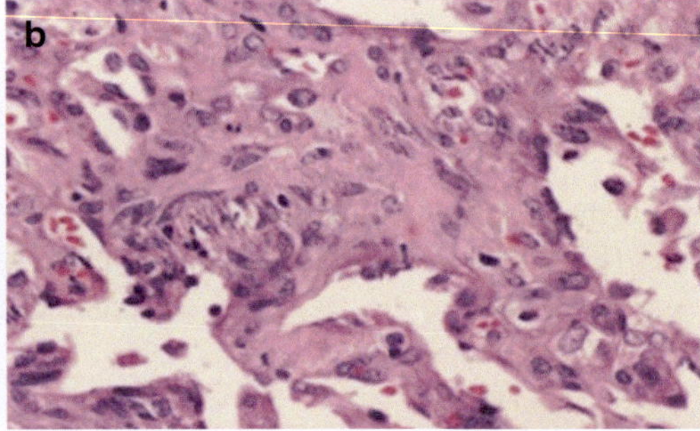

Fig. 12.5 (**a** and **b**) Epithelioid haemangioma with vascular spaces lined by plump epithelioid endothelial cells, H&E ×100

Table 12.1 Differential diagnosis of epithelioid vascular tumours [29]

	EH	EHE	EAS
Clinical	Long and short tubular bones	Long bones	Axial skeleton
Microscopy	Vessel formation prominent	Vessel formation not prominent Polygonal cells, intracytoplasmic vacuoles	Anastomosing vascular channels
IHC	CD31, CD34, ERG, FLI1, FOSB	CAMTA1, ERG, CD31, CD34	CK, CD31, CD34, ERG, FLI1
Molecular	FOS or FOSB rearrangement	WWTR1-CAMTA1 YAP1-TFE3	Limited. No confirmatory test

12.3.1.5 Molecular

Rearrangement of FOS or FOSB is present in these tumours.

12.3.1.6 DD

The differential diagnoses are epithelioid angiosarcoma (EAS) and epithelioid haemangioendothelioma (EHE) [2]. In EH, the atypia is very minimal, mitosis is sparse, necrosis is absent and there will be well-formed vessels. Lobulation is usually seen in benign tumours. The differentiating features in epithelioid vascular tumours are given in Table 12.1.

12.3.1.7 Treatment and prognosis

They are treated by curettage or limited local surgery. Radiation is given to tumours of inaccessible sites. Prognosis is good. Rarely do they recur.

12.4 Malignant Vascular Tumours

Haemangioendothelioma and angiosarcomas of bone are rare and may involve multiple bones.

12.4.1 Epithelioid Haemangioendothelioma (EHE) of Bone

EHE of bone is an uncommon tumour composed of endothelial cells that have epithelial characteristics [8, 19, 38]. It is a low- to intermediate-grade malignant tumour. Vasoformation in these cases is rare.

12.4.1.1 Clinical

It occurs mainly in second to third decades. Pain is the most common clinical presentation. The tumour occurs mainly at or near the ends of bones. The most commonly affected long bones are tibia, femur and humerus. It can affect any portion of the skeleton. A large number of cases are multicentric.

12.4.1.2 Radiology

Lesions are usually lytic with surrounding sclerosis. The features are non-specific (Fig. 12.6a, b). Presence of multiple lytic lesions in one anatomic area may be a clue to the diagnosis. It may show multiple lesions in one single bone or multiple bones of the same limb.

12.4.1.3 Pathology

Grossly, the tumours are soft, nodular with reddish cut surface. Microscopically, cells are in solid sheets and lack the lobulation. Tumour cells are embedded in a myxo-hyaline matrix (Fig. 12.7c). Cells are polygonal with abundant eosinophilic cytoplasm containing single or multiple vacuoles and indented oval nucleus (Fig. 12.6d–g). The cells may have a vacuolated appearance. Intracytoplasmic lumina with erythrocyte is a feature that prompts a diagnosis of tumour of vascular origin (Fig. 12.7c). Sometimes, spindle cells may predominate. The nuclei are round or oval, mildly pleomorphic with large eosinophilic nucleoli. Sparse mitotic activity (1–2/10HPF) is observed. Well-formed vessels are absent. Matrix may resemble cartilage. Sometimes, the matrix undergoes calcification. Eosinophils are sprinkled between tumour

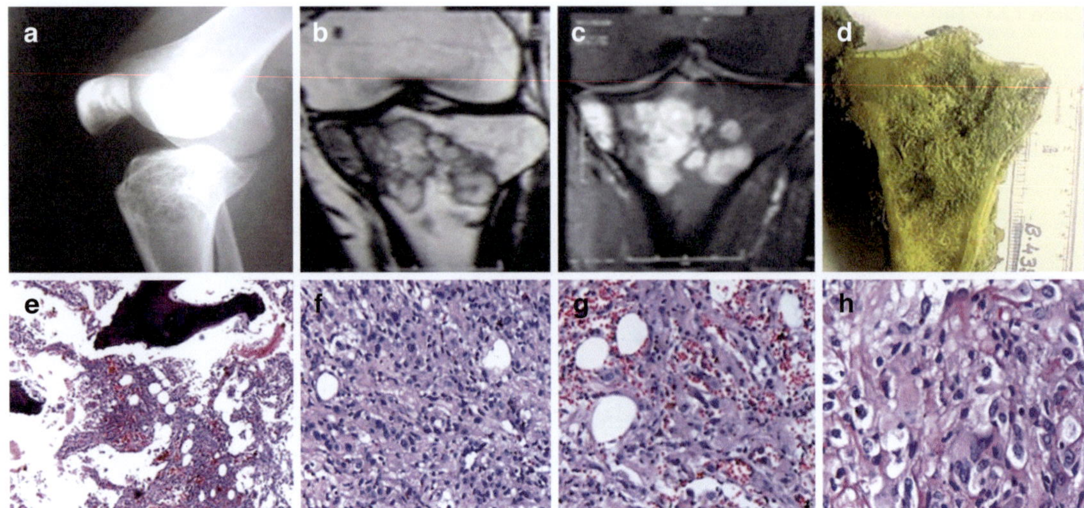

Fig. 12.6 Haemangioendothelioma tibia in a 21-year-old male, radiologically mimicking GCT. (**a**) Plain X-ray and MRI showing lytic lesion involving epiphysis mimicking giant cell tumour. (**b** and **c**) MRI. (**d**) Gross appearance of resected specimen with epi-metaphyseal involvement. (**e**) Scanner view showing sheets of cells, H&E ×40. (**f**) Sheets of epithelioid cells, H&E ×100. (**g**) Extravasated RBCs, H&E ×100. (**h**) High power showing epithelioid cells with abundant cytoplasm, cytoplasmic vacuolation and admixed eosinophils, H&E ×400. IHC for CD31 was strongly positive

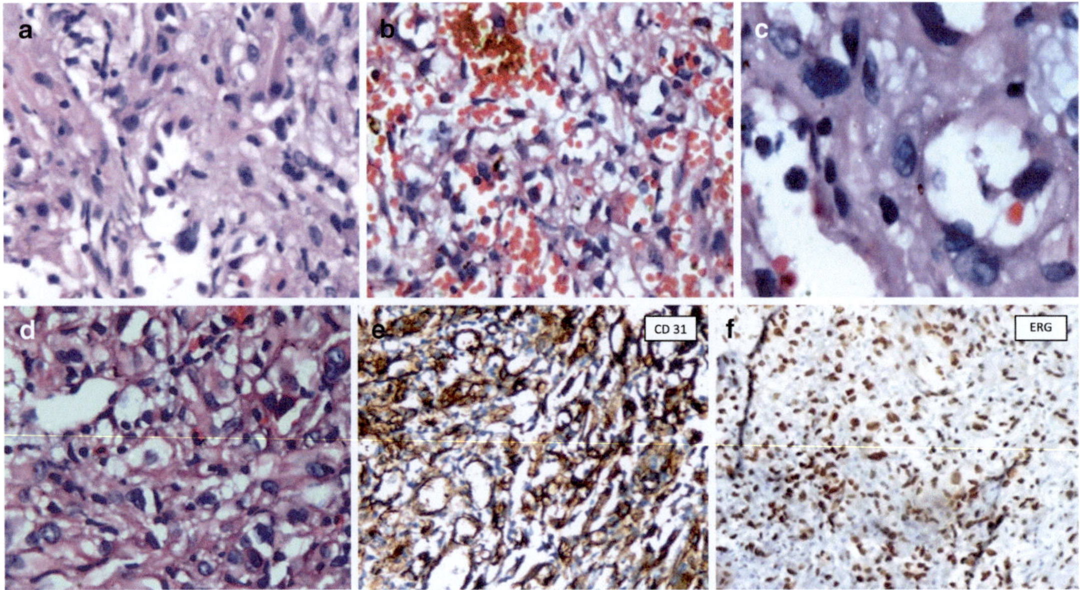

Fig. 12.7 EHE with lumen formation. (**a** and **b**) Note plump endothelial cells projecting into the lumina, H&E ×100. (**c**) Presence of cytoplasmic lumen with RBC in a myxo-hyaline stroma, H&E ×400. (**d**) Sprinkling of eosinophils is a clue for vascular origin, H&E ×250. (**e**) CD31 ×250. (**f**) ERG ×100

cells, a useful clue to suggest vascular origin of the tumour (Fig. 12.7d).

A small group of EHE can show atypical features like nuclear pleomorphism, increased mitotic activity and necrosis. Another group of tumours show large cells with abundant cytoplasm, feathery appearance with moderate nuclear atypia and well-formed vascular lumina. Myxo-hyaline stroma is absent. These tumours show YAP1-TFE3 fusion.

12.4.1.4 IHC

Tumour cells are positive for ERG, CD31 (Fig. 12.7e, f), CD34, FLI1 and other endothelial markers and may show positivity for cytokeratin (Fig. 12.8c) and EMA [22, 27, 29]. EHE with YAP1-TFE3 fusion is positive for TFE3. CAMTA1 is a novel marker which is positive in 85% of cases [47]. It is highly specific.

12.4.1.5 Molecular

WWTR1-CAMTA1 fusion is seen in 95% of cases. Rest 5% shows YAP1-TFE3 fusion.

12.4.1.6 DD

Differential diagnosis includes other epithelioid vascular neoplasms [13, 30]. On a needle biopsy, it is very difficult to differentiate EHE from EA. It is better to give a diagnosis of "malignant epithelioid vascular tumour, at least intermediate grade". Other epithelioid neoplasms like metastatic carcinoma or sarcomas with epithelioid features may cause difficulty [25]. The background myxo-hyaline material may be confused with chondromyxoid fibroma. The typical epithelioid cells with cytoplasmic vacuoles and positivity for vascular markers help in diagnosis.

12.4.1.7 Treatment and Prognosis

Surgical resection is the treatment of choice. Radiotherapy/radiofrequency thermal ablation may be helpful for multicentric disease. Involvement of two or more bones is associated with poor prognosis. EHE has low recurrence rate (13%) and moderate metastatic risk (31%).

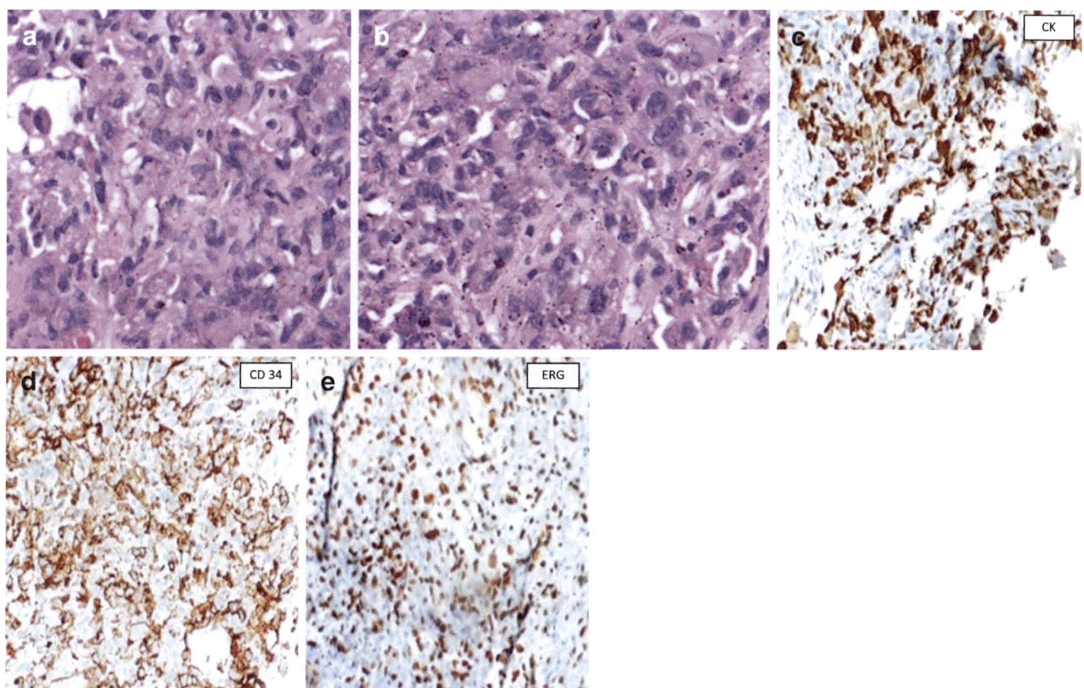

Fig. 12.8 EHE-solid growth pattern without well-formed vascular spaces. (**a**) Epithelioid cells with pleomorphism, H&E X250. (**b**) H&E ×250. (**c**) CK positive ×100. (**d**) CD34 positive ×100. (**e**) ERG showing diffuse nuclear positivity ×100

12.4.2 Primary Pseudomyogenic Haemangioendothelioma of Bone

This entity was previously known as pseudomyogenic variant of epithelioid sarcoma [6]. It is an unusual tumour usually occurring in soft tissue. Recently, Rosenberg et al. described this entity in bone [39]. It is an intermediate-grade malignancy.

12.4.2.1 Clinical

Usually, it occurs in second to fourth decades. Males are commonly affected. 60% of cases occur in less than 30 years age group. They present with progressive localized pain. Multiple discontinuous lesions of the same bone are common. Lower limb bones (40%), vertebrae, pelvis (20%) and upper limb bones (10%) are commonly involved [39–41].

12.4.2.2 Pathology

Ill-defined nodules of spindle and epithelioid cells in sheets and fascicles are seen [42–44]. Neoplastic cells have characteristics of skeletal myocytes. Intracytoplasmic vacuoles and rhabdomyoblast-like cells are noted. No true vasoformation is evident. Reactive bone formation and many osteoclastic giant cells may be present along with mixed inflammatory infiltrate and a myxoid stroma. Mitotic activity is usually sparse (Fig. 12.9).

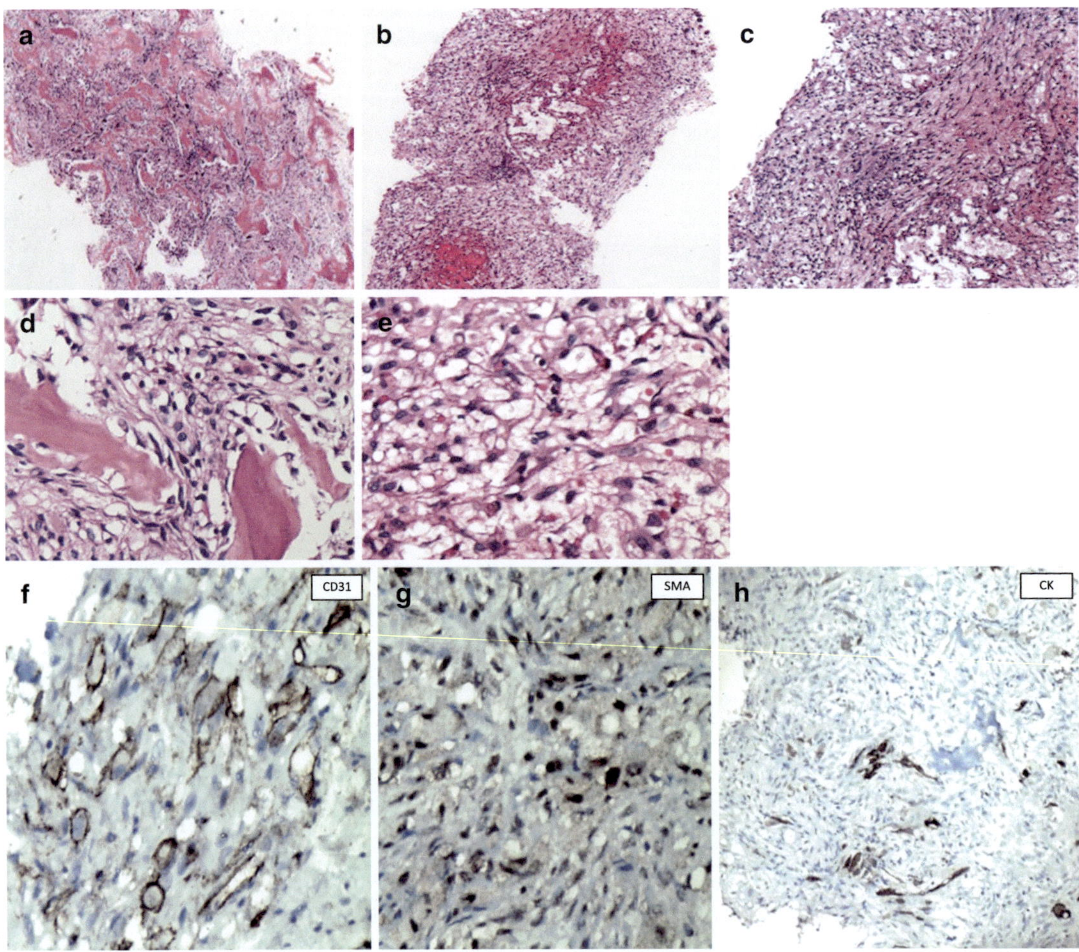

Fig. 12.9 Pseudomyogenic HE. (**a**) Spicules of bone and permeating tumour, H&E ×40. (**b** and **c**) Epithelioid and spindle cells, H&E ×100. (**d** and **e**) H&E ×250. (**f**) CD31 positive ×250. (**g**) SMA-positive areas ×100. (**h**) CK focally positive ×100. Courtesy: This case was contributed by Dr. Nanda Kachare, Aster Medcity, Kochi

12.4.2.3 IHC

Immunohistochemical stains that are positive include CD31, FLI1 and CK (Fig. 12.9). INI1 is retained, and desmin and S100 are negative [45]. A translocation t (7; 19) (q22; q13) is present in these cases (fusion of SERPINE1 and FOSB genes) [46].

12.4.2.4 DD

Differential diagnosis includes other epithelioid vascular tumours. Sometimes, osteoblastoma, giant cell tumour, non-ossifying fibroma, epithelioid sarcoma and metastatic sarcomatoid carcinoma also cause difficulty in differentiation.

12.4.2.5 Prognosis

These cases are shown to have local recurrence and rarely distant metastasis.

12.4.3 Angiosarcoma

Angiosarcomas account for less than 1% of primary malignant bone tumours [3, 9]. Secondary angiosarcomas are reported after radiation for other tumours and also following bone infarction [31]. It is a high-grade malignant neoplasm.

12.4.3.1 Clinical

There is no specific clinical presentation. Pain and swelling are the main complaints. About one-third of the tumours are multifocal [21]. These tumours have a predilection for axial skeleton [28, 35]. Spine and pelvis followed by long bones and small bones of hands and feet are the preferred sites. Multifocality is usually seen in the same topographic area especially in extremities [5, 33].

12.4.3.2 Radiology

Majority of angiosarcomas are purely lytic [4]. Rarely, mixed lytic and sclerotic pattern is observed. They are ill circumscribed. In high-grade cases, cortical destruction and soft tissue extension are seen. Periosteal reaction is absent. Multiple lytic lesions in contiguous bones strongly favour angiosarcomas [5, 33] (Figs. 12.10 and 12.11). In vertebra, the polka-dot appearance can be seen (Fig. 12.12).

12.4.3.3 Pathology

Grossly, tumours are soft, friable, haemorrhagic bright red and sometimes lobulated. Angiosarcoma of bone can be either well-differentiated tumours with well-formed vessels or poorly differentiated tumours [17]. Most of the tumours (>90%) show epithelioid morphology [10, 15]. Cytoplasm contains small one or two vacuoles. Nuclei are vesicular with prominent nucleoli or macronucleoli. Extravasated RBCs and haemosiderin pigment are noted. Solid growth pattern mimics metastatic carcinoma. Some low-grade angiosarcomas may show spindle cells and do not show much cytological atypia. High-grade lesions show interconnecting vessels lined by highly atypical cells

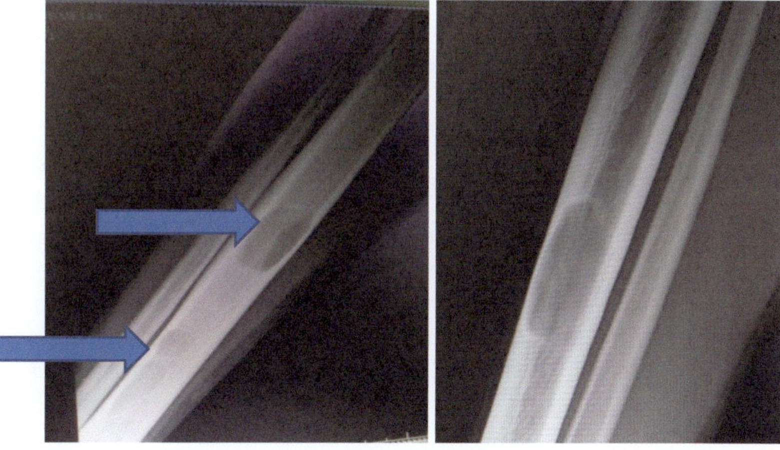

Fig. 12.10 (**a** and **b**) Plain X-ray showing multiple lytic lesions (blue arrow) in the same bone—characteristic of vascular tumours

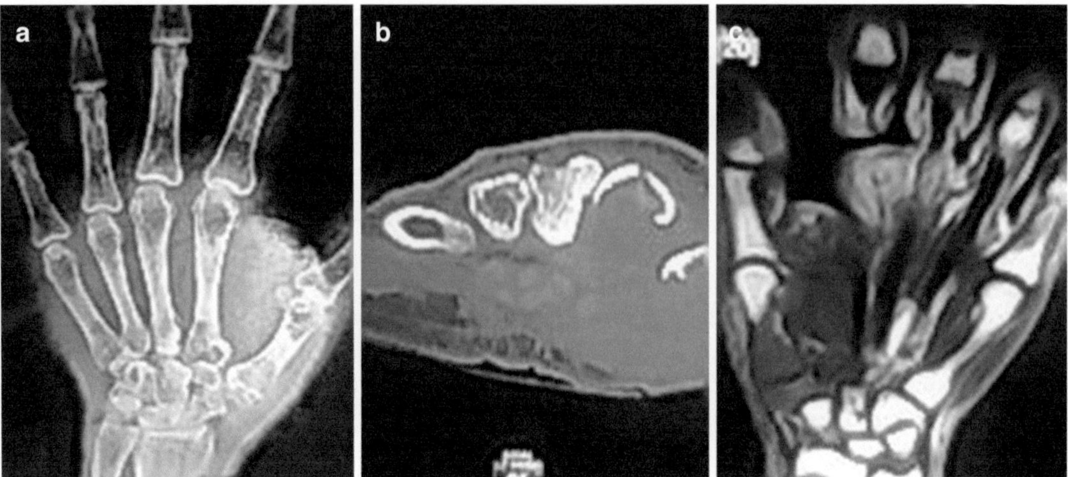

Fig. 12.11 Angiosarcoma of metacarpal bones with soft tissue mass. (**a**) Plain X-ray. (**b** and **c**) MRI

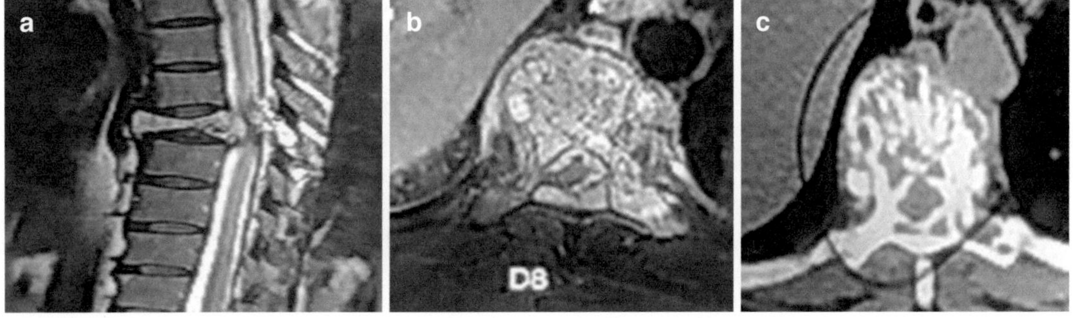

Fig. 12.12 Angiosarcoma of vertebra. (**a–c**) MRI showing destruction of vertebra with coarse trabeculae known as classical polka-dot pattern

or spindling of tumour cells (Fig. 12.13). Vascular spaces anastomose unlike haemangio-endotheliomas. These spaces contain red blood cells. In the absence of vessel formation, the useful diagnostic features are intratumoural haemorrhage and presence of neutrophils. Brisk mitotic activity is seen. Reactive bone formation rimmed by osteoblasts can be a prominent feature. This is seen at the periphery or throughout the lesion. This may confuse with osteoblastoma. Inflammatory cells, especially eosinophils, may be seen throughout the tumour especially in low-grade tumours. Multinucleated giant cells in clusters can be seen. Desmoplastic reaction is absent (Figs. 12.14, 12.15, and 12.16).

12.4.3.4 IHC

Angiosarcomas are positive for cytokeratin, CD31, ERG and FLI1 [14, 32]. CD34 and factor VIII are rarely positive [27, 29]. Other markers which are positive are CK, SMA, D2-40 [16] and EMA.

12.4.3.5 DD

Metastatic carcinoma, especially renal cell carcinoma, is a close differential diagnosis in epithelioid angiosarcomas [35, 37]. But renal cell carcinomas show discrete vascular spaces instead of anastomosing vascular channels. Desmoplastic reaction is common in metastatic carcinoma. Endothelial markers will help in differentiation. Cytokeratin can be positive in both tumours.

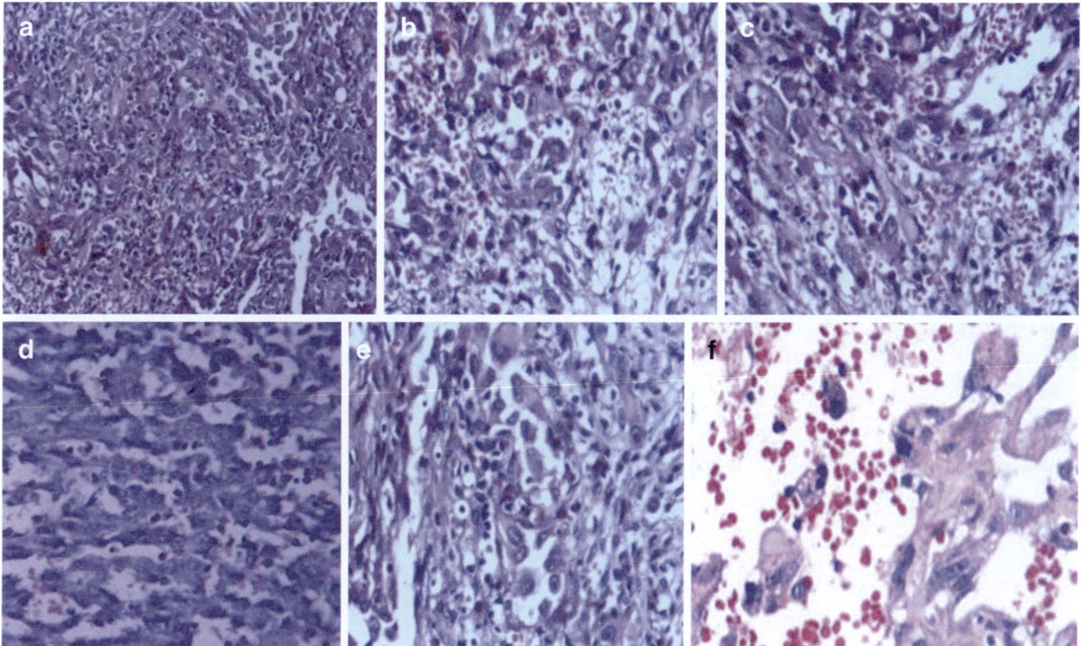

Fig. 12.13 High-grade angiosarcoma metacarpal bones. (**a**) Pleomorphic malignant cells and anastomosing vascular spaces, H&E ×100. (**b–d**) Anastomosing vascular channels filled with blood, H&E ×250. (**e**) Vascular spaces lined by plump highly atypical cells, H&E ×250. (**f**) Extravasated RBCs, H&E ×400

In low-grade angiosarcomas, differential diagnosis includes haemangiomas and bacillary angiomatosis. Differentiation from haemangioma is very difficult. Multicentricity is more common in angiosarcomas. Bacillary angiomatosis is usually seen in immunosuppressed individuals with a proliferation of capillaries. Admixed with this, numerous inflammatory cells, especially neutrophils, and bacterial colonies can be seen.

12.4.3.6 Molecular

There is only limited knowledge on molecular findings in angiosarcomas. Amplification of 2q and 17q described in soft tissue angiosarcomas are described in bone angiosarcomas also [11].

In radiation-induced and lymphedema-associated angiosarcomas, high level MYC amplification is seen on 8q24 [36]. It is absent in primary angiosarcomas. Hence, it is a useful marker for diagnosing these cases.

12.4.3.7 Treatment

Is surgical resection and radiation with or without chemotherapy. Before deciding treatment, multicentricity should be ruled out. Post-radiation sarcomas are reported years after treatment [28].

12.4.3.8 Prognosis

Low-grade angiosarcomas have good prognosis. High-grade tumours have a poor prognosis [26]. Hence, grading of angiosarcoma is important. Verbeke and Bertoni et al. have shown that primary angiosarcoma of bone with more than three mitoses per 10 HPF, prominent nucleoli and less than five eosinophils per 10 HPF has a more aggressive course and worse outcome [35].

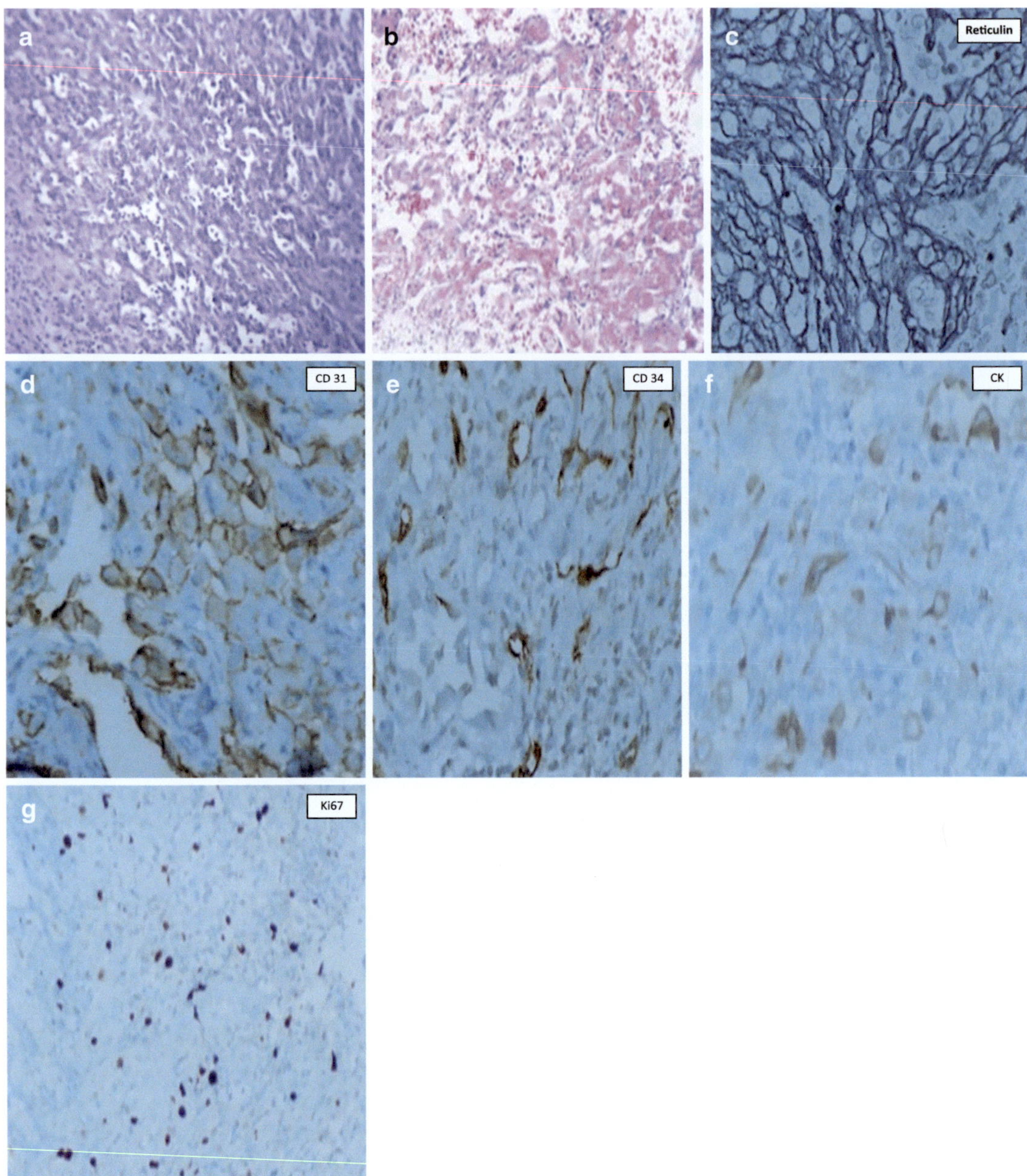

Fig. 12.14 Epithelioid angiosarcoma. (**a** and **b**) Anastomosing vascular channels, epithelioid cells, extravasated RBCs, H&E ×100. (**c**) Reticulin stain highlighting anastomosing vascular channels. (**d**) CD31 ×100. (**e**) CD34 ×250. (**f**) CK ×100. (**g**) high Ki67 index

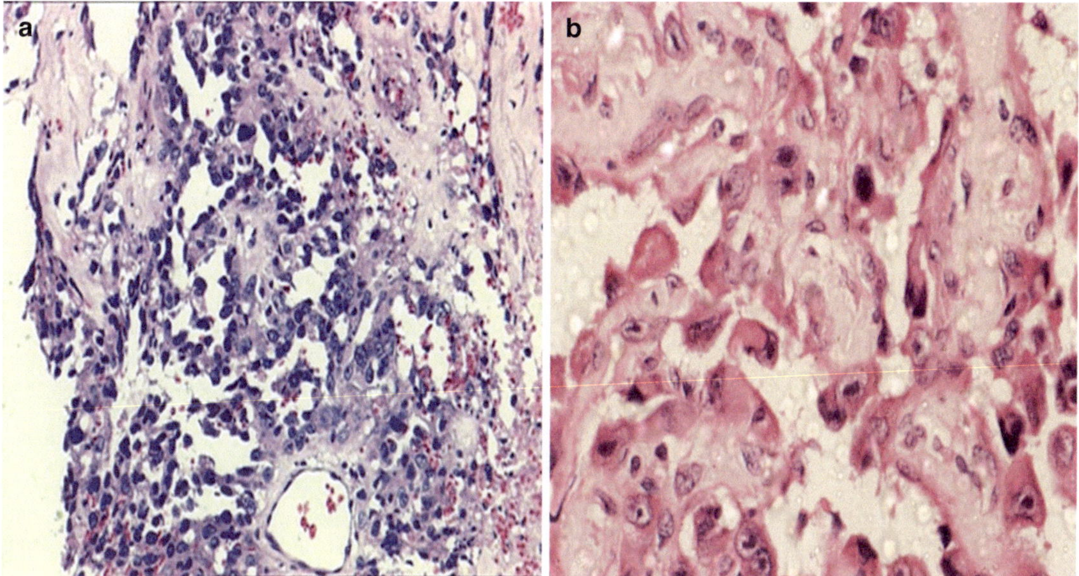

Fig. 12.15 Epithelioid angiosarcoma of humerus. (**a**) Epithelioid cells with anastomosing vascular channels, H&E ×250. (**b**) Vascular spaces lined by plump endothelial cells, H&E ×400

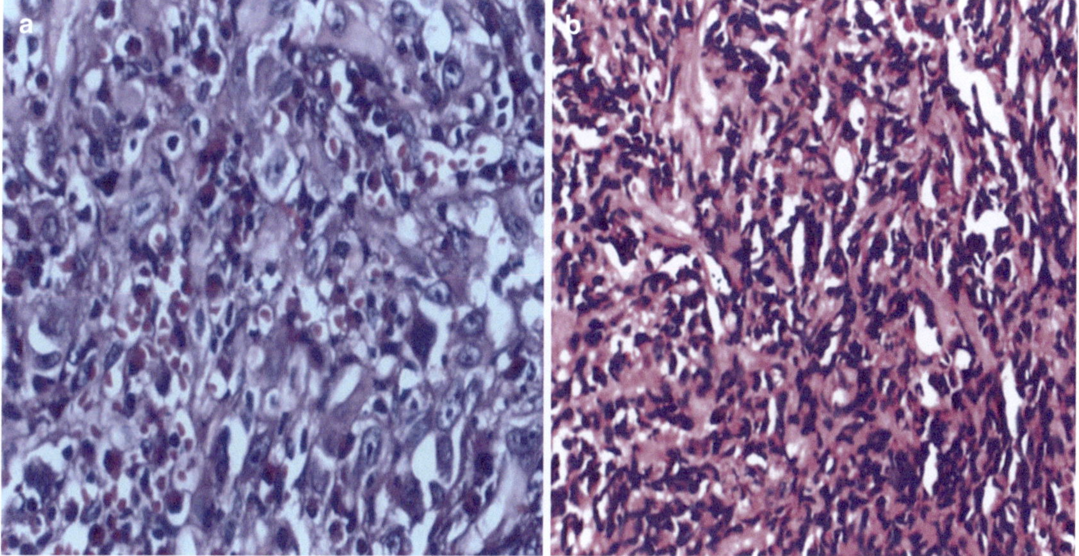

Fig. 12.16 Angiosarcoma. (**a**) Extravasated RBCs, plump cells lining spaces, H&E ×250. (**b**) Spindle cells and anastomosing vascular channels, H&E ×100

Points to Remember

- Vascular tumours of bone can be multifocal.
- Multiple lytic lesions in contiguous bones strongly favour vascular tumours.
- Intracytoplasmic vacuoles, presence of eosinophils and myxoid stroma are features to suspect vascular tumours.
- CD31, ERG, FLI1 and CD34 are common IHC markers for vascular tumours.
- FOS or FOSB is a useful marker for EH.
- WWTR1-CAMTA1 fusion is seen in 95% of cases of EHE.
- Grading of angiosarcoma is important.
- Low-grade AS has a good prognosis.

References

1. Adler CP. Hemangioma of the bone. In Bone diseases. Berlin(Germany) Springer: 2000; 370–5.
2. Deyrup AT, Montag AG. Epithelioid and epithelial neoplasms of bone. Arch Pathol Lab Med. 2007;131:205–16.
3. Antonescu CR, Huang SC, Sung YS, Zhang L, Helmke BM, Kirchner M, Stenzinger A, Mechtersheimer G. Novel GATA6-FOXO1 fusions in a subset of epithelioid hemangioma. Mod Pathol. 2021;34(5):934–41.
4. Merrow AC, Gupta A, Patel MN, Adams DM. Revised classification of vascular lesions from the international society for the study of vascular anomalies: radiologic-pathologic update. Radiographics. 2014;2016(36):1494–516.
5. Balicki D, Buhrmann R, Maclean J, et al. Multicentric epithelioid angiosarcoma of the bone. Pitfalls in clinical and morphological diagnosis. Blood Cells Mol Dis. 1996;22:205–13.
6. Billings SD, Folpe AL, Weiss SW. Epithelioid sarcoma like hemangioendothelioma. Am J Surg Pathol. 2003;27:48–57.
7. Bruder E, Perez-Atayde AR, Jundt G, Alomari AI, Rischewski J, Fishman SJ, Mulliken JB, Kozakewich HP. Vascular lesions of bone in children, adolescents, and young adults. Virchows Arch. 2009;454:161–79.
8. Campanacci M, Boriani S, Giunti A. Hemangioendothelioma of bone: a study of 29 cases. Cancer. 1980;46:804–14.
9. Antonescu C. Malignant vascular tumors—an update. Mod Pathol. 2014;27:S30–8.
10. Deshpande V, Rosenberg AE, O'Connell JX, Nielsen GP. Epithelioid angiosarcoma: a case report with review of literature. Indian J Pathol Microbiol. 2008;51:515.
11. Dunlap JB, Magenis RE, Davis C, Himoe E, Mansoor A. Cytogenetic analysis of a primary bone angiosarcoma. Cancer Genet Cytogenet. 2009;194:1–3.
12. Bruder E, Perez-Atayde AR, Jundt G, Alomari AI, Rischewski J, Fishman SJ, Mulliken JB, Kozakewich HPW. Vascular lesions of bone in children, adolescents, and young adults. A clinicopathologic reappraisal and application of the ISSVA classification. Virchows Archiv. 2009;454:161.
13. Evans HL, Raymond AK, Ayala AG. Vascular tumors of bone: a study of 17 cases other than ordinary hemangioma, with an evaluation of the relationship of hemangioendothelioma of bone to epithelioid hemangioma, epithelioid hemangioendothelioma, and high-grade angiosarcoma. Hum Pathol. 2003;34:680–9.
14. Folpe AL, Chand EM, Goldblum JR, Weiss SW. Expression of Fli-1, a nuclear transcription factor, distinguishes vascular neoplasms from potential mimics. Am J Surg Pathol. 2001;25:1061–6.
15. Hasegawa T, Fujii Y, Seki K, et al. Epithelioid angiosarcoma of bone. Hum Pathol. 1997;28:985–9.
16. Hu X, Edwards J, de Silvio O, Jackson D, Banerji S, Athanasou NA. Expression of a lymphatic endothelial cell marker in benign and malignant vascular tumours. Hum Pathol. 2004;35:857–61.
17. Krishnan Unni K, Inwards CY, Bridge JA, Kindblom L-G, Wold LE. AFIP atlas of tumor pathology series 4-tumors of the bones and joints fascicle 2. Washington, DC: ARP Press; 2005. p. 273–6.
18. Keel SB, Rosenberg AE. Hemorrhagic epithelioid and spindle cell hemangioma: a newly recognized, unique vascular tumor of bone. Cancer. 1999;85: 1966–672.
19. Kleer CG, Unni KK, McLeod RA. Epithelioid hemangioendothelioma of bone. Am J Surg Pathol. 1996;20(11):1301–11.
20. Lawley LP, Cerimele F, Weiss SW, et al. Expression of wilms tumor 1 gene distinguishes vascular malformations from proliferative endothelial lesions. Arch Dermatol. 2005;141(10):1297–300.
21. Meis-Kindblom JM, Kindblom LG. Angiosarcoma of soft tissue: a study of 80 cases. Am J Surg Pathol. 1998;22:683–97.
22. Naeem N, Mushtaq S, Akhter N, Hussain M, Hassan U. Effectiveness of vascular markers (immunohistochemical stains) in soft tissue sarcomas. J Coll Physicians Surg Pak. 2018;28(5):352–6.
23. O'Connell JX, Kattapuram SV, Mankin HJ, Bhan AK, Rosenberg AE. Epithelioid hemangioma of bone. A tumor often mistaken for low-grade angiosarcoma or malignant hemangioendothelioma. Am J Surg Pathol. 1993;17(6):610–7.
24. Nielsen GP, Srivastava A, Kattapuram S, Deshpande V, O'Connell JX, Mangham CD, Rosenberg AE. Epithelioid hemangioma of bone revisited: a study of 50 cases. Am J Surg Pathol. 2009;33(2):270–7.
25. O'Connell JX, Nielsen GP, Rosenberg AE. Epithelioid vascular tumors of bone: a review and proposal of a classification scheme. Adv Anat Pathol. 2001;8(2):74–82.
26. O'Connell JX, Nielsen GP, Rosenberg AE. Epithelioid vascular tumors of bone: a reviewof bone to epithelioid hemangioma, epithelioid hemangioendothelioma, and high-grade angiosarcoma. Hum Pathol. 2003;34:680–9.

27. Ohsawa M, Naka N, Tomita Y, Kawamori D, Kanno H, Aozasa K. Use of immunohistochemical procedures in diagnosing angiosarcoma. Evaluation of 98 cases. Cancer. 1995;75:2867–74.
28. Palmerini E, Maki RG, Staals EL, et al. Primary angiosarcoma of bone: a retrospective analysis of 60 patients from 2 institutions. Am J Clin Oncol. 2014;37(6):528–34.
29. Pusztaszeri MP, Seelentag W, Bosman FT. Immunohistochemical expression of endothelial markers CD31, CD34, von Willebrand factor, and Fli-1 in normal human tissues. J Histochem Cytochem. 2006;54:385–95.
30. Ramkumar S. Epithelioid haemangioma of bone: a case series and comprehensive literature review reappraising the diagnostic classification of all epithelioid vascular neoplasms of bone. Cureus. 2021;13(6):e15371. https://doi.org/10.7759/cureus.15371. PMID: 34094789; PMCID: PMC8168629
31. Rossi S, Fletcher CD. Angiosarcoma arising in hemangioma/vascular malformation: report of four cases and review of the literature. Am J Surg Pathol. 2002;26(10):1319–29.
32. Rossi S, Orvieto E, Furlanetto A, Laurino L, Ninfo V, Dei Tos AP. Utility of the immunohistochemical detection of FLI-1 expression in round cell and vascular neoplasm using a monoclonal antibody. Mod Pathol. 2004;17:547–52.
33. Santeusanio G, Bombonati A, Tarantino U, et al. Multifocal epithelioid angiosarcoma of bone: a potential pitfall in the differential diagnosis with metastatic carcinoma. Appl Immunohistochem Mol Morphol. 2003;11:359–63.
34. Unni KK, Inwards CY, Bridge JA, Kindblom LG, Wold LE. Vascular Tumors. 2005;10:261–79.
35. Verbeke SLJ, Bertoni F, Bacchini P, Sciot R, Fletcher CDM, Kroon HM, Hogendoorn PCW, Bovée JVMG. Distinct histologic features characterize primary angiosarcoma of bone. Histopathology. 2011;58:254–64.
36. Udager AM, Ishikawa MK, Lucas DR, McHugh JB, Patel RM. MYC immunohistochemistry in angiosarcoma and atypical vascular lesions: practical considerations based on a single institutional experience. Pathology. 2016;48(7):697–704.
37. Verbeke SL, Bovée JV. Primary vascular tumors of bone: a spectrum of entities? Int J Clin Exp Pathol. 2011;4(6):541–51.
38. Weiss SW, Ishak KG, Dail DH, Sweet DE, Enzinger FM. Epithelioid hemangioendothelioma and related lesions. Semin Diagn Pathol. 1986;3:259–87.

Primary Pseudomyogenic Haemangioendothelioma of Bone

39. Rosenberg AE, et al. Primary pseudomyogenic hemangioendothelioma of bone. J Surg Pathol. 2016;40:587–98.
40. Bartholomew JR, Tran M. Pseudomyogenic hemangioendothelioma – a rare vascular tumor. Vasc Med. 2020;25(1):93–4.
41. Hornick JL, Fletcher CD. Pseudomyogenic hemangioendothelioma:a distinctive, often multicentric tumor with indolent behavior. Am J Surg Pathol. 2011;35:190–201.
42. Inyang A, Mertens F, Puls F, Sumathi V, Inwards C, Folpe A, Lee C-H, Zhang Y, Symmans P, Rubin B, Nielsen GP, Nguyen V-H, Rosenberg AE. Primary pseudomyogenic hemangioendothelioma of bone. Am J Surg Pathol. 2016;40(5):587–98.
43. Otani S, Nakayama R, Sekita T, et al. Pseudomyogenic hemangioendothelioma of bone treated with denosumab: a case report. BMC Cancer. 2019;19:872.
44. Bharat R, Ashish G, Venkatesh R. A rare case of multifocal pseudomyogenic hemangioendothelioma, involving soft tissues and bone, misdiagnosed as a rhabdomyosarcoma: diagnostic and treatment implications. Indian J Pathol Microbiol. 2016;59(3):382–5.
45. Sun Y, Zhao M, Lao IW, et al. The clinicopathological spectrum of pseudomyogenic hemangioendothelioma: report of an additional series with review of the literature. Virchows Arch. 2020;477:231–40. https://doi.org/10.1007/s00428-020-02753-4.
46. Trombetta D, Magnusson L, von Steyern FV, et al. Translocation t(7;19)(q22;q13)-a recurrent chromosome aberration in pseudomyogenic hemangioendothelioma? Cancer Genet. 2011;204:211–5.
47. WHO Classification of Tumours. Soft tissue and bone tumours, vol. 3. Edited by the WHO Classification of Tumours Editorial Board. 5th ed. IARC; 2020.

Angiomatosis

48. Soler R, Pombo F, Bargiela A, Grana J, Arnal F. Diffuse skeletal cystic angiomatosis:spectrum of vascular tumors: implications in tumor diagnosis. Hum Pathol. 2000;31:1062–7.
49. Yamamoto T, Iwasaki Y, Kurosaka M, Minami R. Angiosarcoma arising from skeletal haemangiomatosis in an atomic bomb survivor. J Clin Pathol. 2001;54(9):716–7.

Massive Osteolysis

50. Shives TC, Beabout JW, Unni KK. Massive osteolysis. Clin Orthop Relat Res. 1993:294.

13 Adamantinoma of Bone

Adamantinomas are rare biphasic tumours (0.4% of all bone tumours), predominantly occuring in the tibia with unknown histogenesis. The name adamantinoma was given to this tumour because of its resemblance to ameloblastoma of jawbones [1]. The epithelial islands with basal palisading admixed with spindle cell stroma are seen in these tumours also. The epithelial islands in these tumours are thought to be traumatic implantation of epithelium from cutaneous surface or congenital rests of epithelium [2, 3]. Some authors are of the opinion that they are sarcomas similar to synovial sarcoma and not an epithelial neoplasm. But the exact pathogenesis of the lesion is still unclear. Since these tumours express vimentin and cytokeratin, a transformation of mesenchymal stem cells to epithelial islands has been implicated in the pathogenesis. Osteofibrous dysplasia is thought to be a precursor lesion of adamantinoma [4].

The adamantinoma group of tumours consists of classic adamantinoma, dedifferentiated adamantinoma, osteofibrous dysplasia-like adamantinoma and OFD. These tumours form a spectrum of tumours of same evolution [1, 4, 5] (Table 13.1). Tibial diaphysis is the preferred site for all the four lesions. Cytokeratin is positive in all the tumours. They have similar immunohistochemical findings. OFD and classic adamantinoma are positive for cytokeratin [7, 8] (AE1/AE3) and CK19 [5] and weakly positive for CK8 and CK18.

Table 13.1 Classification of adamantinoma (WHO 2020) [6]

Intermediate (locally aggressive)
Osteofibrous dysplasia (OFD)-like adamantinoma
Malignant
Classic adamantinoma
Dedifferentiated adamantinoma

13.1 Clinical Features

Adamantinomas predominantly affect females (about 90%) in third and fourth decades [9, 10]. Most of the tumours arise in tibia (>80%) with synchronous involvement of the fibula in 10% of cases. Rarely does it occur in bones of the upper extremities, pelvis and ribs. In young boys, osteofibrous dysplasia with adamantinoma is reported. It presents as painful or painless swelling [3].

13.2 Radiology

Plain X-ray shows eccentric, lytic lesion arising in the cortex with multilobation and scalloping with peripheral sclerosis. They may extend to the medullary cavity and soft tissue. They are located in metaphysis or metadiaphyseal region.

13.3 Pathology

Grossly, they are lobulated, firm and fibrous to soft brain-like mass.

J. Kattoor et al., *Bone Tumors*, https://doi.org/10.1007/978-981-99-4738-6_13

13.3.1 OFD-like Adamantinoma

In this type, OFD-like areas predominate [11]. Epithelial clusters are few in number. The epithelial cells may be detected only by IHC for cytokeratin. This is a locally aggressive type of adamantinoma.

13.3.2 Classic Adamantinoma

In classic adamantinoma, small epithelial islands in a fibrous stroma are seen. These two components vary in amount. The histologic variants of classic adamantinoma [12] are tubular, basaloid, squamous and spindle cell variants. Tubular adamantinomas are composed of epithelial cells arranged in a vascular or glandular pattern due to central discohesion of cells. The basaloid variant shows peripheral palisading and central stellate or spindle cells resembling ameloblastoma of jaw. Some are predominantly spindle cells (spindled variant) having fibrosarcoma-like appearance [13] (Fig. 13.1). But cytokeratin-positive cells will be seen when immunohistochemical stains are done. Anastomosing spaces resembling vascular spaces are seen in some cases. This is also a distinguishing feature from other sarcomas. Some other tumours are predominantly epithelial resembling metastatic carcinoma (basaloid, squamous variants). Rarely, the squamous cells can show malignant features (Fig. 13.2). Typically, epithelial islands have cuboidal epithelium at the

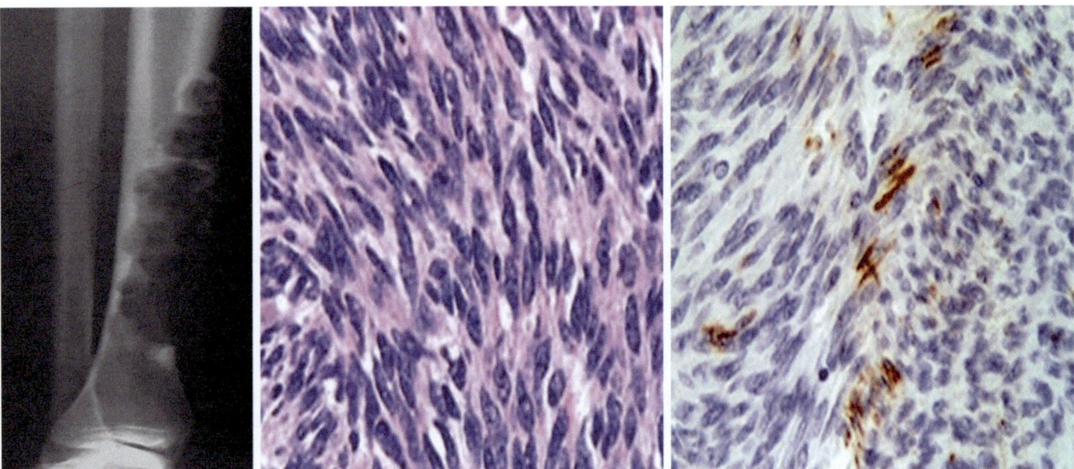

Fig. 13.1 Spindle cell variant of adamantinoma in a 38-year-old female. (**a**) Plain X-ray: showing classical well-circumscribed osteolytic lesion with septation, cortical scalloping and peripheral sclerosis. (**b**) Spindle cells resembling fibrosarcoma, H&E ×400. (**c**) Cytokeratin-positive cells ×250. Classical radiology findings with cytokeratin positivity helped in diagnosis

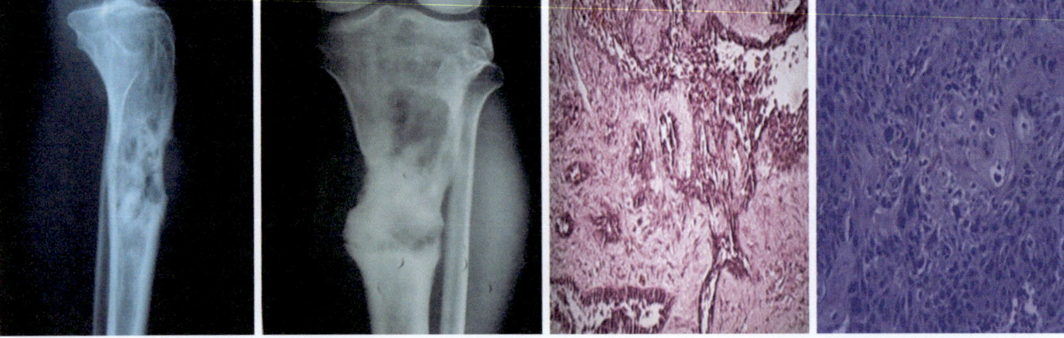

Fig. 13.2 Tibial tumour in a 32-year-old male. (**a** and **b**) Plain X-ray showing metadiaphyseal destructive lesion with patchy sclerosis and cortical destruction. (**c**) Epithelial adamantinoma, H&E ×250. (**d**) Squamous cell carcinoma area, H&E ×250. This patient had squamous cell carcinoma arising in adamantinoma

periphery showing palisading with minimal cytologic atypia. This is helpful in differentiating from metastatic carcinoma.

13.3.3 Dedifferentiated Adamantinoma

Dedifferentiated variant [17, 18] is very rare. It shows sheets of large pleomorphic cells without epithelial differentiation adjacent to foci of classic adamantinoma. Brisk mitotic activity is seen in pleomorphic cells. Osteoid, chondroid or clear cell differentiation is observed in this type.

13.4 IHC and EM

Epithelial cells coexpress keratin, EMA, P63, vimentin and podoplanin [14–16]. Spindle cells are positive for vimentin. Basal epithelial markers like CK5, CK14 and CK19 are positive. CK8 and CK18 are absent. Electron microscopy confirms epithelial features [14].

13.5 DD

The main DD is osteofibrous dysplasia. In OFD, keratin-positive cells are seen singly, whereas in adamantinoma, epithelial cells are seen in nests [5]. Fibrosarcoma and synovial sarcoma are difficult to differentiate when spindle cells predominate. If the epithelioid cells are abundant, it is difficult to differentiate from metastatic carcinoma. Another differential is adamantinoma like Ewing sarcoma. The clinical and radiological appearance will help in differentiation. In difficult cases, EWSR1 fusion transcript by FISH may have to be done.

13.6 Treatment and Prognosis

Chemotherapy and radiation are thought to be ineffective, and amputation was considered the mainstay of treatment. Recently, wide en bloc resection with subsequent reconstruction has been thought to be highly effective for limb preservation. Marginal excision will result in recurrence.

Adamantinoma is a low-grade malignancy. The recurrence rate of OFD-like adamantinomas is less (20%) compared to the classical adamantinomas (90%). The recurrent tumour is usually more aggressive. Long-term follow-up is necessary. Poor prognostic factors include young age at presentation especially in females (<20 years), pain at the time of presentation, short duration of symptoms and lack of squamous differentiation. Lung [19, 20], lymph nodes, brain [21] and bone are the sites of metastasis [22]. Metastatic lesions may have pure spindle cells or pure epithelial cells or a mixture of both. Dedifferentiated adamantinoma behaves aggressively.

Points to Remember

- Adamantinomas are biphasic tumours.
- Tibia is the commonest site.
- Radiologically, cortical lobulated destructive lesion with sclerotic border is seen.
- Morphology patterns include squamous, tubular, basaloid and spindle cell type.
- CK will be positive in these tumours.
- Osteofibrous dysplasia is thought to be a precursor of this tumour.

References

Adamantinoma

1. Hazelbag HM, Taminiau AH, Fleuren GJ, Hogendoorn PC. Adamantinoma of the long bones: a clinicopathological study of thirty-two patients with emphasis on histological subtype, precursor lesion, and biological behavior. J Bone Joint Surg Am. 1994;76:1482–99.
2. Gulia A, Panda PK. Adamantinoma; An update. J Bone Soft Tissue Tumors. 2017;3(2):16–9.
3. Varvarousis DN, Skandalakis GP, Barbouti A, Papathanakos G, Filis P, Tepelenis K, Kitsouli A, Kanavaros P, Kitsoulis P. Adamantinoma: an updated review. In Vivo. 2021;35(6):3045–52.
4. Khanna M, Delaney D, Tirabosco R, et al. Osteofibrous dysplasia, osteofibrous dysplasia-like adamantinoma and adamantinoma: correlation of radiological imaging features with surgical histology and assessment of the use of radiology in contributing to needle biopsy diagnosis. Skeletal Radiol. 2008;37:1077–84.
5. Ishida T, Iijima T, Kikuchi F, Kitagawa T, Tanida T, Imamura T, Machinami R. A clinicopathological and

immunohistochemical study of osteofibrous dysplasia, differentiated adamantinoma, and adamantinoma of long bones. Skeletal Radiol. 1992;21(8):493–502.
6. WHO Classification of Tumours. Soft tissue and bone tumours, vol. 3. Edited by the WHO Classification of Tumours Editorial Board. 5th ed. IARC; 2020.
7. Benassi MS, Campanacci L, Gamberi G, Ferrari C, Picci P, Sangiorgi L, Campanacci M. Cytokeratin expression and distribution in adamantinoma of the long bones and osteofibrous dysplasia of tibia and fibula. An immunohistochemical study correlated to histogenesis. Histopathology. 1994;25:71–6.
8. Hazelbag HM, Fleuren GJ, vd Broek LJ, Taminiau AH, Hogendoorn PC. Adamantinoma of the long bones: keratin subclass immunoreactivity pattern with reference to its histogenesis. Am J Surg Pathol. 1993;17(12):1225–33.
9. Jain D, Jain VK, Vasishta RK, et al. Adamantinoma: A clinicopathological review and update. Diagn Pathol. 2008;3:8.
10. Desai SS, Jambhekar N, Agarwal M, Puri A, Merchant N. Adamantinoma of tibia: a study of 12 cases. J Surg Oncol. 2006;93(5):429–33.
11. Ratra A, Wooldridge A, Brindley G. Osteofibrous dysplasia–like adamantinoma of the tibia in a 15-year-old girl. Am J Orthop. 2015;44(10):E411–3.
12. Czerniak B, Rojas-Corona RR, Dorfman HD. Morphologic diversity of long distribution in adamantinoma of the long bones and osteofibrous dysplasia of epithelial origin. Am J Clin Pathol. 1969;51:786–92.
13. Horvai A, Dashti NK, Rubin BP, et al. Genetic and molecular reappraisal of spindle cell adamantinoma of bone reveals a small subset of misclassified intraosseous synovial sarcoma. Mod Pathol. 2019;32:231–41.
14. Perez-Atayde AR, Kozakewich HP, Vawter GF. Adamantinoma of the tibia an ultrastructural and immunohistochemical study. Cancer. 1985;55:1015–23.
15. Kashima TG, Dhonge A, Taylor R, Flanagan AM, Hogendoorn P, Athanasou NA. Podoplanin expression in adamantinoma of long bones and osteofibrous dysplasia. Virchows Archiv. 2011;459(1):41–6.
16. Rosai J, Pinkus GS. Immunohistochemical demonstration of epithelial differentiation in adamantinoma of the tibia. Am J Surg Pathol. 1982;6(5):427–34.
17. Nouri H, Jaafoura H, Bouaziz M, Ouertatani M, Abid L, Meherzi MH, Ladeb MF, Mestiri M. Dedifferentiated adamantinoma associated with fibrous dysplasia. Orthop Traumatol Surg Res. 2011;97:770–5.
18. Hazelbag HM, Laforga JB, Roels HJ, Hogendoorn PC. Dedifferentiated adamantinoma with revertant mesenchymal phenotype. Am J Surg Pathol. 2003;27(12):1530–7.
19. Ampatzidou F, Pasteli N, Voulioti E, Madesis A, Kilmpasani M, Asteri TH. Lung metastasis from tibial adamantinoma. Greek E-J Perioperat Med. 2018;17(b):42–6.
20. Southam BR, Crawford AH, Billmire DA, Geller J, Von Allmen D, Schumaier AP, Szabo S. Long-term follow-up of adamantinoma of the tibia complicated by metastases and a second unrelated primary cancer: a case report and literature review. Case Rep Orthop. 2018;2018:5493750.
21. Schowinsky JT, Ormond DR, Kleinschmidt-DeMasters BK. Tibial adamantinoma: late metastasis to the brain. J Neuropathol Exp Neurol. 2015;74(1):95–7.
22. De Keyser F, Vansteenkiste J, Van Den Brande P, Demedts M, Van de Woestijne KP. Pulmonary metastases of a tibia adamantinoma: case report and review of the literature. Acta Clin Belg. 1990;45:31–3.

14 Cystic Lesions of Bone

Cystic lesions of bone develop when one or several factors affecting bone remodelling cause increased rate of bone resorption compared to bone formation. Cysts are closed spaces usually filled with fluid or semisolid material. They are incidentally detected or diagnosed when pathological fracture occurs. The true incidence is unknown because many cysts are asymptomatic.

Bone cysts are benign lesions [1]. Any bone can be affected. They are often asymptomatic. Pain, swelling and fractures are the main symptoms.

Bone cysts can be grouped as primary cysts and secondary cysts [1]. Simple bone cyst (unicameral bone cyst), aneurysmal bone cyst, ganglion cyst and epidermal inclusion cyst are the primary bone cysts. When it occurs secondary to other diseases, they are called secondary cysts (Table 14.1).

Table 14.1 Classification of bone cysts

Primary cysts	Secondary cysts
Simple bone cyst (SBC) Aneurysmal bone cyst (ABC) Ganglionic bone cyst Epidermal inclusion cyst	ABC-like cyst Arthritis related-osteoarthritis(degenerative joint disease) and rheumatoid arthritis Post-traumatic cysts Hormonally induced remodelling cysts Haemodialysis-associated cysts

14.1 Simple Bone Cyst (SBC)

SBC, also known as unicameral cyst of bone, usually arises as a result of disturbance in growth of the bone at the epiphyseal line [2]. It is usually unilocular.

14.1.1 Clinical

It is common in the first two decades of life [4]. Upper diaphysis of humerus, proximal femur and proximal tibia are the preferred sites. Pelvic bones and calcaneum are rarely involved and these patients are slightly older. Patients present with pain or pathologic fracture.

14.1.2 Radiology

These are lytic expansile lesions in the medullary cavity, abutting the epiphyseal plate (Fig. 14.1). Cortex is thin. Cortical erosion is seen when there is pathological fracture. Fine trabeculations can be seen within the cyst. If the cyst is seen away from the epiphyseal plate, it is called latent cyst [3]. Cystic cavity may be empty or filled with clear/greenish fluid. Cyst wall may contain ridges or a thin layer of fleshy tissue. When there is

J. Kattoor et al., *Bone Tumors*, https://doi.org/10.1007/978-981-99-4738-6_14

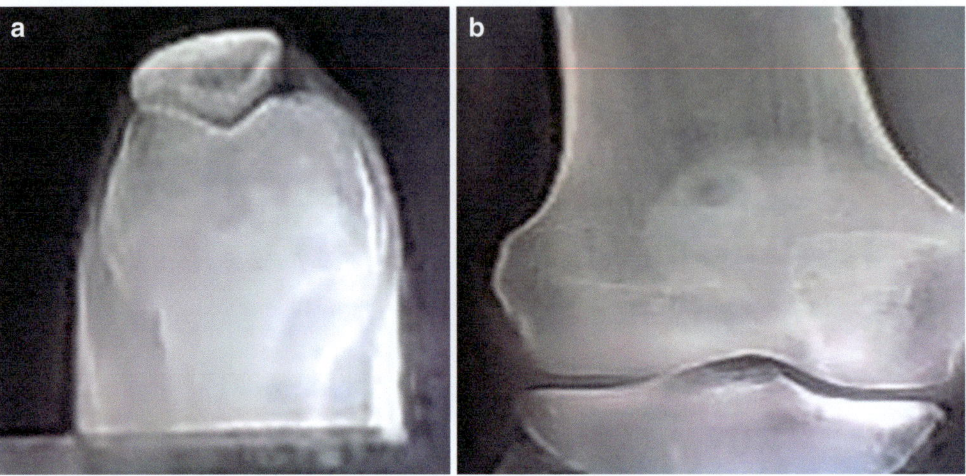

Fig. 14.1 Simple bone cyst patella. (**a** and **b**) Well-defined lytic lesion <0.5 cm

pathological fracture, pieces of broken bone float in cyst fluid, the so-called fallen fragment sign [6] (Fig. 14.2).

14.1.3 Pathology

Histology shows cyst with a fibrous wall. No definite lining cells are seen [3]. Cyst wall may also show an amorphous material (fibrinous deposits), which may calcify and resemble cementum [5] (Fig. 14.3a, b). If the cyst wall is thick, multinucleated giant cells, haemosiderin-laden macrophages and chronic inflammatory cells (Fig. 14.3c, d) are seen. If giant cells are prominent, an erroneous diagnosis of giant cell tumour will be made. If there is a pathological fracture, changes of healing fracture callus with proliferating fibroblasts and reactive bone will be present (Fig. 14.4). If not correlated with radiology, this can be mistaken for osteosarcoma.

14.1.4 Treatment and prognosis

Earlier, these lesions were treated with simple curettage and bone grafting. Recently, intralesional injection of methylprednisolone has been given. Some people suggest that drilling multiple holes in the lesion is therapeutic.

SBC in patients older than 10 years has got a good prognosis [7]. Younger patients (<10 years) and juxta-epiphyseal location are prone for recurrence. Rarely, malignant transformation-like fibrosarcoma developing in SBC has been reported.

Aneurysmal bone cyst is discussed in the chapter on giant cell-rich lesions of bone.

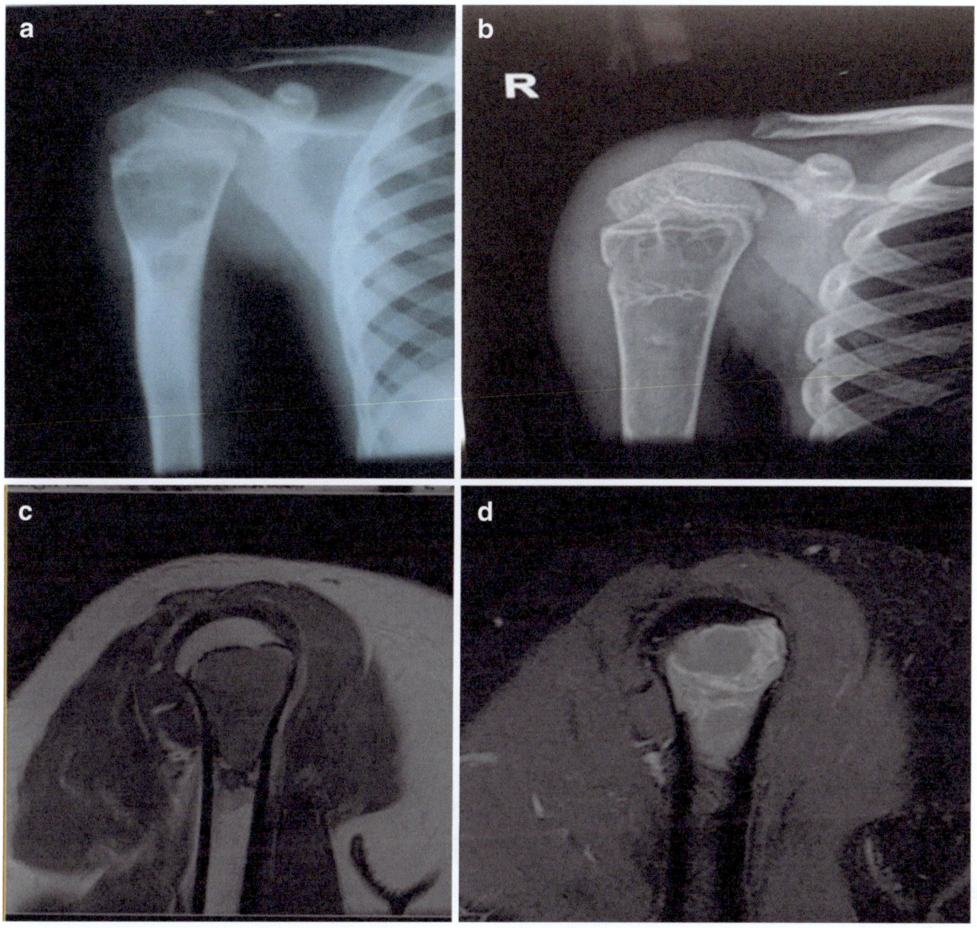

Fig. 14.2 Simple bone cyst humerus with fracture. (**a** and **b**) Plain X-ray showing expansile lytic lesion in the upper humerus with fracture. (**c** and **d**) MRI of same case

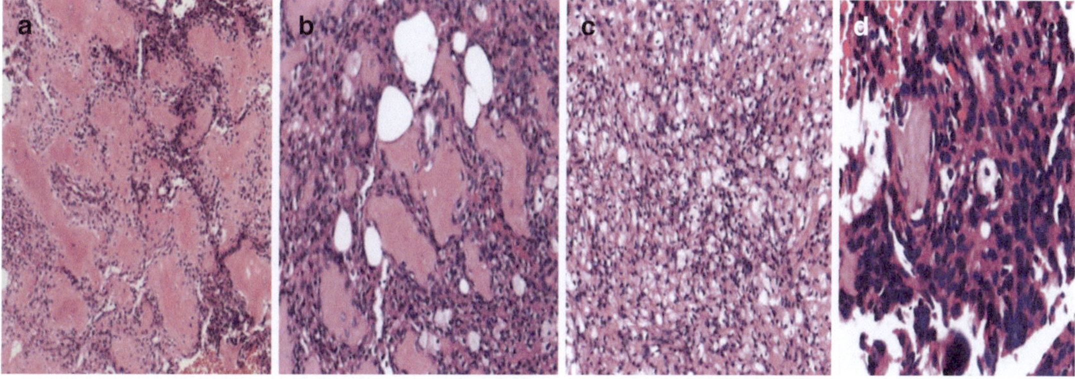

Fig. 14.3 Simple bone cyst. (**a**) Cementum-like material, H&E ×100. (**b**) H&E ×250. (**c**) Foamy macrophages, H&E ×100. (**d**) Inflammatory cells, H&E ×250

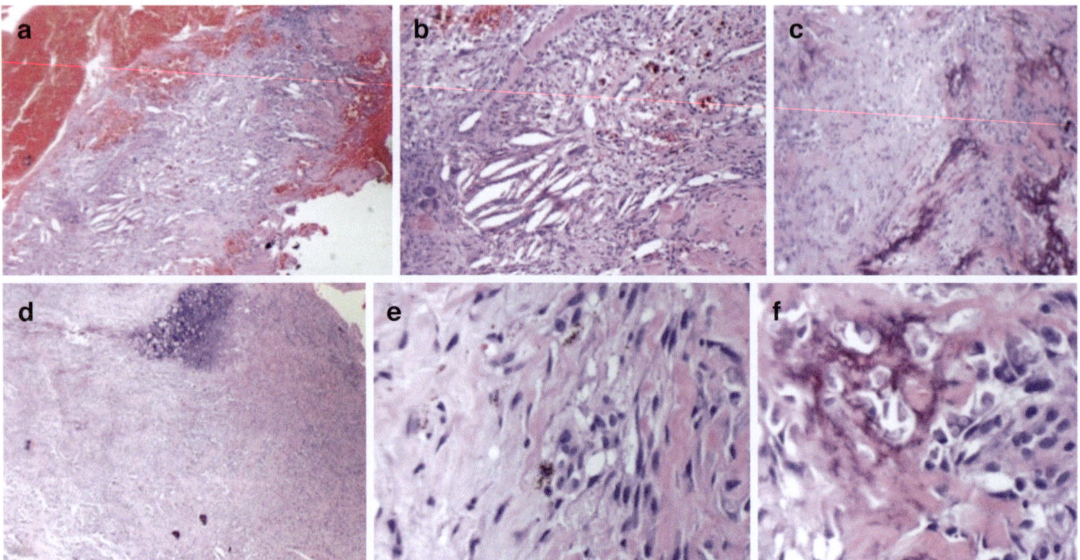

Fig. 14.4 SBC with fracture callus in a 32-year-old male. (**a** and **b**) Show cholesterol clefts, amorphous deposits, haemosiderin-laden macrophages and cleft-like spaces. (**c**–**f**) Last four pictures show healing fracture with zonation of calcifying osteoid, cartilage and fibrous tissue. Plump fibroblasts mimic malignant cells. Callus should not be mistaken for osteosarcoma

14.2 Ganglion Cyst

Ganglion cysts are similar to the ganglion cyst of tendon sheath [8, 9]. These cysts are seen at or near the joints. They are usually single, unilocular filled with mucoid material and have a thick fibrous wall.

14.2.1 Clinical

These lesions are seen in skeletally mature young to middle-aged men. The most common site is hip followed by knee, ankle and wrist.

14.2.2 Radiology

On plain X-ray, they are seen as well-circumscribed lytic lesion extending to the articular cartilage. A sclerotic rim is seen in majority of the cases.

14.2.3 Pathology

The pathogenesis of ganglion cyst is unknown. Grossly, the cysts are with a thick wall containing mucoid material. Sometimes, thin trabeculations can be seen. Microscopically, a thick fibrous wall without a lining and filled with light blue material is seen.

14.2.4 Differential diagnosis

Differential diagnosis is cysts of degenerative joint disease (Figs. 14.5 and 14.6). Histology is same in both, but radiological evidence of degenerative joint disease helps in differentiation.

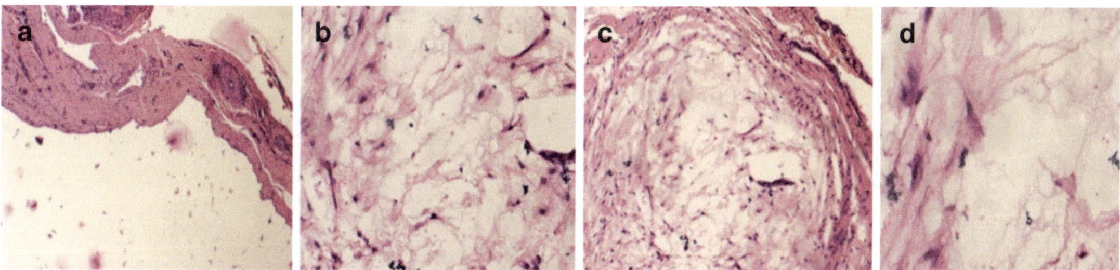

Fig. 14.5 Intraosseous ganglion. (**a**) Thick fibrous wall without lining. (**b–d**) Cyst filled with myxoid material and scattered stellate cells

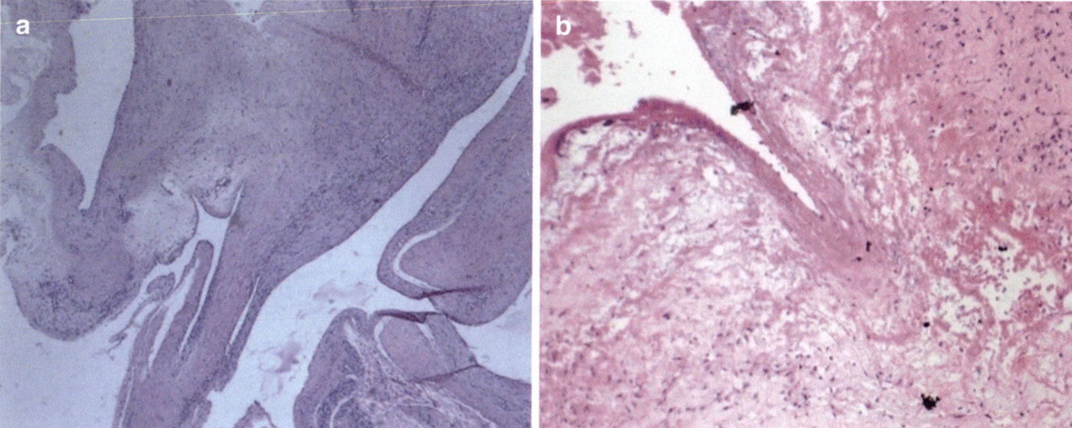

Fig. 14.6 Ganglion cyst. (**a**) Multiloculated pseudocyst. (**b**) With myxoid degeneration

14.3 Synovial Cysts and Meniscal Cysts

Synovial cyst (bursa) occurs due to herniation of the synovial membrane into the intra-articular or periarticular fat tissue, through the joint capsule. They may be seen in continuity to the synovial cavity. Hence, they are lined with synovium.

14.3.1 Clinical

Any joint can be affected. It is described in various joints like knee, spine, shoulder, elbow, hip, hand, foot and ankle. These cysts are seen associated with trauma, degenerative joint disease or inflammatory processes. Baker's cyst and spinal cysts are synovial cysts.

14.3.2 Radiology

Plain X-ray shows an ill-defined or rounded, non-calcified soft tissue mass. The diagnosis is usually straightforward with USG/MRI.

14.3.3 Pathology

The cysts are lined by synovium [26]. The Baker's cyst [24] (popliteal cyst) shows cartilage in the cyst wall. Palisading histiocytes and fibrinoid necrosis may be seen. Associated complications are haemorrhage, inflammation, rupture, presence of intra-articular loose bodies and synovial proliferation.

14.3.4 DD

Ganglion cysts—They do not communicate with synovium and hence they are not lined by synovium.

14.3.5 Treatment

Surgical excision and/or sclerotherapy is the treatment.

Meniscal cysts they are small and mainly present in the lateral aspect of the knee joint. Meniscal cysts are small cysts associated with horizontal meniscal tears [26]. Rarely, it can become very big [25]. They typically involve the lateral aspect of the knee joint.

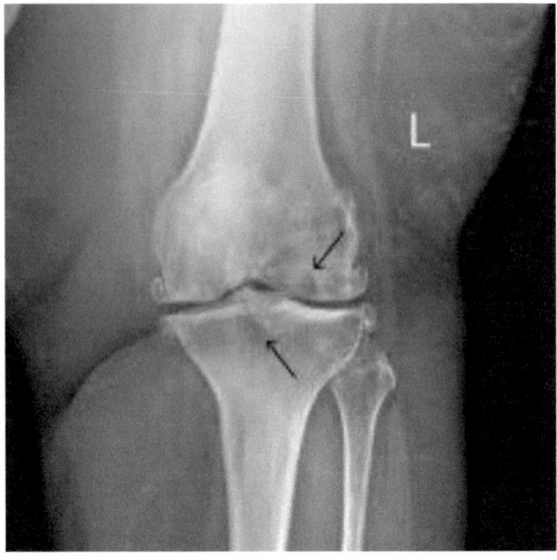

Fig. 14.7 Plain X-ray of subchondral cyst of degenerative joint disease (geode)

14.4 Geodes-Cysts of Degenerative Joint Disease (DJD)

Cysts seen in degenerative joint disease are also called pseudocyst [23]. It is often accompanied by cysts in the juxta-articular bone.

14.4.1 Clinical

They are usually multiple, vary in size and are seen more in weight-bearing bones. Osteophytes and narrowing of joint spaces are seen. These cysts are multilocular and pyriform in shape with a sclerotic rim. They are filled with a degenerative fibromyxoid material. Sometimes, cysts are so extensive and interfere with surgical procedures. When extensive, they mimic neoplasm of bone.

Geodes are also subchondral cysts associated with degenerative joint disease. They are well-defined lytic lesions seen in the periarticular region (Fig. 14.7). As it is seen at the epiphysis, it is mistaken for tumours of epiphysis like chondroblastoma or clear cell chondrosarcoma. The synovial fluid infiltrates to the underlying bone due to degenerative changes in the articular cartilage of the joint.

14.4.2 Pathology

Cyst may have a synovial lining, and cyst wall is fibrous. Fibrosis and fat necrosis may be present in the adjacent marrow.

Egger cysts are acetabular cysts associated with degenerative joint disease. It is seen in the hip joint.

The dorsal cysts are seen in distal interphalangeal joints of middle-aged women. Joint space narrowing and Heberden nodes (osteophytes) are seen associated with it. They are thin-walled and contain a clear fluid.

In rheumatoid arthritis, the synovium of joints in the hands is affected. Inflammation and granuloma formation will be seen.

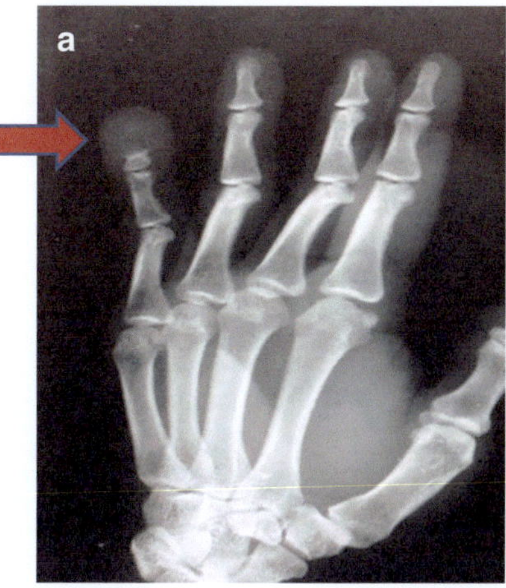

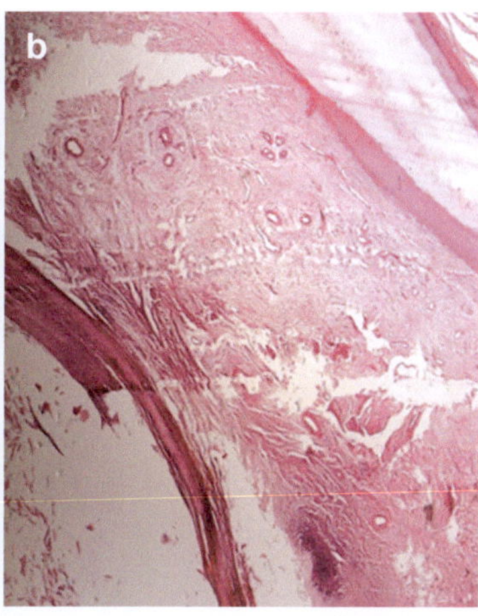

Fig. 14.8 Epidermal inclusion cyst of fifth terminal phalanx. (**a**) Plain X-ray. (**b**) Cyst lined by squamous epithelium with flakes of keratin similar to cutaneous counterpart

14.5 Epidermal Inclusion Cysts

These are rare lesions occurring mainly in young males of second to fourth decades [11]. Bones of skull and phalanges of hand are commonly affected (Fig. 14.8a). Patients usually present with pain and swelling. In the plain X-ray, they are seen as well-defined lytic lesion with sclerotic margins. CT and MRI are not required. Microscopically, the cysts are filled with keratinous material and lined by squamous epithelium (Fig. 14.8b), similar to lesions of skin. Rupture of cysts may cause inflammation. These cases are treated with excision [10].

14.6 Post-traumatic Cysts

In 1981, Pfister-Goedeke and Braune described cystic lesions following fractures. It is thought to be due to subperiosteal haemorrhage infiltrating into bone. Post-traumatic cysts are of two types: transient cortical defects occurring in children [12] and cysts similar to ABC occurring in adults and children (Fig. 14.9). The distal radius is a common site. The cysts regress in 1–2 years [13].

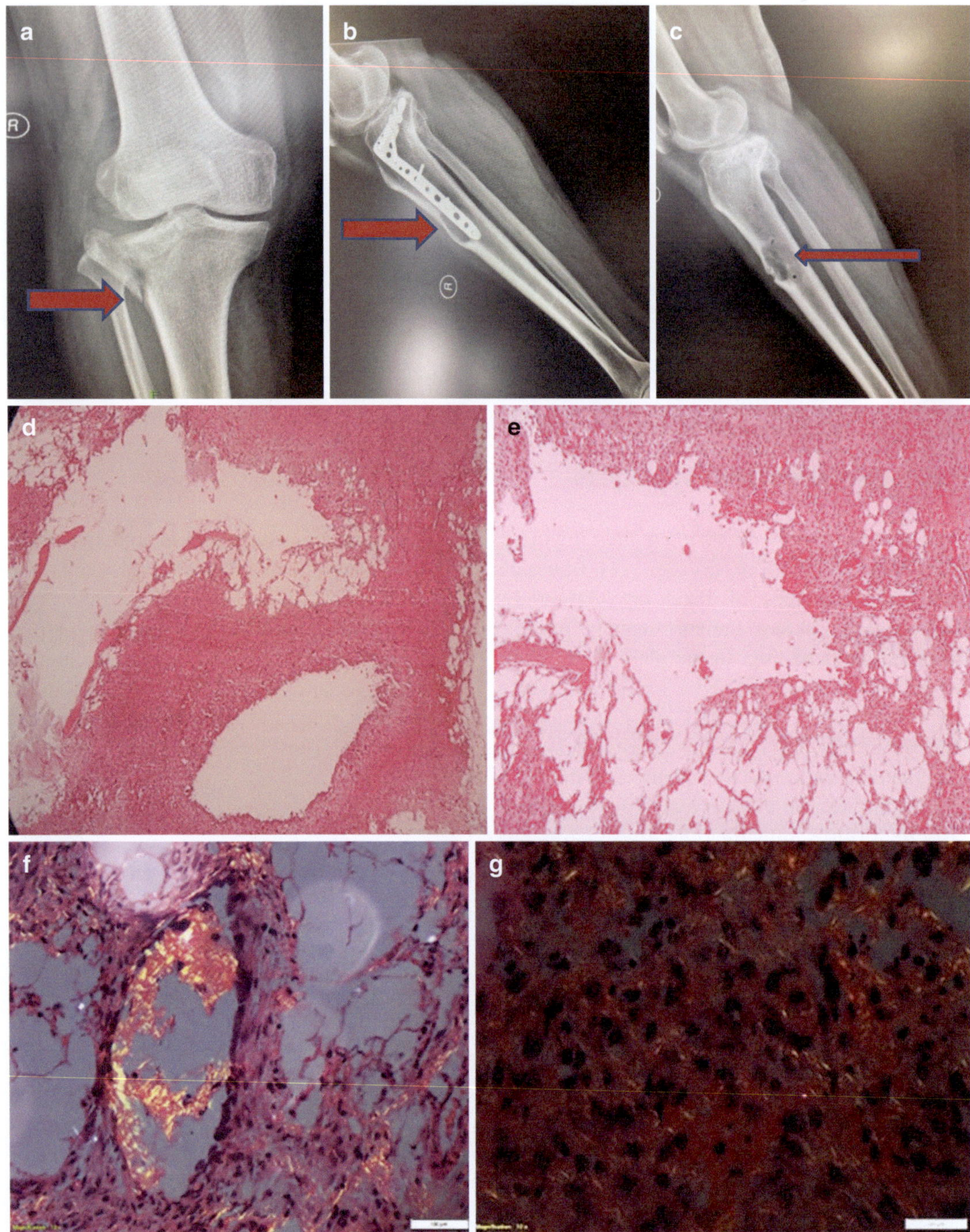

Fig. 14.9 Post-traumatic cyst in a case after implant for fracture correction. (**a–c**) Fracture tibia 3 years back, corrected with fracture reduction and implant (arrows). (**d** and **e**) Cyst developed at the site of implant given to correct fracture. Looks like ABC. Cyst wall showing histiocyte-like cells. (**f** and **g**) Implant material under polarizer. *Courtesy Dr. Jayanthi for contributing this case

14.7 Haemodialysis-Associated Cysts

Subchondral cysts develop due to metabolic disturbances in patients with chronic renal failure undergoing long-term haemodialysis (more than 10 years). They are commonly seen in the wrist, shoulder, hip and patella. These cyst-like lesions contain β_2-microglobulin amyloid [20].

14.8 Hydatid Cyst of Bone

Hydatid disease is produced by the larval stage of the *Echinococcus* tapeworm. Bone hydatid cysts are seen mainly in the vertebrae and pelvic bones [14–16]. It is also seen in the femur, tibia, humerus, skull and ribs. The cyst expands the bone. It can cause cortical destruction and may extend to soft tissue. Radiologically, it appears as unilocular or multilocular cyst [17]. In the vertebra, these cysts are mistaken for osteomyelitis or bone neoplasms.

14.9 Haemophilic Cyst

Due to bleeding occuring into the muscle, under the periosteum or into the bone, a cystic swelling is formed. They present as osteolytic lesion. Destruction of bone is followed by formation of bone or calcification in the adjacent soft tissue. This can resemble osteosarcoma, and hence they are called pseudotumour [21, 22]. The bones most commonly involved are the femur, pelvic bones, tibia and small bones of the hand. Cysts have a fibrous capsule, and the cyst contains clotted blood or toothpaste-like material. Bone fragments, haemosiderin-laden macrophages, new bone formation and multinucleated giant cells may be seen.

14.10 Pseudocyst

Pseudocysts are formed by subperiosteal bleeding resulting in pseudotumours [19]. A large haematoma forms under the periosteum. Periosteum is elevated, and new bone formation occurs.

14.10.1 Pathology

A pseudoencapsulation with fibrous tissue and subperiosteal new bone formation are seen. Inflammatory cells are seen at the edges of haematoma, and the central portion shows necrotic bony trabeculae and cartilage. The bone in contact with blood shows areas of resorption with more number of osteoclastic giant cells, and the bone away from blood shows new bone formation.

14.10.2 Treatment

Conservative management is given. Biopsy may cause severe haemorrhage.

14.11 Miscellaneous Cysts

Intraosseous pneumatocyst usually seen in the sacroiliac joint or spine, subpubic cartilaginous cysts seen in multiparous women, Baker's pseudocyst [18] and carpal bone cysts [19] are the other cysts described in the bone.

Table 14.2 shows features of common cysts of bone. Odontogenic cysts are given in Chap. 19.

Table 14.2 Features of common cystic lesions of bone

Lesion	SBC	ABC	Ganglion cyst and subchondral cyst	Epidermoid cyst	Cystic echinococcosis
Age/sex	<20 years M:F 2:1	<30 years Females	For GC = 40 years For SUBCC= >50 years	More in males	Any age
Common site/location	Long bones proximal humerus, femur Meta/diaphysis	Distal femur proximal tibia, spine, pelvis Meta / diaphysis *GCRG* (so-called *solid ABC*)	Tibia medial malleolus, femur, ulna, hands and feet subchondral cyst epiphyseal	Skull bones and terminal phalanges of hand/toes	Flat bones like vertebra, pelvis and mandible epiphysis
Aetiology	Focal cessation of medullary bone formation	Trauma/tumour-induced anomalous vascular process	GC → unknown SUB CC - with osteoarthritis	Congenital/traumatic implantation	*Echinococcus* tapeworm's larval cystic stage
Radiology and differential diagnosis	Central fusiform Expansion with intact cortex Fallen fragment sign DD: ABC, Brown Tr, NOF, FD	Solitary, expansile eccentric multiloculated lesion, breached cortex, buttress of solid periosteal response. MRI: lobulated, and fluid-fluid levels DD: *SBC, GCT, CMF, NOF, OS*	GC-Eccentric, oval to round, well-defined peripheral location SUBCC-Trabeculated lytic lesion, thin sclerotic rim	Sharply outlined, lytic areas with a sclerotic border	Four different types Single or multiple, uni- or multiloculated, and thin or thick calcified wall MRI: Typical DD: Tuberculosis, metastases and GCT
Gross	Yellowish fluid	Friable spongy haemorrhagic mass	Clear, gelatinous fluid		Pearly white smooth-surfaced cyst
Micro and DD	Thin layer of fibrous tissue with collagen/cementum-like substance DD: ABC	Richly vascular fibrous septa with iron pigment, mitosis, clustered small osteoclasts DD; GCT, OS, haemophilic pseudotumour	Focal areas of mucoid degeneration and patchy dense collagen	Characteristic keratin-filled cyst lined by squamous epithelium	Classical three-layered cyst with brood capsules and scolices = hydatid sand
Comments	Cholesterol clefts, giant cell reaction secondary to intracystic haemorrhage can mimic ABC	33% as solid ABC having expanded fibrous septa. 33% are secondary to GCT/chondroblastoma/fibrous dysplasia/CMF/osteoblastoma/OS/chondro/fibrosarcoma	Usually incidental MRI diagnostic	The radiology DDs: Enchondroma ECRG, acral metastases, subungual melanoma	If the cysts were to rupture while in the body, the patient would go into anaphylactic shock
Prognosis	Spontaneous regression in most. Rarely growth disturbances; recurrence = 10–20%	Intermediate, locally aggressive neoplasm, local recurrence rate up to 30%; USP6 rearrangement of spindle cells used to differentiate primary and solid ABC from the lesions with ABC like changes	Very low rate of recurrence. Curettage if symptomatic	Total **removal** of these **cysts** + washing of the cavity with 0.9% saline may prevent recurrence	Antibody detection by Casoni test, haemagglutination test or antigen detection also an adjunct

Table courtesy: Dr. Jayasree Geothe

Points to Remember

- Primary cysts of bone are expansile lesions.
- Common cysts are simple bone cyst and aneurysmal bone cysts.
- Common site for SBC is humerus.
- SBC shows non-specific histological changes.
- Pathological fracture is common, and fracture callus should not be mistaken as osteosarcoma.
- Ganglion cyst and epidermal inclusion cysts are rare. The latter is mainly seen in terminal phalanx of hand.
- Cysts of degenerative joint disease (geode cyst) are mistaken radiologically for epiphyseal tumours like chondroblastoma or clear cell chondrosarcoma.

References

Simple Bone Cyst

1. Özgün G, Yalçınkaya U, Yazıcı Z, Sarısözen B. Pathological analysis of cystic lesions of the bones: a retrospective single-center 10-year overview. Eur Res J. 2018;4(4):333–42.
2. Cohen J. Etiology of simple bone cyst. J Bone Joint Surg Am. 1970;52(7):1493–7.
3. Jaffe HL, Lichtenstein L. Solitary unicameral bone cyst with emphasis on the roentgen picture, the pathologic appearance, and the pathogenesis. Arch Surg. 1942;44(6):1004–25.
4. Lodwick GS. Juvenile unicameral bone cyst; a roentgen reappraisal. Am J Roentgenol Ther Nucl Med. 1958;80(3):495–504.
5. Mirra JM, Bernard GW, Bullough PG, Johnston W, Mink G. Cementum-like bone production in solitary bone cysts (so-called "cementoma" of long bones): report of three cases—electron microscopic observations supporting a synovial origin to the simple bone cyst. Clin Orthop Relat Res. 1978;135:295–307.
6. Reynolds J. The "fallen fragment sign" in the diagnosis of unicameral bone cysts. Radiology. 1969;92(5):949–53.
7. Wilkins RM. Unicameral bone cysts. J Am Acad Orthop Surg. 2000;8(4):217–24.

Ganglion Cysts

8. Feldman F, Johnston A. Intraosseous ganglion. AJR Am J Roentgenol. 1973;118(2):328–43.
9. Sim FH, Dahlin DC. Ganglion cysts of bone. Mayo Clin Proc. 1971;46(7):484–8.

Epidermoid Cysts

10. Kurosawa K, Kobayashi R, Takagishi K. Distal phalangeal reconstruction for recurrent intraosseous epidermoid cyst of the finger - a case report. Hand Surg. 2011;16:375–7.
11. Wang BY, Eisler J, Springfield D, Klein MJ. Intraosseous epidermoid inclusion cyst in a great toe. A case report and review of the literature. Arch Pathol Lab Med. 2003;127:e298–300.

Post-Traumatic Bone Cyst

12. Pfister-Goedeke L, Braune M. Cyst-like cortical defects following fractures in children. Pediatr Radiol. 1981;11:83–6.
13. Moore TE, King AR, Travis RC, et al. Post-traumatic cysts and cyst-like lesions of bone. Skeletal Radiol. 1989;18:93–7.

Hydatid Cyst

14. Bilhim T, Costa Pereira M, Leal C, Cardoso A. Pelvic cystic bone lesions on MR. Clin Cases. 2010; https://doi.org/10.1594/EURORAD/CASE.8513.
15. Kalinova K, Proichev V, Stefanova P, Tokmakova K, Poriazova E. Hydatid bone disease: a case report and review of the literature. J Orthop Surg. 2005;13:323–5.
16. Loudiye H, Aktaou S, Hassikou H, El-Bardouni A, El-Manouar M, Fizazi M, Tazi A, Hajjaj-Hassouni N. Hydatid disease of bone. Review of 11 cases. Joint Bone Spine. 2003;70:352–5.
17. Torricelli P, Martinelli C, Biagini R, Ruggieri P, De Cristofaro R. Radiographic and computed tomographic findings in hydatid disease of bone. Skeletal Radiol. 1990;19:435–9.

Miscellaneous Cysts

18. Segura J, Palanca D, Bueno AL, Seral B, Castiella T, Seral F. Baker's pseudocyst in the prosthetic knee affected with aggressive granulomatosis caused by polyethylene wear. Chir Organi Mov. 1996;81:421–6.

19. Sanal HT, Chen L, Haghighi P, Trudell DJ, Resnick DL. Carpal bone cysts: MRI, gross pathology and histology correlation in cadavers. Diagn Interv Radiol. 2014;20:503–6.

Haemodialysis Associated Cyst

20. Sargent MA, Fleming SJ, Chattopadhyay C, Ackrill P, Sambrook P. Bone cysts and haemodialysis-related amyloidosis. Clin Radiol. 1989;40(3):277–81.

Haemophilic Cyst

21. Steel WM, Duthie RB. Hemophilic cysts-report of 5 cases. J Bone Joint Surg. 1969;51 B(4):614–26.
22. Khubrani AM, Alshomer FM, Alassiri AH, Al Meshal O. Pseudotumor of hemophilia of the thumb. Saudi Med J. 2020;41(7):763–6.

Geode-Osteoarthritis Related Cyst

23. Guve M, Ozler T, Kocadal O, Ozkan F, Altintas F. An atypically located large subchondral cyst in an osteoarthritic hip joint: A case report. J Med Case Reports. 2013;7:176.

Meniscal and Synovial Cysts

24. Crowell MS, Westrick RB, Fogarty BT. Cysts of the lateral meniscus. Int J Sports Phys Ther. 2013;8(3):340–8.
25. Kim Y, D'Lima DD, Joo Y, et al. Huge intrameniscal cyst successfully treated by open debridement and combined arthroscopic and open repair: a case report. BMC Musculoskelet Disord. 2020;21:190.
26. Saini S, Sinha M, Gulati NS, Das A, Mehndiratta MM. Cytomorphological study of articular and periarticular cystic lesions. Int J Healthcare Biomed Res. 2018;6(4):23–36.

15 Metastatic Tumours of Bone

Metastatic tumours of the bone are more common than the primary tumours of bone. After lung and liver, bone is the third most common site for metastatic carcinoma [1, 2]. Prostate cancer in men and breast cancer in women are the most common types of cancers that metastasize to bones [3]. Any bone may be involved with metastases. The bones near the centre of the body are commonly involved in metastasis. The commonest bone involved is vertebra. Other common sites are pelvic bones, femur, humerus, ribs and skull. It is rare in small bones of hands and feet. If the bones below the mid-forearm or mid-calf are involved, usually the primary will be from the lung, kidney or GIT.

Metastatic bone lesions can be either osteolytic or osteoblastic lesions [4]. Carcinomas of the breast, prostate, lung, thyroid and kidney are the common cancers that metastasize to the bone [1, 5, 6]. Primary breast and prostate cancers metastasizing to the bone are very common [3, 7]. Similarly, lung, thyroid and kidney cancers also frequently spread to the bones [8, 9] (Table 15.1). Patients present with pain, fracture, spinal cord compression and a high calcium blood level [10].

Pathogenesis: A number of mechanisms interact between malignant cells and their microenvironment [11]. Hence, each tumour results in choosing their preferable site for metastasis [12]. Haematogenous spread of metastatic cells occurs due to the proliferation of a single-cell population resulting in micrometastases and then vascularized metastasis [13].

The chemokine receptors, cell adhesion molecules and cell surface receptors produced by the tumour cells attach the cells to the bone matrix, and they start growing in the bone [14]. In osteolytic metastasis, osteoclastic cells get stimulated by some factors produced by the tumour cells. Some of the factors promoting bone metastasis are PTHrP, IL-1, IL-6, prostaglandin E2, TNF and CSF-1. PTHrP is one of the major factors promoting metastasis to bone in breast cancer [15, 16]. Hence, PTHrP-positive tumours mostly develop skeletal metastasis. Carcinomas of bladder, kidney, prostate, cervix and breast express IL-6 [3, 6, 8]. Glioblastoma cells also express IL-6.

Prostate cancer produces blastic bone metastasis [17]. 15–20% of breast cancers also show blastic metastasis. In this type, bone formation is more than bone resorption [5, 18, 19]. Severe bone pain is the main symptom. Since the bone

Table 15.1 Common sites of metastatic tumours in bone

Sites of metastasis
Bones with red marrow • Proximal femur and humerus • Vertebra • Skull • Ribs
Common primaries—breast, prostate, kidney, lung, thyroid
Subungual metastasis—usually metastasis from RCC

J. Kattoor et al., *Bone Tumors*, https://doi.org/10.1007/978-981-99-4738-6_15

produced is of poor quality, pathological fractures are common. In lung and renal metastasis, another type of metastasis called cortical metastasis occurs [20]. In cortical metastasis, the cortex is destroyed without involving the medullary cavity.

Clinical features: Metastatic lesions are single or multiple. When multiple lesions are seen in adults, the usual differential diagnosis is metastasis and myeloma (Table 15.3). The first symptom of bone metastasis is bone pain. The pain is intermittent and is worse at night [10]. It may progressively worsen and become constant. Pathologic fractures are common [21]. Pressure symptoms are common in spine metastasis. Hypercalcaemia due to calcium leak to the blood can be present in some metastatic tumours. This hypercalcaemia in turn can produce other symptoms like constipation, nausea, loss of appetite, extreme thirst, frequent urination, dehydration and fatigue. It can even cause confusion and coma. 25–30% of cases present with metastasis as the initial manifestation. The common occult primaries are lung, liver, pancreas and gastrointestinal tract. Adenocarcinoma accounts for 70% of all cases.

Radiology: They can be lytic or sclerotic or mixed lytic and sclerotic [22] (Table 15.2). Purely lytic lesion with aneurysmal dilatation of bone is more likely to be a metastasis from kidney. Thyroid is another site to be ruled out in such cases. Sclerotic metastasis occurs from prostate in males and breast in females [3].

Bone scan is useful in detecting involvement of other bones [4]. The extent of the disease can be best assessed by CT scan, especially PET-CT and MRI [23, 24]. They also help in the detection of the primary site.

Pathology: Fine needle aspiration cytology (FNAC) or biopsy is performed to confirm metastasis from a known primary [25]. Metastatic adenocarcinomas and squamous cell carcinomas are easy to diagnose. If the primary is unknown, IHC may be required for confirmation [26–28] (Figs. 15.1, 15.2, 15.3, 15.4, and 15.5). Sometimes, the initial presentation may be metastatic lesion, and IHC may help to pinpoint the primary (Fig. 15.6). Even after IHC, the primary may remain unknown [9, 29] (Fig. 15.7). The

Table 15.2 Common metastatic sites in relation to radiology findings

Radiology and common metastatic sites
• **Purely blastic** – Prostate – Stomach – Carcinoid – Medulloblastoma • **Purely lytic** – Renal cell carcinoma (RCC) – Thyroid • **Mixed blastic and lytic** – Breast – Lung – GIT
In any patient >30 years with a malignant solitary or multiple lytic tumours with fusiform bone expansion, consider metastasis from RCC first, metastasis from thyroid second and then other possibilities

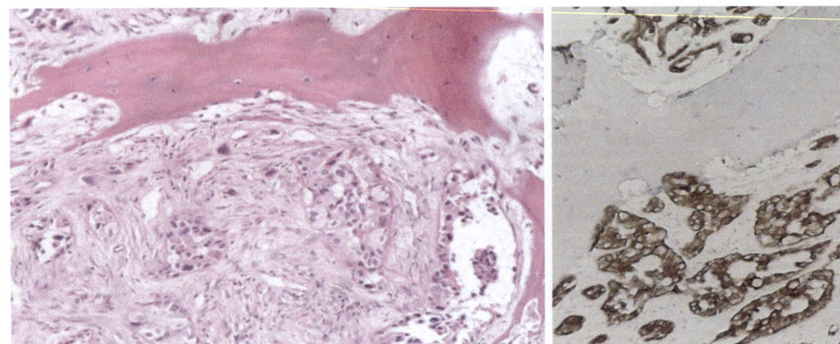

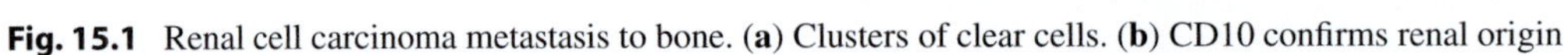

Fig. 15.1 Renal cell carcinoma metastasis to bone. (**a**) Clusters of clear cells. (**b**) CD10 confirms renal origin

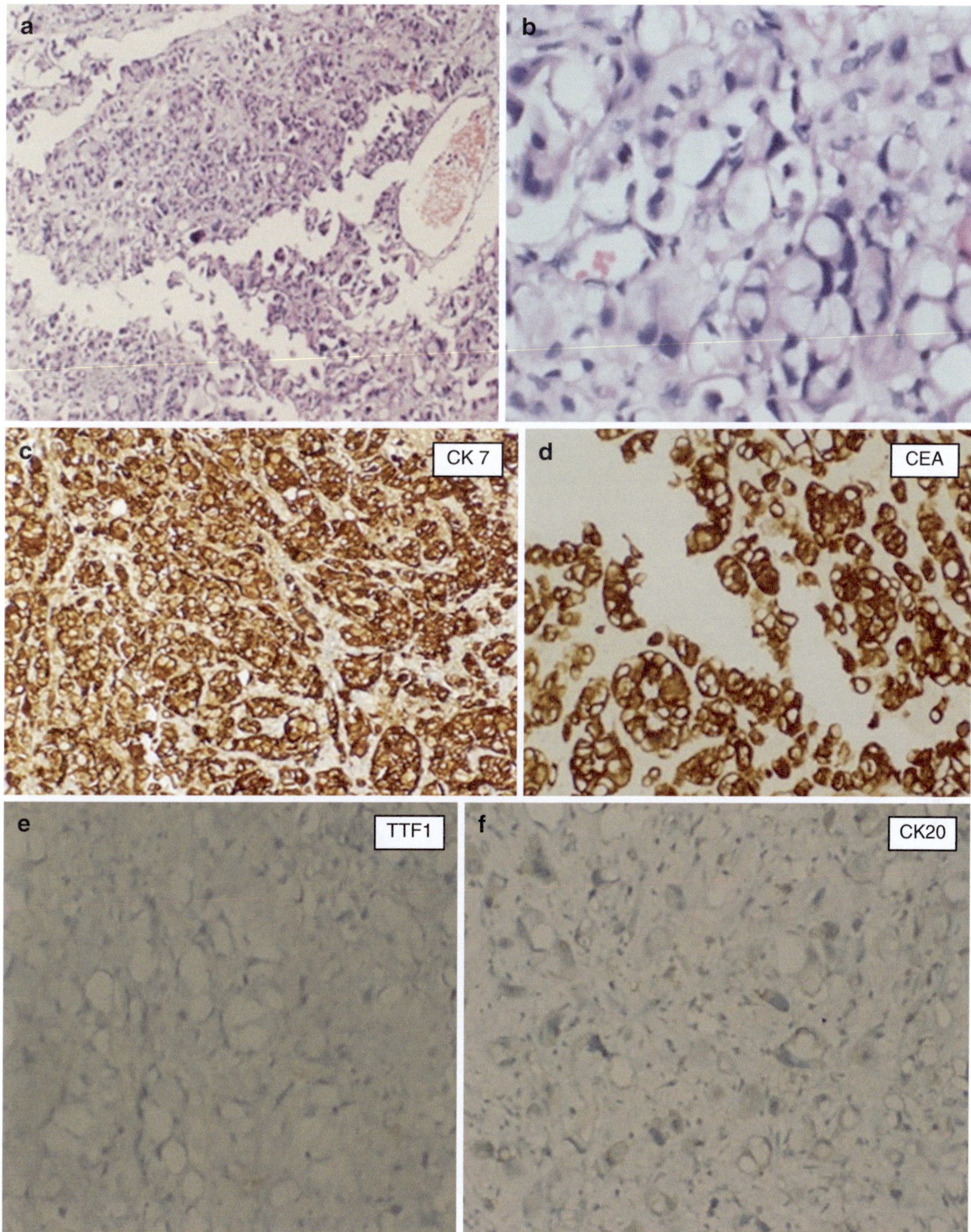

Fig. 15.2 Signet ring cell carcinoma metastasis to bone. (**a** and **b**) Signet ring cells and spicule of bone. (**c** and **d**) CK7 and CEA strongly positive. (**e** and **f**) CK20 and TTF1 negative. Primary was in pancreas with raised serum CA19.9 (>25,000)

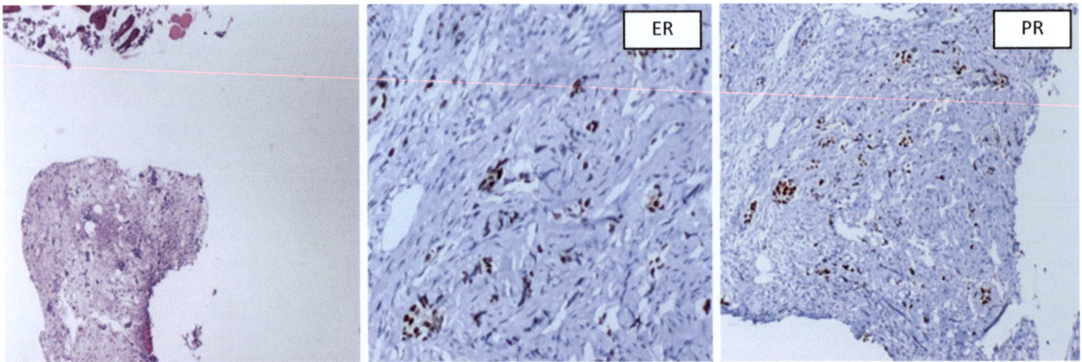

Fig. 15.3 Metastasis from carcinoma breast. (**a**) Needle biopsy showing cluster of cells. (**b** and **c**) ER and PR showing strong nuclear positivity

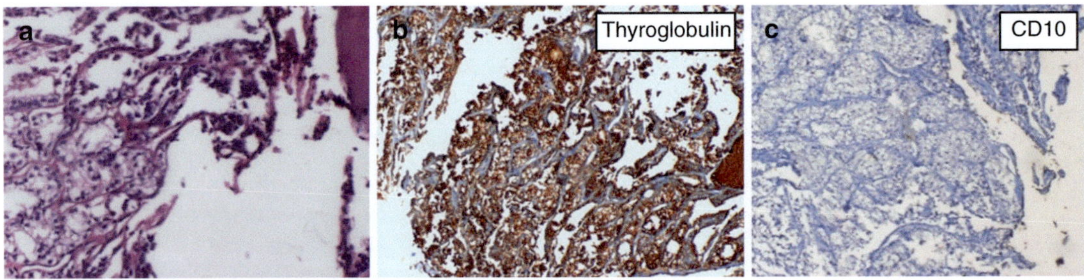

Fig. 15.4 (**a**) Metastatic carcinoma with clear cells—metastasis from thyroid primary. (**b**) Thyroglobulin positive. (**c**) CD10 negative. Differential diagnosis was renal cell carcinoma

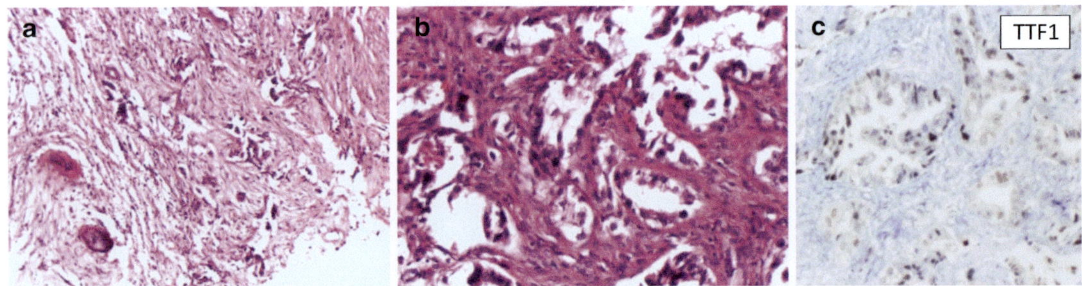

Fig. 15.5 (**a** and **b**) Metastasis from adenocarcinoma. (**c**) TTF1 positive. Metastasis from lung

gene expression profiling can classify the majority of tumour classes both in patients with known primary and in patients with unknown primary. Microarray profiling is another tool to locate primary when it is unknown.

Rarely, a metastatic carcinoma has spindle cells and may be mistaken for a primary bone tumour. This is common for renal cell carcinoma (RCC), which may be sarcomatoid. Reactive osteoid accompanying metastatic carcinoma may be mistaken for osteosarcoma (Fig. 15.8). Some osteosarcomas can be epithelioid also, making differentiation difficult. Some lytic metastases may show increased number of osteoclastic giant cells and are mistaken for giant cell tumour. Sometimes, anaplastic large cell lymphoma (ALCL) can mimic a metastatic carcinoma (Fig. 15.9).

In children, metastasis from neuroblastoma is the commonest (see chapter on malignant round

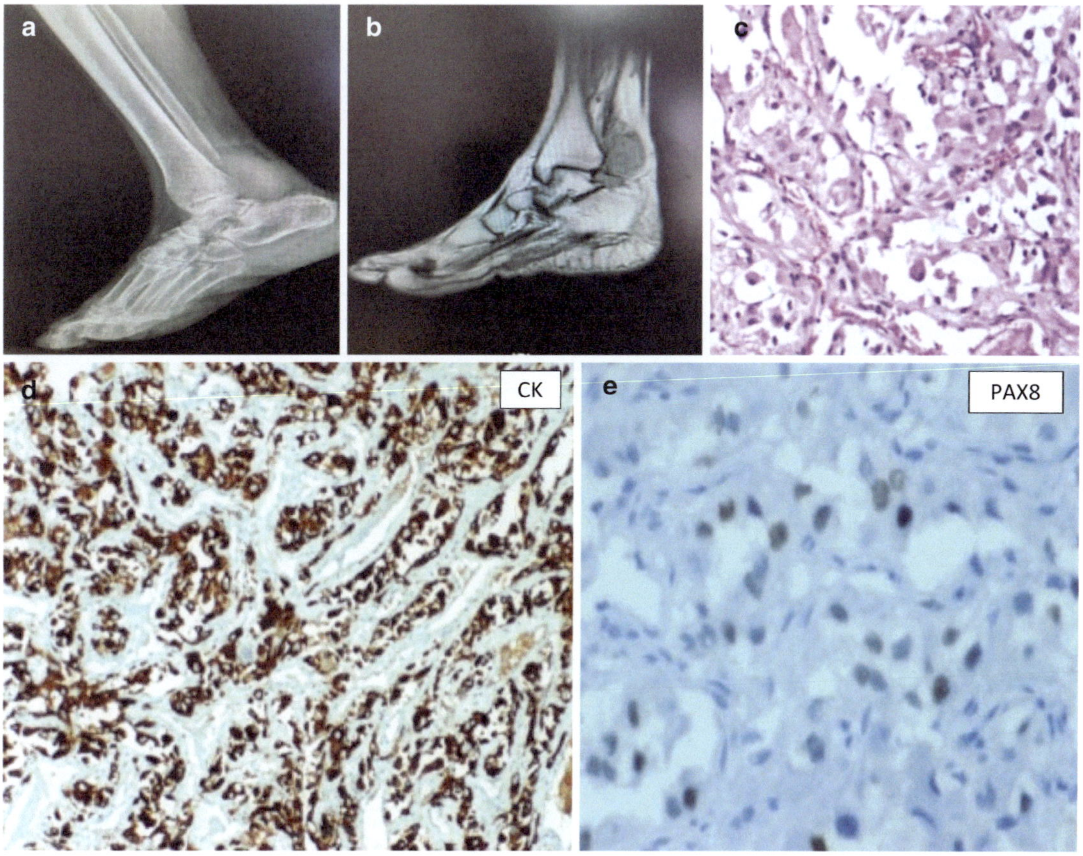

Fig. 15.6 71-Year-old female with lytic lesion at the lower end of the fibula. Referred as clear cell chondrosarcoma. (**a** and **b**) Plain X-ray and MRI showing lytic lesion at the lower end of the fibula. (**c**) Cells with clear cytoplasm. (**d**) CK diffusely strongly positive. (**e**) PAX 8 moderate nuclear positivity. Metastasis from renal cell carcinoma. Ultrasound abdomen revealed renal mass

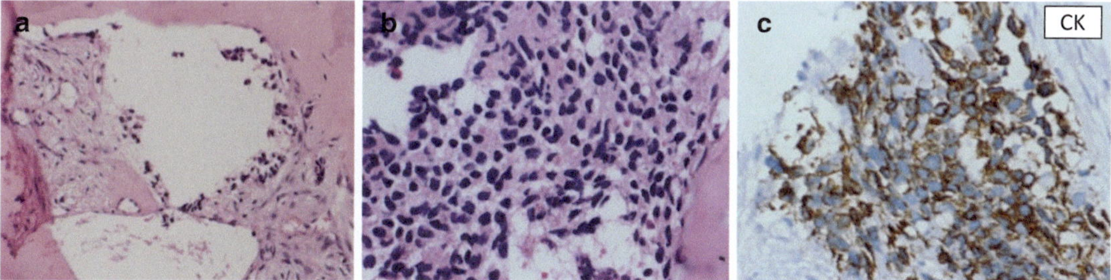

Fig. 15.7 (**a** and **b**) Undifferentiated malignant neoplasm. (**c**) IHC for CK only positive—metastatic carcinoma. LCA, vimentin and S100 negative, ruling out lymphoma, sarcoma and melanoma

cell tumours of bone). Medulloblastomas, Ewing sarcoma and rhabdomyosarcomas are the other malignant round cell neoplasms that can metastasize to bone.

Primary bone tumours like Ewing sarcoma and osteosarcomas can show metastasis to other bones. If the gap between primary diagnosis and development of metastasis is more than 6 months, it is called metastatic. Otherwise, it is called multicentric.

Most lymphomas that involve bone are secondary to lymph node involvement. Hodgkin's disease (HD) usually involves bone in the later stages of the disease [30]. Primary involvement of bone in HD is very rare [3, 10, 18, 31].

Bone metastases occur in almost 10% of sarcomas [32]. Angiosarcoma, dedifferentiated liposarcoma, leiomyosarcoma, undifferentiated sarcoma and alveolar soft part sarcoma (ASPS) are the mesenchymal malignancies that metastasize to the bone. Other rare tumours like haemangiopericytoma of meninges and malignant mixed mullerian tumour (MMMT) of uterus can also metastasize to bone (Fig. 15.10). If a leiomyosarcoma (LMS) of bone is seen, it is mandatory to rule out metastasis from elsewhere. Primary LMS is also reported. Similarly, ASPS can present as bone tumour as its initial presentation, and later the primary will be detected in soft tissue.

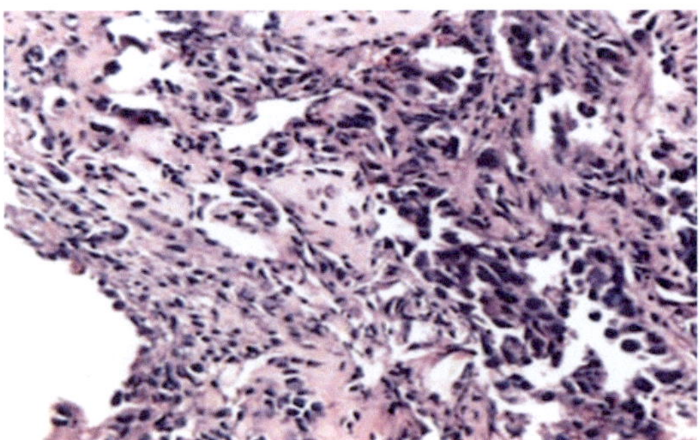

Fig. 15.8 Reactive osteoid in metastatic carcinoma

DD: Metastatic carcinoma becomes a diagnostic problem when it is solitary and mimics primary malignancy of bone [33]. Destructive bone lesion like that seen in renal cell carcinoma (RCC) is likely to be mistaken for primary because of solitary large lytic lesion. When multiple bone lesions are seen in an adult, the differential diagnoses include metastatic carcinoma, myeloma and lymphoma (Table 15.3). Vascular tumours can also be multiple. A clinical history is the most helpful information for the diagnosis. Sheets of histiocytes can be mistaken for clear cell carcinoma metastasis (Fig. . 15.11).

Treatment: It is important to locate primary tumours, especially prostate, thyroid and breast, which are treatable with good prognosis. In case of RCC metastasis, occurring years after the removal of primary tumour, prognosis is good. But those presenting with metastasis at the time of diagnosis will have a poor prognosis. Lung carcinoma with metastasis has poor

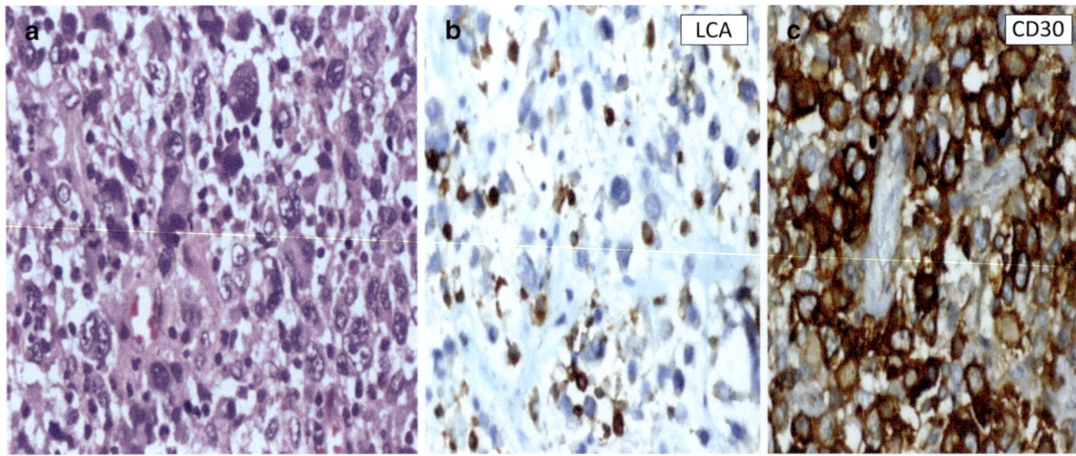

Fig. 15.9 (**a**) ALCL mimicking metastatic carcinoma. (**b**) Tumour cells negative for LCA. (**c**) Diffuse strong positivity for CD30

prognosis. The prognosis depends on the primary site [31]. Recently, bisphosphonates [34] and denosumab [35] are given for metastatic carcinomas with good effect. Bone radiofrequency ablation is a safe and useful treatment in certain metastastatic lesions to relieve pain [29]. Targeted therapy can also be given if the primary is located [36].

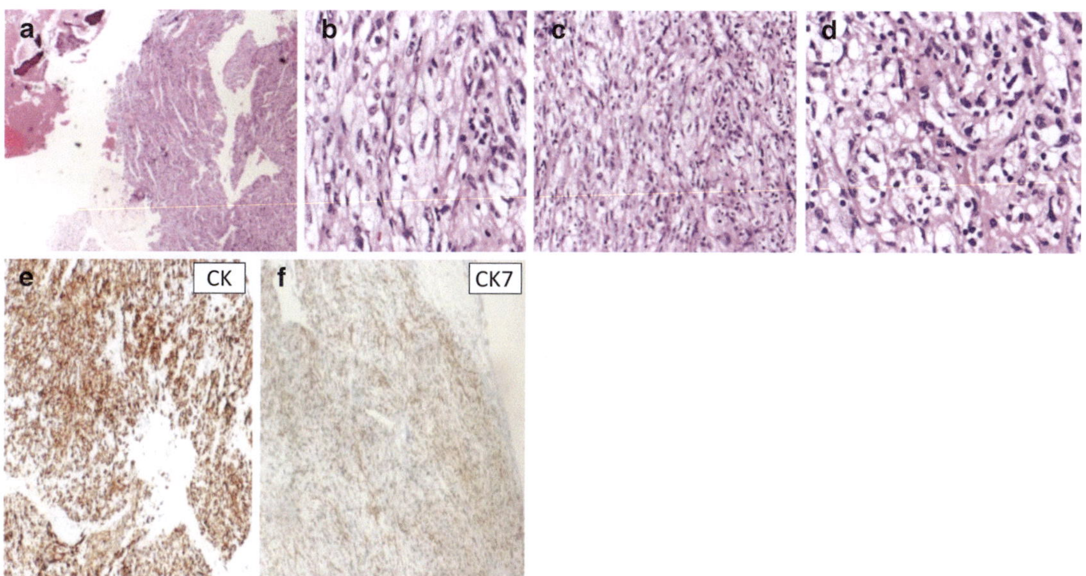

Fig. 15.10 (**a–d**) Metastatic carcinosarcoma vertebra. Search for primary revealed carcinosarcoma of uterus. (**e**) CK diffusely positive. (**f**) CK7—few groups of cells positive

Table 15.3 Differential diagnosis when multiple bone lesions are seen

Multiple bone lesions—differential diagnosis
Metastasis
Myeloma
Lymphoma
Vascular lesions

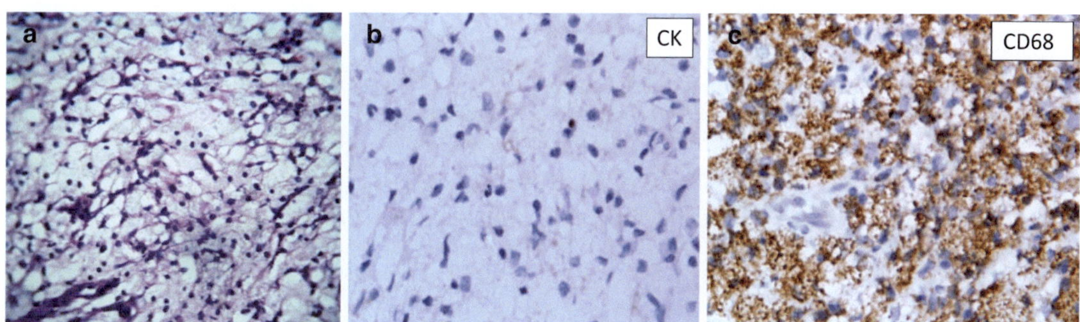

Fig. 15.11 (**a**) Histiocytes at fracture site mimicking metastatic carcinoma. (**b**) CK negative. (**c**) Histiocytic marker CD68 positive

Points to Remember

Most common bone tumours of bone are metastatic tumours.

Multiple bone lesions in elderly—rule out metastasis and myeloma.

Common cancers that metastasize to bone—Ca breast, lung, prostate, kidney and thyroid.

Judicial use of IHC markers helps in locating the primary site.

References

1. Airoldi G. Cancer of unknown primary origin: utility and futility in clinical practice. Ital J Med. 2012;6:315–26.
2. Carlson HR. Carcinoma of unknown primary: searching for the origin of metastases. J Am Acad Phys Assist. 2009;22:18–21.
3. Wang C, Wu G, Shen M, Cui K, Shen Y. Comparison of distribution characteristics of metastatic bone lesions between breast and prostate carcinomas. Oncol Lett. 2013;5:391–7.
4. Kakhki VRD, Anvari K, Sadeghi R, Mahmoudian A-S, Torabian-Kakhki M. Pattern and distribution of bone metastases in common malignant tumors. Nucl Med Rev. 2013;16(2):66–9.
5. Cecchini M, Wetterwald A, Pluijm G, Thalmann G. Molecular and biological mechanisms of bone metastasis. EAU Update Series. 2005;3:214–26.
6. Gottwald L, Dukowicz A, Piekarski J, et al. Bone metastases from gynaecological epithelial cancers. J Obstet Gynaecol. 2012;32:81–6.
7. Morgan JWM, Adcock KM, Donohue RE. Distribution of skeletal metastases in prostatic and lung cancer. Urology. 1990;36:31–4.
8. Chen SC, Kuo PL. Bone metastasis from renal cell carcinoma. Int J Mol Sci. 2016;17(6):987.
9. Khan MN, Sharfuzzaman A, Mostafa MG. Spinal cord compression as initial presentation of metastatic occult follicular thyroid carcinoma. J Neurosci Rural Pract. 2014;5(2):155–9.
10. Coleman RE. Clinical features of metastatic bone disease and risk of skeletal morbidity. Clin Cancer Res. 2006;12:6243s–9s.
11. Macedo F, Ladeira K, Pinho F, Saraiva N, Bonito N, Pinto L, Gonçalves F. Bone metastases: an overview. Oncol Rev. 2017;11:321e.
12. Langley RR, Fidler IJ. The seed and soil hypothesis revisited—the role of tumor-stroma interactions in metastasis to different organs. Int J Cancer. 2011;128:2527–35.
13. Chambers A, Naumov G, Varghese H, et al. Critical steps in hematogenous metastasis: an overview. Surg Oncol Clin N Am. 2001;10:243–55.
14. Muller A, Homey B, Soto H, et al. Involvement of chemokine receptors in breast cancer metastasis. Nature. 2001;410:50–6.
15. Chirgwin JM, Guise TA. Molecular mechanisms of tumor-bone interactions in osteolytic metastases. Crit Rev Eukaryot Gene Expr. 2000;10:159–78.
16. Kang Y, Siegel PM, Shu W, et al. A multigenic program mediating breast cancer metastasis to bone. Cancer Cell. 2003;3:537–49.
17. Mohammad KS, Guise TA. Mechanisms of osteoblastic metastases: role of endothelin-1. Clin Orthop. 2003;415(Suppl):S67–74.
18. Berrettoni BA, Carter JR. Mechanisms of cancer metastasis to bone. J Bone Joint Surg Am. 1986;68:308–12.
19. Boyce BF, Yoneda T, Guise TA. Factors regulating the growth of metastatic cancer in bone. Endocr Relat Cancer. 1999;6:333–47.
20. Deutsch A, Resnick D. Eccentric cortical metastases to the skeleton from bronchogenic carcinoma. Radiology. 1980;137:49–52.
21. Wick MR. Metastases to bones. Seminars in diagnostic pathology. 2014;31(53–6):5.
22. Rosenthal D. Radiologic diagnosis of bone metastases. Cancer. 1997;80:1595–607.
23. Evans A, Robertson J. Magnetic resonance imaging versus radionuclide scintigraphy for screening in bone metastases. Clin Radiol. 2000;55:653.
24. Lawrenz JM, Gordon J, George J, Haben C, Rubin BP, Ilaslan H, Mesko NW, Nystrom LM. Does PET/CT aid in detecting primary carcinoma in patients with skeletal metastases of unknown primary? Clin Orthop Relat Res. 2020;478(11):2451–7.
25. Wedin R, Bauer HC, Skoog L, Söderlund V, Tani E. Cytological diagnosis of skeletal lesions. Fine-needle aspiration biopsy in 110 tumours. J Bone Jt Surg Br. 2000;82(5):673–8.
26. Kandalaft PL, Grown AL. Practical applications in immunohistochemistry: carcinomas of unknown primary site. Arch Pathol Lab Med. 2016;140(6):508–23.
27. Kima LD, Buenob FT, Yonaminea ES, de Prósperob JD, Pozzana G. Bone metastasis as the first symptom of tumors: role of an immunohistochemistry study in establishing primary tumor. Rev Bras Ortop. 2018;53(4):467–71.
28. Park SY, Kim BH, Kim JH, Lee S, Kang GH. Panels of immunohistochemical markers help determine primary sites of metastatic adenocarcinoma. Arch Pathol Lab Med. 2007;131:1561–7.
29. Thacker PG, Callstrom MR, Curry TB, Mandrekar JN. Palliation of painful metastatic disease involving bone with imaging-guided treatment: comparison of patients' immediate response to radiofrequency ablation and cryoablation. Vasc Intervent Radiol. 2011;197(2):510–5.

30. Gaudio F, Pedote P, Asabella AN, Ingravallo G, Sindaco P, Alberotanza V, Perrone T, Laddaga FE, Rubini G, Ianora AAS, Specchia G. Bone involvement in Hodgkin's lymphoma: clinical features and outcome. Acta Haematol. 2018;140:178–82.
31. Hemminki K, Riihimäki M, Sundquist K, Hemminki A. Site-specific survival rates for cancer of unknown primary according to location of metastases. Int J Cancer. 2013;133(1):182–9.
32. Vincenzi B, Frezza AM, Schiavon G, et al. Bone metastases in soft tissue sarcoma: a survey of natural history, prognostic value and treatment options. Clin Sarcoma Res. 2013;3:6.
33. Papagelopoulos P, Savvidou O, Galanis E, et al. Advances and challenges in diagnosis and management of skeletal metastases. Orthopedics. 2009;29(7):609–20.
34. Coleman R, Seaman J. The role of zoledronic acid in cancer: clinical studies in the treatment and prevention of bone metastasis. Semin Oncol. 2001;28:11–6.
35. Steger G, Bartsch R. Denosumab for the treatment of bone metastases in breast cancer: evidence and opinion. Ther Adv Med Oncol. 2011;3:233–43.
36. Ibrahim T, Farolfi A, Mercatali L, et al. Metastatic bone disease in the era of bone-targeted therapy: clinical impact. Tumori. 2013;99:1–9.

16 Rare Tumours of Bone

Certain tumours rarely occur as primary bone tumours. Some are benign, and a few of them are malignant. Benign tumours include schwannoma, lipoma, phosphaturic mesenchymal tumour, mixed tumour and myoepithelioma. Certain soft tissue sarcomas are sometimes seen primarily in bone. These include leiomyosarcoma, clear cell sarcoma and alveolar soft part sarcoma. Malignant counterparts of mixed tumour and myoepithelial tumours are also described primarily in bone. Ependymoma is another tumour rarely seen in bone. A brief description of these tumours is given in this chapter.

16.1 Benign Tumours

16.1.1 Schwannoma

Schwannomas (also called neurilemmomas) are rare tumours occurring in bone (0.2%) [2]. They are slow-growing nerve sheath tumours. The most commonly affected bones are mandible and sacrum [1]. This is because sensory nerves pass through these bones. Long bones and vertebrae can also be involved. The syndromes associated with intraosseous schwannomas are von Recklinghausen's disease and Carney syndrome [6].

16.1.1.1 Clinical

Schwannomas usually occur in adults (the second to fifth decades). They are rare in children. Females are more commonly affected. Pain is the common presenting symptom.

16.1.1.2 Radiology

The radiological findings of the intraosseous schwannomas are non-specific.

Plain X-ray shows a well-defined lytic lesion with thin sclerotic rim. Multiple schwannomas are reported [5]. The radiologic differential diagnosis in long bones includes fibrous dysplasia or non-ossifying fibroma. In metadiaphyseal tumours, simple bone cyst is a differential.

16.1.1.3 Pathology

Primary schwannoma of the bone is rarely encapsulated. Giant schwannomas are described [7]. Histologically, cellular (Antoni A) and loosely arranged (Antoni B) areas are seen (Fig. 16.1a). The palisading seen in soft tissue schwannomas is rarely present in osseous schwannomas. Bone schwannomas are cellular, and Verocay bodies may be absent. Presence of perivascular chronic inflammation is another finding. S100 protein is diffusely and strongly positive in schwannomas (Fig. 16.1b). Cellular, ancient and melanotic variants of schwannomas are also described. Rarely, myxoid schwanno-

J. Kattoor et al., *Bone Tumors*, https://doi.org/10.1007/978-981-99-4738-6_16

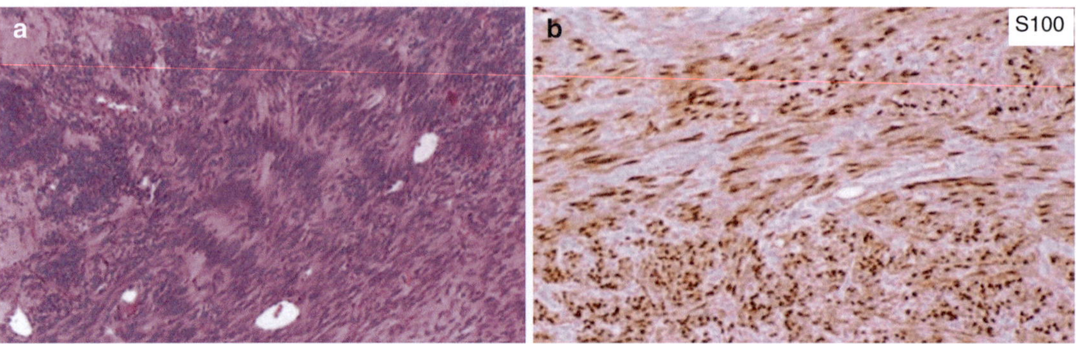

Fig. 16.1 Schwannoma. (**a**) Antoni A and B areas, H&E ×100. (**b**) S100 showing diffuse strong positivity ×100

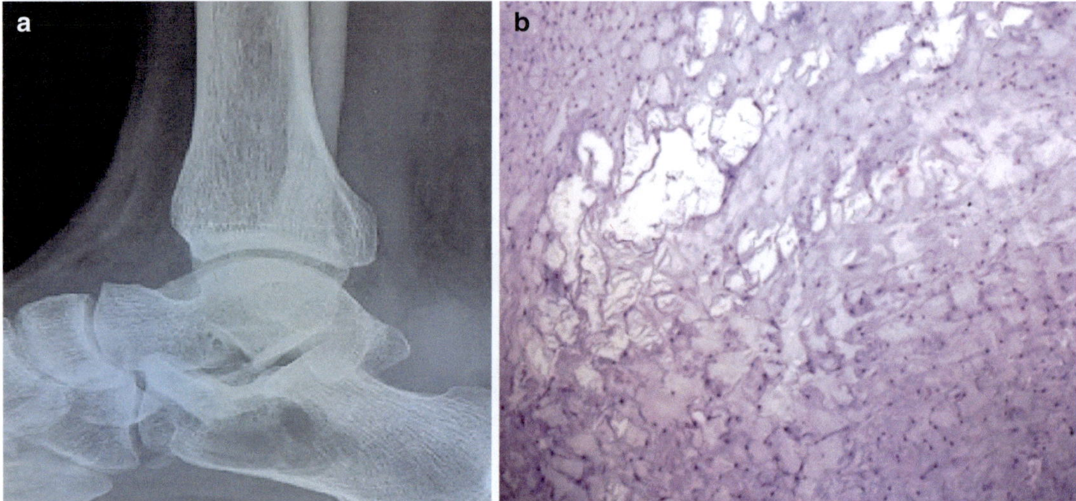

Fig. 16.2 Myxoid schwannoma of talus. (**a**) Plain X-ray showing lytic lesion involving talus. (**b**) Scattered spindle cells in myxoid matrix, H&E ×250

mas composed predominantly of myxomatous stroma may be seen (Fig. 16.2).

16.1.1.4 DD

Desmoplastic fibroma, well-differentiated fibrosarcoma, fibrous dysplasia and non-ossifying fibroma are the main DDs. Diffuse and strong positivity for S100 helps in differentiation.

16.1.1.5 Treatment and Prognosis

Intraosseous schwannomas are treated with local excision alone. Incompletely removed tumours recur. But malignant transformation has not been reported. Schwannomas of the bone behave in a benign manner. Some melanotic schwannomas lacking malignant features may behave like malignant tumours. They can present with metastasis. Hence, a long-term follow-up is recommended.

16.1.2 Lipoma

Intraosseous lipoma is a very rare lesion [9, 11]. Degenerative changes are common with areas of fat necrosis, cystic changes and calcification. Even though primary pleomorphic liposarcoma is reported in bone [10], the entity liposarcoma of bone is removed from the 2020 WHO classification [97].

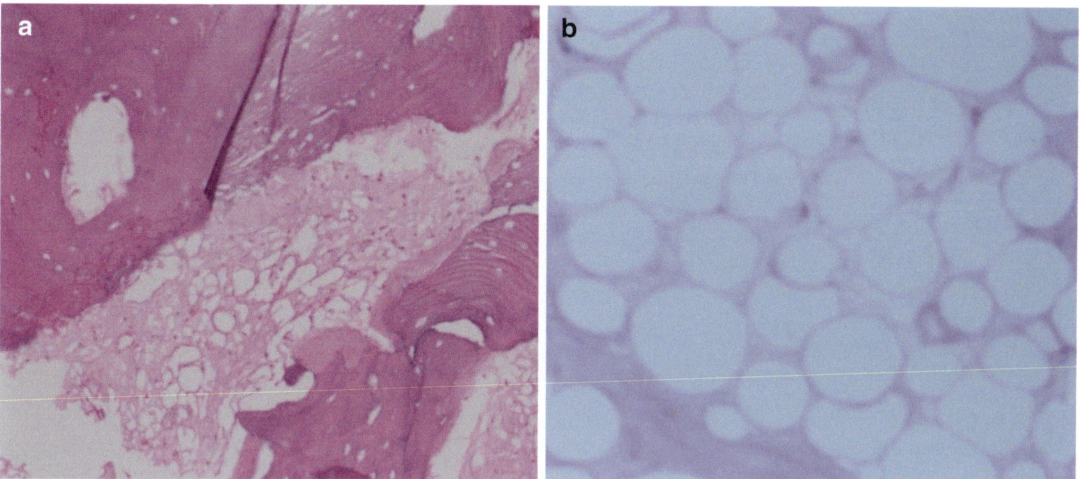

Fig. 16.3 Intraosseous lipoma. (**a**) Mature adipocytes in between bony spicules, H&E ×100. (**b**) Adipocytes with eccentrically placed flat nuclei, H&E ×250. Picture courtesy: Dr. Jayanthi Kamashi

16.1.2.1 Clinical

Pain is the major symptom. Parosteal lipoma presents with painful swelling. It usually occurs in fifth to sixth decades. Males are more affected. It is detected incidentally. Intraosseous lipomas occur mainly in the metaphysis of long bones of lower limb and calcaneum [9, 11]. Other sites are spine, pelvic bone, skull and ribs.

16.1.2.2 Radiology

They are seen as low-density lesions on plain X-ray [12]. Lipomatous nature can be detected on MRI. Calcifications are seen at the margins. In the calcaneum, cystic degeneration can be seen.

16.1.2.3 Pathology

Tumours are 3–5 cm in size, yellowish soft and sometimes gritty. The surrounding bone is sclerotic. Mature adipocytes are seen in lobules (Fig. 16.3). Foamy macrophages, small foci of necrosis and fibrosis can be seen. Parosteal lipoma is seen on the surface. Sometimes, endochondral ossification-like changes are noted in this area. Cells are positive for S100.

16.1.2.4 DD

Bone marrow infarction with dystrophic calcification is a close differential diagnosis. This condition is without a definite mass, and there will be presence of necrotic bone.

16.1.2.5 Treatment and prognosis

Radiological follow-up with conservative treatment is the recommended treatment. Surgery is indicated if the tumour is painful, in the presence of pathological fracture and if histological diagnosis is required. The prognosis is excellent.

16.1.3 Hibernoma

Hibernoma is very rare and usually affects females of 40–80 years of age. It is more common in axial skeleton [14].

16.1.3.1 Radiology

On PET-CT, this lesion shows high uptake. On CT scan, it is seen as sclerotic and ill defined.

16.1.3.2 Pathology

Brown fat cells [13] with multiple vacuoles and scalloping central nuclei are seen (Fig. 16.4). Admixed with these cells, haematopoietic elements are seen. Brown fat marker UCP1 will be positive.

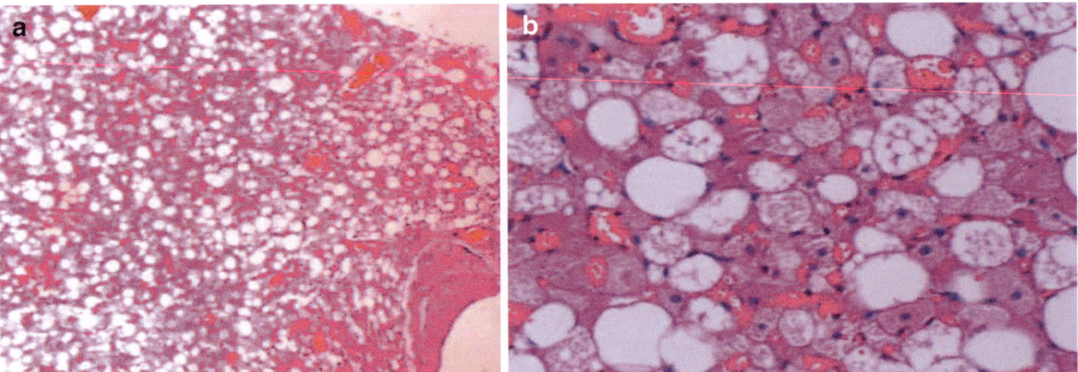

Fig. 16.4 Hibernoma. (**a**) Low power showing immature adipocytes, H&E ×100. (**b**) Immature adipocytes (brown fat) with multiple vacuoles, H&E ×400

16.1.3.3 Treatment

Symptomatic tumours are curetted, and prognosis is good.

16.1.4 Phosphaturic Mesenchymal Tumour

Tumour-induced osteomalacia (TIO) was first described by Prader and colleagues in 1957. Later in 1987, Weidner and Santa Cruz named it as "phosphaturic mesenchymal tumour" (PMT). The fusion of FN1-FGFR1 and FGF1 genes was described in this tumour by Lee and colleagues in 2015 [30].

16.1.4.1 Clinical

The PMT cases commonly occur in bone [23, 24], soft tissue and head and neck (maxillofacial sinuses) [33]. It occurs in middle-aged adults. In the bone, it commonly involves the appendicular skeleton, cranial bones and paranasal sinuses [29]. Sometimes, multiple bones are involved [25]. They present with muscle pain and progressive weakness, which is present for many months. Later, bone pain and fractures occur. Serum levels of FGF23 are increased. Serum FGF23 levels drop rapidly after tumour resection.

16.1.4.2 Radiology

They are lytic on CT scans with matrix formation. On MRI examination, they are solid enhancing.

16.1.4.3 Pathology

The tumours are well circumscribed. Focal cystic change may be present. The cut surface is fleshy and myxoid with brownish areas. This brownish colour is due to the haemorrhagic giant cell areas.

They are composed of fibroblast-like spindled or stellate undifferentiated mesenchymal cells without atypia; microcystic change is admixed with prominent sclerotic matrix with characteristic bluish to hyaline appearance (Fig. 16.5). Scattered osteoclastic giant cells and foci of haemorrhage can be seen. A highly vascular stroma and lattice-like or grungy calcification with smudgy pale blue to purple colour is described. Unusual features are oxalate-like crystals, foci of mature-looking hyaline cartilage and extensive haemorrhage. Haemangiopericytoma-like vascular pattern can be seen. Sometimes, a mixture of fat cells and vessels mimicking angiomyolipoma is seen. Chondromyxoid fibroma-like features and features resembling solid ABC are described. Rarely, secondary aneurysmal bone cyst-like changes are present. In the skull bones, a biphasic pattern with proliferation of epithelium and stroma can be seen.

Less than 10% of PMTs are histologically malignant showing pleomorphism, increased mitosis, necrosis and decreased matrix production. It resembles fibrosarcoma or undifferentiated pleomorphic sarcoma. Benign areas may be seen in some parts of the tumour or in previous biopsy. Sometimes histologically benign PMT can have

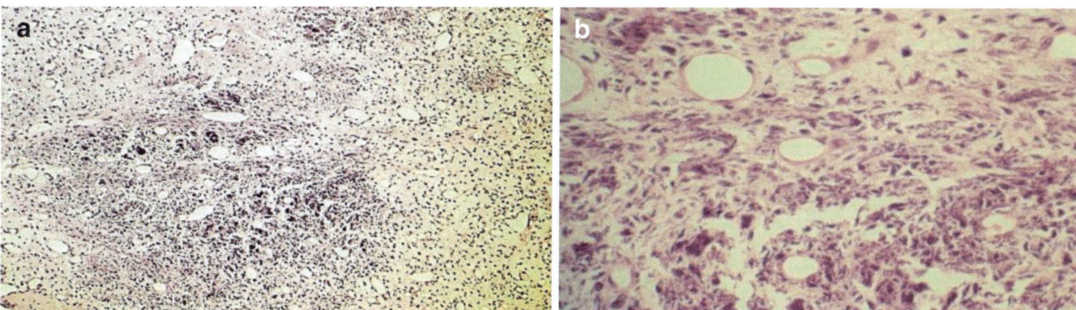

Fig. 16.5 Phosphaturic mesenchymal tumour. (**a** and **b**) Spindle cells, thin-walled blood vessels and sclerotic matrix with bluish appearance, H&E ×100

lung metastases. Malignant PMT can behave aggressively with local recurrence, distant metastasis and poor prognosis.

16.1.4.4 IHC

α-Smooth muscle actin, CD34, S100, synaptophysin, ERG, FLI1 [32], CD56, D2-40 [31] and DOG 1 [26] can show positivity. Recently, SATB2 has shown consistent positivity in PMT. FGF23 by IHC is helpful in diagnosing these tumours.

16.1.4.5 Molecular

FN1-FGFR1 or FN1-FGF1 fusions are identified as molecular markers [28, 30].

16.1.4.6 DD

PMT has a wide range of differentials. It includes solitary fibrous tumours, sinonasal glomangiopericytomas, nasal angiofibromas, giant cell-rich tumours of bone and soft tissue, tenosynovial giant cell tumours (benign and malignant), aneurysmal bone cysts, benign and malignant cartilaginous tumours, benign and malignant osteogenic tumours, spindle cell lipomas, haemangiomas and various neuroendocrine neoplasms. Detection of fibroblast growth factor (FGF23) in the blood or by IHC in the tissue will help in the diagnosis [27].

16.1.4.7 Treatment and Prognosis

PMTs are excised, mainly to relieve the symptoms [34]. Majority is benign, and less than 10% are malignant.

16.1.5 Melanotic Neuroectodermal Tumour of Infancy (MNTI)

This is a rare and unusual tumour usually seen adherent to bone. The common sites are maxilla, mandible [17] and skull bones. There are rare case reports of tumour occurring in long bones like femur [15, 16]. We have seen a case in radius. MNTI has also been reported in the mediastinum, thigh, foot, shoulder and gonads. It is considered to be derived from neural crest.

16.1.5.1 Clinical

It is a tumour of infancy (95%). Females are more affected than males. It presents as a tumour around mouth with a bluish discolouration because of the presence of pigment. Usually, it is a firm tumour which can grow rapidly causing facial disfigurement. Elevated levels of vanillylmandelic acid are seen in these patients.

16.1.5.2 Radiology

Plain X-ray shows lytic and expansile lesions resembling cyst with well-defined margins. Calcifications within the tumour may be present.

16.1.5.3 Pathology

Macroscopically, it has a fibrous appearance with variable pigmentation. Histology shows two type of cells—small blue round cells and large epithelioid cells with melanin granules [19]. Background shows neurofibrillary material. Tumour is arranged in alveolar or tubular pattern (Fig. 16.6).

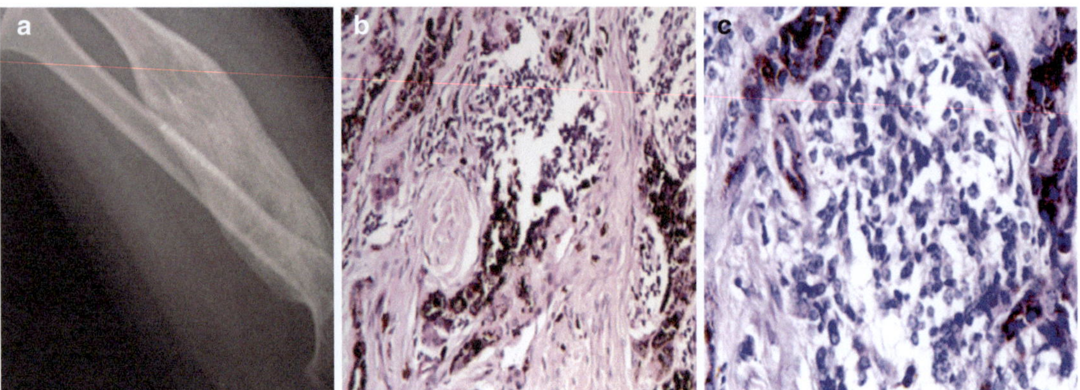

Fig. 16.6 Melanotic neuroectodermal tumour of radius in a 10-month-old baby. (**a**) Plain X-ray showing lytic lesion in radius. (**b**) Round cells with brownish pigment, H&E ×100. (**c**) Neuroblast-like cells admixed with epithelioid cells having melanin granules in the cytoplasm, H&E ×250

16.1.5.4 IHC

They are positive for cytokeratin, EMA and HMB-45 [18]. Round cells are positive for CD57 and show focal positivity for synaptophysin and S100 protein.

16.1.5.5 DD

Other round cell tumours come in the differential diagnosis. But presence of melanin-containing cells on careful examination clinches the diagnosis.

16.1.5.6 Treatment and Prognosis

Some tumours show spontaneous regression. Wide local excision with free surgical margin is the line of treatment. Relapse rate after incomplete excision is between 15% and 45%. Rarely, metastasis can occur to lymph nodes, liver, bone and soft tissue. Chemotherapy is given for recurrent and metastasized tumours. Overall prognosis is good.

16.1.6 Mixed Tumour of Bone

Mixed tumour contains two epithelial components, namely epithelial cells and myoepithelial cells, and a mesenchymal component (Fig. 16.7). It commonly occurs in salivary gland (pleomorphic adenoma) and also in lacrimal gland, lungs, breast, skin and soft tissue. When they occur in bone, it is usually metastatic from primary elsewhere [36, 37]. Rare examples are reported in bone also [38].

Squamous cells, myoepithelial cells and chondroid cells are seen in varying proportions. Cellular atypia, increased mitosis, focal coagulative necrosis and infiltration between bony trabeculae are the features to consider it as a low-grade malignant mixed tumour. A case with chondrosarcoma and squamous cell carcinoma arising in mixed tumour has been reported in the literature.

Metastasizing mixed tumours are extremely rare. Metastasis can occur to lung, bone, lymphnodes and rarely liver. The mandible is the most common site of bone metastasis. Direct infiltration of bone from nail bed of toe is described [35]. Rarely, primary malignant mixed tumour is also described in bone.

16.1.6.1 DD

The differential diagnosis includes metastasis of mixed tumour to bone, chondroid syringoma of skin or primary mixed tumour of soft tissue invading bone. Before giving a diagnosis of primary mixed tumour of bone, rule out benign mixed tumour of skin or salivary gland as they rarely metastasize.

16.1.6.2 Treatment

Resection is recommended for benign mixed tumours of bone.

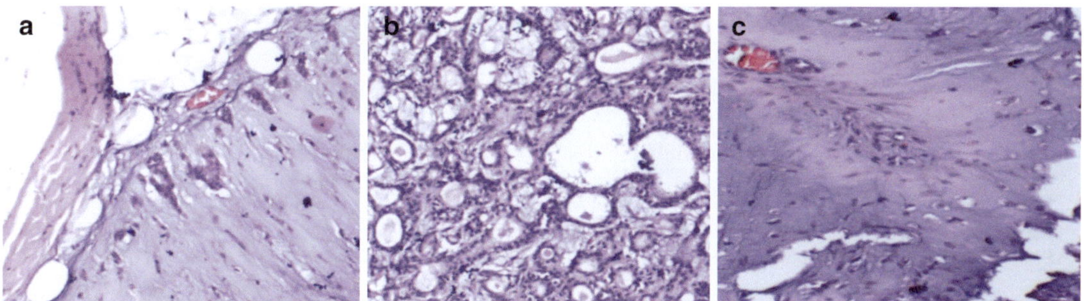

Fig. 16.7 Mixed tumour. (**a**) Encapsulated tumour with epithelial cells in a myxoid stroma, H&E ×100. (**b**) Double-layered epithelium with epithelial and myoepithelial cells lining acini, H&E ×100. (**c**) Predominantly chondromyxoid tissue and few epithelial cells, H&E ×250

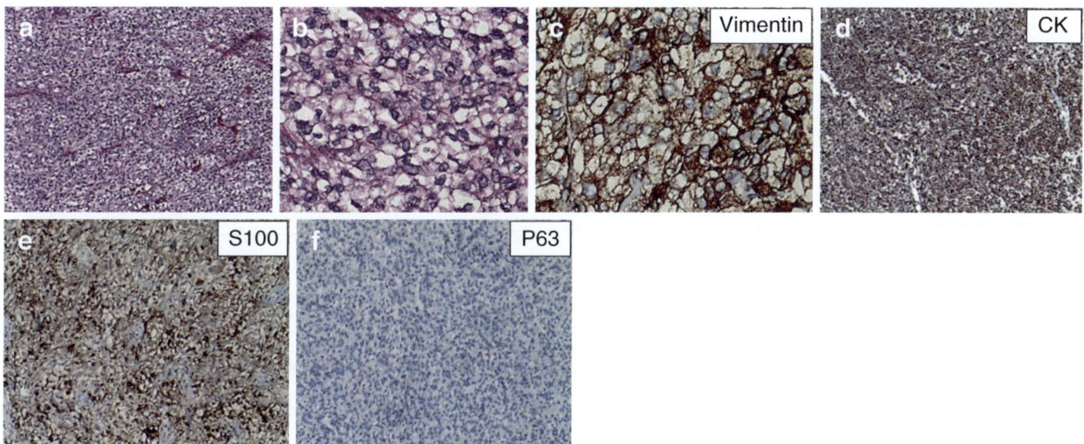

Fig. 16.8 Myoepithelioma of shoulder in a 15-year-old boy*. (**a**) Tumour cells in nests separated by thin vascular channels, H&E ×100. (**b**) Polygonal cells with clear cytoplasm and vesicular nuclei, H&E ×250. (**c**) Vimentin strongly positive ×250. (**d**) CK strongly and diffusely positive ×100. (**e**) S100 positive ×100. (**f**) P63 weakly positive ×100. *This case was contributed by Dr. Nanda Kachare, Consultant Pathologist, Aster Medcity, Kochi

16.1.7 Myoepithelioma of Bone

Primary musculoskeletal myoepithelial tumours (METs) are uncommon [43]. Mixed tumours, parachordomas and myoepitheliomas are a spectrum of tumours having myoepithelial lineage. They have a hyalinized to chondromyxoid stroma. Immunohistochemistry and molecular studies have recently recognized these tumours in various sites. EWSR1 gene rearrangements have been described in these tumours [40].

16.1.7.1 Clinical

They occur in young adults with no specific gender predilection. Ilium [48] and tibia are commonly involved. Other sites reported are humerus [44], ribs [41], spine [45], cuboid bone [49], maxilla [42] and femur [39].

16.1.7.2 Radiology

They are lytic lesions on plain X-ray. Occurrence of a primary intraosseous MET has been attributed to intraosseous displacement of myoepithelial elements during embryogenesis.

16.1.7.3 Pathology

Histologically predominant cells are myoepithelial cells embedded in a hyalinized to chondromyxoid stroma. The cells are polygonal, spindly or plasmacytoid with eosinophilic to clear cytoplasm, embedded in a myxoid, myxochondroid, chondroid and/or osteoid stroma (Fig. 16.8).

16.1.7.4 IHC

By IHC, these tumours are positive for epithelial markers such as EMA and AE1/AE3, along with variable S100, GFAP, p63, calponin and SMA positivity [46]. Brachyury negativity helps in distinguishing it from chordoma. Extensive cortical destruction and tumour necrosis with adjacent tissue infiltration are suggestive of malignancy.

16.1.7.5 DD

Myoepitheliomas lack a definite ductal component. The parachordoma cells have diffuse vacuolization of cytoplasm. Other diagnostic mimics are metastatic carcinomas, chondrosarcoma (skeletal and extraskeletal myxoid type) and other sarcomas exhibiting myxoid change. A wide panel of IHC markers are essential for their distinction.

16.1.7.6 Treatment and Prognosis

Myoepitheliomas are treated with surgery—either curettage or resection. If complete removal is not possible, they can recur. It should be distinguished from myoepithelial carcinoma. Myoepithelial carcinomas have a more tendency for metastasis [39].

16.1.8 Solitary Fibrous Tumour (SFT)

The haemangiopericytoma (HPC) and solitary fibrous tumour were considered as two ends of a group of diseases. In the new WHO (2020) [97], the use of HPC terminology is not recommended, and all these tumours are included in SFT. However, other textbooks describe HPC of bone. HPC is another very rare primary bone tumour. HPC of bone occurs as metastasis from soft tissue HPC or HPC of meninges [50, 52, 53].

SFT of bone can be primary or secondary. Primary SFT of bone is very rare [54]. In 1942, Stout and Murray described this lesion in soft tissue. Occasional solitary bone lesions are reported after this.

16.1.8.1 Clinical

Primary HPC of bone is seen in young and older adults, commonly in the fourth or fifth decade. Ilium is most commonly affected.

16.1.8.2 Radiology

The findings are non-specific and usually seen as expansile lytic lesions.

16.1.8.3 Pathology

Histologically, they resemble soft tissue SFTs. Tumour cells are oval to spindly with ill-defined cytoplasmic borders. They are fairly uniform with minimal atypia, arranged around vascular spaces (Fig. 16.9a, b). Branching vascular spaces are characteristically described as staghorn vascular pattern/HPC pattern (Fig. 16.9c, d). In SFT, this pattern is seen throughout the tumour.

16.1.8.4 IHC

Immunohistochemically, CD34 may show variable positivity (Fig. 16.9e, f). STAT6 is the specific marker for SFT [51, 55].

16.1.8.5 DD

Metastatic SFT of meninges is common and cannot be distinguished from primary SFT. A positive clinical history only helps in differentiation. Other differentials include osteosarcoma, undifferentiated sarcoma, fibrosarcoma, mesenchymal chondrosarcoma, etc. All these tumours can have foci of HPC pattern. Mesenchymal chondrosarcomas contain islands of chondroid tissue.

16.1.8.6 Treatment and prognosis

They are treated by resection and have a good prognosis.

16.1.9 Myxopapillary Ependymoma

Ependymomas are tumours arising from the walls of the brain ventricles or from the spinal cord. Myxopapillary ependymomas occur exclusively in the cauda equina region [86]. There are rare case reports of ependymoma of sacrum [87, 88] and spine [89]. This may be mistaken for chordomas because they may have a myxoid matrix.

16.1.9.1 Clinical

Myxopapillary ependymoma is a subtype of ependymoma. It was reported by Kernohan in 1932. They are seen more often in adults but can

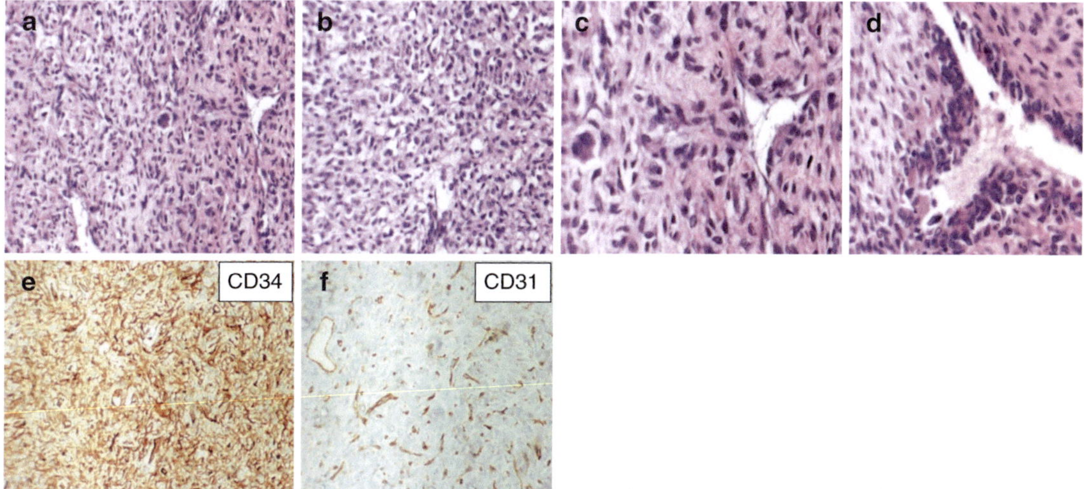

Fig. 16.9 SFT. (**a** and **b**) Short spindly cells in sheets with scattered thin-walled vessels, H&E ×100. (**c**) Staghorn vascular pattern, H&E ×250. (**d**) Cells are oval to spindly arranged around blood vessels, H&E ×400. (**e**) CD 34 is strongly positive ×100. (**f**) CD31 negative in tumour cells ×100

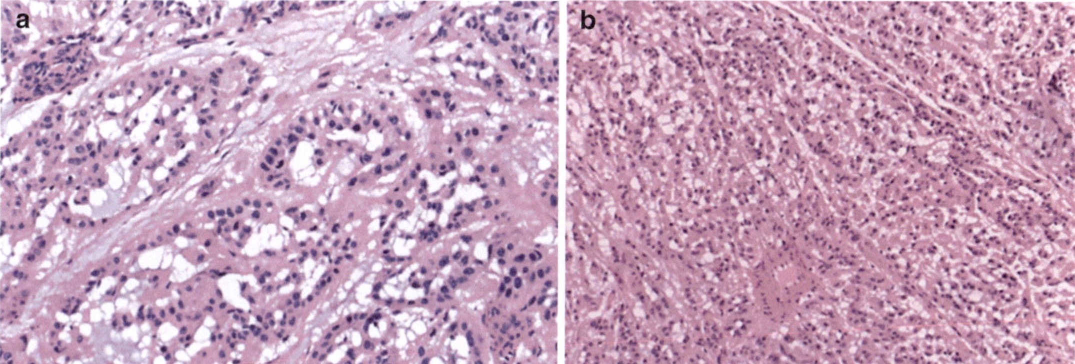

Fig. 16.10 Myxopapillary ependymoma. (**a**) Cells in groups in a myxoid stroma resembling metastatic carcinoma, H&E ×250. (**b**) Cells in cords resembling chordoma, H&E ×100

occur in children also. The presenting symptoms are pain during walking, especially in the calf, which is rapidly relieved by adopting a flexed posture of the hips. These symptoms may mimic lumbar disc disease or spinal tumours.

16.1.9.2 Radiology

The radiology findings of spinal lesions are not specific. MRI is helpful in identifying the extent of the tumour, presence of bone destruction and extension to adjacent soft tissues.

16.1.9.3 Pathology

The tumours are composed of round to oval cells with nuclei arranged around stromal cores in a myxoid background (Fig. 16.10). Histologically, they are considered as benign tumours (WHO grade 1). But they have a tendency for local recurrence.

16.1.9.4 DD

Differential diagnosis includes chordoma and metastatic mucinous carcinoma.

16.1.9.5 Treatment and Prognosis

The treatment is surgical removal. They can recur locally. The prognosis for intradural tumours is good. The extradural tumours have poor prognosis.

16.1.10 Paraganglioma

Paragangliomas arise from chemoreceptor cells. The tumours have an endocrine appearance with cell groups arranged around sinusoidal vessels (zellballen appearance). The cells have granular cytoplasm and centrally placed round nuclei (Fig. 16.11). Paragangliomas of bone are usually metastasis from soft tissue [20, 21]. But rarely, primary paragangliomas of bone can occur [22]. It is reported in sacrum and ilium.

16.1.11 PEComa

Primary PEComas of bone are extremely rare [96].

16.1.11.1 Clinical

It occurs in adults mainly in the fourth or fifth decade. In the reported cases, the bones involved are humerus [91], tibia, talus [93], vertebra, scapula and femur [92]. Craniofacial bone involvement of a paediatric case is also described [90]. Primary PEComa of bone tends to involve lower extremities. Before labelling this tumour as primary of bone, other primary sites like uterus have to be ruled out.

16.1.11.2 Radiology

Primary PEComas of bone present with osteolytic lesions. In aggressive cases, destruction of cortex and infiltration to soft tissue will be present. PET scan is done if metastasis is suspected [94].

16.1.11.3 Pathology

Histologically, the tumours are composed of both epithelioid and spindle cells. They are arranged in nests and around blood vessels (Fig. 16.12). Size more than 5 cm, infiltrative growth pattern with increased cellularity, high nuclear grade,

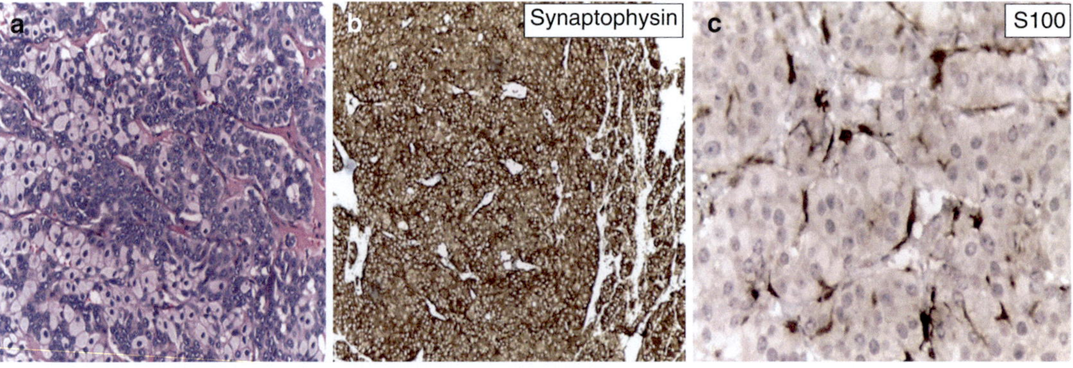

Fig. 16.11 (**a**) Paraganglioma showing zellballen pattern, H&E ×100. (**b**) Strong synaptophysin positivity ×250. (**c**) S100 highlights sustentacular cells ×250

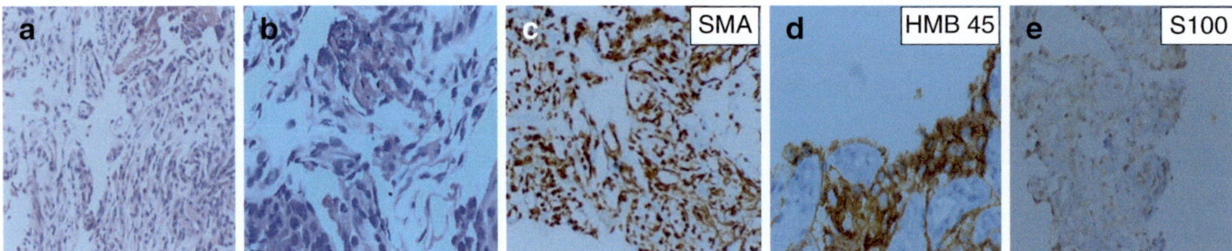

Fig. 16.12 PEComa. (**a**) Shows short spindle and oval cells, H&E ×40. (**b**) Cells with moderate cytoplasm and dense nuclei, H&E ×100. (**c**) SMA ×100. (**d**) HMB45 strongly positive ×250. (**e**) S100 is weakly positive ×40

necrosis and increased mitotic activity (>1/50 HPF) are the features to suggest malignancy.

16.1.11.4 IHC

PEComas are positive for both melanocytic (e.g. HMB45, Melan-A) and myogenic (e.g. smooth muscle actin, desmin) markers. Epithelial markers are negative. TFE3 can be positive.

16.1.11.5 DD

The major differential diagnoses include metastatic clear cell carcinoma (especially renal cell carcinoma), alveolar soft part sarcoma (ASPS), metastatic malignant melanoma and clear cell sarcoma. One case mimicking granular cell tumour is also described [95].

16.1.11.6 Treatment and prognosis

Benign PEComas are treated by resection of involved bone and is curative. In malignant cases, adjuvant chemotherapy and radiotherapy have been tried. Prognosis is variable. Malignant lesions may develop metastasis. Lung and other bones are the sites of metastasis described in reported cases.

16.2 Malignant Tumours

16.2.1 Leiomyosarcoma (LMS)

Primary LMS of bone is a rare neoplasm [56] (<0.7%). It was first described in 1965. The skeletal LMS is aggressive with a 35% overall survival (OS). When LMS occurs in bone, it is usually metastatic. Hence, before giving a diagnosis of primary LMS of bone, metastasis from elsewhere should be ruled out.

16.2.1.1 Clinical

They present with pain, swelling and rarely pathological fracture. Most cases occur in the fifth decade of life. Some cases are seen at sites of prior radiotherapy, bone infarcts, Paget disease of the bone and orthopaedic implant [60]. LMS of bone is thought to be EBV related in immunocompromised patients [64].

16.2.1.2 Radiology

They are osteolytic with wide zone of transition and cortical destruction [59]. There will be no bone matrix production (Fig. 16.13a). Radiologically, some tumours can mimic osteomyelitis [62].

16.2.1.3 Pathology

Morphologically, it shows spindle cells with smooth muscle differentiation showing cytological atypia. The cytoplasm is fibrillary with cigar-shaped nuclei (Fig. 16.13b). Lack of osteoid or chondroid matrix is the specific characteristic of primary bone LMS. Areas of necrosis or haemorrhage can be seen. Primary bone LMS is usually high grade (Fig. 16.14). Epithelioid LMS of bone can also occur [61].

16.2.1.4 IHC

Smooth muscle markers like SMA, desmin and h-caldesmon will be strongly positive. To diagnose LMS, at least two smooth muscle markers should be positive [57] (Fig. 16.13c, d). Among the positive markers of smooth muscle, h-caldes-

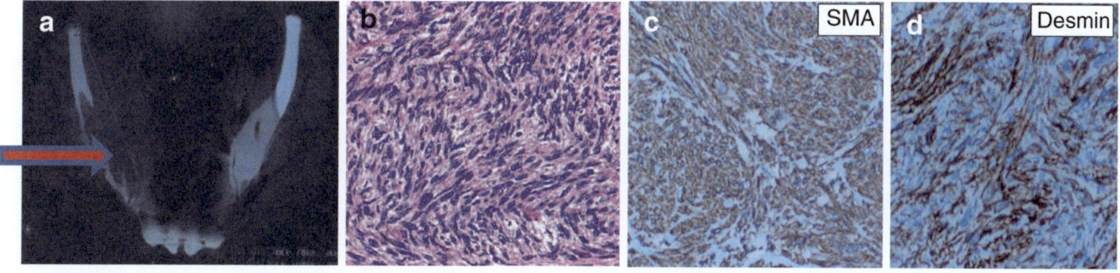

Fig. 16.13 LMS pelvis. (**a**) MRI showing destruction of iliac bone. (**b**) Interlacing bundles of malignant spindle cells, H&E ×250. (**c**) SMA ×250. (**d**) Desmin diffusely and strongly positive ×250

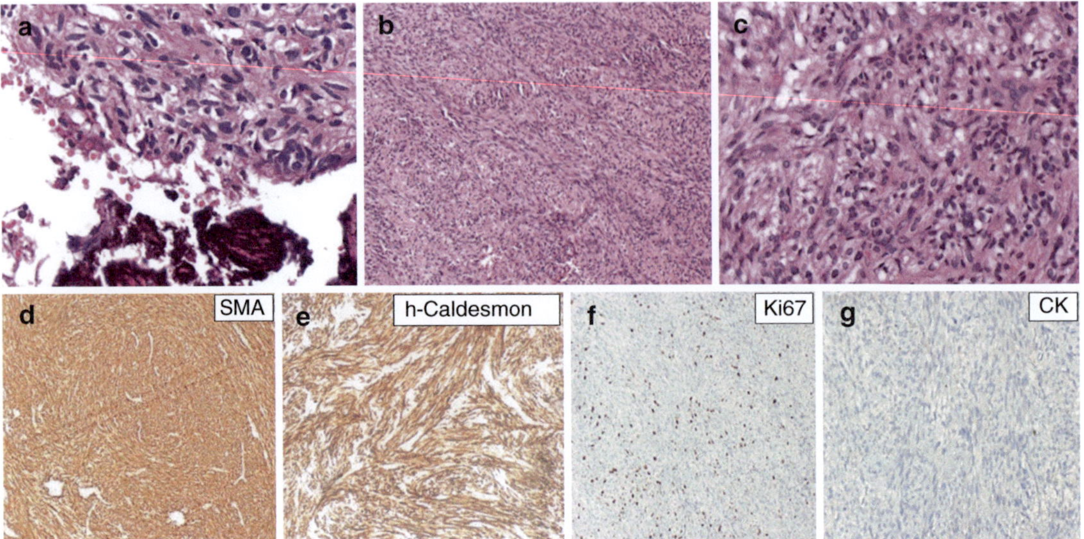

Fig. 16.14 Primary high-grade LMS of tibia. (**a**) Bone fragments and spindle cell sarcoma, H&E ×250. (**b**) Pleomorphic spindle cells in fascicles, H&E ×100. (**c**) Epithelioid cells, H&E ×250. (**d**) SMA ×100. (**e**) H-Caldesmon strongly positive ×250. To call smooth muscle tumour, at least two smooth muscle markers should be positive. (**f**) Ki67 index is high ×100. (**g**) Cytokeratin is negative ×100

mon is more specific, and it is negative in fibroblastic osteosarcoma. Desmin is positive only in 50% of tumours. If ER and PR are positive in a female patient, it suggests uterine origin. CK (30%) and S100 can be positive.

16.2.1.5 DD

The main differential diagnosis is osteosarcoma and fibrosarcoma or a dedifferentiated chondrosarcoma and undifferentiated pleomorphic sarcoma. Due to CK and S100 positivity in primary osseous LMS, diagnostic difficulty can occur especially when desmin is negative [64].

16.2.1.6 Prognosis

Clinical outcome depends on histological grade [58]. High-grade tumours have poor prognosis [63, 65].

16.2.2 Malignant Peripheral Nerve Sheath Tumour (MPNST)

Primary bone malignant peripheral nerve sheath tumour (MPNST) or malignant schwannoma is extremely rare [4]. Majority of these tumours occur in cases with neurofibromatosis-1 (NF-1). Mandible is the most commonly affected bone [1, 8]. Rarely, other bones like maxilla, spine, sternum and long bones of extremities can be the sites. Small bones of hand and foot are rarely affected. As the bone does not contain many sensory nerve fibres, the occurrence of MPNST is very rare in bone. Infiltration from soft tissue MPNST to bone is more common than those arising primarily in bone.

16.2.2.1 Pathology

It is a spindle cell sarcoma with haemangiopericytoma-like vascular pattern and alternating hyper- and hypocellular areas. The cells are pleomorphic spindly with pale cytoplasm and wavy hyperchromatic nuclei. Mitosis can be prominent. Heterologous elements like skeletal muscle, bone, cartilage and angiosarcomatous areas may be present rarely.

16.2.2.2 IHC

S100 shows variable positivity. Some tumours are negative for S100 (Fig. 16.15). Other IHC markers positive in MPNST are SOX10 and GFAP. Complete loss of H3K27me3 is seen in high-grade MPNST.

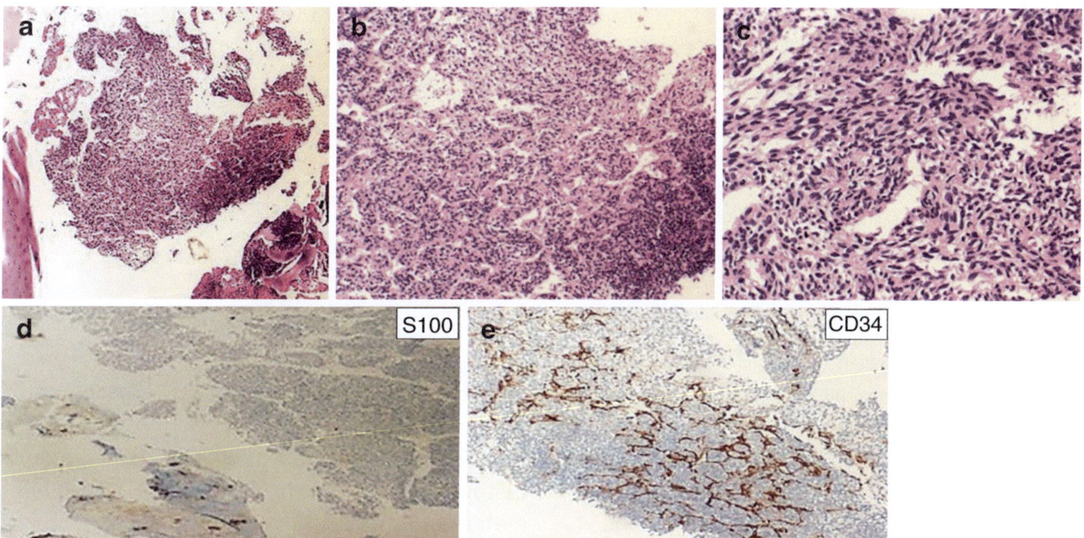

Fig. 16.15 Vertebral metastasis from a known case of MPNST. (**a**) Bone and tumour with spindle cells, H&E ×40. (**b** and **c**) Sheets of malignant spindle cells, H&E ×250. (**d**) S100 was negative ×100. (**e**) CD34 highlights vessels ×100

16.2.2.3 DD

Differential diagnoses include osteosarcoma, clear cell sarcoma and other spindle cell sarcomas such as synovial sarcoma, fibrosarcoma, leiomyosarcoma and undifferentiated sarcoma. The diagnosis of MPNST of bone is considered when it is arising from a nerve in juxtacortical bone, or in a patient with neurofibromatosis.

16.2.2.4 Treatment

The primary treatment is radical wide excision of the tumour. Adjuvant treatment is necessary for high-grade tumours.

16.2.3 Alveolar Soft Part Sarcoma (ASPS)

Alveolar soft part sarcoma (ASPS) is a neoplasm composed of cells with granular cytoplasm arranged in an alveolar pattern [66].

16.2.3.1 Clinical

ASPS is an extremely rare soft tissue sarcoma and accounts for 1% of soft tissue tumours. It usually involves thigh and buttocks of young adults. Its occurrence in bone is either as primary or as metastasis from soft tissue [10]. 10% occur as primary bone tumour. The sites involved are scapula [73], sacrum [74] and vertebra [75]. Patients present with pain and mass or with metastatic disease at presentation [71]. Some cases of soft tissue ASPS are present with synchronous metastasis in bone [68].

16.2.3.2 Radiology

On plain radiographs, soft tissue shadow, with calcification and destruction of bone can be seen [70].

16.2.3.3 Pathology

The cells are epithelioid with abundant granular cytoplasm and vesicular nuclei with prominent nucleolus, in an alveolar pattern [67, 72] (Fig. 16.16). Clear cell change of the cytoplasm can mimic renal cell carcinoma. The cytoplasm contains PAS-positive, diastase-resistant rod-shaped crystalline structures (Fig. 16.16c). Alcian blue and trichrome histochemical stains can also be positive in these crystalline structures. Mitotic activity is sparse. Presence of necrosis is rare.

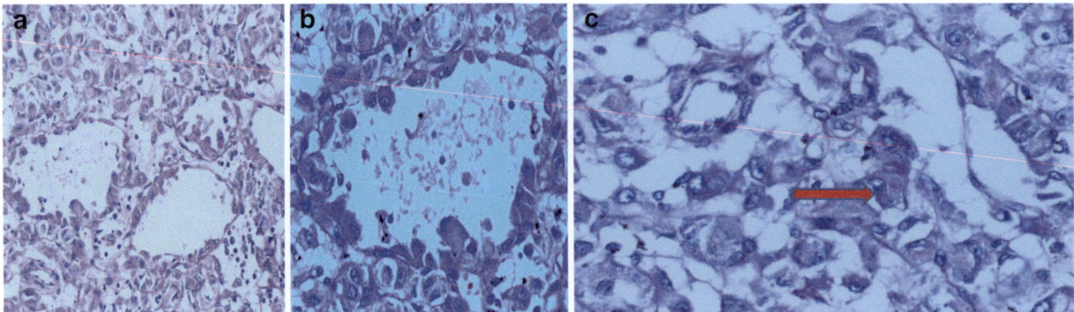

Fig. 16.16 ASPS. (**a**) Cells in alveolar pattern, H&E ×250. (**b**) Cells with abundant eosinophilic cytoplasm and vesicular nuclei with prominent nucleolus, H&E ×400. (**c**) PAS-positive crystalline structures (red arrow), PAS ×400

16.2.3.4 IHC

TFE3 is a highly sensitive and specific marker of the ASPS.

16.2.3.5 Molecular

TFE3 gene rearrangement or ASPSCR1-TFE3 fusion protein demonstration is helpful for the diagnosis of ASPS [69].

16.2.3.6 DD

ASPS can be confused with alveolar rhabdomyosarcoma, paraganglioma, metastatic renal cell carcinoma, metastatic hepatocellular carcinomas and endocrine neoplasias.

16.2.3.7 Treatment and Prognosis

The treatment is excision with adequate surgical margins. Although adjuvant chemotherapy and radiotherapy are used, their effectiveness is debatable. Metastases from ASPS generally go to lung, brain and surrounding bones. A better prognosis is seen in young patients with small size of the tumour.

16.2.4 Clear Cell Sarcoma

Clear cell sarcoma (CCS) or melanoma of soft parts of bone is a rare tumour. It can also occur rarely in gastrointestinal tract or head and neck. This soft tissue sarcoma is thought to arise from neural crest cells. By immunohistochemistry, both CCS and malignant melanoma share same markers. But CCS lacks melanoma-associated BRAF mutations. A specific translocation t (12; 22) (q13; q12) is observed in CCS82. It occurs due to fusion of EWS (22q12) and ATF1 (12q13) genes. Hence, CCS is considered as a distinct neoplasm.

16.2.4.1 Clinical

Primary CCS of the bone is extremely rare. The sites of bone reported are jaw [78], scapula [85], vertebra [76], pubic bone[83], metatarsals [80], ribs [77], radius, sacrum [84] and humerus [81]. It can also occur in tendons [79]. Pain and tenderness are the main symptoms. There is a slight female predominance.

16.2.4.2 Pathology

Grossly, these tumours are well defined or encapsulated. The cells are polygonal or spindly, arranged in nests or fascicles. Cells have abundant cytoplasm (Fig. 16.17). Some tumours exhibit marked pleomorphism, solid pattern and myxoid stroma (Fig. 16.18a).

16.2.4.3 IHC

Clear cell sarcomas are strongly positive for S100 protein, HMB-45 and Melan-A (Fig. 16.18b, c), similar to melanomas.

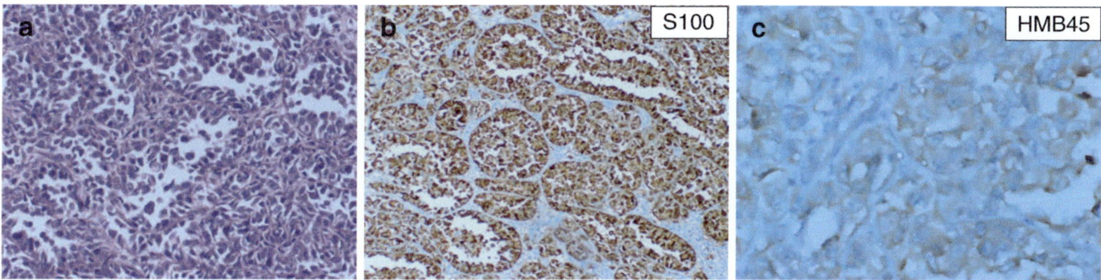

Fig. 16.17 (**a**) Clear cell sarcoma in a nested pattern, H&E ×100. (**b**) S100 strongly positive ×250. (**c**) HMB45 weakly positive ×250

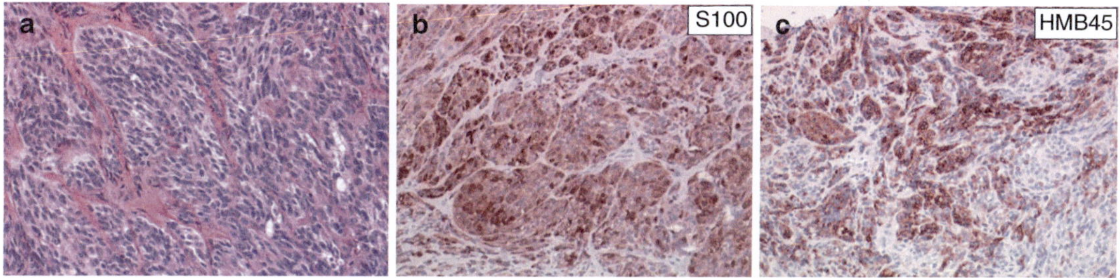

Fig. 16.18 (**a**) Clear cell sarcoma with spindle cell pattern, H&E ×250. (**b**) S100 ×250. (**c**) HMB45 ×250

16.2.4.4 DD

Before labelling a tumour as clear cell sarcoma arising in bone, one should rule out a primary clear cell sarcoma/melanoma elsewhere.

16.2.4.5 Molecular

t (12; 22) (q13; q12) translocation is a specific translocation present in clear cell sarcoma in 50–75% of cases.

16.2.4.6 Prognosis

This tumour is very rare, and hence its metastatic potential is unknown.

16.2.5 Malignant Mixed Tumour

Malignant mixed tumour occurring in bone is usually metastasis from other sites [81–83]. Primary malignant mixed tumours are extremely rare. The features of malignancy are cellular atypia, increased mitosis, cartilage consistent with grade 1 chondrosarcoma and presence of necrosis, and infiltration between pre-existing bony trabeculae.

16.2.6 Malignant Myoepithelial Tumour (Myoepithelial Carcinoma)

Primary intraosseous myoepithelial carcinomas are rare tumours [39]. It can mimic conventional osteosarcoma, myoepithelial carcinoma of salivary gland and epithelial/cartilaginous differentiation in clear cell chondrosarcoma.

Radiology: They present with a lytic lesion with cortical destruction.

Pathology: Malignant myoepithelial tumour (MET) or myoepithelial carcinoma cells have moderate nuclear atypia. The tumour cells infiltrate into soft tissue (Fig. 16.19). Mitotic activity and necrosis may not be evident. Myoepithelial markers like P63, CK 5/6 and SMA will be positive. Most malignant tumours are INI1 negative [47].

Primary sclerosing epithelioid fibrosarcoma is given in Chap. 6.

Primary DSRCT of bone is described in Chap. 8.

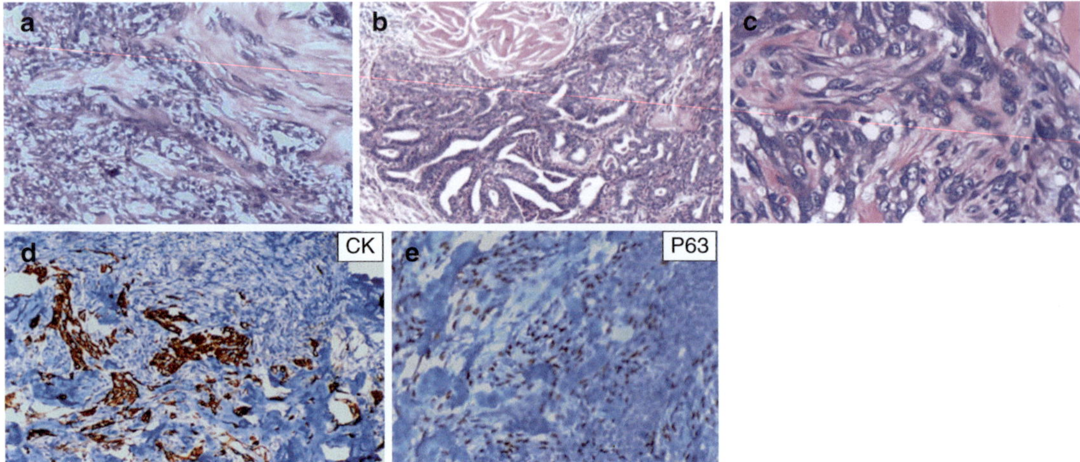

Fig. 16.19 (**a**) Myoepithelial carcinoma. Epithelioid and spindle cells infiltrating soft tissue, H&E ×100. (**b**) Cells infiltrating muscle ×100. (**c**) H&E ×400. (**d**) CK ×100. (**e**) P63 ×100. Myoepithelial markers are positive

Points to Remember

- Common soft tissue tumours like schwannoma and lipoma can rarely present as primary osseous tumours.
- Malignant tumours like leiomyosarcoma, synovial sarcoma and clear cell sarcoma can occur in bone as primary tumours.
- When these tumours are encountered, remember to rule out primary elsewhere in the soft tissue, before labelling them as primary of bone.

References

Schwannoma and MPNST

1. Bullock MJ, Bedard YC, Bell RS, et al. Intraosseous malignant peripheral nerve sheath tumor: report of a case and review of the literature. Arch Pathol Lab Med. 1995;119:367–70.
2. Ida CM, Scheithauer BW, Yapicier O, et al. Primary schwannoma of the bone: a clinicopathologic and radiologic study of 17 cases. Am J Surg Pathol. 2011;35(7):989–97.
3. Ida CM, Scheithauer BW, Yapicier Ö, Carney JA, Wenger DE, Inwards CY, Bertoni F, Spinner RJ, Unni KK. Primary schwannoma of the bone: a clinicopathologic and radiologic study of 17 cases. Am J Surg Pathol. 2011;35:989–97.
4. Devnani B, Biswas A, Bakhshi S, Khan SA, Mridha AR, Agarwal S. Primary intraosseous malignant peripheral nerve sheath tumor of metacarpal bones of the hand in a patient without neurofibromatosis 1: report of a rare case. Indian J Med Paediatr Oncol. 2017;38(2):232–5.
5. Wang G, Wen X, Qu L, Qi X, Yang C. Intraosseous schwannoma involving multiple bones of the foot: a case report. J Foot Ankle Surg. 2016;55(1):201–6.
6. Jangam SS, Ingole SN, Deshpande MD, Ranadive PA. Solitary intraosseous neurofibroma: report of a unique case. Contemp Clin Dent. 2014;5:561–3.
7. Li KH, Yang Q, Gao BB, et al. Giant intraosseous schwannoma of the calcaneus. Int J Clin Exp Med. 2016:6897–901.
8. Sestan B, Miletic D, Jonjic N, Gulan G. Intraosseous epithelioid malignant schwannoma. Orthopedics. 2007;30:67–9.

Lipoma and Liposarcoma

9. Campbell RS, Grainger AJ, Mangham DC, Beggs I, Teh J, Davies AM. Intraosseous lipoma: report of 35 new cases and a review of the literature. Skelet Radiol. 2003;32(4):209–22.
10. Tiemeier GL, Brown JM, Pratap SE, McCarthy C, Kastrenopoulou A, Bradley K, Wilson S, Orosz Z, Gibbons CLMH, Oppermann U, Athanasou NA. Pleomorphic liposarcoma of bone: a rare primary malignant bone tumour. Clin Sarcoma Res. 2018;8:2.
11. Kang HS, Kim T, Oh S, Park S, Chung SH. Intraosseous lipoma:18 years of experience at a single institution. Clin Orthop Surg. 2018;10:234–9.

12. Kim JW, Kim SJ, Kim GE, Ki SY, Lee SJ, Park JG. Radiologic findings of intraosseous lipoma of long bones. J Korean Soc Radiol. 2016;75(4):313–21.

Hibernoma

13. Enerback S. Brown adipose tissues in humans. Int J Obes. 2010;34(Suppl 1):S43–6.
14. Vlychou M, Teh J, Whitwell D, Athanasou NA. Intraosseous hibernoma: a rare adipocytic bone tumour. Skelet Radiol. 2016;45:1565–9.

Melanotic Neuroectodermal Tumour of Infancy (MNTI)

15. Bhardwaj N, Yadav R, Sampath Kumar V, Khan SA. Melanotic neuroectodermal tumour of infancy presenting as a lytic lesion in femur: a rare tumour at a rare site with an unusual behaviour. BMJ Case Rep. 2019;12(10):e231959.
16. Elli M, Aydin O, Pinarli FG, Dagdemir A, Dabak N, Selcuk MB, Acar S. Melanotic neuroectodermal tumor of infancy of the femur. Pediatr Hematol Oncol. 2006;23(7):579–86.
17. Hoshina Y, Hamamoto Y, Suzuki I, et al. Melanotic neuroectodermal tumor of infancy in the mandible. Report of a case. Oral Surg Oral Med Oral Pathol Oral Radiol Endod. 2000;89:594–9.
18. Nelson ZL, Newman L, Loukota RA, Williams DM. Melanotic neuroectodermal tumor of infancy - an immunohistochemical and ultrastructural study. Br J Oral Maxillofac Surg. 1995;33:375–80.
19. Rege JD, Shet T, Sawant HV, Naik LP. Cytologic diagnosis of a melanotic neuroectodermal tumor of infancy occurring in the cranial bones. Diagn Cytopathol. 1999;21(4):280–3.

Paraganglioma

20. Ayala-Ramirez M, Palmer JL, Hofmann MC, de la Cruz M, Moon BS, Waguespack SG, Habra MA, Jimenez C. Bone metastases and skeletal-related events in patients with malignant pheochromocytoma and sympathetic paraganglioma. J Clin Endocrinol Metab. 2013;98(4):1492–7.
21. Duet M, Herman P, Wassef M, Huy PTB, Laredo J-D. Bone metastases from head and neck paragangliomas: uncommon MR findings in an uncommon condition—report of three cases. J Magn Reson Imaging. 2006;24:428–33.
22. Srilatha PS, Rao L. Locally aggressive primary intraosseous paraganglioma of sacrum. J Clin Diagn Res. 2017;11(9):ED09–11.

Phosphaturic Mesenchymal Tumour (PMT)

23. Agaimy A, Michal M, Chiosea S, Petersson F, Hadravsky L, Kristiansen G, Horch RE, Schmolders J, Hartmann A, Haller F, Michal M. Phosphaturic mesenchymal tumors: clinicopathologic, immunohistochemical and molecular analysis of 22 cases expanding their morphologic and immunophenotypic spectrum. Am J Surg Pathol. 2017;41(10):1371–80.
24. Folpe AL. Phosphaturic mesenchymal tumors: a review and update seminars in diagnostic. Pathology. 2019;3:260–8.
25. Arai R, Onodera T, Terkawi MA, Mitsuhashi T, Kondo E, Iwasaki N. A rare case of multiple phosphaturic mesenchymal tumors along a tendon sheath inducing osteomalacia. BMC Musculoskelet Disord. 2017;18:79.
26. Creytens D, Van Dorpe J. DOG1 expression in phosphaturic mesenchymal tumour. J Clin Pathol. 2016;69:1037–8. https://doi.org/10.1136/jclinpath-2016-203893.
27. Feng J, Jiang Y, Wang O, et al. The diagnostic dilemma of tumor induced osteomalacia: a retrospective analysis of 144 cases. Endocr J. 2017;64:675–83.
28. Houang M, Clarkson A, Sioson L, et al. Phosphaturic mesenchymal tumors show positive staining for somatostatin receptor 2A (SSTR2A). Hum Pathol. 2013;44:2711–8.
29. Schmolders J, Hartmann A, Haller F, Michal M. Phosphaturic mesenchymal tumors clinicopathologic, immunohistochemical and molecular analysis of 22 cases expanding their morphologic and immunophenotypic spectrum. Am J Surg Pathol. 2017;41:1371–80.
30. Lee JC, Su SY, Changou CA, et al. Characterization of FN1-FGFR1 and novel FN1-FGF1 fusion genes in a large series of phosphaturic mesenchymal tumors. Mod Pathol. 2016;29:1335–46.
31. Tajima S, Fukayama M. Possibility of D2-40 as a diagnostic and tumor differentiation- suggestive marker for some of phosphaturic mesenchymal tumors. Int J Clin Exp Pathol. 2015;8:9390–6.
32. Tajima S, Takashi Y, Ito N, et al. ERG and FLI1 are useful immunohistochemical markers in phosphaturic mesenchymal tumors. Med Mol Morphol. 2016;49:203–9.
33. Wu H, Bui MM, Zhou L, Li D, Zhang H, Zhong D. Phosphaturic mesenchymal tumor with an admixture of epithelial and mesenchymal elements in the jaws: clinicopathological and immunohistochemical analysis of 22 cases with literature review. Mod Pathol. 2019;32:189–204.
34. Zuo Q, Wang H, Li W, et al. Treatment and outcomes of tumor-induced osteomalacia associated with phosphaturic mesenchymal tumors: retrospective review of 12 patients. BMC Musculoskelet Disord. 2017;18:403.

Mixed Tumour

35. Barreto CA, Lipton MN, Smith HB, Potter GK. Intraosseous chondroid syringoma of the hallux. J Am Acad Dermatol. 1994;30:374–8.
36. Jacobson ES, Jacobson HG, Batsakis JG. Malignant mixed tumor of parotid gland with a solitary metastasis to the radius. J Oral Surg. 1973;31:539–42.
37. Parikh HK, Parikh DM. Malignant mixed tumor of the salivary gland with bone metastasis: a case report and literature review. Indian J Cancer. 1991;28:171–5.
38. Zhansan S, Li Z, Liu B. Primary malignant mixed tumor of bone: a case report. Int J Clin Exp Pathol. 2015;8(7):8433–7.

Myoepithelioma and Myoepithelial Carcinoma

39. Alberghini M, Pasquinelli G, Zanella L, Pignatti G, Benini S, Bacchini P, et al. Primary malignant myoepithelioma of the distal femur. APMIS. 2007;115:376–80.
40. Antonescu CR, Zhang L, Chang NE, Pawel BR, Travis W, Katabi N, et al. EWSR1-POU5F1 fusion in soft tissue myoepithelial tumors. A molecular analysis of sixty-six cases, including soft tissue, bone, and visceral lesions, showing common involvement of the EWSR1 gene. Genes Chromosomes Cancer. 2010;49:1114–24.
41. Biradar P, Menon S, Patil A, Karimundakal G, Jambhekar N. Primary myoepithelial carcinoma of rib bone: morphology, immunohistochemical evaluation and diagnostic dilemma in an unusual case. J Can Res Ther. 2015;11:647.
42. Ferretti C, Coleman H, Altini M, Meer S. Intraosseous myoepithelial neoplasms of the maxilla: diagnostic and therapeutic considerations in 5 South African patients. J Oral Maxillofac Surg. 2003;61:379–86.
43. Kurzawa P, Kattapuram S, Hornicek FJ, Antonescu CR, Rosenberg AE, Nielsen GP. Primary myoepithelioma of bone: a report of 8 cases. Am J Surg Pathol. 2013;37:960–8.
44. Park JS, Ryu KN, Han CS, Park YK. Malignant myoepithelioma of the humerus with a satellite lesion: a case report and literature review. Br J Radiol. 2010;83:e161–4.
45. Ghermandi R, Pala E, Gambarotti M, Colangeli S, Boriani S. Myoepithelioma of the spine: first case in the literature. Eur Rev Med Pharmacol Sci. 2014;18(Suppl 1):66–71.
46. Rekhi B, Desai SS, Gulia A, Puri A, Jambhekar NA. Intraosseous myoepithelioma: a rare, distinct tumor entity. Indian J Pathol Microbiol. 2014;57:269–71.
47. Rekhi B, Sable M, Jambhekar NA. Histopathological, immunohistochemical and molecular spectrum of myoepithelial tumours of soft tissues. Virchows Arch. 2012;461:687–97.
48. Rekhi B, Amare P, Gulia A, Baisane C, Patil A, Agarwal S, et al. Primary intraosseous myoepithelioma arising in the iliac bone and displaying trisomies of 11, 15, 17 with del (16q) and del (22q11) – A rare case report with review of literature. Pathol Res Pract. 2011;207:780–5.
49. Xuemei D, Wang D, Li B, Chang H, Shen D. Clinicopathological features of primary myoepithelial carcinoma inside oblique eminence of cuboid bone: a case report. Int J Clin Exp Med. 2018;11(6):6327–31.

Solitary Fibrous Tumour/HPC

50. Ambrosini-Spaltro A, Eusebi V, Stacchiotti S. Meningeal hemangiopericytomas and solitary fibrous tumour presenting with a single bone metastasis: report of six cases and literature review. Clin Sarcoma Res. 2016;6:16–22.
51. Doyle LA, Vivero M, Fletcher CD, et al. Nuclear expression of STAT6 distinguishes solitary fibrous tumor from histologic mimics. Mod Pathol. 2014;27:390–5.
52. Han N, Kim H, Min SK, et al. Meningeal solitary fibrous tumors with delayed extracranial metastasis. J Pathol Transl Med. 2016;50(2):113–21.
53. Hoshi M, Araki N, Naka N, et al. Bone metastasis of intracranial meningeal hemangiopericytoma. Int J Clin Oncol. 2005;10:208–13.
54. Suarez-Zamora DA, Rodriguez-Urrego PA, Soto-Montoya C, Rivero-Rapalino O, Palau-Lazaro MA. Malignant solitary fibrous tumor of the humerus: a case report of an extremely rare primary bone tumor. Int J Surg Pathol. 2018;26(8):772–6.
55. Yoshida A, Tsuta K, Ohno M, et al. STAT6 immunohistochemistry is helpful in the diagnosis of solitary fibrous tumors. Am J Surg Pathol. 2014;38:552–9.

Leiomyosarcoma

56. Antonescu CR, Erlandson RA, Huvos AG. Primary leiomyosarcoma of bone: a clinicopathologic, immunohistochemical, and ultrastructural study of 33 patients and a literature review. Am J Surg Pathol. 1997;21:1281–94.
57. Rekhi B, Kaur A, Puri A, Desai S, Jambhekar NA. Primary leiomyosarcoma of bone—a clinicopathologic study of 8 uncommon cases with immunohistochemical analysis and clinical outcomes. Ann of Diagn Pathol. 2011;15(3):147–56.
58. Brewer P, Sumathi V, Grimer RJ, et al. Primary leiomyosarcoma of bone: analysis of prognosis. Sarcoma. 2012;2012:636849.

59. Cui J, Chen H, Hao D, Liu J, Hou F, Xu W. Imaging features of primary leiomyosarcoma of bone. Int J Clin Exp Med. 2017;10(7):10846–51.
60. Zumárraga JP, Arouca MM, Baptista AM, Caiero MT, Rubio DE, Pires O, de Camargo. Primary leiomyosarcoma of bone: clinicopathologic and prognostic factors analysis in a single institution. Acta Ortop Bras. 2019;27(3):152–5.
61. Lopez-Barea F, Rodriguez-Peralto JL, Sanchez-Herrera S, Gonzalez-Lopez J, Burgos-Lizaldez E. Primary epithelioid leiomyosarcoma of bone. Case report and literature review. Virchows Arch. 1999;434:367–71.
62. Lopez-Barea F, Rodriguez-Peralto JL, Sanchez-Herrera S, Gonzalez-Lop Chow LT. Metatarsal leiomyosarcoma masquerading as acute osteomyelitis—a diagnostic trap unveiled by vigilant clinical, radiologic and pathologic analysis. Foot (Edinb). 2016;27:10–5.
63. Adelani MA, Schultenover SJ, Holt GE, Cates JMM. Primary leiomyosarcoma of extragnathic bone: clinicopathologic features and reevaluation of prognosis. Arch Pathol Lab Med. 2009;133(9):1448–56.
64. Wang GY, Lucas DR. Primary leiomyosarcoma of bone: review and update. Arch Pathol Lab Med. 2019;143:1332–7.
65. Rajendra R, Pollack S, Rodler ET, Conrad EU, Davidson DJ, Chai X, Jones RL. Outcome of leiomyosarcoma of bone: a single center experience. J Clin Oncol. 2013;31(15_suppl):–e21502.

Alveolar Soft Part Sarcoma

66. Folpe AL, Deyrup AT. Alveolar soft-part sarcoma: a review and update. J Clin Pathol. 2006;59:1127–32.
67. Pena-Burgos EM, Pozo-Kreilinger JJ, Tapia-Viñe M, Redondo A, Mendiola-Sabio M, Ortiz-Cruz EJ. Primary intraosseous alveolar soft part sarcoma: report of two cases with radiologic-pathologic correlation. Ann Diagn Pathol. 2023;62:152078. https://doi.org/10.1016/j.anndiagpath.2022.152078. ISSN 1092-9134
68. Gavriilidis P, Themeli I, Nikolaidou A. Alveolar soft-part sarcoma with synchronous bone metastasis: rare manifestation of one of the least common soft-tissue sarcomas. Hippokratia. 2013;17(2):192.
69. Ladanyi M, Lui MY, Antonescu CR, Krause-Boehm A, Meindl A, Argani P, et al. The der(17)t(X;17)(p11;q25) of human alveolar soft part sarcoma fuses the TFE3 transcription factor gene to ASPL, a novel gene at 17q25. Oncogene. 2001;20:48–57.
70. Lorigan JG, O'Keeffe FN, Evans HL, Wallace S. The radiologic manifestations of alveolar soft-part sarcoma. AAJR Am J Roentgenol. 1989;153:335–9.
71. Ohshika S, Kawai A. A case of an alveolar soft part sarcoma with secondary scapular involvement. Jpn J Clin Oncol. 2012;42:463.
72. Park YK, Unni KK, Kim YW, Han CS, Yang MH, Wenger DE, et al. Primary alveolar soft part sarcoma of bone. Histopathology. 1999;35:411–7.
73. Yavuz A, Göya C, Bora A, Beyazal M. Primary alveolar soft part sarcoma of the scapula. Case Rep Oncol. 2013;6:356–61.
74. Zadnik PL, Yurter A, DeLeon R, Molina CA, Groves ML, McCarthy E, Sciubba DM. Alveolar soft-part sarcoma in the sacrum: a case report and review of the literature. Skelet Radiol. 2014;43:115–20.
75. Zhu FP, Lu GM, Zhang LJ, Wang JD, An XJ, Dong YC. Primary alveolar soft part sarcoma of vertebra: a case report and literature review. Skelet Radiol. 2009;38:825–9.

Clear Cell Sarcoma

76. Ramoh CN, Zou Y, Hamzah F, Yu L, Zhu Y. Clear cell sarcoma of lumbar vertebra: A case report on how imaging improved diagnostics after initial suspicions. Am J Diagn Imaging. 2020;6(1):7–14.
77. Hersekli MA, Ozkoc G, Bircan S, Akpinar S, Ozalay M, Tuncer I, Tandogan RN. Primary clear cell sarcoma of rib. Skelet Radiol. 2005;34:167–70.
78. Inoue S, Chepeha DB, Lucas DR, Faisal S, Stewart RC, Mushtaq R, et al. Clear cell sarcoma of the jaw: a case report and review of the literature. J Pediatr Hematol Oncol. 2013;35:402–5.
79. Kawai A. Clear cell sarcoma of tendons and aponeuroses: a study of 75 patients. Cancer. 2007;109(1):109–16.
80. Licata L, Fenga D, Speciale G, Rosa MA. Clear cell sarcoma of metatarsus. Folia Med. 2014;56(4):271–4.
81. Liu X, Zhang H, Dong Y. Primary clear cell sarcoma of humerus: case report. World J Surg Oncol. 2011;9:163.
82. Sandberg AA, Bridge JA. Updates on the cytogenetics and molecular genetics of bone and soft tissue tumors: clear cell sarcoma (malignant melanoma of soft parts). Cancer Genet Cytogenet. 2001;130:1–7.
83. Nakayama S, Yokote T, Iwaki K, Akioka T, Miyoshi T, Hirata Y, Takayama A, Nishiwaki U, Masuda Y, Tsuji M, Hanafusa T. A rare case of primary clear cell sarcoma of the pubic bone resembling small round cell tumor: an unusual morphological variant. BMC Cancer. 2012;12:538–42.
84. Zhang W, Shen Y, Wan R, Zhu Y. Primary clear cell sarcoma of the sacrum: a case report. Skelet Radiol. 2011;40:633–9.
85. Zhang X, Hu C, Cai L. A giant clear cell sarcoma on right scapular: a case report. Acta Orthop Traumatol Turcica. 2016;50:473–6.

Myxopapillary Ependymoma

86. Biagini R, Demitri S, Orsini U, Bibiloni J, Briccoli A, Bertoni F. Osteolytic extra-axial sacral myxopapillary ependymoma. Skelet Radiol. 1999;28:584–9.

87. Gupta R, Rishi A, Suri V, Sharma MC, Gupta A, Garg A. Sacral myxopapillary ependymoma with extensive osteolysis. J Neuro-Oncol. 2007;86(3):349–52.
88. Shors SM, Jones TA, Jhaveri MD, Huckman MS. Best cases from the AFIP: myxopapillary ependymoma of the sacrum. Radiographics. 2006;26(Suppl 1):S111–6.
89. Strojnik T, Bujas T, Velnar T. Invasive myxopapillary ependymoma of the lumbar spine: a case report. World J Clin Cases. 2019;7(10):1142–8.

PEComa of Bone

90. Diab J, O'Neill T, Moore L, Santoreneos S, Flapper W. An index case of primary osseous PEComa in a paediatric craniofacial skeleton. Eur J Plast Surg. 2019;42:629–32.
91. Zhong J, Yangfan H, Si L, Xing Y, Geng J, Jiao Q, Zhang H, Yao W. Primary perivascular epithelioid cell tumor (PEComa) in bone: a review of the literature and a case arising in the humerus with multiple metastases. J Bone Oncol. 2021;26:100336.
92. Lao IW, Yu L, Wang J. Malignant perivascular epithelioid cell tumor (PEComa) of the femur: a case report and literature review. Diagn Pathol. 2015;10:54.
93. Gebhart M, Coltofeanu A. PEComa of the talus: a unique case of a soft tissue tumor within bone. Acta Chir Belg. 2019;119(2):118–22.
94. Rakheja R, Abikhzer G, Alabed YZ, Nahal A, Lisbona R. The appearance of osseous PEComa on F-18 FDG PET/CT. Clin Nucl Med. 2012;37(2):190–2.
95. Sadigh S, Shah P, Weber K, Sebro R, Zhang PJ. Primary malignant perivascular epithelioid cell neoplasm (PEComa) of the bone mimicking granular cell tumor in core biopsy: a case report and literature review. Oncol Lett. 2018;15(3):2946–52.
96. Yamashita K, Fletcher CD. PEComa presenting in bone: clinic-pathologic analysis of six cases and literature review. AJSP. 2010;34:1622–9.
97. WHO Classification of Tumours. Soft tissue and bone tumours, vol. 3. Edited by the WHO Classification of Tumours Editorial Board. 5th ed. IARC; 2020.

17 Tumour-Like Lesions of Bone

There are many lesions affecting bones, which are mistaken for tumours, both clinically and radiologically [1]. The lesions which were considered tumours of undetermined neoplastic nature in 2013 WHO like aneurysmal bone cyst, chondromesenchymal hamartoma of chest wall, simple bone cyst, fibrous dysplasia and osteofibrous dysplasia, LCH, Erdheim-Chester disease and Rosai-Dorfman disease are now considered as neoplasms of bone in the fifth edition of the WHO [106]. Tumour-like lesions such as exuberant callus, myositis ossificans, giant cell reparative granuloma, periosteal desmoid, xanthoma of bone, epidermoid cyst and cyst of degenerative joint disease are already dealt with in other chapters. This chapter mainly includes Paget disease, osteomyelitis, hamartomas, hyperparathyroidism and certain other rare lesions which mimic tumours.

17.1 Paget Disease of Bones

Paget disease of bone (PDB) is the second most common bone remodelling disease after osteoporosis [2]. It was described by Sir James Paget. The disease is more prevalent in the United Kingdom and Western Europe. The disease is uncommon in India, African blacks, China, Japan, Southeast Asia and Scandinavia. The family history is positive in 15–30% of cases [9]. There is sevenfold risk in first-degree relatives of patients with PDB.

17.1.1 Pathogenesis

Increased osteoclastic bone resorption, increased and disorganized bone formation and increased vascularity of bone cause skeletal manifestations in PDB. The osteoclasts contain more nuclei than normal. They are increased in size and number. The bone is a mosaic of woven and lamellar bone. Inclusion bodies are present in the nuclei in these cases. Hence, a viral aetiology has also been suggested. Paget disease is thought to be due to infection by paramyxovirus like mumps, measles and rubella. Infection may be present for many years before the occurrence of symptoms [5, 7, 11]. Other viral infections suggested to cause PDB include respiratory syncytial virus and canine distemper virus. But some studies have shown that PDB does not have any abnormalities of immune response to antibodies of measles or other paramyxoviruses. Increased dietary calcium intake, vitamin D deficiency and excessive biomechanical loading of affected bones are thought to be factors causing PDB.

PDB is a disease of the osteoclasts. Increased sensitivity to factors like 1,25-dihydroxy vitamin D and receptor activator of NF-kB ligand (RANKL) promotes bone resorption. Genetic factors are considered in the pathogenesis of this disease. SQSTM1 mutation is seen associated with severely affected cases.

J. Kattoor et al., *Bone Tumors*, https://doi.org/10.1007/978-981-99-4738-6_17

17.1.2 Clinical

The disease occurs in middle to old-aged individuals. It is unusual before 40 years of age. It affects either a single bone (monostotic) or multiple bones (polyostotic). The pelvis, femur, spine, skull and tibia are commonly affected. The clavicles, ribs, scapulae and bones of upper limb are less affected. PDB rarely involves the small bones. Most of the patients are asymptomatic. Bone pain, if present, is worse at night. Bowing of long bones, enlargement of the skull and frontal bossing are features of this disease. The bowing of long bones occurs anteriorly and laterally. Presence of fissure fractures causes sudden increase in pain.

17.1.3 Laboratory findings

There will be increase in serum total and bone-specific alkaline phosphatase (BSAP) levels. Vitamin D deficiency and hypercalcaemia can be seen in patients with PDB. Hyperparathyroidism has to be ruled out in these cases. Raised urinary hydroxyproline and proline levels, due to increased osteoclastic activity, can be present [6]. These are reliable markers for the activity of the disease.

17.1.4 Radiology

Plain X-ray shows lytic lesions in the early phase [10]. The lesion usually extends to the end of bone. The lytic lesion is a V-shaped lesion in the long bones, which is also known as "blade of grass" appearance. The bone is widened, and there will be bowing of bone (Fig. 17.1a, b). Cortical and medullary bones are thickened (Fig. 17.1c). Increased bone resorption results in increased bone formation, and a picture of mixed lytic and sclerotic areas may be observed (Figs. 17.1d and 17.2). Osteolytic lesions in the skull are described as osteoporosis circumscripta. Later, there is increased osteoblastic activity with enlargement of the skull and a classic "cotton wool" appearance (Fig. 17.3). Involved vertebrae may be completely sclerotic (ivory vertebra). On bone scan, they show increased uptake.

17.1.5 Histopathology

In PDB, the osteoclasts are increased in number and size. The number of nuclei in each giant cell is also increased. The osteoclasts are seen in lacunae near the trabeculae. The bony trabeculae are thickened and irregular resulting in irregular blue cement lines, which are very characteristic of

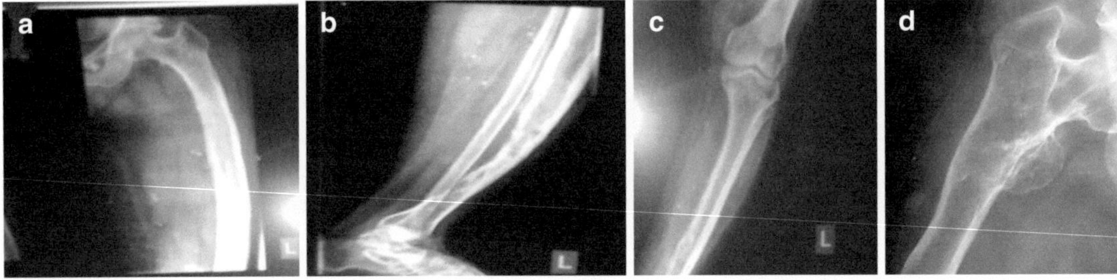

Fig. 17.1 Paget disease of bone. (**a** and **b**) Plain X-ray showing bowing of tibia and femur in a 62-year-old female. (**c**) Thickening of tibial cortex. (**d**) Irregular lytic and sclerotic areas with severe osteoporosis

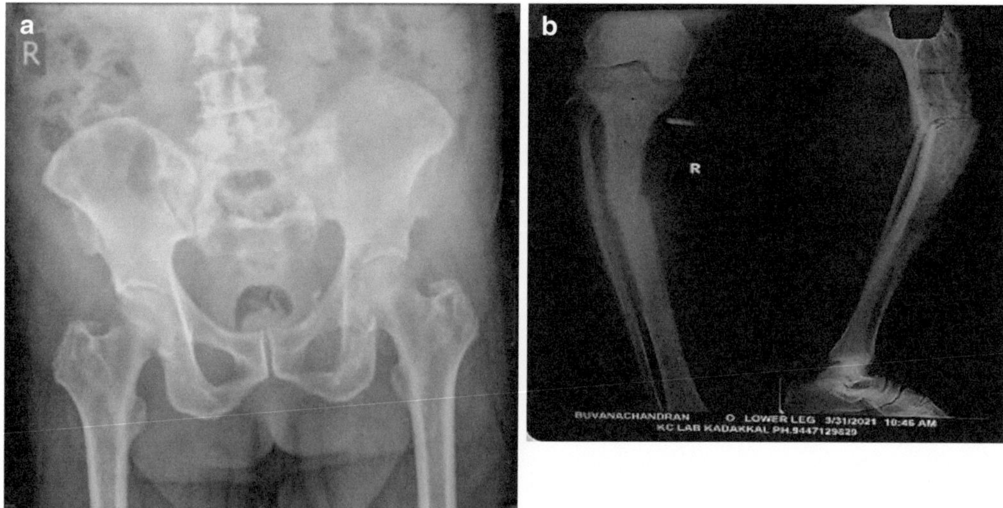

Fig. 17.2 Paget disease of bone. (**a**) Pelvis and (**b**) tibia with fracture

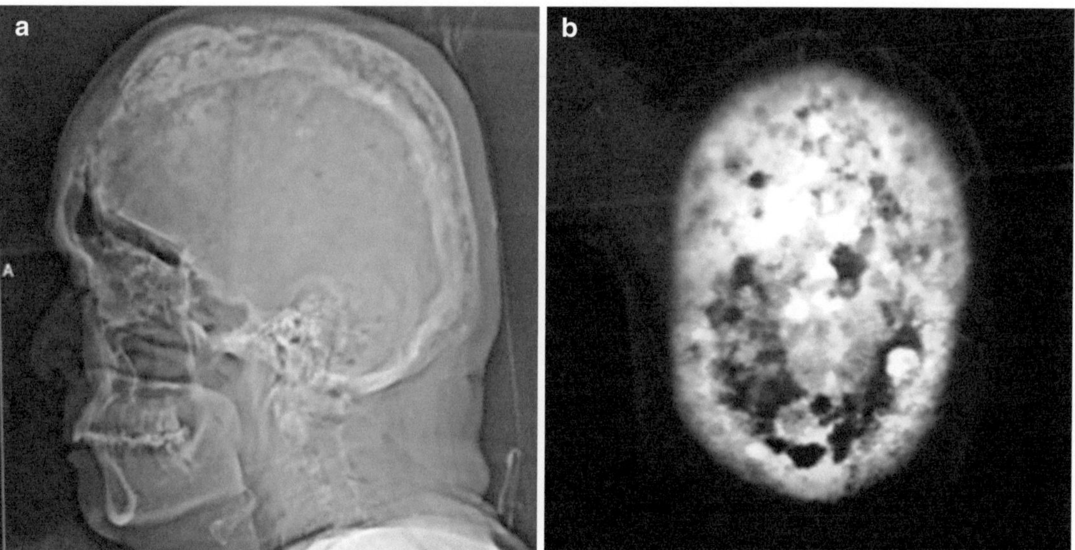

Fig. 17.3 Paget disease in an 82-year-old male. (**a** and **b**) Cotton wool appearance of skull in Paget disease. He also had osteosarcoma of skull bone

Paget disease (Fig. 17.4a, b). In the later stages of mixed osteolytic-osteoblastic phase, new bone formation (woven bone) can be noted [8].

Pagetoid bone can be seen in other conditions like osteosarcoma and other bone forming tumours. Hence while diagnosing PDB, radiological correlation is mandatory.

PDB has a risk of developing sarcomas—osteosarcomas or other sarcomas like chondrosarcoma or fibrosarcoma. The common bones affected are femur, pelvic bones, humerus, tibia and skull (Fig. 17.5). These patients have a poor prognosis. Skeletal or extraskeletal benign giant cell tumours have also been reported.

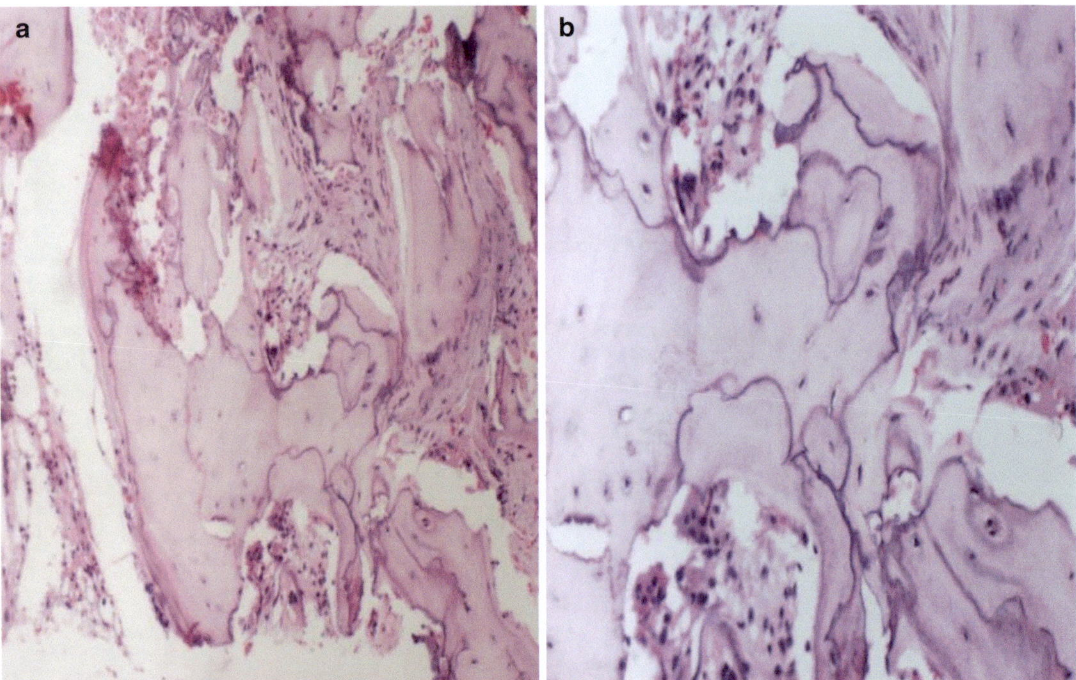

Fig. 17.4 PDB. (**a**) Thickened bony trabeculae with cement lines, H&E ×100. (**b**) Increased number of osteoclastic giant cells adjacent to bony trabeculae, H&E ×250

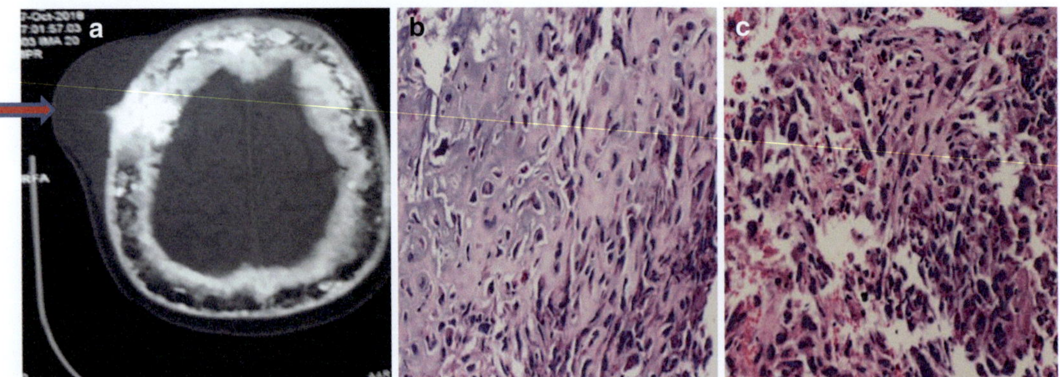

Fig. 17.5 Osteosarcoma in Paget disease of skull in an 82-year-old male. (**a**) MRI: Typical cotton wool appearance of skull with growth protruding outside (red arrow). (**b**) Chondroblastic osteosarcoma with high grade (grade 3) hyaline cartilage with peripheral spindling of cells, H&E ×250. (**c**) Pleomorphic malignant cells, H&E ×250

17.1.6 Treatment

Paget disease of bone is treated with nitrogen-containing bisphosphonates [4]. Denosumab may also be effective in treating Paget disease of bone [3]. Surgery may be required in cases with complications like stenosis and fractures.

17.2 Osteomyelitis

In acute or chronic osteomyelitis, alterations in radiologic images may simulate bone tumours [15, 16, 20].

17.2.1 Clinical

Clinically, osteomyelitis can have systemic symptoms like fever, leucocytosis or increased ESR as in Ewing sarcoma.

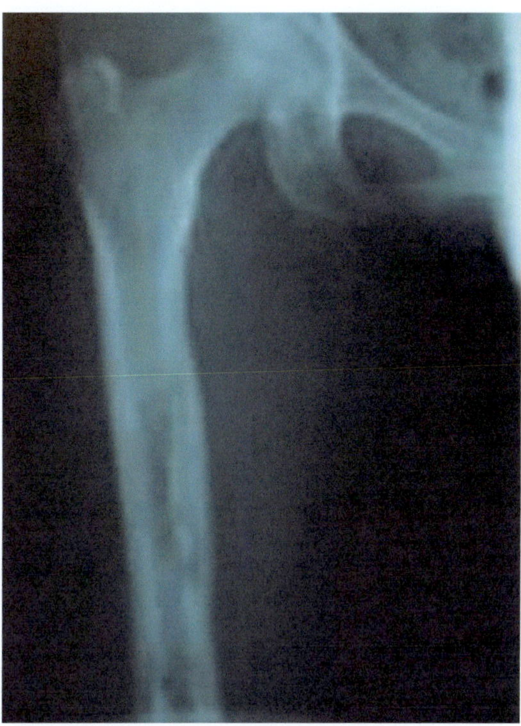

Fig. 17.6 Osteomyelitis of femur. Periosteal reaction and permeative lesion resembling Ewing sarcoma

17.2.2 Radiology

Radiographic changes of osteomyelitis include lytic area with periosteal elevation in multiple layers (onion-peel appearance) and soft tissue swelling. Hence it is often mistaken for Ewing sarcoma [25] (Fig. 17.6). In the chronic phase of osteomyelitis, the radiographic picture can simulate osteosarcoma or giant cell tumour with geographic areas of destruction. MRI is found to be useful to differentiate osteomyelitis from tumours [19, 31]. An inner hyperintense ring and a granulation tissue lining the cavity are thought to be the most important findings to differentiate an abscess from a tumour. This is known as "penumbra sign". Sometimes, the cortex shows dense thickening (Fig. 17.7a).

17.2.3 Pathology

A polymorphous population of inflammatory cells admixed with capillaries and necrotic bone will be seen (Fig. 17.7b–d). When plasma cells predominate, kappa and lambda stain will identify the polyclonal nature of plasma cells, thus ruling out plasmacytoma. Similarly, if eosinophils predominate with a mixture of histiocytes, LCH may be the differential diagnosis. IHC for CD1a will help in differentiation. Mixture of inflammatory cells can be seen in SHML, Hodgkin and non-Hodgkin lymphoma [32]. All these have to be carefully excluded before a diagnosis of osteomyelitis is given [13].

17.2.4 Subacute Osteomyelitis

Subacute osteomyelitis (Brodie's abscess) is a distinct entity and is different from other forms of osteomyelitis. A radiolucent area surrounded by dense zone resembles osteoid osteoma.

Osteomyelitis can be caused by different types of bacteria and fungi. Specific chronic infections like tuberculosis, actinomycosis, coccidioidomycosis or blastomycosis are often seen (Fig. 17.11).

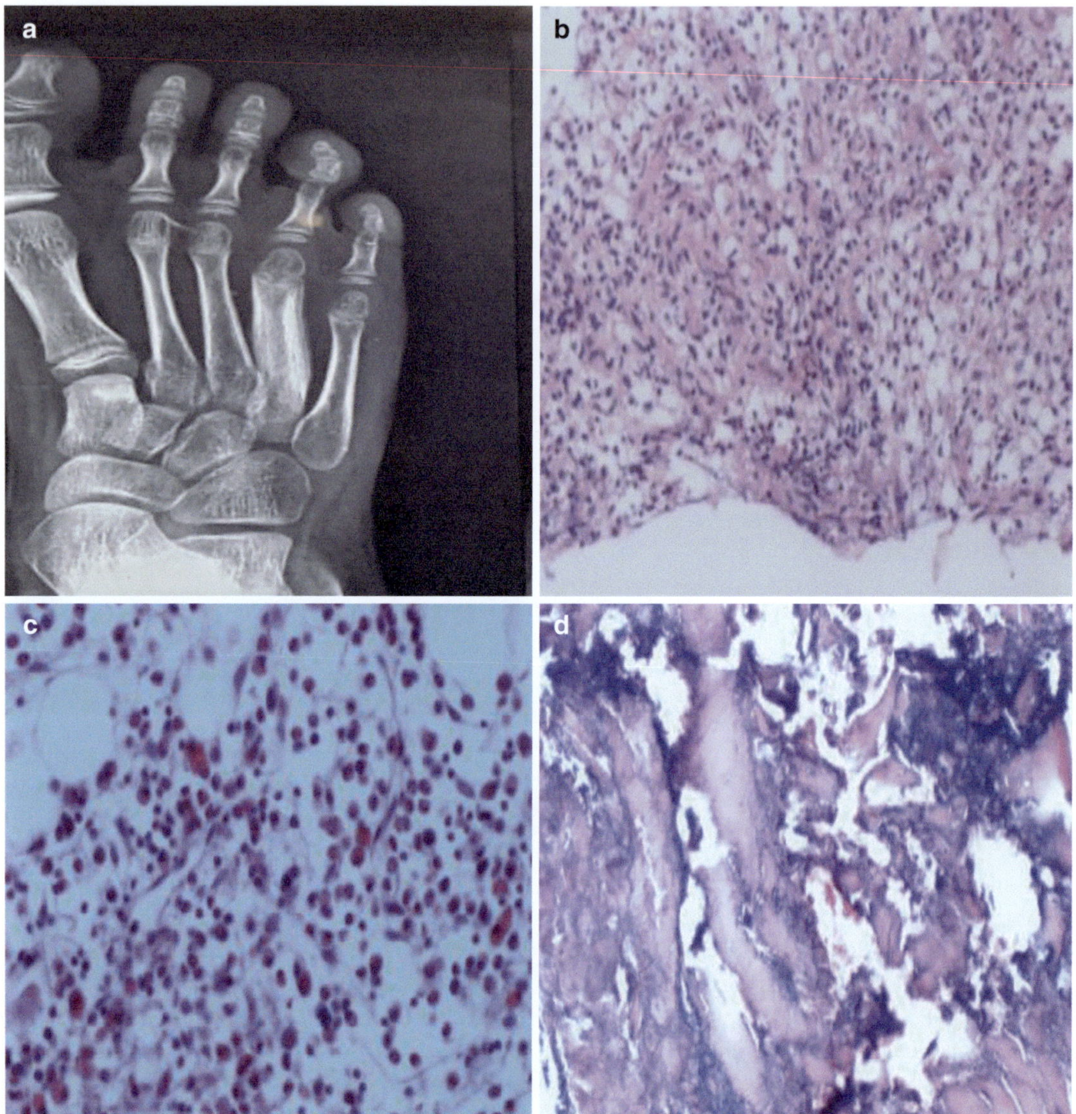

Fig. 17.7 Osteomyelitis of fourth metatarsal. (**a**) Plain X-ray showing thickened cortex of fourth metatarsal bone. (**b**) Sheets of inflammatory cells, H&E ×40. (**c**) Chronic inflammatory cells, H&E ×100. (**d**) Necrotic bone with empty osteocytes (devoid of nuclei), H&E ×250

Tuberculous infection of bone is another great mimicker of bone tumour [17, 34]. Fever and pain can be absent in these cases. Any bone can be affected. Spinal involvement by tuberculosis differs from bacterial spinal infection. The disc spaces remain normal for a long time. The involvement of adjacent bones with narrowing of joint space is a useful finding to suspect infective aetiology. Microscopy shows granulomas with caseation necrosis (Fig. 17.8).

17.2.5 Sclerosing Osteomyelitis

Garre described a **sclerosing osteomyelitis** that causes thickening of bone without abscess formation. Sclerosis of bone may mimic a tumour on radiograph. A biopsy becomes mandatory in difficult situations. While taking biopsy, it is important that a sample should be taken for culture to identify the organism (Figs. 17.9 and 17.10).

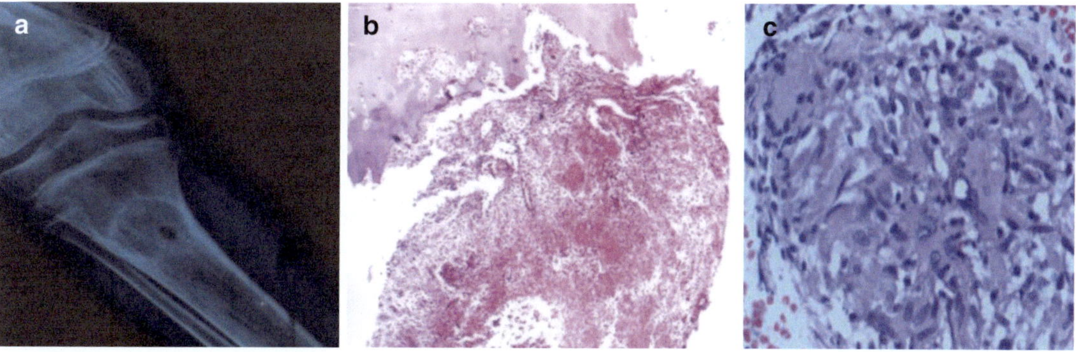

Fig. 17.8 Tuberculous osteomyelitis in a boy having acute lymphoblastic leukaemia. (**a**) Radiology shows thickening of cortex with a lytic lesion in the upper tibia. (**b**) Section from bone showing necrotizing granuloma, H&E ×100. (**c**) Granuloma with epithelioid cells and Langhans giant cells, H&E ×250

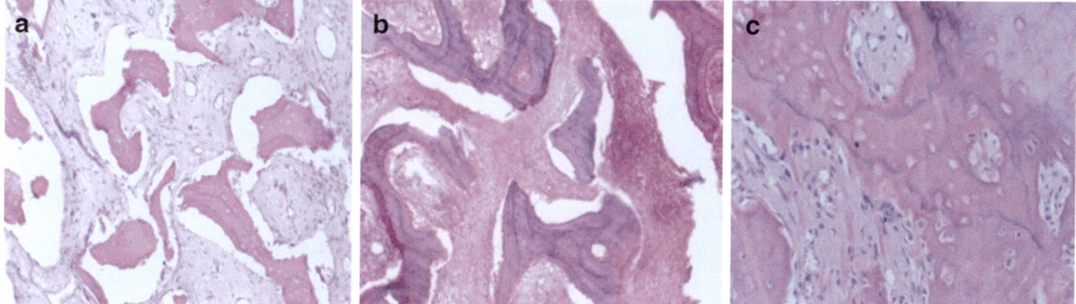

Fig. 17.9 Garre's osteomyelitis in mandible in a 13-year-old girl. (**a**, **b**, **c**) Note the thickened bony trabeculae with cement lines, immature woven bone and intervening fibrotic stroma

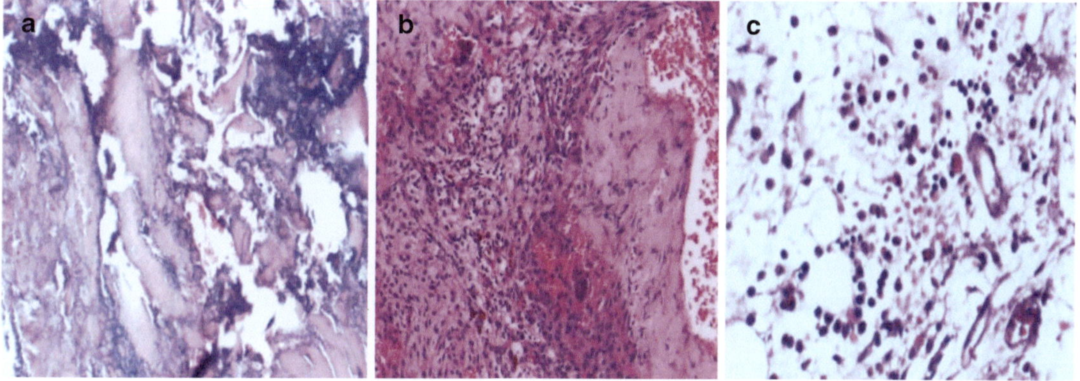

Fig. 17.10 Sclerosing osteomyelitis in a 9-year-old girl. (**a**) Thickening of bone, necrotic bone

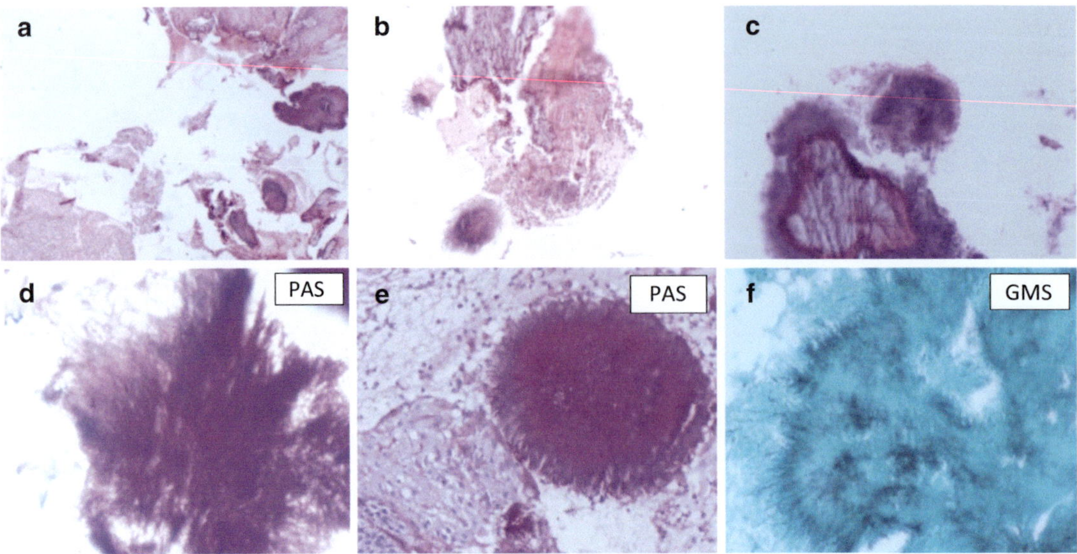

Fig. 17.11 Actinomycotic infection of mandible in a patient with osteoradionecrosis and osteomyelitis. (**a–c**) Necrotic bone and actinomycotic colonies, H&E ×40. (**d**, **e**) PAS stain highlighting the organism with Splendore-Hoeppli phenomenon, PAS ×250. (**f**) Gomori methenamine silver (GMS) ×400

Some of the other reported organisms causing osteomyelitis are actinomycosis [14, 18, 23] (Fig. 17.11), aspergillosis [22], cryptococcosis [26], candida [28] and syphilis [29].

Sinus tract of osteomyelitis can be a site of malignancy [24, 27]. Squamous cell carcinoma can develop in a sinus tract [12, 21]. Other tumours that are described in a setting of osteomyelitis are osteosarcoma [31], fibrosarcoma [30], lymphoma [33] and plasmacytoma [35].

17.3 Hamartoma

The word hamartoma is derived from two Greek words (hamartia and oma). In this lesion, there is an overgrowth of mature tissues that normally occur in that area or organ, but with disorganization. One element of tissue may predominate. They may be epithelial, mesenchymal or mixed.

There are two hamartomas described in bone. They are

1. Nasal chondromesenchymal hamartoma
2. Mesenchymal hamartoma of chest wall

17.3.1 Nasal Chondromesenchymal Hamartoma (NCMH)

In the sinonasal region, the common hamartomatous lesion mimicking bone tumour is nasal chondromesenchymal hamartoma (NCMH).

17.3.1.1 Clinical

Nasal chondromesenchymal hamartomas are common in infants [36] (less than 3 months of age). It can also occur in older children [42] with chronic sinusitis. Pleuropulmonary blastoma is seen associated with NCMH. The mass arises from nasal septum or vestibule and rarely involves sinuses. Clinical features are nasal obstruction, epistaxis and persistent rhinorrhoea [43]. The pathogenesis is poorly understood.

17.3.1.2 Pathology

NCMH is firm and white, with areas resembling cartilage [39]. Microscopically, fibroblasts lie in a hyaline cartilaginous background (Fig. 17.12). Sometimes, bone or bony islands are seen.

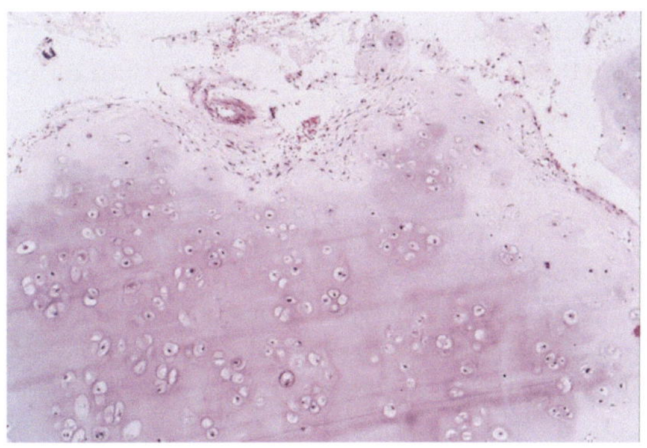

Fig. 17.12 NCMH-cartilage admixed with fibrous tissue at the periphery, H&E ×100

17.3.1.3 DD

NCMH is a benign lesion, and it should not be mistaken for aggressive lesions like chondroblastic osteosarcoma or chondrosarcoma, which is more common in nasal bone.

17.3.2 Mesenchymal Hamartoma of the Chest Wall (MHCW)

MHCW is a very rare benign tumour of bone. McLeod and Dahlin called it hamartoma of the chest wall. MHCW involves the ribs as expansile lytic lesions [44]. They occur in infants. Males are more affected. These lesions should not be mistaken for aggressive bone tumours because these tumours may show plump fibroblasts and cellular cartilage.

17.3.2.1 Clinical

80% of cases present at birth or in early infancy. They are usually solitary. Rarely, it can be bilateral or multicentric [37]. Child presents with respiratory distress. The swelling is subcutaneous, immobile and hard. Deformity of ribs can be present.

17.3.2.2 Radiology

Plain X-ray shows expansile lesion with well-defined sclerotic margins. Secondary aneurysmal bone cyst formation can be present. Chondroid popcorn-like calcifications may be seen [41]. Rib destruction may or may not be present. Radiologically, malignant tumours like congenital neuroblastoma, Ewing sarcoma and malignant teratoma are the differential diagnoses.

17.3.2.3 Pathology

Grossly, they are well circumscribed, solid and cystic. Microscopically, small round to oval cells admixed with osteoclastic giant cells and islands of hyaline cartilage are seen. Sometimes, cells are spindly [40]. Cartilage shows increased cellularity [38]. Aneurysmal bone cyst-like changes may also be seen.

17.3.2.4 DD

The differential diagnosis includes malignant tumours with high-grade cartilage-like chondroblastic osteosarcoma or benign tumours like osteochondromas. Chondrosarcomas occur in adults, at the periphery of the ribs, and grow rapidly with cortical destruction. The cartilage in MHCW resembles benign articular cartilage or cartilage in enchondral ossification.

17.3.2.5 Treatment and Prognosi

Spontaneous regression is seen in bilateral tumours. Conservative management is given in asymptomatic patients. But growing lesions are excised. MHCW stops growing within the first year of life. Malignant transformation in MHCW is very rare. Prognosis of these lesions is good, and it is important that it should not be overtreated.

17.4 Calcifying Pseudoneoplasm

Calcifying pseudoneoplasms of the neuraxis (CAPNON) are rare tumours [45]. The pathogenesis is unknown. It can occur anywhere within the neuraxis [46]. These lesions are considered non-neoplastic synovial cysts of a joint of the degenerated intervertebral disc.

Clinically and radiologically, they are benign lesions that mimic ossified vascular lesions [47]. They can arise anywhere along the CNS. It is most common in spine in proximity to a disc space [49]. It can also occur in orbit, brain [48] and long bones.

17.4.1 Radiology

It shows a calcified extradural mass.

17.4.2 Pathology

Histologically vague granulomas with palisading histiocytes and giant cells are seen. Calcification is seen in the centre. Both immature and mature bone with trabeculae and lacunae containing osteocytes may be present.

17.4.3 Treatment

Surgical removal is the treatment [50].

17.5 Osteonecrosis

Infarction of bone is the death of bone tissue due to loss of blood supply. Bone infarct commonly occurs in the femoral head [52] after high-dose corticosteroid therapy (avascular necrosis) or it can be idiopathic. It is also common in caisson workers after decompression sickness and also in sickle cell anaemia cases. Alcohol abuse, pancreatitis, organ transplant, haemodialysis [57], radiation therapy, etc. can cause bone infarct. Bisphosphonates can cause radio necrosis of jaw [58, 59]. Diabetes, Gaucher disease and HIV infection can also lead on to bone necrosis. Legg–Calvé–Perthes syndrome is osteonecrosis of femoral head, and it occurs in children. Other bones like scaphoid bone (Preiser disease), navicular bone (Köhler disease) and lunate bone (Kienböck disease) are also affected.

Ischemic death of the cellular elements of the bone and marrow is called as bone infarct or osteonecrosis. The lesions involving metaphysis and diaphysis are called bone infarcts, and those involving epiphysis are called avascular necrosis. Some use both terms as synonyms.

17.5.1 Clinical

Pain is the presenting complaint. Limitation in movement can occur. Femur, humerus, knees [53], shoulders, ankles and jaws are commonly involved.

17.5.2 Radiology

Bone scan and MRI are the best modalities for diagnosis [55]. Radiograph shows an area of lucency surrounded by hazy sclerosis. In late stages, articular cortex will collapse. Idiopathic bone infarct usually involves metaphysis of long bones. In early lesions, no visible lesion is evident on radiographs. Later, an area of sclerosis appears at the periphery of lesion. This is mistaken for a cartilage tumour.

17.5.3 Pathology

Grossly, a crescentic yellow area is seen near articular cartilage [54]. Cartilage may lift off from bone. Histologically, nonviable bony trabeculae with empty lacunae are seen. But over-decalcification can also give an appearance similar to this. Marrow may show evidence of fat necrosis (Fig. 17.13). Later stages show foci of calcification or fibrosis replacing necrosed fat of marrow. The collagenized tissue can be demonstrated by trichrome stain (Fig. 17.13d–f). Secondary aneurysmal bone cyst can be an associated finding. Osteomyelitis can develop around areas of necrosis [56].

Rarely, malignancies are reported in association with infarcts. Osteosarcoma, fibrosarcoma and undifferentiated sarcomas [51] are reported.

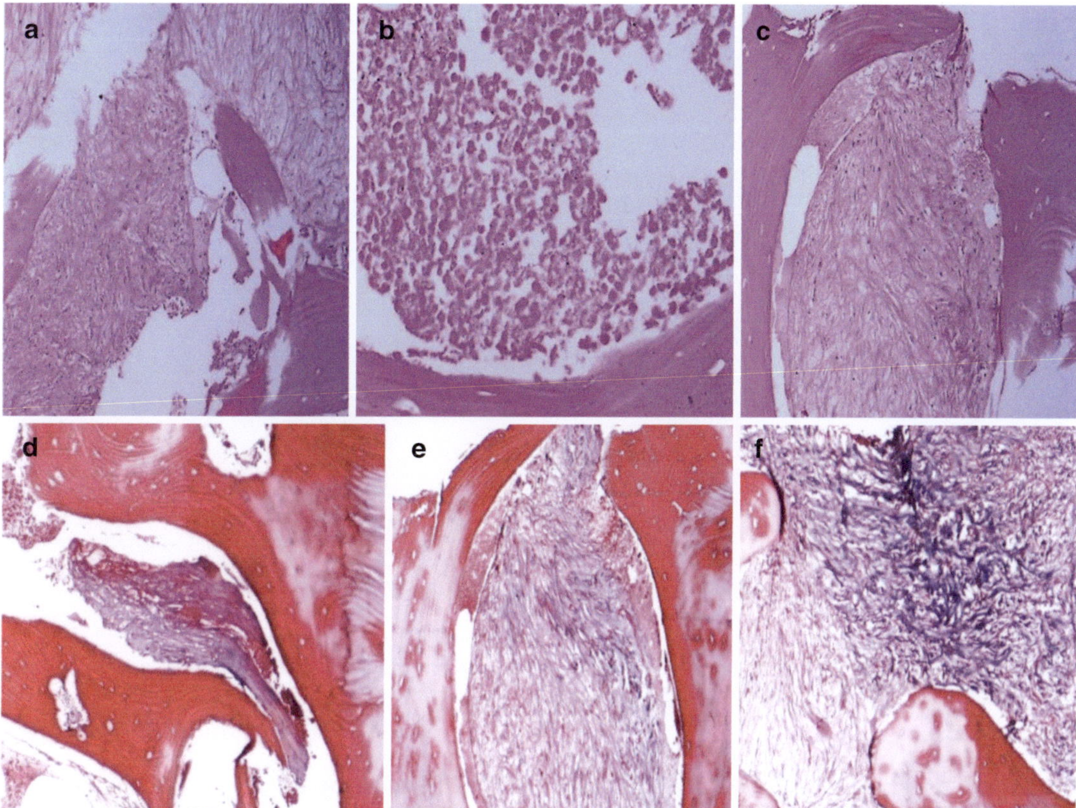

Fig. 17.13 Bone infarction/avascular necrosis. (**a** and **b**) Bone with necrotic marrow, H&E ×100. (**c**) Fibrous tissue, H&E ×100. (**d**) Trichrome stain showing blue-coloured collagen replacing marrow space ×40. (**e**) Trichrome ×100. (**f**) Trichrome ×250

17.5.4 Treatment

Femoral head necrosis if extensive and associated with impending fracture may require total hip replacement therapy. No treatment is required in other sites.

17.6 Hyperparathyroidism (HPT)

HPT occurs due to hyperplasia or neoplasm of parathyroid. Primary [63] and secondary HPT can occur in renal diseases. Bony changes can be seen in both primary and secondary HPT. It can affect any bone [60].

17.6.1 Radiology

Brown tumour of HPT produces lytic lesion. Typical subperiosteal resorption can be seen in phalanges of hand [61, 62]. Multiple bones can be involved [64]. MRI is useful in the diagnosis [65].

17.6.2 Pathology

Histologically, brown tumour shows clusters of osteoclastic giant cells in a fibrous stroma (Fig. 17.14). Haemosiderin-laden macrophages may be seen. HPT should be suspected when a giant cell tumour occurs in an unusual location

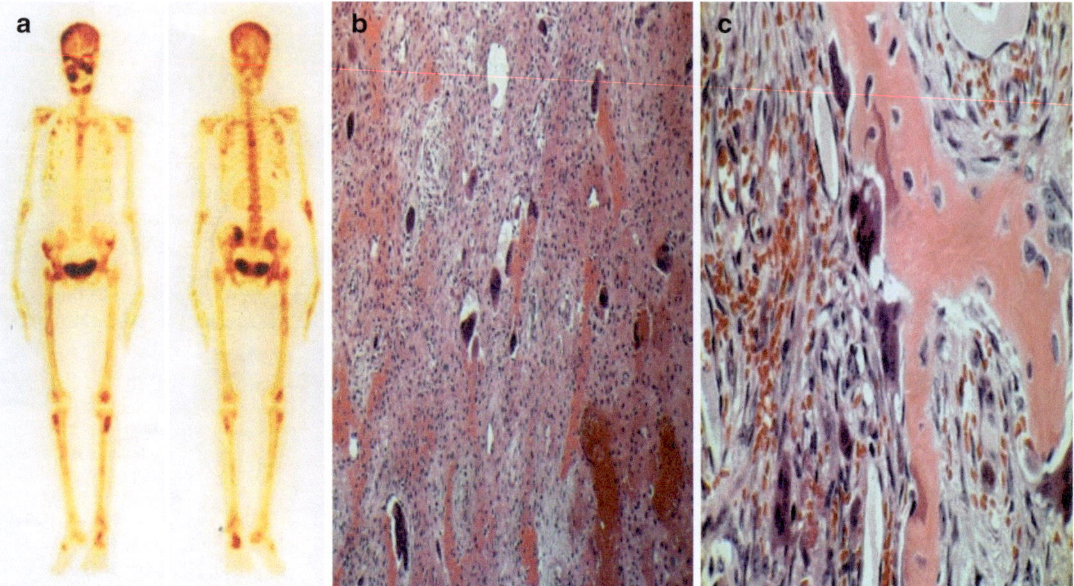

Fig. 17.14 Brown tumour of HPT. Biopsy from nasal mass. (**a**) Bone scan showing increased uptake in multiple bones. (**b** and **c**) Clusters of giant cells in a spindle cell stroma. Osteoclasts are seen very close to bony trabeculae, H&E ×100. FNA from tibia showed giant cell-rich lesion in this case

like ribs or metaphysis of long bones. Also, if giant cell-rich lesions are seen in multiple bones, HPT should be ruled out. Increased osteoclastic and osteoblastic activity is seen in the bony trabeculae. Reactive osteoid as in solid ABC may be observed.

17.7 Mastocytosis

Mast cell disease (MCD) affects one or more organs. It is characterized by accumulation of neoplastic mast cells (MCs) in the affected organs.

17.7.1 Clinical Features

The symptoms are non-specific [66]. The patients present with urticaria pigmentosa, unexplained flushing, hypotension and abdominal cramps. If there is no clinical suspicion, it will end in wrong diagnosis. Skeletal lesions occur in 70–75% of patients with systemic mastocytosis [71].

17.7.2 Radiology

When bone is involved, both lytic and sclerotic bone lesions are seen [70]. Fractures of the bones are commonly encountered [72]. The bones of axial skeleton, pelvis and proximal ends of long bones are commonly affected. The lesions are mistaken for metastasis [67], Paget disease, hyperparathyroidism, lymphoma and myelofibrosis [68].

17.7.3 Pathology

The bony trabeculae are thickened. The paratrabecular region will be infiltrated by mast cells, which are small oval cells seen in aggregates and giving a micro-granulomatous appearance [69]. Eosinophils are usually seen admixed with these cells (Fig. 17.15a and b). Mast cells stain positive with toluidine blue (metachromatic stain), Giemsa, etc. (Figs. 17.15c and 17.16). Immunohistochemistry for CD117 will be positive. CD25 is another marker of diagnostic value [73].

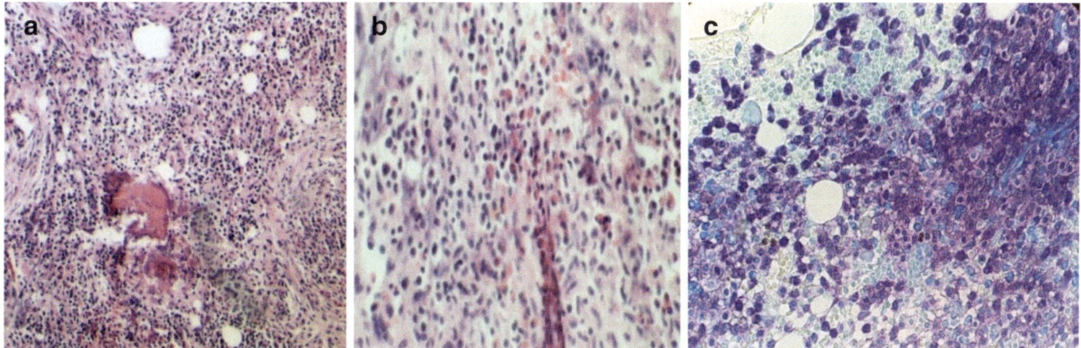

Fig. 17.15 Mastocytosis. (**a** and **b**) Mast cells admixed with eosinophils, H&E ×100. (**c**) Toluidine stain shows metachromatic granules ×250

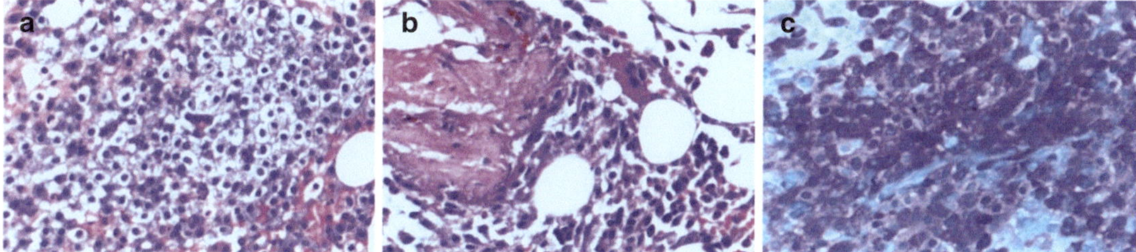

Fig. 17.16 Mastocytosis of bone marrow. (**a**) Cells with clear cytoplasm, H&E ×250. (**b**) Foci of spindle cells, H&E ×250. (**c**) Toluidine blue showing metachromatic granules ×250

17.7.4 Prognosis

Systemic mastocytosis may be associated with haematological malignancies like leukaemia. Patients usually die due to malignancy.

17.8 Subungual Keratoacanthoma (SUKA)

Subungual keratoacanthoma (SUKA) is a form of keratoacanthoma, which grows rapidly [74]. It is rare. It behaves in an aggressive manner [76].

17.8.1 Clinical

They are painful hyperkeratotic masses under the nail plate [77]. It causes destruction of underlying bone. It has a predilection for first three fingers of the hand. It is solitary or multiple. Sometimes, they can be hereditary. It usually occurs in middle-aged men. Trauma and human papillomavirus infection are suggested aetiological factors.

17.8.2 Radiology

X-ray shows erosion of distal phalanx due to pressure from the tumour [75]. The differential diagnoses include squamous cell carcinoma, epidermal cyst, intraosseous ganglion and glomus tumour.

17.8.3 Pathology

A large crater-like squamo-proliferative lesion similar to the cutaneous counterpart with connection to epidermis is seen. It consists of lobules and nests of glassy squamous epithelium with numerous dyskeratotic cells with minimal cytological atypia and low mitotic activity. The lesion is well demarcated.

17.8.4 DD

Differential diagnosis is squamous cell carcinoma of nail bed, which is usually infiltrative.

17.8.5 Treatment and Prognosis

It is a self-limiting disease. It can undergo spontaneous regression [78]. In some cases, conservative surgery may be required.

17.9 Stress Fracture, Insufficiency Fracture and Avulsion Injury

17.9.1 Stress Fracture

A stress fracture happens from repetitive trauma. It is a very small crack in the bone and is commonly seen in athletes, especially long-distance runners [79]. Stress fractures are usually associated with repetitive activities like jogging and marching. Stress injuries can be found in the tibial shaft and metatarsals.

17.9.1.1 Radiology

Plain X-ray is negative, but a hot bone scan and increased signals on MRI will be observed. CT scan shows fractures which are not evident on plain radiographs (Fig. 17.17).

17.9.1.2 Pathology

Biopsy shows woven bone with calcification in the bone marrow spaces, and they appear as permeative lesions [80]. They show reactive new bone mimicking osteosarcoma. But cellular areas are absent. Careful examination under low power shows typical zonation of bone, cartilage and fibroblastic proliferation from outside to inside (Figs. 17.17c, d and 17.18).

17.9.1.3 DD

In needle biopsy, osteosarcoma is the closest differential diagnosis. Typical history of stress and presence of zonation are helpful features for ruling out malignancy. A proper history, radiology and a careful histological examination are required for proper diagnosis. Histologically, newly formed trabeculae are not packed and are separated by marrow. Lack of mass lesion on radiology is another clue.

17.9.1.4 Treatment

Conservative management is given.

17.9.2 Insufficiency Fracture

An insufficiency fracture is due to osteoporosis. The sacral ala and pubic ramus are sites of insufficiency fractures. Increased uptake on bone scans and a linear sclerosis of sacral ala or lytic lesion of pubic rami simulating metastatic carcinoma are seen. Patients may give a history of malignancy and radiation therapy to pelvis. Biopsy shows reactive new bone formation.

17.9.3 Avulsion Fracture

Avulsion injury occurs in young adults in the ischial tuberosity or tibial tubercle. Patients with avulsion injury usually complain of sudden and severe pain. They are young and healthy. Exuberant callus formation will mimic a neoplasm. Radiology shows a mass near the ischial tuberosity. Serial radiology pictures have to be examined to arrive at a proper diagnosis.

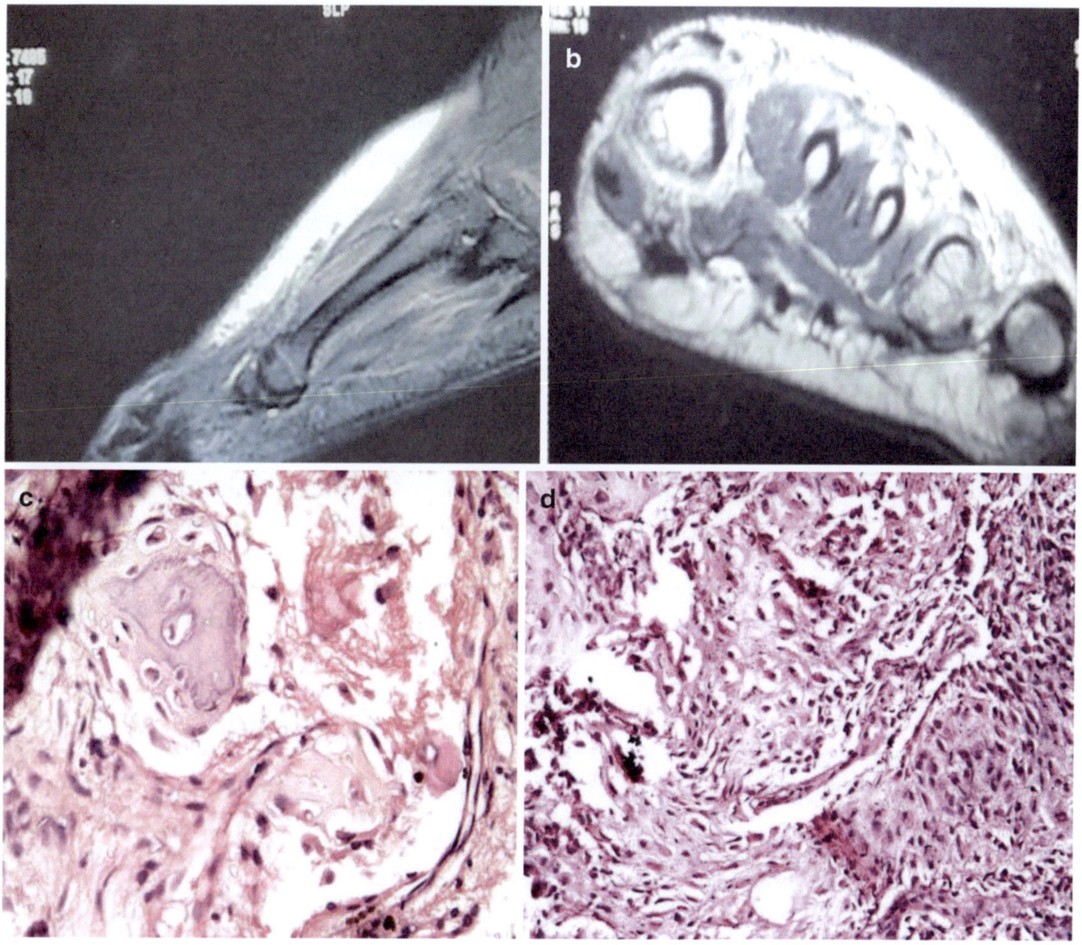

Fig. 17.17 Stress fracture in an 8-year-old girl who is a dancer. (**a** and **b**) MRI showing fracture of the fourth metatarsal. (**c** and **d**) Typical zonation—outer bone, inner cartilage and fibrous tissue, H&E ×100

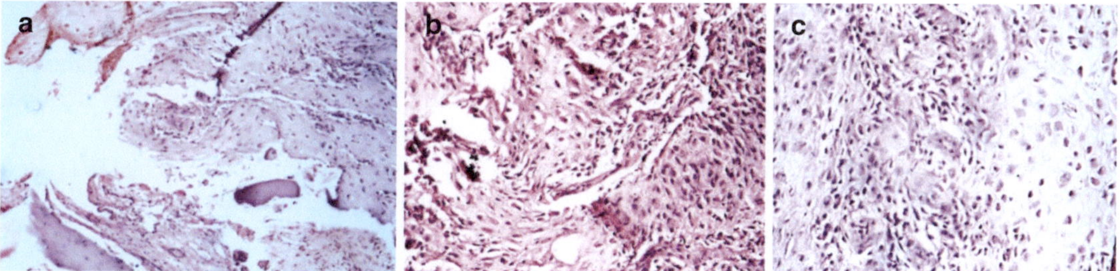

Fig. 17.18 Fracture callus mimicking osteosarcoma. (**a**) Bone with cellular spindle cells, H&E ×40. (**b**) Spindle cells with osteoid, H&E ×100. (**c**) Cellular cartilage, H&E ×250

17.10 Transient Osteoporosis

In this condition, patients present with immense pain [81]. Radiographs show severe osteoporosis of femoral head, which shows increased uptake on bone scan, thus simulating a neoplasm [84]. It resembles avascular necrosis [82, 83]. Treatment is supportive, and patients fully recover.

17.11 Traumatic Osteolysis

There is unilateral or bilateral loss of portion of lateral ends of clavicle [89]. Other bones reported are acetabulum [85], pubic bone [86], skull bones [87] and humerus [88]. Patient experiences severe pain. This is due to physical activity. Biopsy is not required. Cessation of the activity which caused the condition will result in complete cure.

17.12 Sternocostoclavicular Hyperostosis

Sternocostoclavicular hyperostosis (SCCH) is a chronic inflammatory disorder [90].

17.12.1 Clinical

The clinical symptoms are erythema, swelling and throbbing pain of the sternoclavicular joint. SCCH occurs in adults and is more common in females. Other joints may also be affected. Hence, it has to be differentiated from the seronegative spondyloarthropathies and infectious osteomyelitis.

17.12.2 Radiology

Radiological manifestations are seen in the sternum, clavicles, upper ribs and spine. Local to diffuse ossification and hyperostosis are seen [91]. Bony overgrowth involving the medial end of the clavicle and sternum along with soft tissue calcification of periarticular tissues can be seen. The first rib may also be involved. Unilateral involvement is uncommon.

17.13 Neuropathic Joint

Conditions like diabetic neuropathy, syringomyelia and syphilis cause neuropathic joint. This is due to repeated trauma. Patients present with swelling near affected joint. Calcific debris is seen in the joint. In later stages, bone near the affected joint disappears and thus gives an appearance of a neoplasm [92, 93, 94]. Microscopically, features similar to degenerative joint disease like debris from articular cartilage and bone are seen. In fact, neuropathic joint is a severe form of degenerative joint disease.

17.14 Melorheostosis

Melorheostosis is a rare bone dysplasia seen mainly in children [102]. Cortical hyperostosis occurs in one or multiple bones. There will be soft tissue calcification or ossification. This is described as "dripping candle wax" appearance of the cortex [95]. The lower extremities are more affected [100]. The affected bone is clearly demarcated from the uninvolved bone [101]. Soft tissue involvement is seen in 25% [97].

17.14.1 Pathology

There is a mixture of osteoid, chondroid and fibrovascular tissue. Mutations in *MAP2K1* have recently been identified as a cause of melorheostosis [99].

17.14.2 Treatment and Prognosis

Melorheostosis is incurable. Denosumab and bisphosphonates are tried in some cases [98]. Osteosarcoma developing in melorheostosis bones is reported [96].

17.15 Osteopetrosis

Osteopetrosis is an extremely rare inherited disorder. It is also known as marble bone disease. The bones are hard and become denser. Based on age and clinical features, three clinical forms, namely infantile, intermediate and adult-onset types, are described. It is an extremely rare inherited disorder and occurs following consanguineous marriages. It has an autosomal recessive inheritance.

17.15.1 Clinical

Patients present with failure to thrive and growth retardation. Bones become harder, denser and break. Hence, it is known as "brittle bone disease". Stunted growth, deformities, increased incidence of fractures, blindness, facial paralysis and deafness due to cranial nerve entrapment are all described. Pancytopenias due to bone marrow failure occur. Extramedullary haematopoiesis results in hepatosplenomegaly, hypersplenism and haemolysis. Failure of bone remodelling leads to haematopoietic failure. The presence of renal acidosis and calcification of brain along with osteopetrosis is seen in marble brain syndrome [105].

17.15.2 Radiology

Generalized osteosclerosis with uniformly sclerotic or alternating sclerotic and lucent bands, club-like bone or appearance of bone within bone and fractures are seen. Thickened and dense skull, especially the skull base, and extremely dense vertebrae with alternating bands, named as rugger-jersey sign, are seen [103]. Radiological findings are enough to arrive at a diagnosis (Fig. 17.19a–e).

17.15.3 Lab Findings

Laboratory signs include hypocalcaemia, elevated parathormone and increased acid phosphatase.

17.15.4 Pathology

Bone biopsy is not essential for diagnosis. But it is useful to predict the likelihood that bone marrow transplant (BMT) will succeed. If bone marrow is crowded, response to BMT is poor. In case a biopsy is taken, especially when there is pancytopenia and clinical suspicion of leukaemia, islands of cartilage within mature bone, woven bone and either normal or increased or decreased number of osteoclasts are seen [104] (Fig. 17.19f–h).

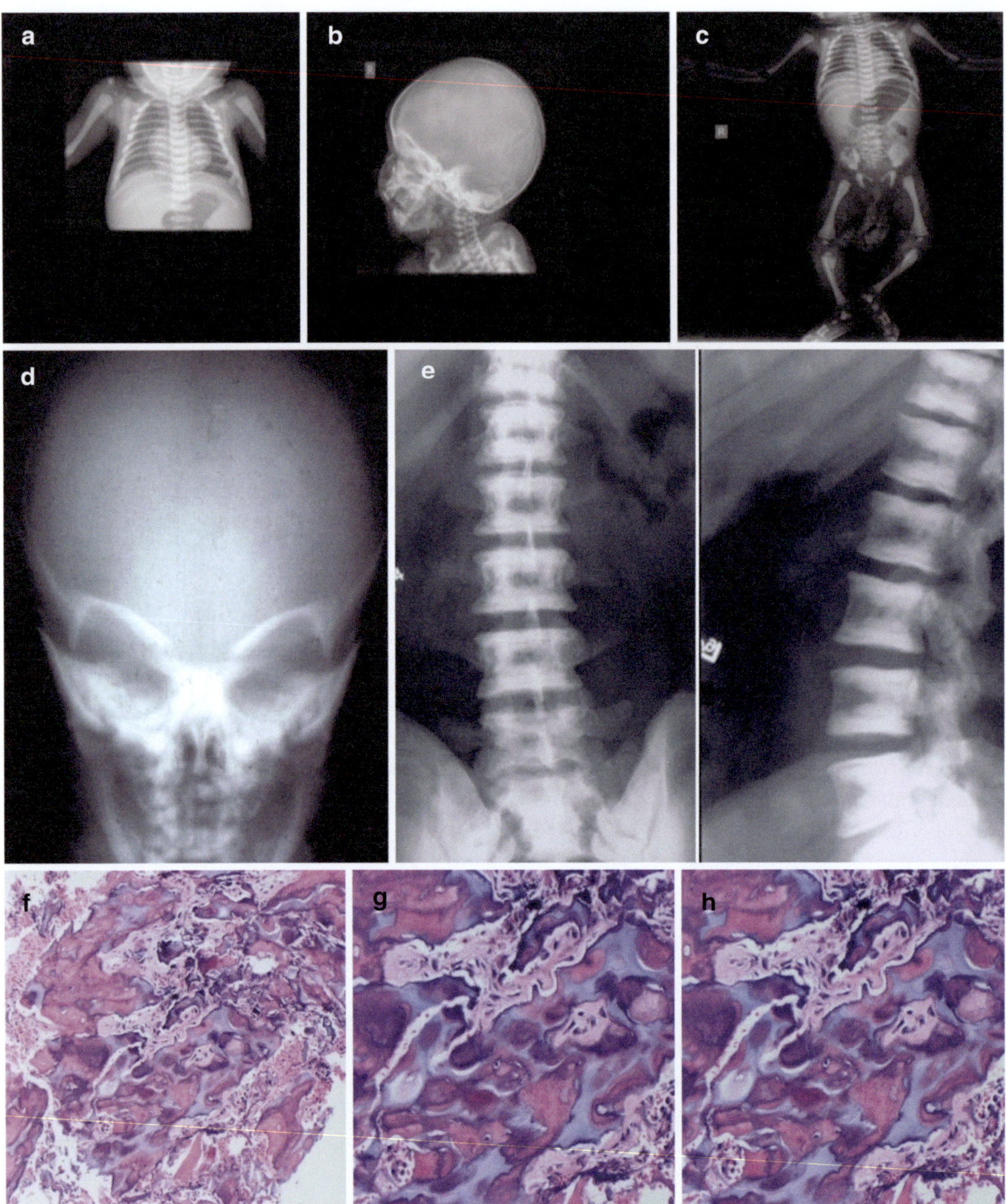

Fig. 17.19 Osteopetrosis in a 6-month-old baby who presented with pancytopenia. (**a–e**): Radiology showing generalized osteosclerosis-sclerotic ribs, skull base and alternating bands in vertebrae. (**f–h**) Islands of cartilage within mature bone or woven bone and scattered osteoclastic giant cells, H&E ×250

17.15.5 DD

Differential diagnosis includes hypervitaminosis D, hypoparathyroidism, myeloproliferative disease, paediatric lead toxicity and pseudohypoparathyroidism.

17.15.6 Treatment

Treatment is bone marrow transplant.

Points to Remember

- Radiological correlation is a must to rule out tumour-like lesions.
- Pagetoid bone can be seen in osteoid-producing tumours like osteosarcoma.
- Radiology of osteomyelitis can mimic Ewing sarcoma or lymphoma.
- Giant cell-rich lesions involving multiple bones—always rule out hyperparathyroidism.
- If osteomyelitis is suspected by clinical/radiological findings, a sample should be sent for culture at the time of biopsy.
- Avascular necrosis and insufficiency/avulsion/stress fractures can mimic tumours. Hence, a proper clinical history and radiology findings are important to diagnose these cases.
- Osteopetrosis can be diagnosed by radiology images. Biopsy is not.

References

Tumour-Like Lesions of Bone

1. Fabrizio Remotti MD, Frieda Feldman MD. Nonneoplastic lesions that simulate primary tumors of bone. Arch Pathol Lab Med. 2012;136:772–88.

Paget Disease of Bone

2. Britton C, Walsh J. Paget disease of bone-an update. Aust Fam Physician. 2012;41:100–3.
3. Hirao M, Hashimoto J. Denosumab as the potent therapeutic agent against Paget's disease of bone. Clin Calcium. 2011;21:1231–8.
4. Licata AA. Discovery, clinical development, and therapeutic uses of bisphosphonates. Ann Pharmacother. 2005;39:668–77.
5. Kurihara N, Hiruma Y, Yamana K, Michou L, Rousseau C, Morissette J, Galson DL, Teramachi J, Zhou H, Dempster DW, Windle JJ, Brown JP, David Roodman G. Contributions of the measles virus nucleocapsid gene and the SQSTM1/p62P392L mutation to Paget disease. Cell Metab. 2011;13(1):23–34.
6. Ralston SH. Clinical practice. Paget's disease of bone. N Engl J Med. 2013;368:644–50.
7. Rebel A, Basle M, Pouplard A, Malkani K, Filmon R, Lepatezour A. Towards a viral etiology for Paget's disease of bone. Metab Bone Dis Relat Res. 1981;3:235–8.
8. Seton M. Paget disease of bone: diagnosis and drug therapy. Cleve Clin J Med. 2013;80:452–62.
9. Seton M, Choi HK, Hansen MF, Sebaldt RJ, Cooper C. Analysis of environmental factors in familial versus sporadic Paget's disease of bone: The New England registry for Paget disease of bone. J Bone Miner Res. 2003;18:1519–24.
10. Moore TE, Kathol MH, El-Khoury GY, Walker CW, Gendall PW, Whitten CG. Unusual radiological features in Paget's disease of bone. Skelet Radiol. 1994;23(4):257–60.
11. Visconti MR, Usategui-Martín R, Ralston SH. Antibody response to paramyxoviruses in Paget's disease of bone. Calcif Tissue Int. 2017;101(2):141–7.

Chronic Osteomyelitis

12. Alami M, Mahfoud M, El Bardouni A, Berrada MS, YaacoubiM E. Squamous cell carcinoma arising from chronic osteomyelitis. Acta Orthop Traumatol Turc. 2011;45(3):144–8.
13. Barakat A, et al. Chronic osteomyelitis: a review on current concepts and trends in treatment. Orthop Trauma. 2019;33:181–7. https://doi.org/10.1016/j.mporth.2019.03.005.
14. Bartkowski SB, Zapala J, Heczko P, Szuta M. Actinomycotic osteomyelitis of the mandible: review of 15 cases. J Craniomaxillofac Surg. 1998;26:63–7.
15. Cabanela ME, Sim FH, Beabout JW, Dahlin DC. Osteomyelitis appearing as neoplasms. A diagnostic problem. Arch Surg. 1974;109:68–72.
16. Cottias P, Tomeno B, Anract P, Vinh TS, Forest M. Subacute osteomyelitis presenting as a bone tumour. A review of 21 cases. Int Orthop. 1997;21:243–8.
17. Lebowitz D, Wolter L, Zenklusen C, Chouiter A, Malinverni R. TB determined: tuberculous osteomyelitis. Am J Med. 2014;127(3):1–4.
18. Gannepalli A, Ayinampudi BK, Baghirath PV, Reddy GV. Actinomycotic osteomyelitis of maxilla

presenting as oroantral fistula: a rare case report. Case Rep Dent. 2015;2015:689240.
19. Grey AC, Davies AM, Mangham DC, Grimer RJ, Ritchie DA. The 'penumbra sign' on T1-weighted MR imaging in subacute osteomyelitis: frequency, cause and significance. Clin Radiol. 1998;53:587–92.
20. Huang PY, Wu PK, Chen CF, Lee FT, Wu HT, Liu CL, Chen TH, Chen WM. Osteomyelitis of the femur mimicking bone tumors: a review of 10 cases. World J Surg Oncol. 2013;22(11):283.
21. JoLi Q, Cui H, Dong J, et al. Squamous cell carcinoma resulting from chronic osteomyelitis: a retrospective study of 8 cases. Int J Clin Exp Pathol. 2015;8(9):10178–84.
22. Koehler P, Tacke D, Cornely OA. Aspergillosis of bones and joints a review from 2002 until today. Mycoses. 2014;57:323–35.
23. Lau L, Darraj M, Keynan Y. Mandibular Actinomyces osteomyelitis mimicking osteosarcoma. JMM Case Rep. 2016;3(6):e005073. https://doi.org/10.1099/jmmcr.0.005073:1-3.
24. McGrory JE, Pritchard DJ, Unni KK, Ilstrup D, Rowland CM. Malignant lesions arising in chronic osteomyelitis. Clin Orthop Relat Res. 1999;362:181–9.
25. McCarville MB, Chen JY, Coleman JL, Li Y, Li X, Adderson EE, Neel MD, Gold RE, Kaufman RA. Distinguishing osteomyelitis from Ewing sarcoma on radiography and MRI. AJR Am J Roentgenol. 2015;205(3):640–50.
26. Medaris LA, Ponce B, Hyde Z, et al. Cryptococcal osteomyelitis: a report of 5 cases and a review of the recent literature. Mycoses. 2016;59:334–42.
27. Moura DL, Ferreira R, Garruço A. Malignant transformation in chronic osteomyelitis. Rev Bras Ortop. 2017;52(2):141–7.
28. Neofytos D, Huprikar S, Reboli A, et al. Treatment and outcomes of Candida osteomyelitis: review of 53 cases from the PATH Alliance(R) registry. Eur J Clin Microbiol Infect Dis. 2014;33:135–41.
29. Park KH, Lee MS, Hong IK, et al. Bone involvement in secondary syphilis: a case report and systematic review of the literature. Sex Transm Dis. 2014;41:532–7.
30. Puri A, Parasnis AS, Udupa KV, Duggal A, Agarwal MG. Fibroblastic osteosarcoma arising in chronic osteomyelitis. Clin Radiol. 2003;58(2):170–2.
31. Reinehr T, Burk G, Michel E, Andler W, Davies AM, Grimer R. The penumbra sign in subacute osteomyelitis. Eur Radiol. 2005;15:1268–70.
32. Shimose S, Sugita T, Kubo T, Matsuo T, Nobuto H, Ochi M. Differential diagnosis between osteomyelitis and bone tumors. Acta Radiol. 2008;49(8):928–33.
33. Badam TK, Devadoss S, Balaji M, Devadoss A, Rajasekharan PN. Primary bone lymphoma mimicking as osteomyelitis: an unusual presentation. J Orthop Oncol. 2016;2(2):1–5. https://doi.org/10.4172/2472-016X.1000111.
34. Thawani M, Hale E, Habte-Gabr E. Multifocal tubercular osteomyelitis: a case with atypical manifestations. Tuberc Res Treat. 2011;2011:483802. https://doi.org/10.1155/2011/483802.
35. Yang XW, Zhou GC, Long ZS, Gong FP, Chen G. Solitary bone plasmacytoma of the tibia presenting as chronic osteomyelitis: a rare case report and literature review. Medicine (Baltimore). 2023;102(12):e33307.

Hamartoma

36. Ünal A, Kum RO, Avcı Y, Ünal DT. Nasal chondromesenchymal hamartoma, a rare pediatric tumor: Case report. Turk J Pediatr. 2016;58(2):208–11.
37. Altaner S, Yoruk Y, Bilgi S, Puyan FO, Doganay L, Kutlu K. Multifocal mesenchymal hamartoma of the chest wall. Respirology. 2006;11(3):334–8.
38. Amstalden EM, Carvalho RB, Pacheco EM, Oliveira-Filho A, Stragea-Neto L, Rosenberg AE. Chondromatous hamartoma of the chest wall: description of 3 new cases and literature review. Int J Surg Pathol. 2006;14:119–26.
39. Fedda F, Boulos F, Sabri A. Chondro-osseous respiratory epithelial adenomatoid hamartoma of the nasal cavity. Int Arch Otorhinolaryngol. 2013;17(2):218–21.
40. Gambarotti M, Righi A, Vanel D, Cocchi S, Benini S, Elli FM, Mantovani G, Ruggieri P, Boriani S, Donati DM, Sbaraglia M, Dei Tos AP, Picci P. Fibrocartilaginous mesenchymoma of bone: a single-institution experience with molecular investigations and a review of the literature. Histopathology. 2017;71(1):134–42.
41. Groom KR, Murphey MD, Howard LM, Lonergan GJ, Rosado-de-Christenson ML, Groom KR, Murphey MD, Howard LM. Mesenchymal hamartoma of the chest wall: radiologic manifestations with emphasis on cross-sectional imaging and histopathologic comparison. Radiology. 2002;222(1):205–11.
42. Ozolek JA, Carrau R, Barnes EL, Hunt JL. Nasal chondromesenchymal hamartoma in older children and adults series and immunohistochemical analysis. Arch Pathol Lab Med. 2005;129:1444–50.
43. Mason KA, Navaratnam A, Theodorakopoulou E, Chokkalingam PG. Nasal Chondromesenchymal hamartoma (NCMH): a systematic review of the literature with a new case report. J Otolaryngol Head Neck Surg. 2015;44(1):28.
44. Yeshvanth S, et al. Mesenchymal hamartoma of the chest wall- mimicker of malignancy. J Cancer Res Ther. 2011;7(4):496–8.

Calcifying Pseudoneoplasm of Bone

45. Bertoni F, Unni KK, Dahlin DC, et al. Calcifying pseudoneoplasms of the neural axis. J Neurosurg. 1990;72:42–8.

46. Brasiliense LB, Dickson DW, Nakhleh RE, Tawk RG, Wharen R. Multiple calcifying pseudoneoplasms of the neuraxis. Cureus. 2017;9(2):e1044. Published 2017 Feb 21. https://doi.org/10.7759/cureus.1044.
47. Gross JM, Broski SM, Howe BM, Folpe AL. Paraspinal pseudoneoplasms: a series of 58 consultation cases emphasizing the importance of pathology-radiology correlation. Hum Pathol. 2020;103:14–24.
48. Kerr EE, Borys E, Bobinski M, Shahlaie K. Posterior fossa calcifying pseudoneoplasm of the central nervous system. J Neurosurg. 2013;118:896–902. https://doi.org/10.3171/2013.1.JNS121755.
49. Saha A, Arevalo-Perez J, Peck KK, Rosenblum M, Bilsky M, Lis E, Karimi S. Calcifying pseudoneoplasm of the spine: imaging and pathological features. Neuroradiol J. 2018;31(4):440–4.
50. Stienen MN, Abdulazim A, Gautschi OP, Schneiderhan TM, Hildebrandt G, Lücke S. Calcifying pseudoneoplasms of the neuraxis (CAPNON): clinical features and therapeutic options. Acta Neurochir (Wien). 2013;155:9–17.

Osteoradionecrosis

51. Alhamdan HA, Alrifai OI, Shaheen MF, Pant R, Altayeb MA. Bone infarct transformation into undifferentiated pleomorphic sarcoma in sickle cell disease: a case report. Int J Surg Case Rep. 2020;77:243–8.
52. Barille MF, Wu JS, McMahon CJ. Femoral head avascular necrosis: a frequently missed incidental finding on multidetector CT. Clin Radiol. 2014;69:280–5.
53. Graham P. Avascular necrosis and bone infarcts of the knee. Orthop Nurs. 2020;39(1):59–61.
54. Dermawan JK, Goldblum A, Reith JD, Kilpatrick SE. Accurate and reliable diagnosis of avascular necrosis of the femoral head from total hip arthroplasty specimens requires pathologic examination. Am J Clin Pathol. 2021;155(4):565–74.
55. Manenti G, Altobelli S, Pugliese L, et al. The role of imaging in diagnosis and management of femoral head avascular necrosis. Clin Cases Miner Bone Metab. 2015;12:31–8.
56. Blacksin MF, Finzel KC, Benevenia J. Osteomyelitis originating in and around bone infarcts. Am J Roentgenol. 2001;176(2):387–91.
57. Langevitz P, Buskila D, Stewart J, Sherrard DJ, Hercz G. Osteonecrosis in patients receiving dialysis: report of two cases and review of the literature. J Rheumatol. 1990;17(3):402–6.
58. Pires FR, Miranda A, Cardoso ES, et al. Oral avascular bone necrosis associated with chemotherapy and bisphosphonate therapy. Oral Dis. 2005;11:365–9.
59. Yarom N, Shapiro CL, Peterson DE, Van Poznak CH, Bohlke K, Ruggiero SL, Migliorati CA, Khan A, Morrison A, Anderson H, Murphy BA, Alston-Johnson D, Mendes RA, Beadle BM, Jensen SB, Saunders DP. Medication-related osteonecrosis of the jaw: MASCC/ISOO/ASCO clinical practice guideline. J Clin Oncol. 2019;37(25):2270–90.

Hyperparathyroidism

60. Marcocci A, Cianferotti L, Cetani F. Bone disease in primary hyperparathyroidism. Therap Adv Musculoskeletal Dis. 2012;4(5):357–68.
61. Chang CY, Rosenthal DI, Mitchell DM, Handa A, Kattapuram SV, Huang AJ. Imaging findings of metabolic bone disease. Radiographics. 2016;36(6):1871–87.
62. Bennett J, Suliburk JW, Morón FE. Osseous manifestations of primary hyperparathyroidism: imaging findings. Int J Endocrinol. 2020;2020:3146535. https://doi.org/10.1155/2020/3146535.
63. Walker MD, Silverberg SJ. Primary hyperparathyroidism. Nat Rev Endocrinol. 2018;14(2):115–25.
64. Vaishya R, Amit K, Singh H. Multiple "brown tumors" masquerading as metastatic bone disease. World Neurosurg. 2019;12:e431.
65. Hong WS, Sung MS, Chun K-A, et al. Emphasis on the MR imaging findings of Brown tumor: a report of five cases. Skelet Radiol. 2011;40(2):205–13.

Mastocytosis

66. Pardanani A, Akin C, Valent P. Pathogenesis, clinical features, and treatment. advances in mastocytosis. Best Pract Res Clin Haematol. 2006;19(3):595–615.
67. Barer M, Peterson LFA, Dahlin DC, Winkleman RK, Stewart J. Mastocytosis with osseus lesions resembling metastatic malignant lesions in bone. J Bone Joint Surg. 1968;50-A:142–52.
68. Horny HP, Sotlar K, Valent P. Differential diagnoses of systemic mastocytosis in routinely processed bone marrow biopsy specimens: a review. Pathobiology. 2010;77(4):169–80.
69. Horny HP, Valent P. Diagnosis of mastocytosis: general histopathological aspects, morphological criteria, and immunohistochemical findings. Leuk Res. 2001;25:543–51.
70. Huang TY, Yam LT, Li CY. Radiological features of systemic mast-cell disease. Br J Radiol. 1987;60:765–70.
71. Mallya KP, Belurkar S, Kurian A, Rao L, Singhania B. Systemic mastocytosis: predominantly involving the bone, a case report. J Clin Diagn Res. 2013;7(10):2276–7. https://doi.org/10.7860/JCDR/2013/5669.3493.
72. Pescador D, Parrilla CM, Lorenzo JA, Fernández T, Montesdeoca A, Blanco J. Bone involvement in systemic mastocytosis: multiple osteoporotic vertebral

fractures. Case report and review. Ann Spine Res. 2018;1(1):1004.
73. Sotlar K, Horny HP, Simonitsch I, Krokowski M, Aichberger KJ, Mayerhofer M, Printz D, Fritsch G, Valent P. CD25 indicates the neoplastic phenotype of mast cells: a novel immunohistochemical marker for the diagnosis of systemic mastocytosis (SM) in routinely processed bone marrow biopsy specimens. Am J Surg Pathol. 2004;28(10):1319–25.

Subungual Keratoacanthoma

74. Baran R, Goettmann S. Distal digital keratoacanthoma: a report of 12 cases and a review two cases with a review of the literature. Dermatol Surg. 2001;27:575–9.
75. Choi JH, Shin DH, Shin DS, Cho KH. Subungual keratoacanthoma: ultrasound and magnetic resonance imaging findings. Skelet Radiol. 2007;36(8):769–72.
76. Cunha N, André J, Sass U, Richert B. Subungual solitary angiokeratoma simulating a squamous cell carcinoma. Skin Appendage Disord. 2018;4:152–5.
77. Miroux Catarino A, Catorze MG, Viana I. Subungual Keratoacanthoma: a rare variant of Keratoacanthoma. J Portug Soc Dermatol Venereol. 2018;76(4):425–8.
78. Sinha A, Marsh R, Langtry J. Spontaneous regression of subungual keratoacanthoma with reossification of underlying distal lytic phalanx. Clin Exp Dermatol. 2005;30(1):20–2.

Stress Fracture

79. Schilcher J, Bernhardsson M, Aspenberg P. Chronic anterior tibial stress fractures in athletes: no crack but intense remodeling. Scand J Med Sci Sports. 2019;29:1521–8. https://doi.org/10.1111/sms.13466.
80. Patel DS, Roth M, Kapil N. Stress fractures: diagnosis, treatment, and prevention. Am Fam Physician. 2011;83(1):39–46.

Transient Osteoporosis

81. Aprato A, Conti A, Triolo P, Piana R, Masse A. Transient osteoporosis of the hip: state of the art and review of literature. Fortune J Rheumatol. 2019;1(3):021–7.
82. Balakrishnan A, Schemitsch EH, Pearce D, McKee MD. Distinguishing transient osteoporosis of the hip from avascular necrosis. Can J Surg. 2003;46(3):187–92.
83. Rader CP. Transient osteoporosis and osteonecrosis of the femoral head. Risk factors, classification and differential diagnosis. Orthopade. 2007;36:423–9.
84. Yamaguchi R, Yamamoto T, Motomura G, et al. Radiological morphology variances of transient osteoporosis of the hip. J Orthop Sci. 2017;22:687–92.

Traumatic Osteolysis

85. Alexa O, Malancea RI, Puha B, Popescu D, Veliceasa B. Rapidly progressive Osteolysis of the femoral head following an acetabular fracture - case report. J Surg [Jurnalul de chirurgie]. 2017;13(2):81–4.
86. Hall FM, Goldberg RP, Kasdon EJ, Glick H. Post-traumatic osteolysis of the pubic bone simulating a malignant lesion. J Bone Joint Surg. 1984;66(1):121–6.
87. Saoji K, Jaju V, Apte A, Dahiphale DB. Post traumatic giant scalp lesion with large osteolytic lesions of the skull: a case report. Int J Curr Med Appl Sci. 2017;16(2):100–3.
88. Noman S, Faiz S, Khan SA, Sattar A. Massive osteolysis in distal shaft of Humerus: a case report on vanishing bone disease. J Coll Physicians Surg Pak. 2018;28(Special Supplement 3 of Case Reports):S164–5.
89. Smart MJ. Traumatic osteolysis of the distal ends of the clavicles. J Can Assoc Radiol. 1972;23:264–6.

Sternoclavicular Hyperostosis

90. Edwin J, Ahmed S, Verma S, Tytherleigh-Strong G, Karuppaiah K, Sinha J. Swellings of the sternoclavicular joint: review of traumatic and non-traumatic pathologies. EFORT Open Rev. 2018;3(8):471–84.
91. Fritz P, Baldauf G, Wilke HJ, Reitter I. Sternocostoclavicular hyperostosis: its progression and radiological features. A study of 12 cases. Ann Rheum Dis. 1992;51:658–64.
92. Yachoui R, Kreidy M, Parker BJ. Treatment-refractory Sternocostoclavicular hyperostosis. Clin Med Res. 2017;15(1–2):37–40.

Neuropathic Joint

93. Anderson JJ, Woelffer KE, Holtzman JJ, Jacobs AM. Bisphosphonates for the treatment of Charcot neuroarthropathy. J Foot Ankle Surg. 2004;43:285–9.
94. Jones EA, Manaster BJ, May DA, Disler DG. Neuropathic osteoarthropathy: diagnostic dilemmas and differential diagnosis. Radiographics. 2000;20:S279–93.

Melorheostosis

95. Bansal A. The dripping candle wax sign. Radiology. 2008;246(2):638–40.

96. Bostman OM, Holmstrom T, Riska EB. Osteosarcoma arising in a melorheostotic femur: a case report. J Bone Joint Surg Am. 1987;69:232–7.
97. Boulet C, Madani H, Lenchik L, Vanhoenacker F, Amalnath DS, de Mey J, De Maeseneer M. Sclerosing bone dysplasias: genetic, clinical and radiology update of hereditary and nonhereditary disorders. Br J Radiol. 2016;1062:20150349.
98. Byberg S, Abrahamsen B, Kassem M, Ralston S, Schwartz P. Clinical improvement in a patient with monostotic melorheostosis after treatment with denosumab: a case report. J Med Case Rep. 2018;12:278.
99. Fratzl-Zelman N, Roschger P, Kang H, Jha S, Roschger A, Blouin S, Deng Z, et al. Melorheostotic bone lesions caused by somatic mutations in *MAP2K1* have deteriorated microarchitecture and periosteal reaction. J Bone Miner Res. 2019;34(5):883–95.
100. Jain VK, Arya RK, Bharadwaj M, Kumar S. Melorheostosis: clinicopathological features, diagnosis, and management. Orthopedics. 2009;32(7):512–20.
101. Jha S, Laucis N, Kim L, Malayeri A, Dasgupta A, Papadakis GZ, Karantaras A, Torres M, Bhattacharyya T. CT analysis of anatomical distribution of melorheostosis challenges the sclerotome hypothesis. Bone. 2018;117:31–6.
102. Smith GC, Pingree MJ, Freeman LA, Matsumoto JM, Howe BM, Kannas SN, Pyfferoen MD, Struss LT, Wenger DE, Amrami KK, Matsumoto M, Jurisson ML. Melorheostosis: a retrospective clinical analysis of 24 patients at the mayo clinic. PM&R. 2017;9:283–8.

Osteopetrosis

103. Wittenberg A. The rugger jersey spine sign. Radiology. 2004;230(2):491–2.
104. Del Fattore ACA, Teti A. Genetics, pathogenesis and complications of osteopetrosis. Bone. 2008;42:19–29.
105. Jacquemin C, Mullaney P, Svedberg E. Marble brain syndrome: osteopetrosis, renal acidosis and calcification of the brain. Neuroradiology. 1998;40:662–3.
106. WHO Classification of Tumours. In Soft Tissue and Bone Tumours. WHO Classification of Tumours, vol. Volume 3. Edited by the WHO Classification of Tumours Editorial Board. 5th ed. IARC; 2020.

18 Tumours and Tumour-Like Lesions of Synovium

The synovium is a thin special membrane lining the inner surface of the joint capsule. It also lines fat pads, intra-articular ligaments, bursae and tendon sheaths (Fig. 18.1). Some intra-articular structures such as the articular cartilage, menisci, labra and bare bone areas are not covered by the synovium. The fibrous capsule of the joint is in continuity with the outer surface of sub-intima. The porous synovial lining allows diffusion of the nutrients to the avascular cartilage, thereby probably contributing to the accumulation of immune complexes, bacterial cell walls and other inflammatory material in the joint [1].

Synovial diseases are classified as arthropathies and tumours. This chapter gives a brief description of common tumours and tumour-like lesions of synovium. Tenosynovial giant cell tumour, synovial haemangioma, lipoma arborescens, fibroma, synovial chondromatosis, synovial chondrosarcoma, synovial osteochondroma, intra-articular synovial sarcoma, nodular fasciitis and tumour-like lesions of synovium are discussed here.

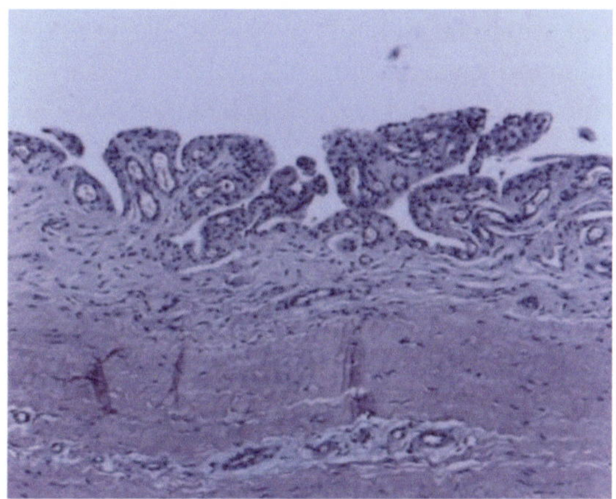

Fig. 18.1 Synovial lining composed of macrophage-like type A synovial cells and fibroblast-like type B synoviocytes supported with sub-intima, H&E ×100

18.1 Benign Tumours and Tumour-Like Lesions of Synovial Tissue

Majority of tumours involving the joint space are likely to be direct extension of neoplasms from the adjacent bones. The primary benign tumours greatly outnumber their malignant counterparts. The tenosynovial giant cell tumour (TSGCT) and synovial chondromatosis (SCh) are two uncommon benign diseases that are unique to the synovium, and only the TSGCT is considered prototypical. The main clinical symptoms of all of these lesions, such as pain, swelling, effusion and joint locking, are not specific [1–3].

18.1.1 Tenosynovial Giant Cell Tumour (TSGCT)

Giant cell tumour of tendon sheath renamed as TSGCT is the most common benign tumour of the tendon sheath and synovium as they share some histologic features. They are predominantly

J. Kattoor et al., *Bone Tumors*, https://doi.org/10.1007/978-981-99-4738-6_18

Table 18.1 Features of localized and diffuse type of TSGC tumours

	Localized type	Diffuse type
Site	Fingers (85%) Others: wrist, ankle, knee, elbow, shoulder	Knee (75%) Ankle, elbow, foot, spinal facets, temporomandibular joint
Age	30–50 years	Younger age
Clinical	Painless, solid slow growing, well circumscribed/lobulated, rarely erodes bone and skin	Painful infiltrative mass with joint effusion and villous pattern for intra-articular type Multinodular, infiltrating in extra-articular to subcutaneous/muscle tissue
Size	0.5–4 cm	>5 cm
Microscopy	Partly capsulated predominance of smaller cells, large cells with plenty of giant cells, mitosis <4/10 HPF	Expansile sheets of large cells alternate with loose zones, more cleft-like spaces, sparse giant cells mitosis >5/10 HPF
IHC	Larger cells: clusterin and desmin positive Smaller cells: CD68, CD45, CD163 +ve Osteoclasts: CD68, CD45, TRAP +ve	Larger cells: clusterin and desmin +ve Smaller cells: CD68, CD45, CD163 +ve Osteoclasts: CD68, CD45, TRAP +ve
Treatment	Excision	Total synovectomy
Prognosis	Benign with possible recurrence in 4–30% but nondestructive	Locally aggressive, with multiple recurrence rate. 18–46% and 33–50%, respectively, for intra- and extra-articular forms

intra-articular and locally aggressive characterized by both inflammatory and neoplastic properties. They do not metastasize.

In WHO soft tissue tumours (2020) [10], it is classified under fibrohistiocytic tumours. Current concept is to classify them as TSGCT, localized and diffuse forms, depending on their growth characteristics. Localized types include giant cell tumours of tendon sheath (nodular tenosynovitis—extra-articular), whereas diffuse type encompasses diffuse-type giant cell tumour. The earlier terminology of "pigmented villonodular tenosynovitis" (PVNS) is no longer used. TGCT-D and TGCT-L share common pathogenesis and histology, but they are clinically distinct lesions (Table 18.1). The localized tumours are smaller, indolent and most frequent in the hands, whereas diffuse tumours affect larger joints of younger patients and are larger in size (>5 cm), often intra-articular and locally aggressive with infiltrative growth pattern and with higher tendency to recur. The diffuse form of the tumour has no capsule. They grow in expansive sheets with more frequent cleft-like spaces and have more haemosiderin and villous architecture of hyperplastic synovium. A vague zoning phenomenon is seen in diffuse type, in which the cells at the periphery of the nodules have smaller nuclei and more cytoplasm [4].

18.1.1.1 Pathophysiology

The IHC staining pattern of clusterin shows that the mononuclear cells are similar to normal synoviocytes. This is the evidence supporting synovial differentiation of tenosynovial giant cell tumours. Cytogenetic and molecular analyses show that diffuse-type giant cell tumour and giant cell tumour of tendon sheath belong to the same biologic continuum [5]. TSGCT was originally believed to be reactive but is now considered neoplastic with demonstration of a translocation between chromosomes 1p13 and 2q35 in which the gene encoding colony-stimulating factor-1 (CSF1) is fused to collagen VI α-3 (COL6A3) gene. This translocation leads to overexpression of CSF1, which in turn recruits non-neoplastic inflammatory cells through paracrine activation of the CSF1 receptor. This phenomenon has been observed in some other tumours too and termed as landscape effect [6–9].

18.1.2 Tenosynovial Giant Cell Tumour-Localized Type (TSGCT-L)

Intra-articular TSGCT was formerly known as localized PVNS, and extra-articular TSGCT was formerly known as nodular tenosynovitis/giant cell tumour of tendon sheath.

18.1.2.1 Clinical features

They typically affect smaller joints, commonest site being those of the hands and feet (85%) and also in locations like wrist, ankle, knee, hip and elbow. Usually, it occurs in the age group of 30–50 years. There is a female predominance. Rarely it can involve knee joint when it should be differentiated from diffuse-type TSGCT.

18.1.2.2 Pathology

Grossly, it is characterized by a well-circumscribed single, small, slow-growing, firm, lobulated, nontender, pedunculated mass, with a diameter of 0.5–4 cm. They are attached to the synovium and have whitish, yellowish or tan, red-brown variegated cut surface (Fig. 18.2a).

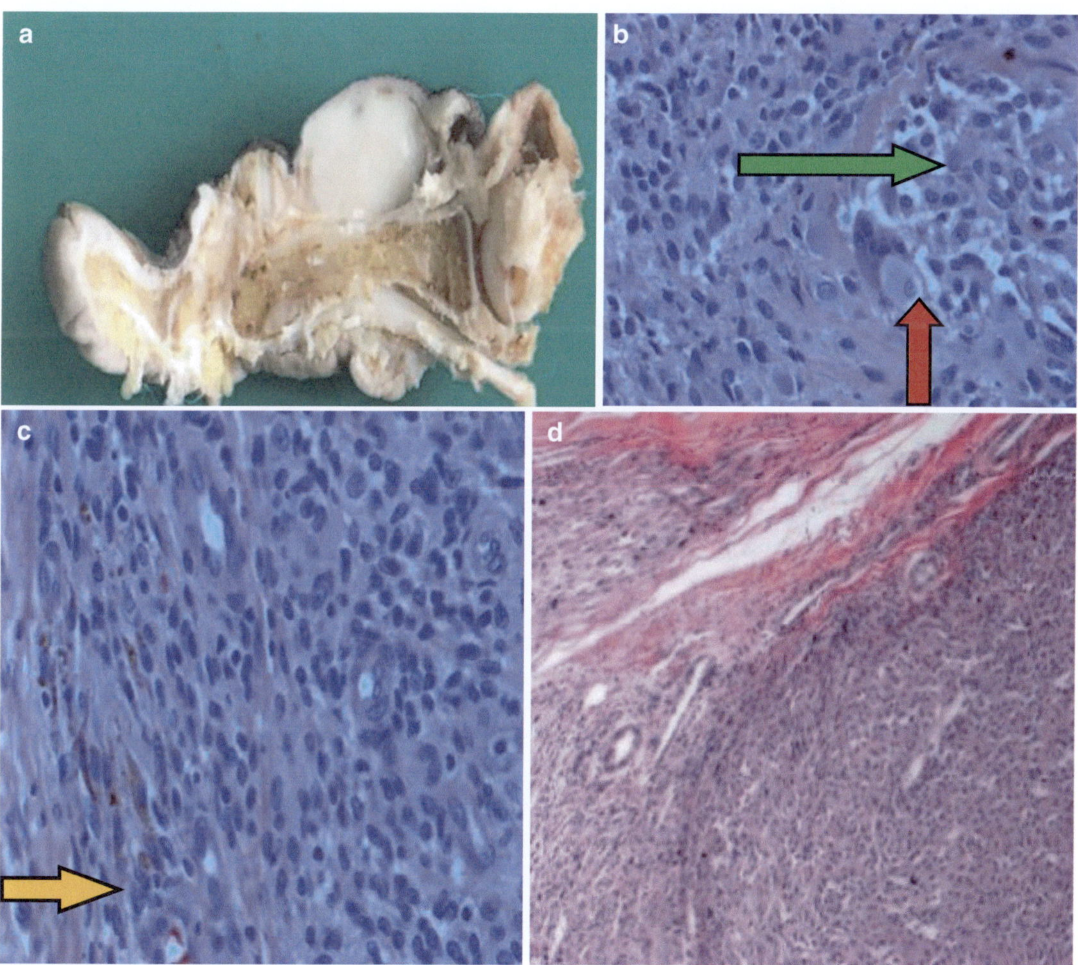

Fig. 18.2 Localized GCT. (**a**) GCT finger. Excised specimen of well-defined nodule with whitish cut surface. (**b**) Two types of cells—large cells with abundant cytoplasm (red arrow) and small histiocyte-like cells (green arrow) and hyalinized stroma in between, H&E ×250. (**c**) Haemosiderin-laden cells (yellow arrow), H&E ×100. (**d**) Lobulated tumour infiltrating periosteum, H&E ×100

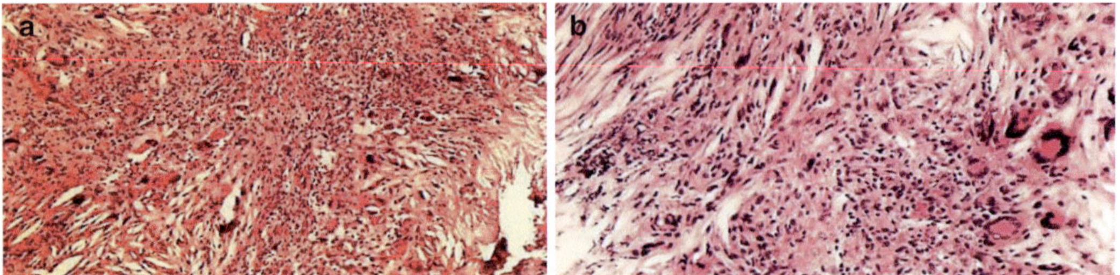

Fig. 18.3 TSGCT. (**a** and **b**) Osteoclastic giant cells mixed with cholesterol clefts, H&E ×100

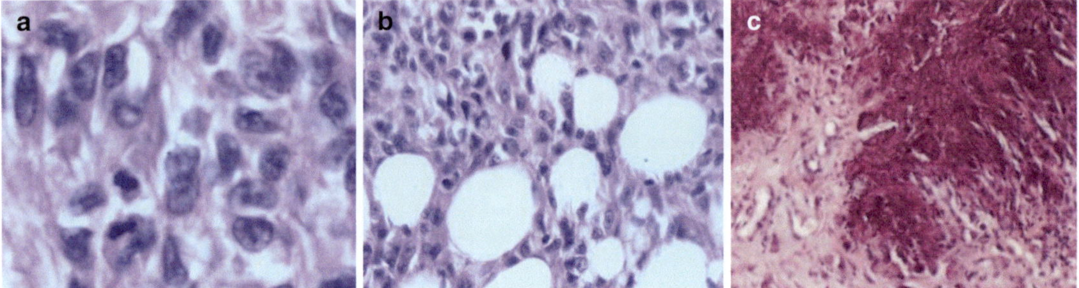

Fig. 18.4 (**a**) Mitosis in TSGCT, H&E ×400. (**b**) Fat infiltration in TSGCT, H&E ×250. (**c**) Extensive calcification in TSGCT, H&E ×100

Microscopy: It shows a moderately cellular neoplasm with fibrous bands separating them into lobules. Large clefts and pseudoglandular or alveolar spaces lined by synovial cells are seen. Two types of mononuclear cells, large polygonal epithelioid type cells and small histiocyte-like cells in variable proportions, are seen (Fig. 18.2b). Variable proportions of osteoclast-like giant cells, foamy histiocytes, siderophages and inflammatory cells are seen admixed with mononuclear cells (Figs. 18.2 and 18.3). Haemosiderin-containing cells, xanthoma cells and cholesterol clefts are often localized at the periphery of the lesion. Mitosis is usually less than 3–5/10 HPF and may reach up to 20/10 HPF (Fig. 18.4a). Atypical mitosis is absent. Cartilaginous and osseous metaplasia is a rare focal finding. Some tumours show extensive calcification (Fig. 18.4c). Long-standing tumours show extensive hyalinization, which may be morphologically mistaken for osteosarcoma (Fig. 18.5).

18.1.2.3 IHC

The mononuclear cells are positive for CD68 and smooth muscle actin (SMA) (Fig. 18.6), which depicts a mixed histiocyte and fibroblastic/myofibroblastic immunophenotype.

18.1.2.4 DD

Soft tissue giant cell tumours—Usually occur in the superficial or deep soft tissue of the hand or arm, but not related to tendon sheath. Microscopic and immunophenotypic profiles are similar to giant cell tumour of bone. But they lack heterogeneity, which is the hallmark of nodular tenosynovitis. Periphery of the lesion shows metaplastic bone.

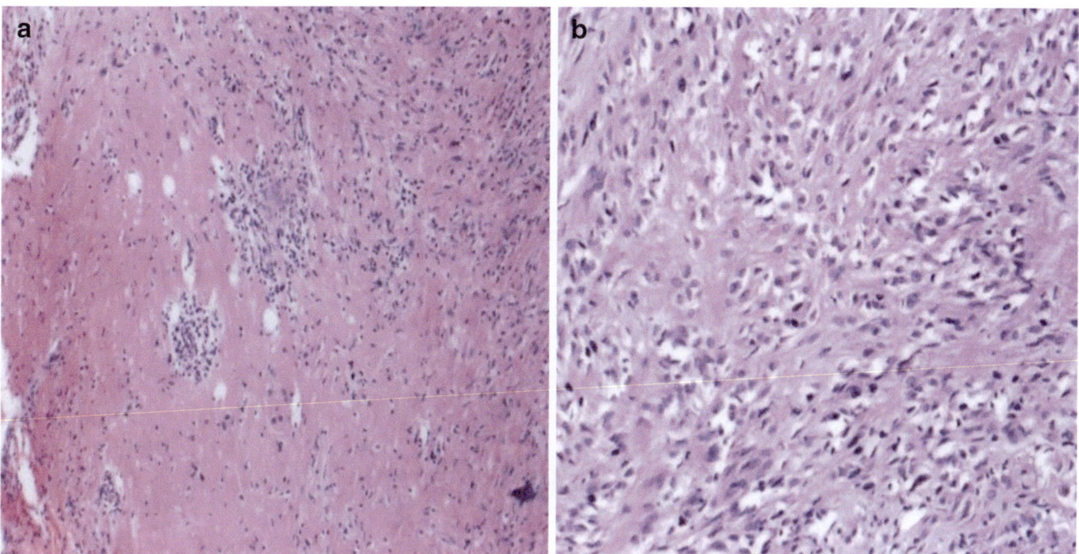

Fig. 18.5 TSGCT. (**a** and **b**) Abundant eosinophilic matrix (hyalinization) seen in long-standing lesions. It should not be mistaken for osteosarcoma, H&E ×100

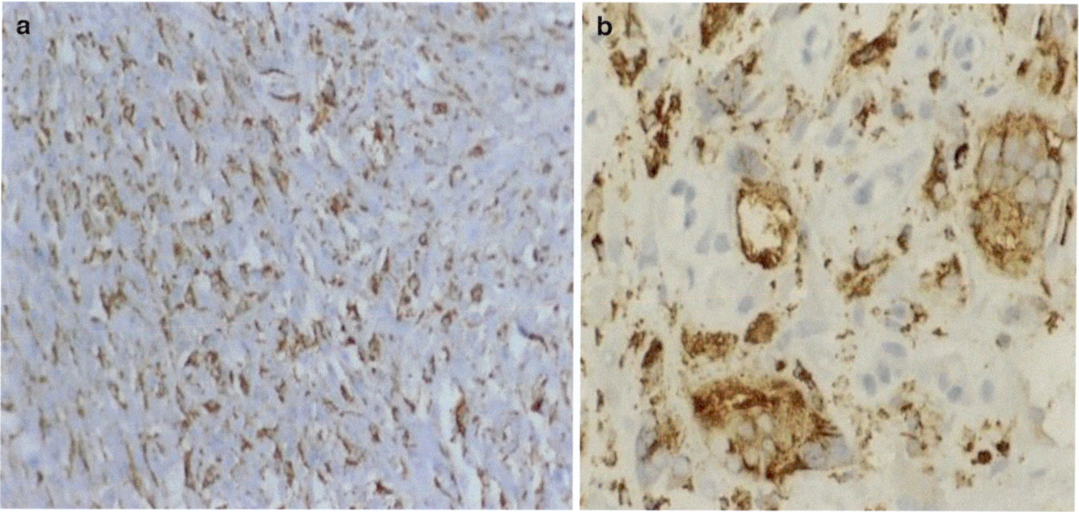

Fig. 18.6 IHC in TSGCT. (**a**) CD68 positive in stromal cells ×100. (**b**) CD68 in giant cells ×250

Osteosarcoma: Long-standing tumours may show pink hyaline material, which may be mistaken for osteosarcoma. TSGCT may also show mitosis, periosteal infiltration and adjacent fat infiltration, which should not be taken as signs of malignancy.

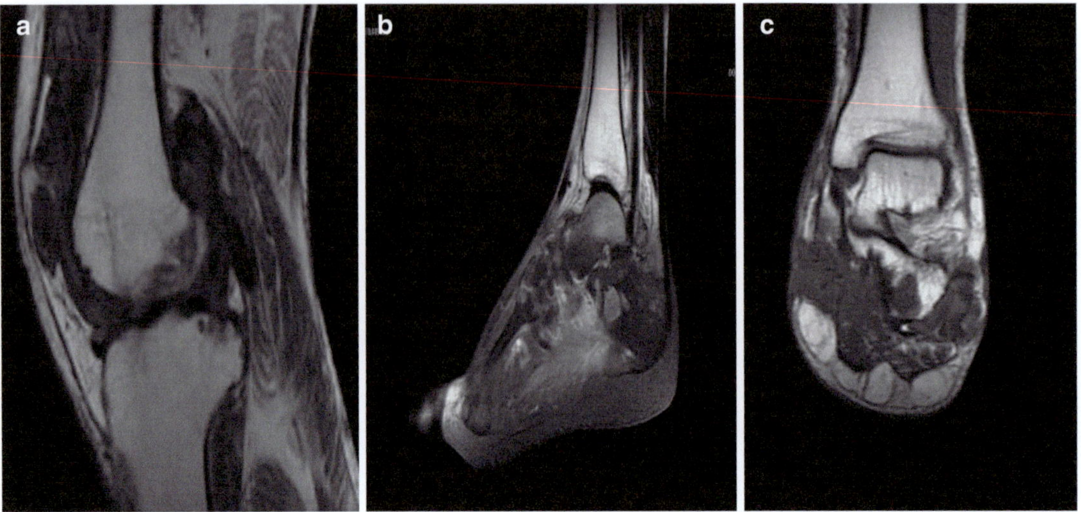

Fig. 18.7 Diffuse TSGCT knee joint. (**a**) Erosion into bone on either side of the joint. (**b** and **c**) Diffuse TSGCT of ankle joint

18.1.2.5 Treatment and Prognosis

Tumours are excised completely. Recurrences occur in 4–30% of cases, but usually are nondestructive and controllable with re-excision.

18.1.3 Tenosynovial Giant Cell Tumour-Diffuse Type (TSGCT-D)

18.1.3.1 Diffuse TSGCT-Intra-articular (Previous Terminology Pigmented Villonodular Synovitis, PVNS)

Clinical Features

Presents as long-standing painful mass, or limitation of movement. The usual age group is second–fourth decades. It is almost always monoarticular and affects large joints such as the knee, shoulder, hip and also temporomandibular joint, calcaneonavicular, mid-tarsal and interphalangeal joints. This is a slowly progressive destructive condition of the synovium and will result in significant morbidity if left untreated [8].

Radiology

They occur as ill-defined periarticular masses or as cystic lesions in the bones on either side of the joint. They are often associated with degenerative joint disease. Destruction of joint with erosion into bone on either side of the joint is typical (Fig. 18.7).

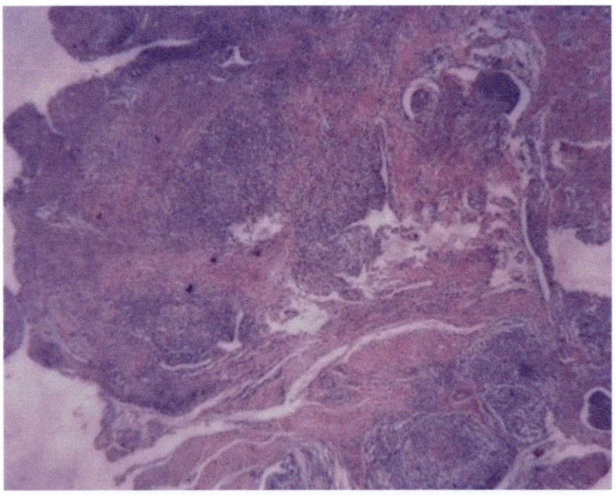

Fig. 18.8 Diffuse TSGCT—nodular infiltrate of the synovium with thick villous excrescences and zonation as the cells at the periphery of the nodules have smaller nuclei and more cytoplasm, H&E ×100

Pathology

Gross: Synovium is thickened and golden yellow to dark rusty brown with diffuse nodularity. They are large (>5 cm), firm or sponge-like. Villous-like excrescences (better appreciated if the specimen is immersed in water) is seen in intra-articular tumours. The synovial fluid may be haemorrhagic.

Microscopy: A nodular infiltrate of the synovium with thick villous excrescences and zonation is seen (Fig. 18.8). Two types of mono-

Fig. 18.9 Diffuse TSGCT: Two types of cells. (**a**) Histiocyte-like small cells and large cells with abundant cytoplasm admixed with haemosiderin-laden macrophages, H&E ×250. (**b**) Eosinophilic matrix resembling osteoid and scattered giant cells, H&E ×250. (**c**) Giant cells are less in number compared to localized form, H&E ×250

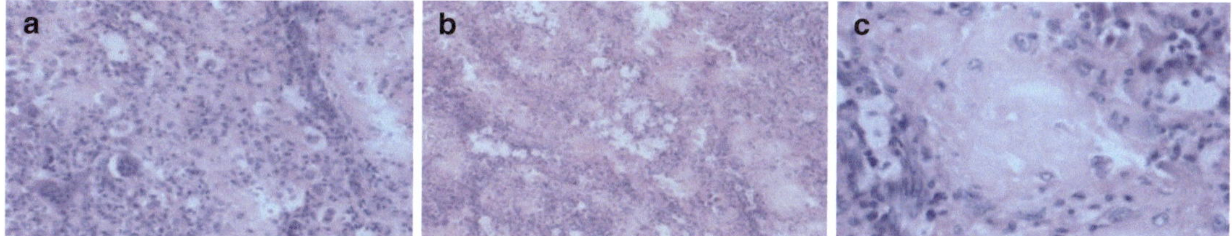

Fig. 18.10 Diffuse TSGCT. (**a**) Osteoclastic giant cells, H&E ×100. (**b**) Foamy macrophages, H&E ×100. (**c**) Hypocellular zones with hyalinization, H&E ×250

nuclear cells are seen—small and large cells, which vary in number. Small histiocyte-like cells with angulated nuclei and nuclear grooves are seen towards periphery of nodules. Larger epithelioid cells are round with thick nuclear membrane, abundant amphophilic cytoplasm and indistinct cytoplasmic processes with peripheral rim of haemosiderin granules. Scattered osteoclastic giant cells (less in number) are seen (Fig. 18.9). Mitosis is usually >5/10 HPF (up to 20/10 HPF). Fibrosis and areas of hyalinization are seen (Fig. 18.10). Spindling of mononuclear cells may be observed. Stroma can show myxoid change [10].

DD

1. Degenerative joint disease—hyperplasia of synovium, no proliferation of synovial cells.
2. Osteosarcoma (OS)—comes as DD if there is increased matrix and sheets of large cells, but OS shows definite atypia.
3. Haemosiderotic synovitis: associated with haemophilia and intra-articular bleeding. The synovium shows a diffuse brown-rusty discoloration with fine villous projections, but the larger nodules and thickened fronds of PVNS do not occur. The haemosiderin is primarily seen in synovial lining cells. Florid mononuclear or giant cell proliferation do not occur.

Molecular

Translocation involving chromosome 1 is usually seen [9].

Treatment and Prognosis

First line of management is wide excision. Recurrences are common, but malignant transformation is very rare.

18.1.3.2 Tenosynovial Giant Cell Tumour-Diffuse Type, Extra-Articular

Presence of an infiltrative, extra-articular mass with or without involvement of the adjacent joint with possible invasion of bones, and more varied histologic pattern, is the typical presentation of this entity, which makes it a real diagnostic challenge for both radiologist and pathologist.

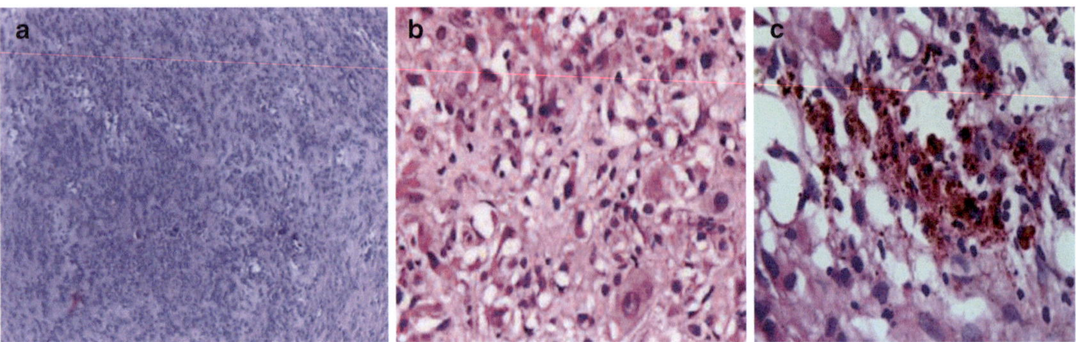

Fig. 18.11 TSGCT-D. (**a**) Cellular tumour in expansive sheets, H&E ×100. (**b**) Expansive sheets of large cells alternate with loose zones and sparse giant cells, H&E ×250. (**c**) Haemosiderophages, H&E ×250

Pathology

Gross: It presents as larger firm/spongy multinodular tumours, >5 cm with variegated yellow brown cut surface, located in periarticular region of knee. Rarely do they occur in the intramuscular or subcutaneous regions of thigh/foot. It lacks the villous architecture of PVNS.

Microscopy: Variably cellular tumour similar to TSGCT-L, but grows in expansive sheets with more frequent cleft-like spaces, lesser number or absent giant cells, variable fibrosis and mitotic activity (5–20/10 HPF) (Fig. 18.11).

Treatment

Total synovectomy for the diffuse form of TSGCT is required. Meticulous dissection and wide excision are required to tackle smaller satellite lesions extending into the surrounding tendon sheath and synovium.

Since TSGCT overexpresses colony-stimulating factor 1 (CSF1), an FDA-approved drug, pexidartinib which inhibits colony-stimulating factor-1 receptor (CSF1R), shows a good tumour response and is considered as a treatment for TGCT in patients with severe morbidity or functional limitations and in cases not amenable to surgery [9].

Prognosis

The diffuse form is often locally aggressive. Even though local recurrence can occur in 9–44% of cases, especially in extra-articular forms, the long-term prognosis is generally excellent.

18.2 Malignant Tenosynovial Giant Cell Tumour

Malignant TSGCT is a synovial based sarcoma with coexisting typical TSGCT, or a recurrent malignant tumour in a previously diagnosed case of typical benign TSGCT. The sarcomatous component shows fibrosarcomatous, myxosarcomatous and malignant fibrous histiocytoma-like features or giant cell tumour-like patterns. Metastatic lesions in lung or lymph nodes have also been reported. Most of the reported malignant cases had multiple local recurrences or widespread bony metastases after primary local excision. Microscopic features are sheets of atypical spindly cells with more than 20 mitoses/10 HPF including atypical mitosis, necrosis, myxoid change and loss of zoning phenomenon [10, 11].

18.3 Synovial Chondromatosis (SCh)

Synovial chondromatosis is a benign neoplasm of synovial tissue, first described by Laennec in 1813. It occurs within the articular joints and also in bursa or tendon sheath. Both primary and secondary types exist. The secondary type is more common than primary type and can be multiarticular. Primary SCh is formation of multiple similarly sized cartilaginous nodules in the subsynovial tissue of a joint (intra-articular), which is almost always monoarticular, or in tendon sheath or bursa (extra-articular).

18.3.1 Clinical Feature

Gradual onset of pain, stiffness, crepitus locking and limitation of movement or palpable enlarging mass around the joint are the typical presenting symptoms. Most examples of SCh involve major joints, most commonly the knee (50%). It can affect any synovial joint. A marked male predominance is seen, and the patients are usually young adults (second to seventh decades). Polyarticular involvement is more frequent in familial cases, in secondary forms and in patients with associated syndromes. Extra-articular (tenosynovial or bursal) chondromatosis is most commonly seen in the hands, feet, wrists, ankles and rarely spine.

Clinically and pathologically, three characteristic phases are recognized [12]:

1. Active intrasynovial disease, without loose bodies
2. Active intrasynovial proliferative lesions and free loose bodies
3. Multiple free osteochondral bodies without demonstrable intrasynovial disease

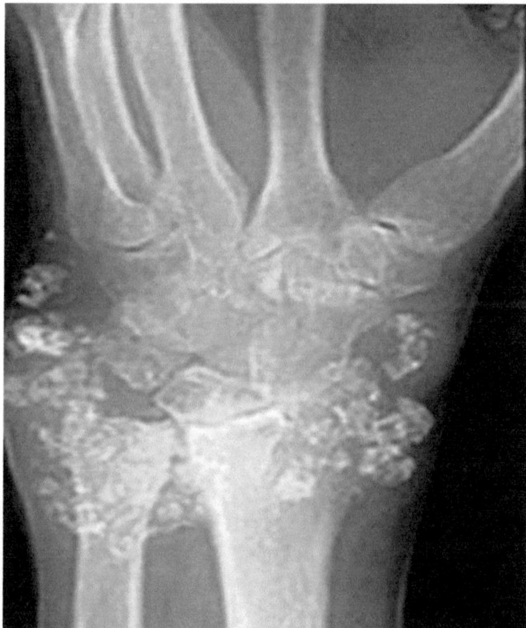

Fig. 18.12 Synovial chondromatosis wrist. Plain X-ray with multiple chondroid type of calcification with intra-articular rings and arcs

18.3.2 Radiology

Radiographic features of synovial chondromatosis are pathognomonic, as multiple intra-articular cartilaginous bodies with "ring-and-arc" feathery chondroid calcification (Fig. 18.12). Extrinsic erosion of nearby bones of the joint is seen in 20–50% of cases [13]. The involved bones can be at risk for developing a pathologic fracture. Chondroid nodules may be seen floating freely in the joint cavity (Fig. 18.13).

18.3.3 Pathology

Gross: Diffuse involvement of the joint surface seen as few to numerous bluish white, multilobulated, almost similar sized nodular projections of hyaline cartilage covered by hyperplastic synovial lining (Fig. 18.14). These glistening white nodules give a "cobblestone" appearance to the synovium.

Microscopy: The proliferating cartilage nodules are seen in lobules with clustering of chon-

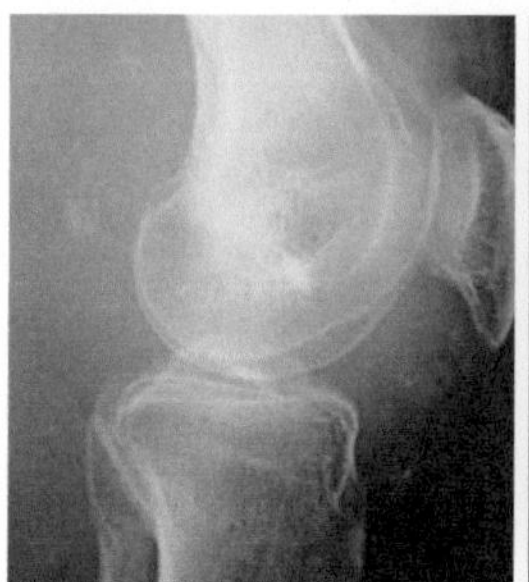
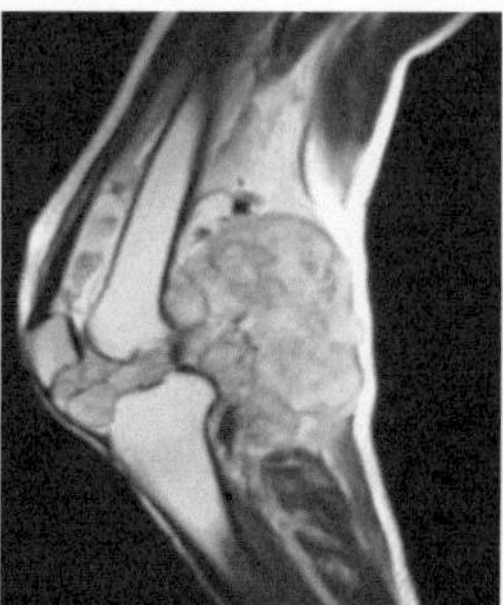
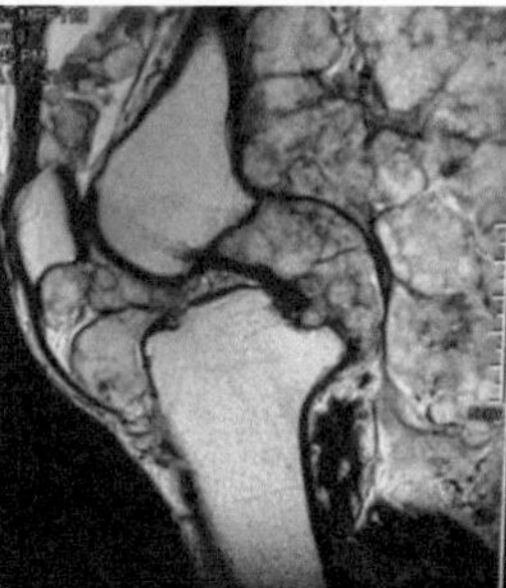
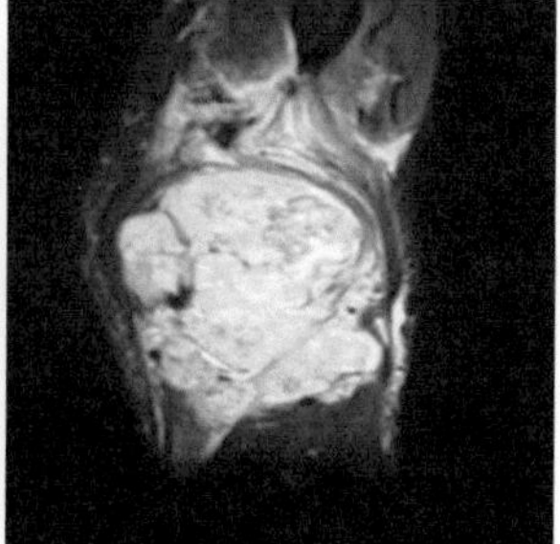

Fig. 18.13 SCh knee in a 65-year-old male with chondrosarcomatous transformation

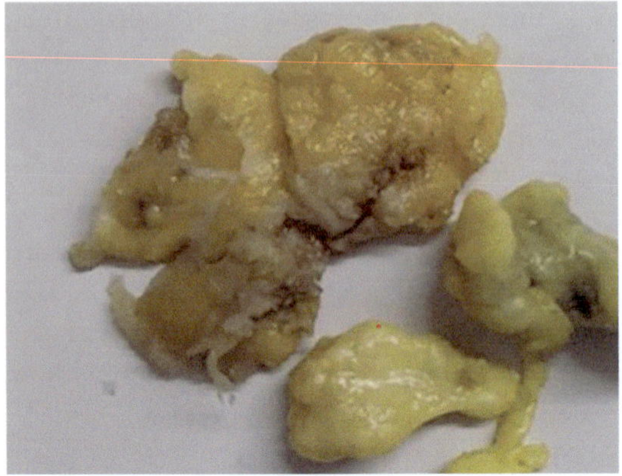

Fig. 18.14 SCh-synovectomy specimen with multiple large pedunculated/sessile chondroid/osteocartilaginous nodules covered by a thickened synovium (intrasynovial phase)

drocytes, which is a sign of benignity (Figs. 18.15 and 18.16). Endochondral ossification is common, but myxoid change is unusual. Chondrocytes with moderate or marked atypia and double-nucleated cells can be seen. When the SCh exhibits aggressive clinical, radiographic or histologic features, differentiation from synovial chondrosarcoma (SCHS) can be challenging [14].

18.3.4 DD

1. Osteocartilaginous loose bodies in degenerative joint disease:

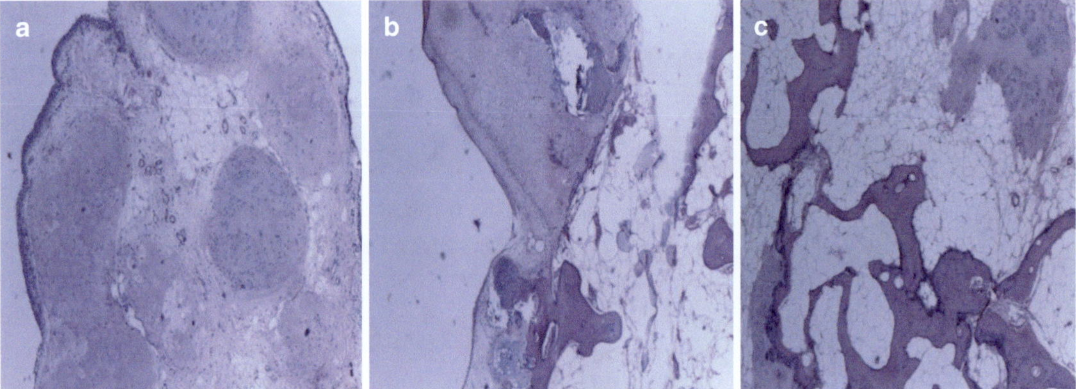

Fig. 18.15 SCh. (**a**) Synovial nodules with clustering of chondrocytes, H&E ×40. (**b**) Focal ossification, H&E ×40. (**c**) Minimal infiltration into underlying bone is permissible with preservation of characteristic clustering of chondrocytes, H&E ×40

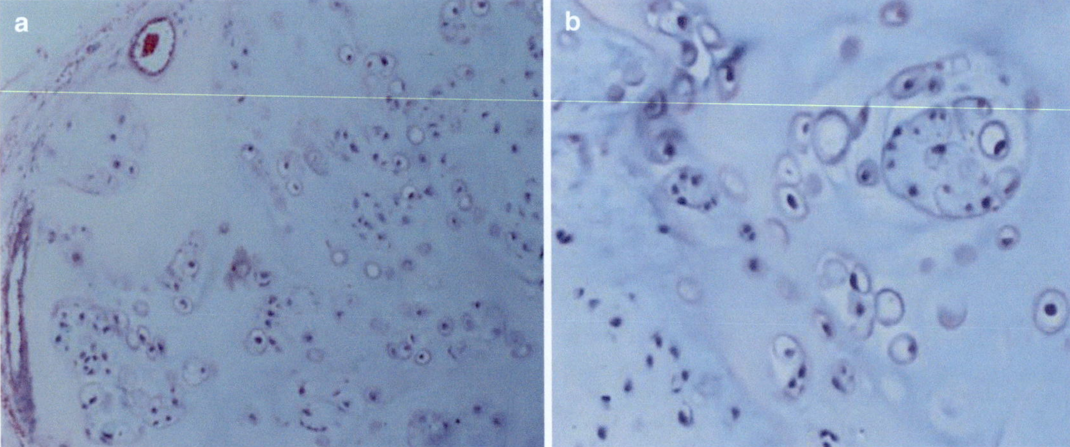

Fig. 18.16 SCh. (**a**) Lobules of hyaline cartilage, H&E ×100. (**b**) Clustering of chondrocytes, H&E ×250

- Grossly, white and firm, fewer in number, smaller and float freely in the joint cavity
- Lacks clustering and nuclear changes of chondrocytes
- Cartilage arranged in layers—tree bark appearance

2. Juxta-articular chondroma:

- Well-circumscribed mineralized mass
- Radiologically fully mineralized resembling extra patella
- Proliferation of cartilage, focal clustering, trabecular bone formation

3. Chondrosarcoma:

- Mostly malignancy in synovial chondromatosis
- Marked myxoid change of the matrix
- Loss of clustering, sheets of chondrocytes
- Crowding and spindling of nuclei

18.3.5 Molecular

Recurrent FN1-ACVR2A rearrangements (fusion between fibronectin 1 (FN1) and activin receptor 2A (ACVR2A)) are seen in 57% of synovial chondromatosis and in 75% of chondrosarcoma secondary to synovial chondromatosis.

18.3.6 Treatment and Prognosis

It is a self-limited process that may recur locally. Recurrence rates range from 3% to 23%; higher rate is seen in tenosynovial cases. In asymptomatic patients, invasive procedures should be avoided as there is a possibility that the nodules may spontaneously get resorbed over time. If gross examination at the time of surgery shows multiple free osteochondral bodies (the disease is in the third phase), then synovectomy may not be necessary. Secondary synovial chondromatosis has indolent course, treated with simple removal of loose bodies and correction of the underlying cause.

18.3.7 Malignant transformation of SCh

Secondary synovial chondrosarcoma (SCHS) has been reported in 1–10% of patients with Sch and is very difficult to distinguish from benign disease itself [13]. Average time to develop malignancy is 11.2 years. Many experts are of the opinion that a history of rapid deterioration in a long-standing case or rapid recurrence after synovectomy may indicate malignant transformation. The criteria to document malignant transformation of an SCh include a pre-existing histologically proven SCh with recurrent tumour as SCHS or coexistence of both areas of SCh and SCHS in the same resected specimen. The only MRI criterion of malignancy is the invasion of the tumour into the bone medullary canal. Superficial erosion of bone can occur in Sch. Morphologically, lack of lobulation with sheets of atypical chondrocytes, lack of clustering of chondrocytes and extensive myxoid changes of matrix are seen (Fig. 18.17). IDH mutations are not present in synovial chondromatosis, whereas IDH1 or IDH2 mutations have been reported in 50–80% of chondrosarcomas [14, 15].

18.3.8 Features of Malignancy in Synovial Chondromatosis [14]

- Sheets of chondrocytes without lobular architecture
- Marked myxoid change of the matrix
- Lack of clustering of cells
- Crowding and spindling of nuclei

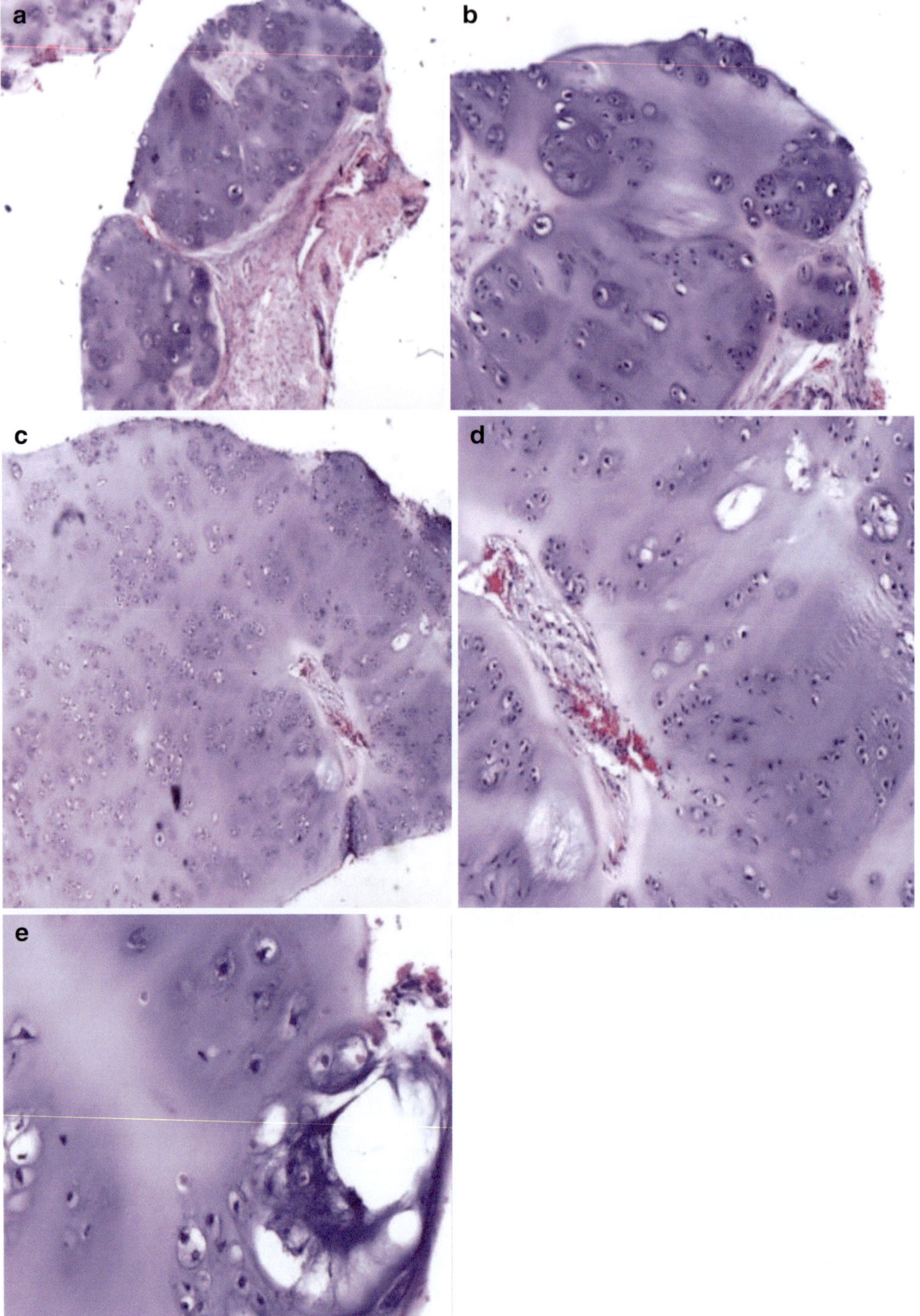

Fig. 18.17 Synovial chondromatosis knee joint in a 65-year-old male. (**a**) Lobules of hyaline cartilage with clustering of chondrocytes, H&E ×40. (**b**) H&E ×250. Malignant transformation was seen in the same case. (**c**) Lobules of cellular cartilage with lack of lobulation, H&E ×100. (d) Lack of clustering of chondrocytes, H&E ×100. (**e**) Pleomorphism of chondrocytes, double-nucleated cells with extensive myxoid change (**c**, **d** and **e** represent areas of malignant transformation)

18.4 Synovial Chondrosarcoma (SCHS)

SCHS arising from the synovial membrane is very rare. It may arise as a primary synovial tumour or as malignant transformation of synovial chondromatosis.

18.4.1 Clinical

Rapid recent progression of symptoms, recurrence within 12 months after resection, soft tissue infiltration of tumour and larger tumour size are the factors which favour SCHS. Even though knee joint is affected commonly, rarely other joints such as the hip, elbow or ankle are affected.

18.4.2 Radiology

Both synovial chondromatosis and synovial chondrosarcoma can have overlapping features on radiographs and MRI. Extra-capsular extension and metaplastic chondroid features are non-specific. The development of destructive changes around the affected joint favours synovial chondrosarcoma [15]. But care should be taken to differentiate these destructive changes from periarticular erosions that can present in synovial chondromatosis. In patients with documented primary synovial chondromatosis, recently detected soft tissue mass and destructive changes in the adjacent bones and the joint should alert one to the development of a secondary synovial chondrosarcoma. Intramedullary infiltration is the only sign of malignancy in a few cases. Radiologically, a permeative and destructive pattern rather than an erosive pattern is suspicious for malignancy.

To differentiate benign from malignant chondroid tumours is difficult based on pathology alone. A diagnosis of benign or even low-grade synovial tumour should be viewed with high suspicion in the setting of a massive tumour. Large size is a strong indicator of aggressive and malignant behaviour. At the interface between tumour and healthy bone, SCh seems to erode the bone with "pushing margins" [12], while the SCHS shows a permeative behaviour with typical "filling up" of marrow spaces. The distinguishing features of synovial chondrosarcoma are arrangement of tumour cells in sheets, loss of the "clustering" growth pattern, extensive myxoid change in the matrix, areas of necrosis, spindling of tumour cells at the periphery of chondroid lobules and permeation of bone trabeculae [14–16]. Pulmonary metastasis may develop.

18.4.3 Treatment and Prognosis

The extent of the disease determines the type of surgery. Radiological correlation with open biopsy is recommended prior to radical surgical resection/amputation in cases with suspicious features of malignancy. The behaviour is similar to skeletal chondrosarcoma with around 30% having metastatic disease.

18.5 Synovial Haemangioma

This is a solitary benign lesion which can be localized or diffuse.

18.5.1 Clinical Feature

Most common presentation is recurrent painless monoarticular atraumatic bloody joint effusions in the knee joints of children and adolescents [17]. Elbow, wrist, ankle and tendon sheaths are also affected. It is usually associated with an adjacent cutaneous or deep soft tissue haemangioma.

18.5.2 Pathogenesis

It is unclear. They are thought to be reactive/vascular malformation/neoplastic.

18.5.3 Radiology

It shows pathognomonic features of haemangioma with phleboliths.

18.5.4 Pathology

Gross: Soft, mahogany brown doughy mass with villous hyperplasia of overlying synovium.

Microscopy: Most common type is cavernous haemangioma, followed by lobular capillary haemangioma, arteriovenous haemangioma or venous haemangioma containing variable amounts of adipose, fibrous and muscle tissue, along with intravascular thrombi [18]. The overlying hyperplastic synovium may show abundant iron deposition in chronic cases from repeated injury and haemarthrosis (Fig. 18.18).

18.5.5 Prognosis

Localized type has good prognosis. Recurrence rate is low. Diffuse type is difficult to resect arthroscopically and has greater chance of recurrence [19].

A comparison of synovial chondromatosis, synovial haemangioma and lipoma arborescens is given in Table 18.2.

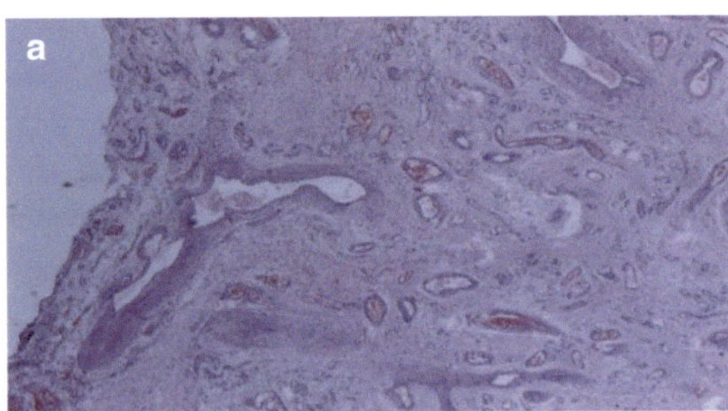

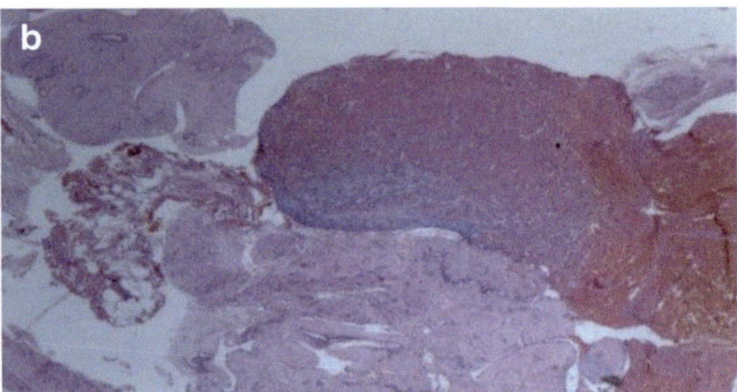

Fig. 18.18 (**a**) Arteriovenous haemangioma covered by synovium, H&E ×100. (**b**) With evidence of organizing haematoma, H&E ×250

Table 18.2 Key points on synovial chondromatosis (Syn.chondromatosis), synovial haemangioma (Syn.haemangioma) and lipoma arborescens

Common features of	Syn.chondromatosis	Syn.haemangioma	Lipoma arborescens
Site of involvement	Knee	Knee	Supra-patellar pouch
Clinical feature	Crepitus, locking, restricted joint movement	Recurrent, painless monoarticular atraumatic bloody joint effusion	Progressive pain and intermittent episodes of joint effusion
Age group and sex	Second to seventh decades Male	Children and adolescents	Second to third decade, male
Types	Primary/secondary, intra/extra-articular, mono/polyarticular	Localized or diffuse	Primary/secondary Mono/polyarticular
Macroscopy	Loose body, cobblestone	Soft, mahogany brown doughy mass with villous hyperplasia of synovium	Intra-articular fatty mass lesions
Microscopy	Clustering and nodular proliferation of chondrocytes, superficial erosion of bone	Cavernous/capillary/AV haemangioma, phleboliths and iron deposition	Villous lipomatous proliferation of synovium
IHC and molecular marker	Recurrent FN1-ACVR2A rearrangements		
Worrisome features	Invasion of the bone medullary cavity, lack of lobulation and clustering, presence of sheets of spindly chondrocytes and extensive myxoid changes of matrix	High recurrence for diffuse type	Surgical resection (synovectomy) for symptomatic lipoma

18.6 Lipoma Arborescens

Lipoma arborescens/diffuse lipoma of joint are a chronic, slowly progressive benign intra-articular lesion characterized by villous lipomatous proliferation of the synovium [20]. This can be primary or secondary. Primary type is idiopathic. Albert Hoffa, a German surgeon, first described it in 1904 (Hoffa's disease). It is usually a monoarticular disease which occurs in young males between the second and third decades of life. Secondary type is a pseudotumour of synovium. It is more common, may be bilateral and involving multiple joints and possibly due to inappropriate fat deposition and is usually seen in elderly patients. It is associated with degenerative diseases, trauma, meniscal injury, rheumatoid arthritis, psoriasis, diabetes mellitus or synovitis.

18.6.1 Clinical Feature

Progressive pain accompanied by intermittent episodes of joint effusion. There may be intermittent worsening of pain and swelling resulting from trapping of hypertrophied fatty villi in between the moving joint surfaces. The suprapatellar pouch of the knee joint is usually involved. Other involved joints are shoulder, hip, elbow, ankle and wrist, periarticular bursae and tendon sheaths.

18.6.2 Radiology

Radiographs and USG images of the lesion are characteristic with absence of any bony or articular surface erosion. Lucent soft tissue mass is seen in the periarticular tissue. On ultrasonography, the villous fatty projections of lipoma arborescens typically display a high echo pattern, similar to that of adjacent subcutaneous fat, like any other fat-containing lesion. MR imaging of lipoma arborescens shows villous or nodular foci in both T1- and T2-weighted images, which is similar to the adjacent fat and distinguishes it from other intra-articular mass-like lesions.

18.6.3 Microscopy

Shows villous lipomatous proliferation of synovium with papillaroid structures. They are lined by synovium, and the stroma contains lobules of adipocytes [21]. Osseous and chondroid metaplasia can occur (Figs. 18.19 and 18.20).

18.6.4 Treatment and Prognosis

An intra-articular injection of corticosteroids may give temporary relief of symptoms. The definitive treatment for symptomatic lipoma is surgical resection (synovectomy) by open

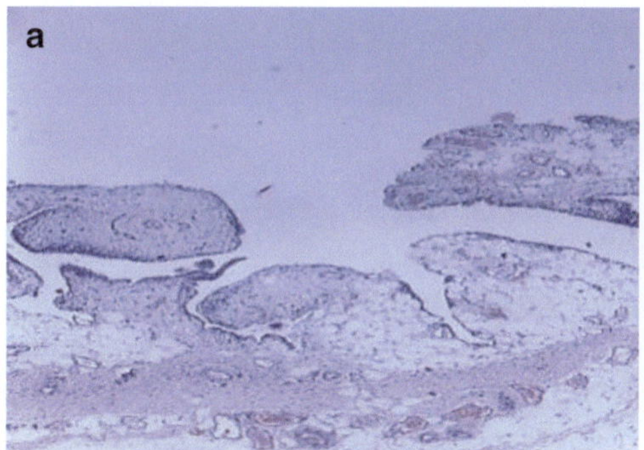

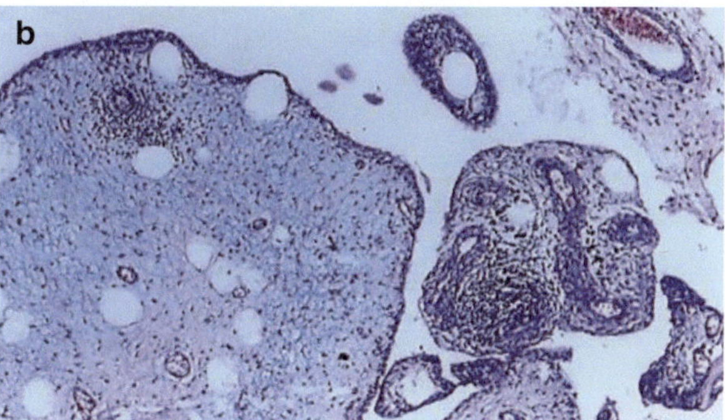

Fig. 18.19 Lipoma arborescens. (**a**) Papillaroid structures lined by synovium with stromal adipocytes, H&E ×40. (**b**) H&E ×100. Primary and secondary lipoma arborescens can be differentiated only by eliciting associated pathology

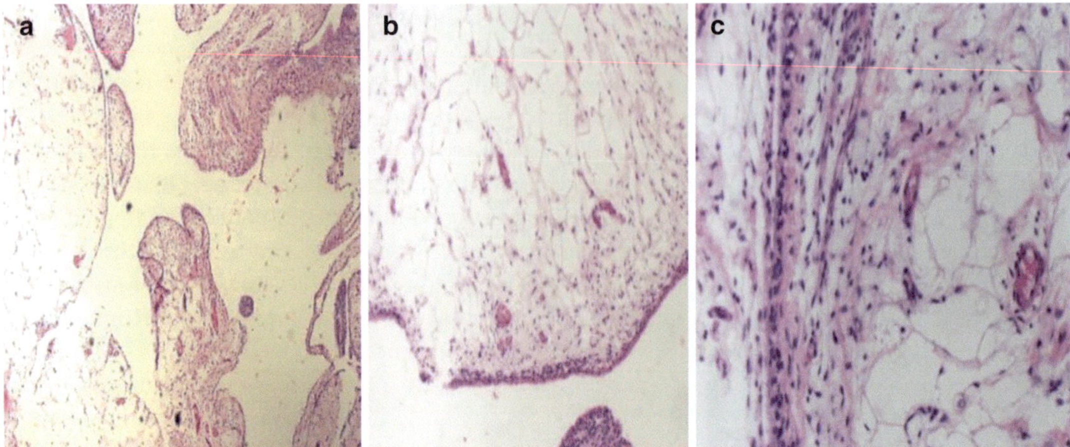

Fig. 18.20 Synovial lipoma. (**a** and **b**) Adipocytes in lobules beneath synovial lining, H&E ×40. (**c**) Synovial lining and adipocytes under the lining epithelium, H&E ×100

arthrotomy or arthroscopy. Recurrence after synovectomy is very rare. In asymptomatic patients, a conservative treatment is indicated [22].

18.7 Nodular Fasciitis

Nodular fasciitis is a benign reactive myofibroblastic proliferation, which typically occurs in young adults with a history of a rapidly growing mass in the subcutaneous tissue, dermis, muscle or intravascular locations in the upper extremities, trunk and head and neck region. Interestingly, nodular fasciitis has also been reported in intra-articular location [23], parotid gland and urinary bladder.

18.7.1 Clinical

Intra-articular nodular fasciitis most frequently occurs in the knees and shoulders. The age range is between 10 and 50 years.

18.7.2 Pathology

Gross: It is seen as a polypoid mass with smooth external surface and a tan-white homogeneous soft cut surface.

Microscopy: It is similar to its more common soft tissue counterpart. These are non-encapsulated and well-circumscribed variably cellular spindle cell lesion centred directly underneath the synovium and arranged in a "tissue culture-like" fashion with accompanying extravasation of red blood cells [23] (Fig. 18.21). A greater tendency for stromal hyalinization and adjacent haemosiderin deposition may be seen. They stain positive for SMA, and Ki-67 is low (around 10%).

18.7.3 Treatment and Prognosis

Excision appears to be curative. They generally do not recur.

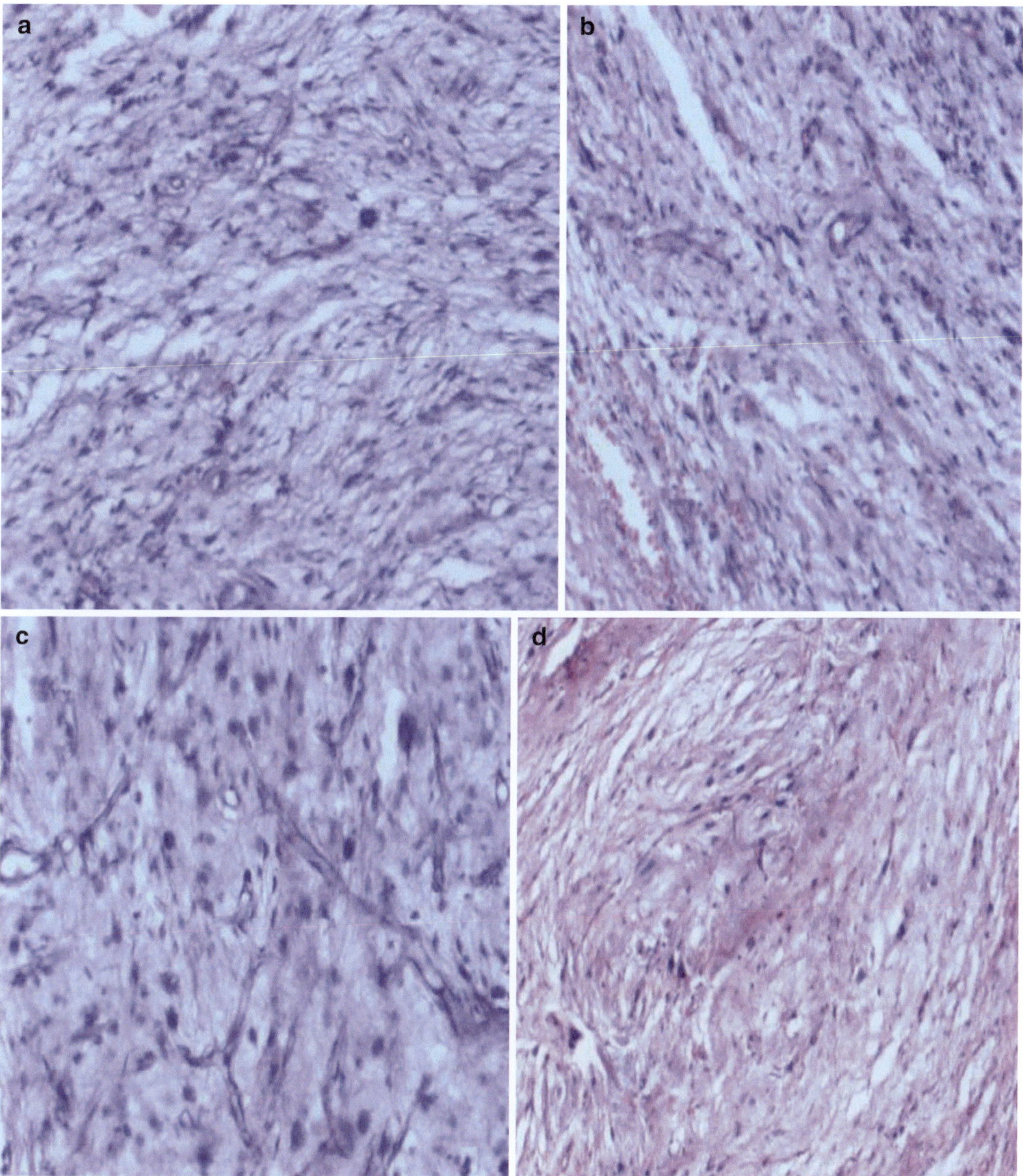

Fig. 18.21 Nodular fasciitis. (**a–d**) Variably cellular "tissue culture-like" spindle cell lesion with extravasation of red blood cells, H&E ×100

18.8 Tenosynovial Fibroma/ Fibroma of Tendon Sheath

Tenosynovial fibroma is a benign, uncommon tumour.

18.8.1 Clinical Features

Most common in adult men. It is more commonly seen in the hands than in the feet, rarely in the toes, knee (posterior joint capsule, posterior cruciate ligament, supra-patellar pouch), radio-ulnar joint, temporomandibular joint and shoulder joint [24, 25].

18.8.2 Pathology

Gross: It is a well-circumscribed, multinodular, dense, fibrous tumour attached to tendon or tendon sheath with a diffuse pearly white lobulated appearance. Size varies from 0.5 to 5.5 cm. Cleft-like spaces are seen.

Microscopy: It shows hypocellular and collagenous lesion with spindle- or stellate-shaped fibroblasts, a partly myxoid stroma and slit-like vessels. Clefting or pseudovascular spaces may be seen. Focal hypercellularity with a tissue culture-like appearance resembling nodular fasciitis is seen in some tumours [26] (Fig. 18.22).

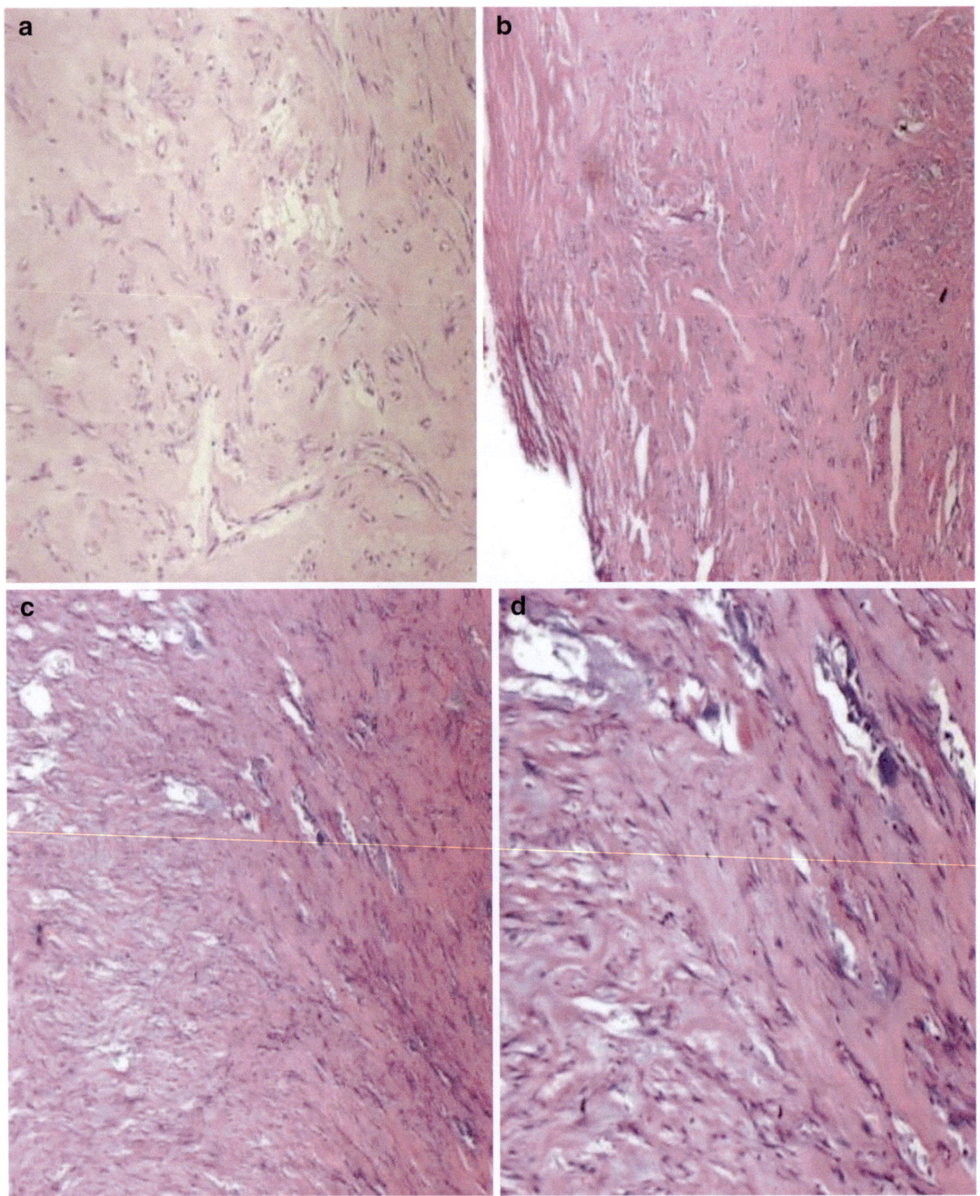

Fig. 18.22 Fibroma of tendon sheath. (**a** and **b**) Hypocellular collagenous lesion, H&E ×40. (**c**) Spindle cells with slit-like vessels, H&E ×100. (**d**) H&E ×250

18.8.3 IHC and Molecular

There is no specific IHC for fibroma. FOSL1 is usually negative compared to its positivity in desmoplastic fibroblastoma. Cellular fibromas of tendon sheath may show USP6 rearrangement as seen in nodular fasciitis [27].

18.8.4 Treatment and Prognosis

Excision appears to be curative with a recurrence rate of 5–10% [27].

18.9 Intra-articular Osteochondromas

Osteochondromas, also termed exostoses, are commonest benign osseous growths that are capped with hyaline cartilage with endochondral ossification in between. They typically occur extra-articularly around the growth plate of long bones in children and typically grow away from the nearby joint. These tumours are seen rarely intra-articularly and are often misdiagnosed, as they are only detectable through imaging or arthroscopic exploration. The osteochondromas arising from the neck of the femur and the talus could be totally intra-articular as these are located within the joints. The knee is also a common location for intra-articular osteochondromas due to the large size of the joint capsule. In contrast to the extra-articular osteochondromas, the intra-articular osteochondromas show thinner layers of fibrous perichondrium and a cartilage cap, with a thicker layer of bone. If they are pedunculated, they may get fractured and become intra-articular loose bodies. Possibility of associated hereditary multiple osteochondromas (HMO), an autosomal dominant bone disorder, can also occur [28].

18.10 Intra-articular Synovial Sarcoma

Synovial sarcoma (SS) is a high-grade sarcoma with variable epithelial differentiation. It is the second common sarcoma of soft tissue in children and young adults, after rhabdomyosarcoma. The "SS" has been proposed to originate from myogenic cell lines, not from synovium. But the name is derived due to its morphological similarity to the embryonic synovium. It may occur at any site. The most common sites are periarticular regions. It also occurs in sites where no synovial tissue is present, e.g. parapharyngeal or abdominal locations. The most frequent site is the lower (62%) and upper (21%) extremities [29]. Less common sites include the head and neck, thorax, pelvis and paravertebral regions.

Approximately 3–5% of SS cases have been estimated to be intra-articular where the most challenging differential diagnosis is localized TSGCT [30, 31].

18.10.1 Clinical

These present as large calcified mass with joint effusion in young males. Most tumours are more than 5 cm in size.

18.10.2 Pathology

Microscopy: As with the soft tissue counterpart, these tumours can also have biphasic, monophasic (purely epithelioid or fibroblastic) appearance with poorly differentiated myxoid, ossifying and calcifying areas. Cells are short spindly, cellular with a haemangiopericytic vasculature in between. Biphasic type shows epithelioid cell clusters, sometimes in glandular pattern (Fig. 18.23). Poorly differentiated SS is often confused with other small round cell tumours (Fig. 18.24).

18.10.3 IHC

Vimentin is positive. Both cytokeratin and EMA are positive in the epithelial areas and in the spindle cell component. Synovial sarcomas express CD99 and BCL2, whereas CD34 is almost always absent (Fig. 18.25a, b). Transducin-like enhancer of split 1 (TLE-1) is a good marker for the diagnosis of synovial sarcoma. Diffuse strong nuclear positivity is seen (Fig. 18.25c). Recently, SS18-

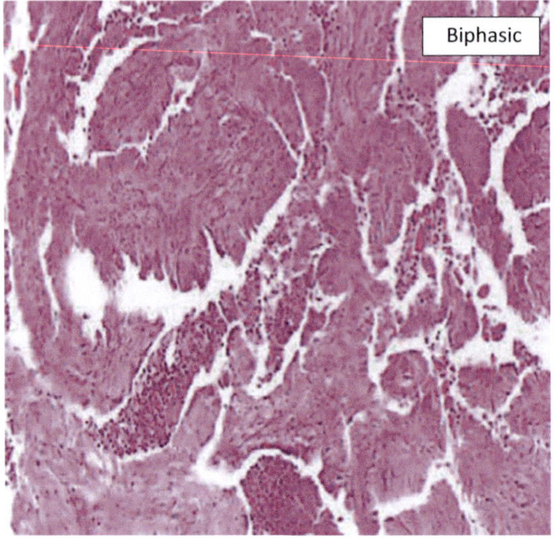

Fig. 18.23 Biphasic synovial sarcoma: epithelioid and spindle cells, H&E ×100

SSX antibody is available with 95% sensitivity and 100% specificity for the diagnosis of synovial sarcoma.

18.10.4 Molecular

A specific chromosomal translocation t(X; 18) (p11; q11) is present in about 90% of cases. SS18-SSX1/2/4 gene fusion is detected commonly by FISH, RT-PCR and NGS methods. The degree of epithelial differentiation is decided by the translocation partner through inhibition of snail or slug genes leading to derepression of E-cadherin. Stronger E-cadherin and extracellular matrix protein MMP2 expression leads to biphasic morphology. SS18-SSX1 translocation is a poor prognostic factor.

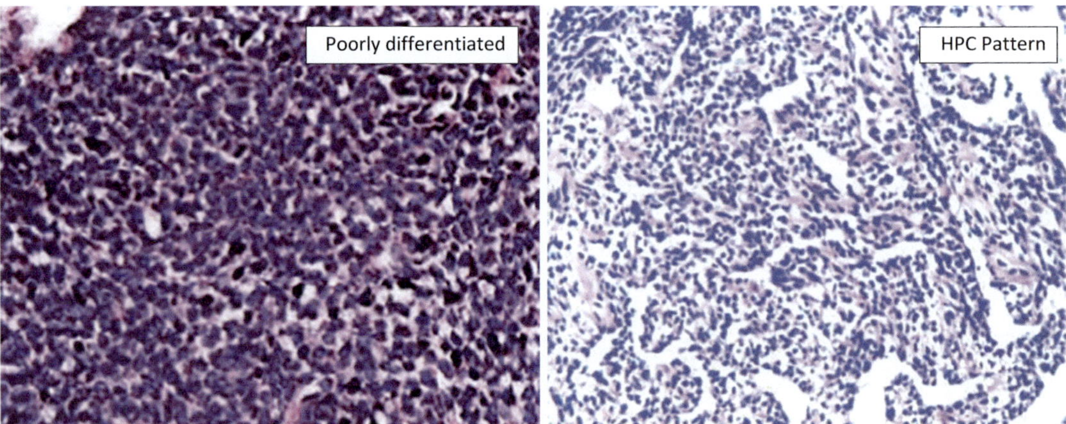

Fig. 18.24 Synovial sarcoma: monophasic. (**a**) Cellular short spindly cells, H&E ×100. (**b**) Haemangiopericytomatous vascular pattern, H&E ×100

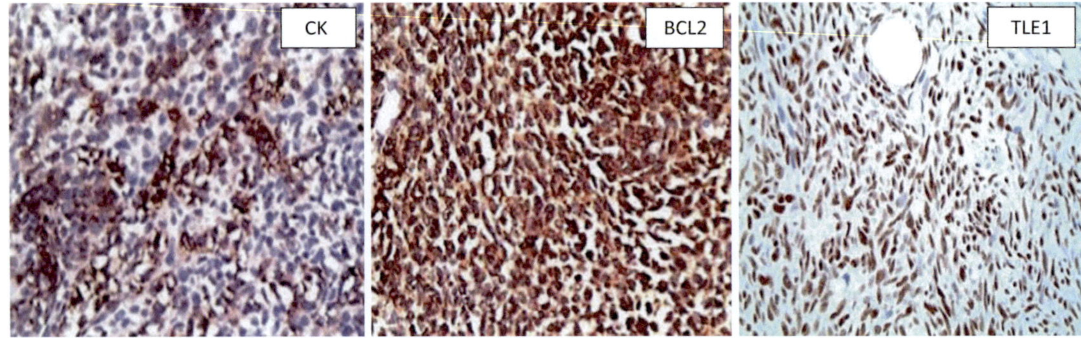

Fig. 18.25 IHC. (**a**) Cytokeratin (AE1/AE3) ×100. (**b**) BCL2 ×100. (**c**) TLE-1 positive ×100. TLE-1 shows diffuse and strong nuclear positivity

18.10.5 Treatment and Prognosis

Wide local excision with negative margins is required. About 50% of patients develop metastasis; most common sites are the lungs and lymph nodes followed by bones, which may occur even after 5–10 years. The adverse prognostic factors are larger tumour size, presence of metastasis at the time of diagnosis and high histological grade with positive margins [29].

18.11 Tumour-Like Lesions of Synovium

Cysts and crystal deposition diseases constitute the tumour-like lesions. Cysts, synovial (bursal cysts), ganglion and meniscal cysts, are described in Chap. 17.

18.11.1 Crystal Deposition Diseases

The common crystal deposition diseases that affect joints are gout (monosodium urate crystal deposition disease), calcium pyrophosphate dihydrate crystal deposition disease (CPPD), calcium hydroxyapatite crystal deposition disease and mixed calcium phosphate crystal deposition disease. Chondrocalcinosis is widespread calcification of articular cartilage, which usually is indicative of CPPD crystal deposition and may involve fibrocartilage or hyaline cartilage.

18.11.1.1 Gout Arthritis Divitum (Disease of Kings)

Gout is a metabolic disorder caused by hyperuricaemia leading to supersaturation and precipitation of monosodium urate (MSU) crystals in joints, bones and soft tissues resulting in inflammation and tissue damage [32]. Gout is historically known as "the disease of kings" or rich man's disease or king of pains. It is a disease known since the time of the ancient Egyptians and is a destructive chronic inflammatory disease characterized by recurrent flares of acute monoarthritis. The inflammatory process is self-limited, on average within 1–2 weeks.

Primary gout—metabolic disease (90%): Idiopathic with overproduction of uric acid or known enzyme defects.

Secondary gout (10%): Increased nucleic acid turnover due to leukaemia/lymphoma and chronic renal disease.

Clinical Features

Gout can present as asymptomatic hyperuricaemia, acute arthritis often with excruciating pain, erythema, swelling and exquisite tenderness, chronic tophaceous arthritis, monoarthritis of first metatarso-phalangeal joint (podagra) and gouty nephropathy [33].

Pathogenesis

Hyperuricaemia results from deregulation of renal and gut excretion of urate due to genetic or environmental factors. Synovial fluid having a low pH is a poor solvent of MSU crystals. Before plasma gets supersaturated, the synovial fluid is supersaturated. It is deposited mainly in peripheral joints, such as the foot where the temperature is low. So, the manifestations of gout commonly occur in foot. The accumulation of urate crystals in soft tissues and joints activates monocytes and macrophages. These macrophages ingest the crystals by phagocytosis. The pro-inflammatory cytokines and chemokines are released, resulting in an acute inflammatory reaction with infiltration of neutrophils into the joints. NLRP3 inflammasome and interleukin-1β play an important role in the initiation of acute gout flares. Repeated attacks of acute arthritis cause formation of tophi in synovial membranes and periarticular tissue, which eventually damages joints. Since inflammasome and interleukin 1 (IL-1) are involved in the pathogenesis of inflammation in gout, it can be treated with appropriate drugs because these lesions are intolerant to routine anti-inflammatory therapies [34].

Radiology Findings

Tophi are radiolucent. Peculiar clasp-like erosion or rat-bite erosions are seen. It is known as Granger's overhanging edges and sclerotic margins. On ultrasonography, the double-contour sign and the snowstorm appearance of crystals within synovial fluid are seen.

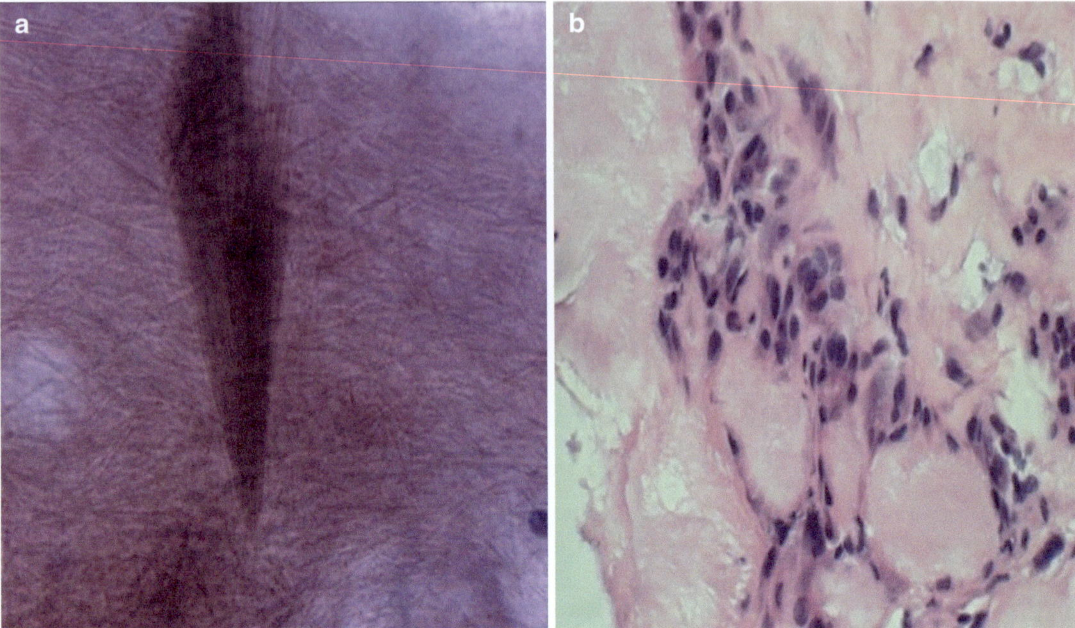

Fig. 18.26 Gout. (**a**) Cytology of gout nodule showing broom-like crystals, Pap ×100. (**b**) Gouty tophi surrounded by giant cells, H&E ×400. These crystals have negative birefringence on polarized light

Pathology

The tophus, which is the pathognomonic hallmark of this disorder, commonly occurs at the first metatarso-phalangeal joint. Other areas are Achilles tendon, peroneal tendon, helix of the ear, olecranon bursa and finger pad and also as subcutaneous nodules in the hands, elbows and feet.

Gross: Appear as variably sized irregular, nodular, plaque-like, fungiform exophytic firm, gritty or semi-solid, cheesy to gelatinous or chalky white nodule.

Microscopy: The crystals dissolve readily in water-based solutions; however, fixation in alcohol will help to preserve the crystals. Alternatively, thickly sectioned, unstained and cover-slipped sections may allow the crystal to be visualized. Staining with non-aqueous alcoholic eosin gives a negative birefringence of these crystals. This is a useful adjunct to the routine H&E stain for differentiating MSU crystals from positive birefringence of rhomboid- to rod-shaped pleomorphic CPPD crystals in pseudogout [35]. It can also be differentiated from the psammoma body-like calcospherites of CHA crystals without birefringence in tumoural calcinosis. Tophus is an aggregate of MSU crystalline material as acellular zone surrounded by a corona zone consisting of foreign body-type multinucleated giant cells, histiocytes, fibroblasts, lymphocytes and plasma cells. The inflamed synovium shows small clusters of MSU crystals, which are slender, long and needle-like. They are negatively birefringent with pannus formation and show destruction of the underlying bone [36] (Fig. 18.26).

18.11.1.2 Calcium Pyrophosphate Dihydrate Crystal Deposition Disease (CPPD)

Synonyms: Pseudogout, chondrocalcinosis

Calcium and pyrophosphate crystal precipitates in the joint spaces. It gets deposited within the synovium and articular cartilage, causing a destructive inflammatory reaction and symptomatic joint effusion.

Clinical Features

Symptoms and age group same as osteoarthritis. Occasional flare similar to gout is observed. Patello-femoral joint is most frequently affected, which is a characteristic feature of CPPD arthritis.

Pathogenesis

The pathogenesis of CPPD disease is not well understood. There are sporadic, hereditary and secondary types of CPPD. The secondary form occurs in hyperparathyroidism, haemochromatosis, hypomagnesaemia, hypophosphatasia, gout, X-linked hypophosphataemic rickets, hypothyroidism, ochronosis and diabetes.

Radiology Findings

White lines of chondrocalcinosis result from calcification of articular cartilage, capsule or synovium, Achilles tendon or plantar fascia. The confirmation of diagnosis is done by demonstration of CPP crystals in tissue or synovial fluid by X-ray diffraction, Fourier transform infrared [FTIR] spectroscopy, etc.

Pathology

It shows calcification of joint cartilage which enlarges into large chalky white friable masses. It is distinguishable from gout by their positive birefringence under polarized light [37]. Histologically, the lesions sometimes have cellular atypia in chondrocytes, suggestive of a malignant cartilage tumour mimicking soft tissue chondrosarcoma (Fig. 18.27). Septic arthritis can coexist with these crystal deposition diseases. Other differentials include trauma, bleeding, polymyalgia rheumatica and other crystal deposition diseases.

Points to Remember

- TSGCT is the most common benign tumour of the tendon sheath and synovium.
- TSGCT shows *CSF1* overexpression or 1p13 (*CSF1*) rearrangements.
- The localized TSGCT, previously known as giant cell tumour of tendon sheath, is most frequent in the hands, is small in size and is indolent.
- The diffuse TSGCT, previously known as pigmented villonodular synovitis, affects larger joints of younger patients and is larger in size (>5 cm), often intra-articular and locally aggressive with infiltrative growth pattern and with higher tendency to recur.
- Malignant TSGCT is a synovial based sarcoma with coexisting typical TSGCT, or a recurrent malignant tumour at the site of previous typical benign TSGCT.
- Synovial chondromatosis (SCh) is an uncommon benign disease unique to the synovium.
- Rarely, SCh can become malignant. Histological features are loss of clustering and lobular architecture, marked myxoid change of the matrix, sheeting, crowding or spindling of chondrocytes.
- Recurrent FN1-ACVR2A rearrangements (fusion between fibronectin 1 (FN1) and activin receptor 2A (ACVR2A)) are seen in 57% of synovial chondromatosis and in 75% of chondrosarcoma secondary to synovial chondromatosis. IDH mutations are not present in synovial chondromatosis, whereas IDH1 or IDH2 mutations have been reported in 50–80% of chondrosarcomas.

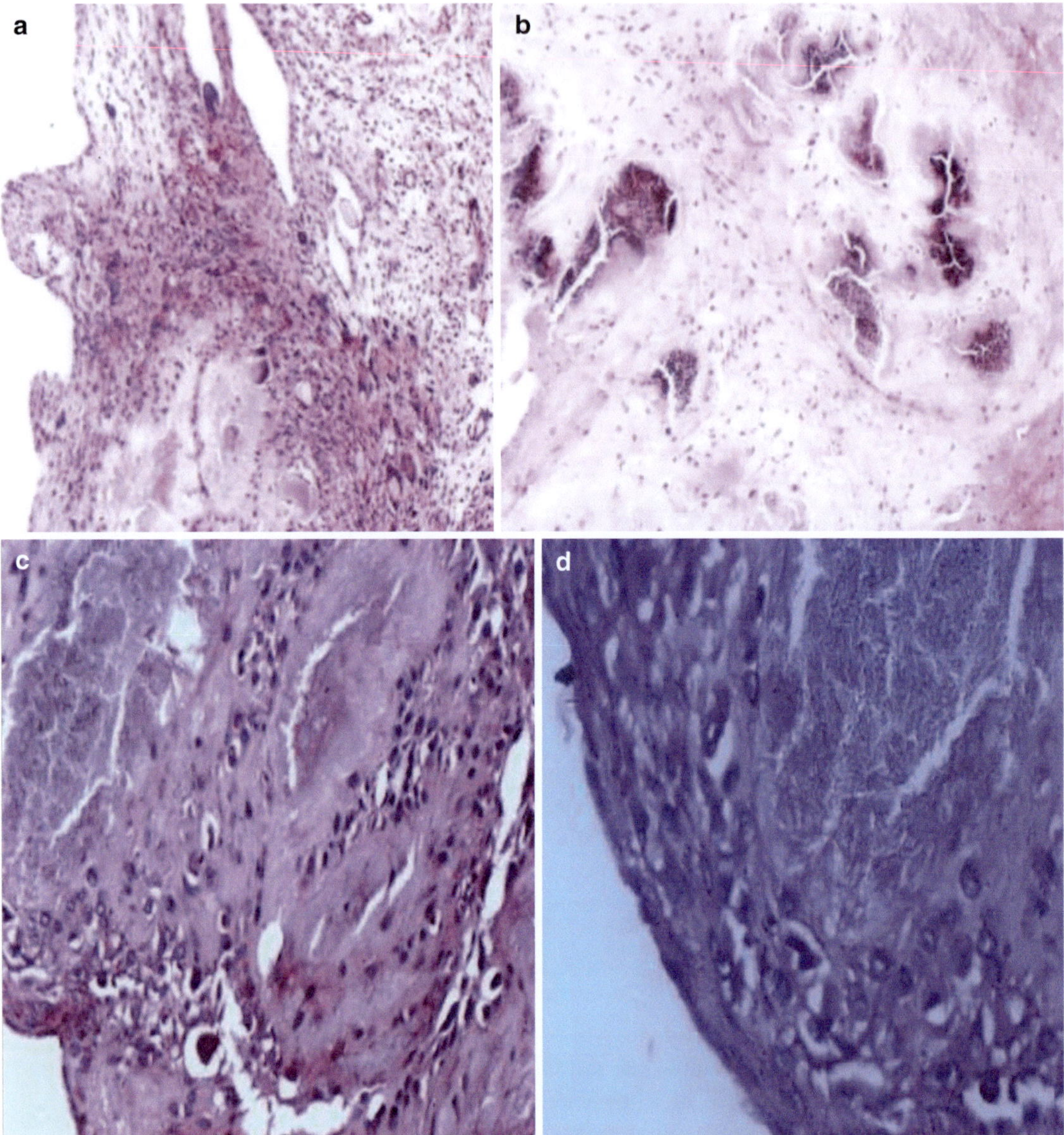

Fig. 18.27 CPPD. (**a**) Scanner view showing inflammatory cells and foreign body giant cells around crystalline structures, H&E ×40. (**b**) Multiple calcified foci with crystalline structures in a myxohyaline stroma, H&E ×100. (**c** and **d**) High power showing the crystalline structure, H&E ×250. These crystals show positive birefringence under polarized light

References

1. Bullough PG. In: Bullough PG, editor. Orthopaedic pathology. 5th ed. Mosby, Inc.; 2010. p. 232–3593.
2. Resnick D. Common disorders of synovium-lined joints: pathogenesis, imaging abnormalities, and complications. Am J Roentgenol. 1988;151:1079–93.
3. Narváez JA, Narváez J, Ortega R, De Lama E, Roca Y, Vidal N. Hypointense synovial lesions on T2-weighted images: differential diagnosis with pathologic correlation. Am J Roentgenol. 2003;181(3):761–9.

TSGCT

4. Abdul-Karim FW, el-Naggar AK, Joyce MJ, Makley JT, Carter JR. Diffuse and localized tenosynovial giant cell tumor and pigmented villonodular synovitis: a clinicopathologic and flow cytometric DNA analysis. Hum Pathol. 1992;23(7):729–35.
5. Boland JM, Folpe AL, Hornick JL, Grogg KL. Clusterin is expressed in normal synoviocytes and in tenosynovial giant cell tumors of localized and diffuse types: diagnostic and histogenetic implications. Am J Surg Pathol. 2009;33(8):1225–9.
6. Lucas DR. Tenosynovial giant cell tumor: case report and review. Arch Pathol Lab Med. 2012;136(8):901–6.
7. Ottaviani S, Ayral X, Dougados M, Gossec L. Pigmented villonodular synovitis: a retrospective single-center study of 122 cases and review of the literature. Semin Arthritis Rheum. 2011;40(6):539–46.
8. Somerhausen NS, Fletcher CD. Diffuse-type giant cell tumor: clinicopathologic and immunohistochemical analysis of 50 cases with extraarticular disease. Am J Surg Pathol. 2000;24(4):479–92.
9. West RB, Rubin BP, Miller MA, Subramanian S, Kaygusuz G, Montgomery K, Zhu S, Marinelli RJ, De Luca A, Downs-Kelly E, Goldblum JR, Corless CL, Brown PO, Gilks CB, Nielsen TO, Huntsman D, van de Rijn M. A landscape effect in tenosynovial giant-cell tumor from activation of CSF1 expression by a translocation in a minority of tumor cells. Proc Natl Acad Sci U S A. 2006;103(3):690–5.
10. WHO Classification of Tumours. In Soft Tissue and Bone Tumours. WHO Classification of Tumours, vol. 3. Edited by the WHO Classification of Tumours Editorial Board. 5th ed. IARC; 2020.

Malignant TSGCT

11. Li CF, Wang JW, Huang WW, et al. Malignant diffuse-type tenosynovial giant cell tumors: a series of 7 cases comparing with 24 benign lesions with review of the literature. Am J Surg Pathol. 2008;32(4):587–99.

Synovial Chondromatosis

12. Milgram JW. Synovial osteochondromatosis: a histopathological study of thirty cases. J Bone Joint Surg Am. 1977;59(6):792–801.
13. Norman A, Steiner GC. Bone erosion in synovial chondromatosis. Radiology, 1986;161:749–52.
14. Ng VY, Louie P, Punt S, Ernest U. Conrad malignant transformation of synovial chondromatosis: a systematic review. Open Orthop J. 2017;11(Suppl-3, M7):517–24.

Synovial Chondrosarcoma

15. Bertoni F, Unni KK, Beabout JW, Sim FH. Chondrosarcomas of the synovium. Cancer. 1991;67(1):155–62.
16. Biazzo A, Confalonieri N. Synovial chondrosarcoma. Ann Transl Med. 2016;4(15):280.

Synovial Haemangioma

17. Bawa AS, Garg R, Bhatnagar K, Singal S. Synovial hemangioma of the knee management and excellent outcome 2 years after arthroscopic synovectomy in a 25-year-old male with a 20-year history. J Orthop Case Rep. 2017;7(3):17–20. https://doi.org/10.13107/jocr.2250-0685.786.
18. Rajni, Khanna G, Gupta A, Gupta V. Synovial hemangioma: a rare benign synovial lesion. Indian J Pathol Microbiol. 2008;51:257–8.
19. Yilmaz E, Karakurt L, Ozdemir H, Serin E, Incesu M. Dizde yaygin sinovyal hemanjiyom: Olgu sunumu [Diffuse synovial hemangioma of the knee: a case report]. Acta Orthop Traumatol Turc. 2004;38(3):224–8.

Lipoma Arborescens

20. Kamran F, Kavin K, Vijay S, Shivanand G. Bilateral lipoma arborescens with osteoarthritis knee: case report and literature review. J Clin Orthop Trauma. 2015;6(2):131–6.
21. Rao S, Rajkumar A, Elizabeth MJ, Ganesan V, Kuruvilla S. Pathology of synovial lipomatosis and its clinical significance. J Lab Physicians. 2011;3(2):84–8.
22. Sanamandra SK, Ong KO. Lipoma arborescens. Singap Med J. 2014;55(1):5–11.

Nodular Fasciitis

23. Wang W, Huang Y, Wang C, et al. Intra-articular nodular fasciitis: a rare lesion case report and an updated review of the literature. BMC Musculoskelet Disord. 2019;20:5.

Fibroma of Tendon Sheath

24. Al-Qattan MM. Fibroma of tendon sheath of the hand: a series of 20 patients with 23 tumours. J Hand Surg Eur. 2014;39:300–5.
25. Chung EB, Enzinger FM. Fibroma of tendon sheath. Cancer. 1979;44:1945–54.
26. Carter JM, Wang X, Dong J, Westendorf J, Chou MM, Oliveira AM. USP6 genetic rearrangements in cellular fibroma of tendon sheath. Mod Pathol. 2016;29(8):865–9.
27. Srivastava P, Srivastava S. Fibroma of flexor tendon sheath of finger: a rare tumor of hand-revisited. J Neoplasm. 2018;3(1):1. https://doi.org/10.21767/2576-3903.100026.

Intra-articular Osteochondroma

28. Kong M, Cao L, Zhang Q, Fang Y, Zhao C, Gu H, Zhang S, Chen Y, Wu J, Bi Q. Identification of a rare case of intra-articular osteochondroma manifesting as three loose bodies in a patient with hereditary multiple osteochondromas: a case report. Oncol Lett. 2015;10(2):798–80.

Intra-articular Synovial Sarcoma

29. A.H. Krieg, F. Hefti, B.M. Speth et al Synovial sarcomas usually metastasize after >5 years: a multicenter retrospective analysis with minimum follow-up of 10 years for survivors Ann Oncol 2011;22(2) : 458–467.
30. Friedman MV, Kyriakos M, Matava MJ, McDonald DJ, Jennings JW, Wessell DE. Intra-articular synovial sarcoma. Skelet Radiol. 2013;42(6):859–67.
31. Nordemar D, Öberg J, Brosjö O, Skorpil M. Intra-articular synovial sarcomas: incidence and differentiating features from localized pigmented villonodular synovitis. Sarcoma. 2015;2015:903873. https://doi.org/10.1155/2015/903873.

Crystal Deposition Diseases

32. Dalbeth N, Merriman TR, Stamp LK. Gout. Lancet. 2016;388(10055):2039–52.
33. Grassi W, De Angelis R. Clinical features of gout. Reumatismo. 2012;63(4):238–45.
34. Hügle T, Krenn V. Histo-Pathophysiologie der Gichtarthritis [Histopathophysiology of Gout]. Ther Umsch. 2016;73(3):137–40. German. PMID: 27008445. https://doi.org/10.1024/0040-5930/a000769.
35. Marson P, Pasero G. Some historical remarks on microcrystalline arthritis (gout and chondrocalcinosis). Reumatismo. 2012;63(4):199–206. https://doi.org/10.4081/reumatismo.2011.199. PMID: 22303526
36. Towiwat P, Chhana A, Dalbeth N. The anatomical pathology of gout: a systematic literature review. BMC Musculoskelet Disord. 2019;20:140.
37. Shidham V, Chivukula M, Basir Z, et al. Evaluation of crystals in formalin-fixed, paraffin-embedded tissue sections for the differential diagnosis of pseudogout, gout, and tumoral calcinosis. Mod Pathol. 2001;14:806–10.

19 Odontogenic Tumours

The different epithelial odontogenic tumours can be classified into ameloblastomas, adenomatoid odontogenic tumours, calcifying epithelial odontogenic tumours, odontogenic ghost cell tumours, squamous odontogenic tumours, ameloblastic fibromas, ameloblastic fibro-odontomas or odontomas [1, 2]. The classification of odontogenic tumours is given in Table 19.1.

Table 19.1 WHO 2017 classification of odontogenic tumours [1]

2017 WHO classification
Epithelial origin
Ameloblastoma
Ameloblastoma unicystic type
Ameloblastoma extraosseous/peripheral type
Metastasizing (malignant) ameloblastoma
Squamous odontogenic tumour
Calcifying epithelial odontogenic tumour
Adenomatoid odontogenic tumour
Mixed origin
Ameloblastic fibroma
Primordial odontogenic tumour
Odontoma, complex type
Odontoma, compound type
Dentinogenic ghost cell tumour
Mesenchymal origin
Odontogenic fibroma
Odontogenic myxoma/myxofibroma
Cementoblastoma
Cemento-ossifying fibroma
Malignant odontogenic tumours
Ameloblastic carcinomas
Primary intraosseous carcinoma, NOS
Sclerosing odontogenic carcinoma
Clear cell odontogenic carcinoma
Ghost cell odontogenic carcinoma
Odontogenic sarcomas
Odontogenic carcinosarcoma

19.1 Epithelial Tumours

19.1.1 Ameloblastoma

Ameloblastomas are benign locally aggressive tumour of odontogenic epithelium and have a tendency for recurrence if not adequately removed. Ameloblastoma accounts for 1% of all jaw tumours and cysts and 18% of all odontogenic tumours [1, 2]. It is the second most common odontogenic tumour.

19.1.1.1 Clinical

Ameloblastoma is a disease of the elderly and usually seen in the fourth and fifth decades of life [3, 4]. 80% of the tumour occurs in mandible and 20% in maxilla. Maxillary ameloblastoma is mostly seen in the posterior molar region. In the mandible, posterior mandible is commonly affected. Ameloblastic carcinomas are commonly seen in maxilla. But unicystic ameloblastoma occurs in younger age group, usually in the second decade of life. Tooth extraction, dental caries and trauma are thought to be factors which predispose to this tumour. Ameloblastomas are slow-growing tumours and remain asymptomatic

J. Kattoor et al., *Bone Tumors*, https://doi.org/10.1007/978-981-99-4738-6_19

until a swelling is noticed. Most patients present with swelling and facial asymmetry [5]. When tumour grows, it forms a hard swelling and causes cortical bone thinning, and an eggshell crackling can be elicited. Since slow growing, it sometimes leads to reactive bone formation with gross enlargement and distortion of the jaw.

19.1.1.2 Radiology

The tumour arises in the bone and is incidentally discovered on dental or plain X-rays. It is a lytic lesion with scalloped boundaries with a soap bubble appearance, which is characteristic of multilocular variant. In the unicystic variant, resorption of tooth roots and impacted molars are seen. CT and MRI can be used to plan the surgery. Magnetic resonance imaging (MRI) helps the detection of a typical lesion arising from the maxilla and extending to the orbit, paranasal sinuses, base of the skull and also soft tissue/marrow extension.

19.1.1.3 Pathology

Different clinicopathological subtypes are solid/multicystic, unicystic, desmoplastic and peripheral types. Ameloblastomas are cystic or solid grossly.

19.1.1.4 Microscopy

Ameloblastomas are mainly divided into four types depending upon the morphological pattern. They are follicular, plexiform, acanthomatous and granular types (Fig. 19.1). Rare variants are clear cell, desmoplastic, basal cell, papilliferous and keratoameloblastoma types. The follicular type consists of epithelial cells similar to enamel in a fibrous stroma. The peripheral cells are columnar to cuboidal with palisading pattern of nuclei (Fig. 19.1g). There are angular cells which are loosely arranged in the centre resembling stellate reticulum, which often show cystic change. In the plexiform type, there are anastomosing strands of ameloblastomatous epithelium with cyst-like stromal degeneration [6–8]. The stellate reticulum is inconspicuous. The desmoplastic ameloblastoma shows cuboidal to flat peripheral cells with spindle-shaped cells in the centre in a densely collagenous stroma. An ameloblastoma may contain mixed histopathological types.

19.1.1.5 Unicystic Ameloblastoma

Unicystic ameloblastoma is a variant of intraosseous ameloblastoma. This occurs with a single cystic cavity, with or without luminal proliferation. It is usually associated with unerupted tooth, most often mandibular third molar. In one-third of cases, cortical perforation is seen. Even though it presents as a monocystic lesion, sometimes the entire lumen is filled with the thickenings. The two histopathological subtypes are luminal and intraluminal type. In the luminal type, cyst is lined focally by ameloblastomatous epithelium. The intraluminal type has extensions of the lining epithelium into the lumen in a plexiform pattern [6–8]. The entire lesion has to be carefully examined before a definitive diagnosis. Some may have a mural component, and these behave aggressively. Enucleation is the treatment. These cases need a long-term follow-up as they may recur even 10 years after initial treatment.

19.1.1.6 Extraosseous or peripheral ameloblastoma

These tumours occur in the soft tissues of gingiva and show microscopic features of ameloblastoma. It is a benign tumour. It occurs between 9 and 92 years with a slight male preponderance. The lingual aspect of mandible is the common site. It also occurs in mandibular retromolar area and maxillary tuberosity. It shows a smooth or papillary granular surface and can present as a sessile exophytic lesion. Duration may be as long as 20 years.

Radiology

A superficial erosion or bony depression with cupping or saucerization is seen.

Pathology

Grossly, it appears as a firm mass with occasional tiny cystic spaces. Histopathology resembles intraosseous type, and differential diagnoses are basal cell carcinoma of oral mucosal origin, skin

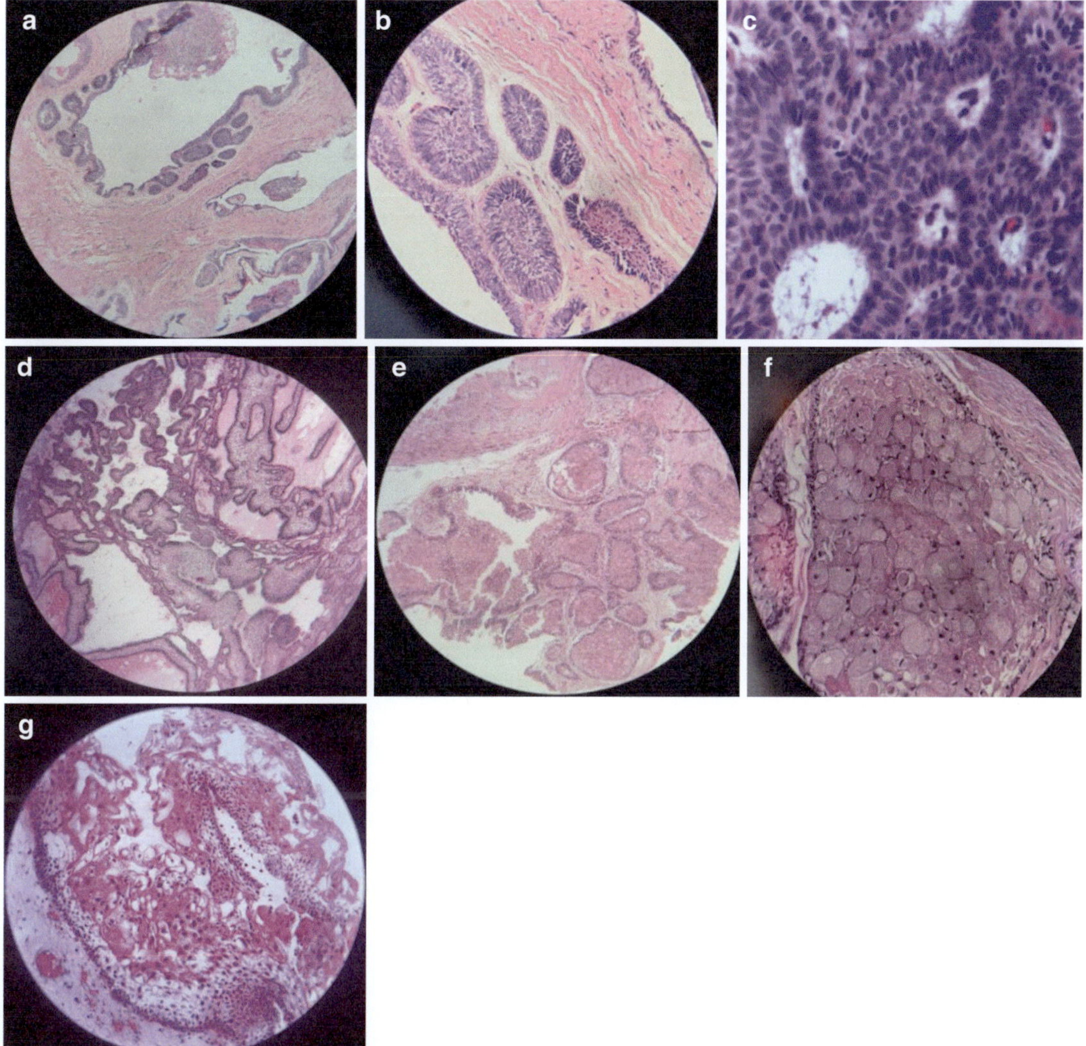

Fig. 19.1 Ameloblastoma: (**a** and **b**) Follicular type, H&E ×100. (**c**) High power showing peripheral palisading of cells, H&E ×400. (**d**) Plexiform type, H&E ×100. (**e** and **f**) Granular cell type, H&E ×100. (**f**) H&E ×250. (**g**) Acanthomatous type, H&E ×100. Picture courtesy: Dr. Heera, Professor of Oral Pathology

appendage tumours and salivary gland tumours with a peripheral palisading pattern. Wide excision with free margins is curative. Recurrence is rare.

19.1.1.7 Metastasizing ameloblastoma

The primary site is usually mandible than the maxilla, and primary lesion is solid/multicystic variant. It metastasizes despite its benign histological appearance. The commonest metastatic site is lung followed by lymph nodes and bone. It is usually diagnosed after the occurrence of metastatic deposits, and there will be a long latent period before metastasis. A few cases recur after repeated surgical intervention.

19.1.1.8 Treatment

As ameloblastoma is a benign, locally aggressive tumour with a high recurrence rate, the treatment may be conservative or radical. The conservative treatment consists of enucleation associated with curettage, the use of adjuvant therapies such as Carnoy's solution and cryotherapy. The radical treatment consists of resection and bone reconstruction [10].

19.1.1.9 Prognosis

Conventional ameloblastomas have a significantly higher recurrence rate (17%). The unicystic type has only 9.1% recurrence rate. Based on the histology, there is no difference in recurrence rates.

19.1.2 Squamous Odontogenic Tumour (SOT)

Squamous odontogenic tumour is a rare benign epithelial odontogenic tumour with tumour cells showing squamous differentiation. Its appearance can be mimicked in varying degrees by some other tumours [1, 11].

19.1.2.1 Clinical

SOTs mainly occur in adult males (mean age 38 years). Usually, they present as single intraosseous tumours. There is a predilection for anterior maxilla and posterior mandible, usually behind the canines. Multifocal and extraosseous tumours are also reported. Most patients are young and asymptomatic. It is a slow-growing tumour, and affected teeth may become loose. Most of them present as unilocular radiolucencies and can show continuity with one or more tooth roots [1, 12].

19.1.2.2 Radiology

They can mimic severe bone loss due to periodontal disease. Sometimes, they present as a triangular cyst, with the base of the triangle towards the root apices [13]. Root resorption is rare.

19.1.2.3 Pathology

Most lesions are curetted. The characteristic features are multiple, circumscribed, rounded or more irregular islands of squamous epithelium in a cellular fibrous stroma. The islands are typically surrounded by flattened or round epithelial cells. A jigsaw-puzzle architecture is seen. Foci of keratin or parakeratin and calcifications, globular eosinophilic structures or microcysts may form within the island. Mitosis is rarely encountered. Occasionally, the tumour is continuous with and appears to be arising from the surface epithelium [12–14]. Ameloblastic differentiation in the form of peripheral columnar cells with palisaded nuclei is absent in SOTs.

19.1.2.4 Pathogenesis

The origin is thought to be from rests of Malassez or from other residual odontogenic rests. NOTCH receptors and their ligands are considered to play a role in the differentiation of SOTS.

19.1.2.5 DDs

The tumour can be misdiagnosed as acanthomatous or desmoplastic variants of ameloblastoma, but SOTs lack peripheral palisading with reverse nuclear polarity. The walls of odontogenic cysts may show microscopic features similar to SOTs and have been called SOT-like proliferations [15].

19.1.2.6 Treatment and Prognosis

They have been removed conservatively by surgery, and recurrence is rare [16].

19.1.3 Calcifying Epithelial Odontogenic Tumour (Pindborg Tumour)

Calcifying epithelial odontogenic tumour (CEOT) is a benign rare epithelial odontogenic tumour accounting for less than 1% of specimens submitted to oral pathology laboratories. It secretes an amyloid protein that tends to calcify. CEOT is called as Pindborg tumour as Pindborg was first to describe it in detail in 1958 [17]. Intraosseous tumours accounted for nearly 88% of all reported cases, while those combined with adenomatoid odontogenic tumours and extraosseous tumours accounted for 6% each.

19.1.3.1 Clinical

Compared to maxilla, the mandible is affected twice. There is a predilection for the body of the mandible and the molar region, and most of them (50–60%) are associated with an embedded tooth [18]. It grows slowly producing bony expansion [18].

19.1.3.2 Radiology

They can be mixed lytic and radiopaque or purely radiolucent [19]. The degree of calcification corresponds to the age of the lesion. The radio-opacities are frequently uniformly distributed throughout the lesion to give the so-called driven snow appearance. The margins are well defined mimicking a dentigerous cyst.

19.1.3.3 Pathology

The tumours are solid with variable amounts of calcification. The microscopy shows different patterns like small islands, cords or trabeculae or large sheets of epithelioid polyhedral cells with abundant well-defined cytoplasm. Some tumours show intercellular bridges. The nuclei are pleomorphic with giant nuclei, and the mitotic rate is very low. A unique extracellular odontogenic amyloid protein provisionally called "AODAM" is secreted by the tumour cells. The eosinophilic material is seen as rounded masses, which stain positively for amyloid. These masses coalesce and calcify in concentric rings called Liesegang rings when more protein is secreted (Fig. 19.2). Along with routine haematoxylin and eosin stains, amyloid protein can be demonstrated using Congo red stain and modified Gallego's stain [20]. The neoplasm can infiltrate adjacent bone mimicking a poorly differentiated carcinoma. Various amounts of glycogen can accumulate focally or in a diffuse manner causing clear cell change, and it is called a clear cell variant. Variable amounts of Langerhans cells have been reported in CEOTs. The hybrid lesion with adenomatoid odontogenic tumour (AOT) has been described, and it behaves more like AOTS.

PTCH mutations have been reported in CEOTs. A malignant counterpart of calcifying epithelial odontogenic tumour has been reported by Basu et al. Non-calcifying Pindborg tumour is very rare [21].

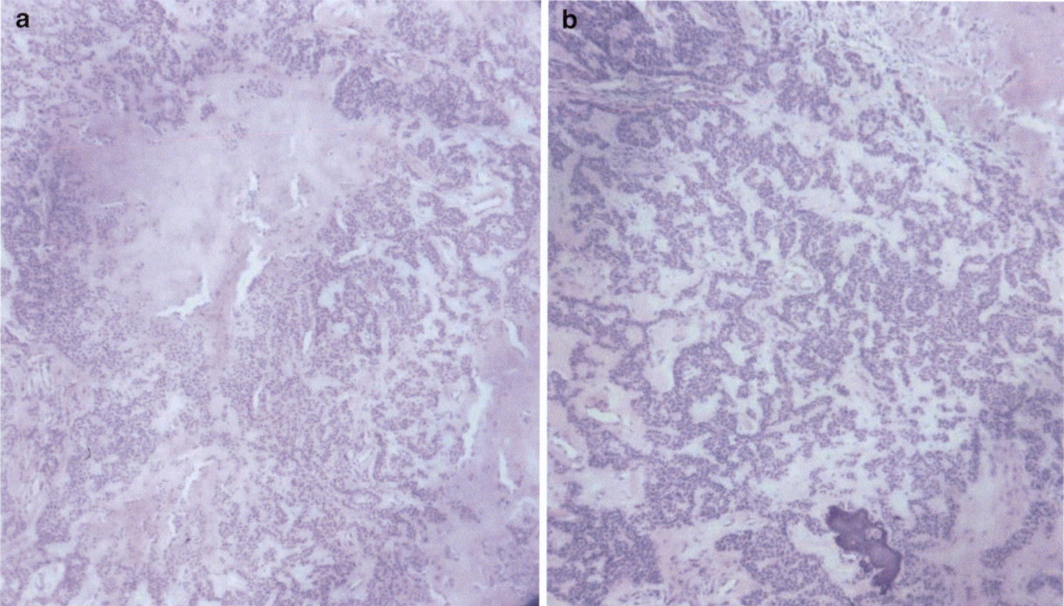

Fig. 19.2 Pindborg tumour: (**a**) Cords and trabeculae of polyhedral epithelial cells with amyloid-like eosinophilic material, H&E ×100. (**b**) Focus of calcification, H&E ×100

19.1.3.4 DD

Calcifying epithelial odontogenic tumours must be differentiated from CEOT-like areas found in follicles of unerupted teeth. The absence of peripheral palisading and the presence of amyloid-like protein are the factors which help to differentiate it from ameloblastoma. The cytological atypia can mimic malignancy, but the lack of mitosis, low Ki-67 proliferation index and presence of calcifying amyloid favour CEOT. Clear cell variant mimics clear cell odontogenic carcinoma or metastatic clear cell carcinoma. But clear cell odontogenic carcinoma has a different immunophenotype and shows the EWSR1 and ATF1 gene rearrangement.

19.1.3.5 Treatment and Prognosis

Most cases of CEOTs are treated with excision with a margin of normal bone [22]. As non-calcifying Pindborg tumour is believed to be an aggressive variant, a definitive resection of the tumour with tumour-free surgical margins and long-term follow-up is recommended [22]. Since CEOTs infiltrate medullary bone, overall recurrence rate is about 15%.

19.1.4 Adenomatoid Odontogenic Tumour (AOT)

Adenomatoid odontogenic tumour (AOT) is an uncommon benign odontogenic tumour showing duct-like structures and is associated with an impacted tooth, usually canine. It affects young people. AOT represents 3–7% of all odontogenic tumours and is considered to be a hamartomatous lesion. The tumour is referred to as "two-thirds tumour". It occurs in the maxilla in about 2/3 cases, about 2/3 cases are in young females, 2/3 cases are associated with impacted tooth and in 2/3 cases affected tooth is canine [12]. AOT shows cytological features similar to various components of enamel organ, dental lamina, reduced enamel epithelium and its remnants [23]. Most of the AOTs (more than 95%) are intraosseous, but extraosseous variants have been described.

19.1.4.1 Radiology

It mimics a dentigerous cyst. Usually, the lesion is unilocular and radiolucent with fine snowflake calcifications. The presence of calcifications helps to differentiate it from dentigerous cyst. It can progress to produce cortical expansion, but perforation is rare [24].

19.1.4.2 Pathology

AOTs are smooth rounded symmetrical encapsulated masses. Grossly, it is seen as solid growth or with a single large cystic space, or as multiple small cystic spaces. The tumour is composed of spindle-shaped or polygonal cells in sheets and whorls with scanty stroma. The amorphous eosinophilic material is seen between the epithelial cells and also in the centre of rosette-like structures. The duct-like structure is lined by a single row of columnar epithelial cells with the nuclei polarized away from the central lumen. Tumour masses of spindle-shaped cells in rosettes and irregular streams with duct-like spaces showing palisaded nuclei are characteristic of adenomatoid odontogenic tumour (Fig. 19.3). The lumen is sometimes empty. Dystrophic calcification is usually seen within the lumen of duct-like structures or in the stroma in AOTs [1, 2, 25]. The stroma is typically loose with scanty cellular elements but may show numerous thin-walled blood vessels sometimes. Occasionally, tumour can be cystic with tumour forming part of the cyst wall. The KI-67 index and BCL2 index are low compared to solid ameloblastoma. There is strong cytoplasmic expression of beta-catenin, but no molecular anomaly has been detected within the beta-catenin gene. The cell of origin of AOT is from the epithelium of dental lamina complex or its remnants.

19.1.4.3 Treatment and prognosis

These lesions shell out easily, and enucleation is almost curative. Recurrence rates are exceedingly low.

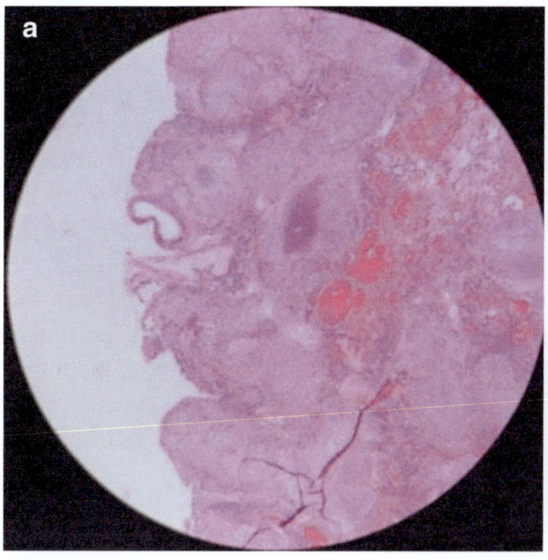

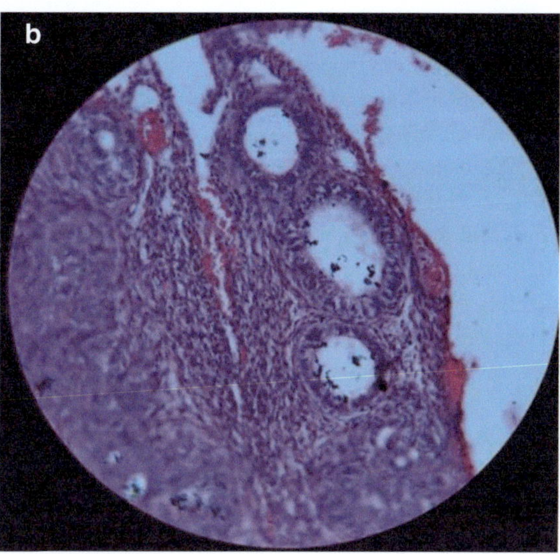

Fig. 19.3 Adenomatoid odontogenic tumour. (**a** and **b**) Tumour masses of spindle-shaped cells in rosettes and irregular streams with duct-like spaces showing palisaded nuclei pushed away from the lumen, H&E ×100. Picture courtesy: Dr. Heera, Professor of Oral Pathology

19.2 Mixed Origin

19.2.1 Ameloblastic Fibroma

Ameloblastic fibroma is a rare, benign, true mixed tumour composed of epithelial and mesenchymal tissue. The epithelium is similar to odontogenic epithelium, and mesenchymal tissue resembles dental papilla. No dental hard tissues are present [26]. It constitutes about 1.5–6.5% of all odontogenic tumours [1, 2].

19.2.1.1 Clinical

Ameloblastic fibroma presents before the end of odontogenesis (younger than 20 years). Male-to-female ratio is 1.4:1. The commonest site of occurrence is the posterior area of the mandible. The peripheral (extraosseous) form is an extremely rare lesion [27]. They are slow-growing painless tumours, which can rarely attain remarkable size causing facial deformity. Its clinical behaviour is in the nature between hamartoma and true neoplasm. It is postulated that if left untreated an ameloblastic fibroma could develop eventually into an odontoma. The age at presentation of ameloblastic fibroma and the odontoma are different. The degree of differentiation is also different. Ameloblastic fibromas, ameloblastic fibrodentinomas and ameloblastic fibro-odontomas form a spectrum of the same lesion. They mature and become odontoma. This "continuum concept" is not well accepted.

19.2.1.2 Radiology

Ameloblastic fibromas are incidentally detected, and majority present as well-defined small unilocular radiolucency [28]. In large-sized lesions, they occur as multiloculated tumours. In 80% of the cases, an impacted tooth may be found. But root resorption and cortical perforation are not present.

19.2.1.3 Pathology

The tumour is an encapsulated solid tumour with smooth outer surface. The capsule can be collagenous. The epithelium consists of narrow, elongated strands of two parallel and tight layers of cuboidal to columnar cells. The epithelium is sharply circumscribed by a basal membrane and forms islands, strands or cauliflower-like proliferations in loose but cellular fibromyxoid connective tissue. Between the peripheral cuboidal cells, a stellate reticulum-like area is seen. The epithelial component can also resemble the follicular stage of the enamel organ. Rarely, there is formation of dental hard tissues, and it can reach a large size. BRAF V600E mutation is seen in rare cases.

19.2.1.4 Treatment and Prognosis

Small asymptomatic cases are removed conservatively. Radical treatment is opted for large destructive tumours. Recurrence is reported in 16% of cases. Sarcomatous change is rare and seen in recurrent tumours [29].

19.2.2 Primordial Odontogenic Tumour (POT)

Primordial odontogenic tumour (POT) is a new emerging entity in 2017 WHO classification of head and neck tumours [1, 2]. It is one of the rare types of mixed epithelial and mesenchymal odontogenic tumour (MOT) and was first described in 2014. POT is composed of dental papilla-like myxoid connective tissue with a delicate membrane of ameloblastic epithelium covering it [30].

19.2.2.1 Clinical

It usually occurs in the first and second decades of life. Most common site is molar tooth of the mandibular region.

19.2.2.2 Radiology

It appears as a well-demarcated radiolucency with unerupted tooth, usually the third mandibular tooth. It can cause displacement and resorption of adjacent tooth.

19.2.2.3 Pathology

On gross examination, it appears as a well-defined multilobular solid firm myxoid mass with a slippery outer surface. Cystic change is uncommon. Usually, it is associated with an embedded tooth.

Histologically, the periphery of the tumour shows a covering by ameloblastic epithelium, consisting of a single layer of columnar cells with typical reverse nuclear polarity. Most of the tumour consists of loose and myxoid fibrous tissue, including spindle cells. The nests of the epithelium contain stellate reticulum between the columnar cells [31, 32]. The peripheral portion of the connective tissue shows dentine. This represents an association between tumour and adjacent tooth. Treatment of choice is enucleation.

19.2.3 Odontomas

Odontomas are the most common odontogenic tumours in the mixed epithelial and mesenchymal tumour-like malformations (hamartomas). They are composed of dental soft and hard tissues like teeth. Once fully calcified, they do not develop further, but may erupt into the mouth like teeth.

19.2.3.1 Clinical

Odontomas are typically seen in children (first and second decades). Both sexes are equally affected. Even though the aetiology is unknown, a possible factor considered is genetic mutation in a tooth germ. They are classified into complex odontomas and compound odontomas [33]. Complex odontomas occur in posterior mandible and anterior maxilla. The compound odontomas are encountered in the anterior maxilla. They are usually asymptomatic. Sometimes, trauma and eruption can cause inflammation leading on to impaction, imposition, malformation or deviation of adjacent teeth. Cyst formation is another rare complication. In patients with Gardner's syndrome, it can be multifocal, but it is very rare [34].

19.2.3.2 Radiology

Odontomas are detected by chance in a routine radiograph or as swelling of the jaw when they are large enough. It is usually associated with an unerupted tooth. Radiologically, odontomas are located over the crown or between the roots of an impacted tooth. It is well defined and radiopaque surrounded by a thin soft tissue capsule. The radiopaque substance is irregular in compound odontomas with numerous tooth-like structures. In complex odontoma, it is a disorganized mass of calcification.

19.2.3.3 Pathology

Grossly, they vary in size from <1 cm to 6 cm. Compound odontomas appear as a cluster of white tooth-like structures or denticles of varying sizes and shapes. But complex odontomas present as a white amorphous bony hard mass. Both these types have a capsule or capsule-like soft tissue surrounding them. Odontoma consists of dentin and enamel. Compound odontomas consist of multiple rudimentary teeth showing dentin, cementum, enamel matrix and pulp. Complex odontoma shows disorganized enamel, dentin or pulpal tissue, which is seen around clefts or hollow circular structures [35]. Periphery shows a thin layer of cementum (Fig. 19.4). Immature connective tissue with cords and strips of ameloblastic epithelium forms the soft tissue capsule.

Sometimes, an ameloblastoma may arise in association with an odontoma. These were called odonto-ameloblastoma previously, but the entity does not exist now. They probably represent immature stages of complex odontomas.

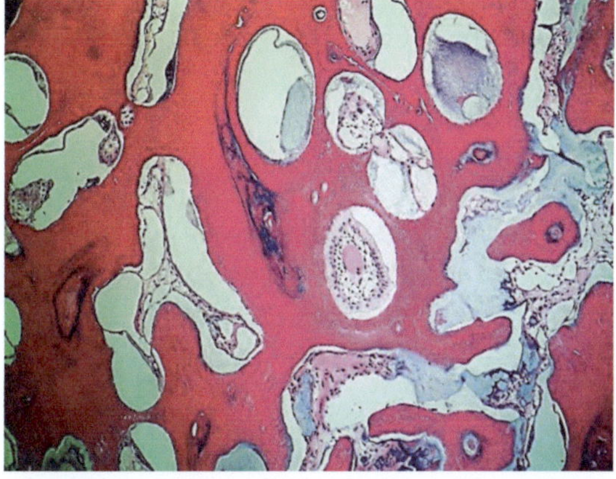

Fig. 19.4 Odontoma: Enamel epithelium surrounded by cementum-like material within the bony trabeculae, H&E ×100

19.2.3.4 Treatment and Prognosis

Treatment is conservative surgery [36]. Recurrence is rare after complete surgery. Prognosis is excellent.

19.2.4 Dentinogenic Ghost Cell Tumour

Dentinogenic ghost cell tumour is a benign, locally aggressive odontogenic neoplasm of maxilla and mandible with a predominantly solid pattern of growth.

19.2.4.1 Clinical

It has a wide age range between 11 and 79 years with peak incidence between the fourth and sixth decades. It is seen slightly predominant in males. It usually presents as intraosseous tumours in posterior maxilla and mandible and is rarely reported as gingival or alveolar mucosal tumour. It usually presents as painless swelling. The extraosseous type presents as a sessile sometimes pedunculated exophytic soft tissue nodule.

19.2.4.2 Pathogenesis

Wnt signalling pathway may have a role in the development similar to calcifying odontogenic cyst since beta-catenin gene mutations and beta-catenin overexpression are also identified in DGCT [37].

19.2.4.3 Radiology

Majority present as radiopaque lesions with well-defined borders and a mixed radio density due to varying levels of calcification. Rarely are they associated with odontomas, similar to calcifying odontogenic cyst [37].

19.2.4.4 Pathology

Gross: It usually presents as a solid tumour.

Microscopically, it consists of sheets of anastomosing cords and strands of odontogenic epithelium (ameloblastic-like areas with palisading of basaloid cells) admixed with ghost cells, which are anucleate epithelial cells with pale clear cytoplasm. It represents the location of a previously resorbed nucleus or organelles. Minor cysts may form inside these epithelial islands. These epithelial cells are interspersed with islands of swirling cells with squamous differentiation. Odontogenic epithelial cells demonstrate round uniform basophilic nuclei and pale eosinophilic to clear cytoplasm. The background shows stellate reticulum-like proliferation and varying levels of dentinoid and cementum-like calcified collagenous matrix [38]. Mitosis is usually rare.

19.2.4.5 DD

The differential diagnosis includes ameloblastoma, calcifying odontogenic cyst, craniopharyngioma and ghost cell odontogenic carcinoma.

19.2.4.6 Treatment and prognosis

Wide local excision is done for intraosseous tumours, while more conservative excision is done for extraosseous type. Long-term follow-up is advised for these tumours as late recurrence can occur.

19.3 Tumours of Mesenchymal Origin

19.3.1 Odontogenic Fibroma

Odontogenic fibromas are rare, benign mesenchymal odontogenic tumour consisting of mature fibrous tissue with variable amounts of inactive-appearing odontogenic epithelium. The two common variants are

- Central or intraosseous type
- Peripheral or extraosseous type, seen in tooth-bearing region of the jaws

Peripheral type is more common than central type.

19.3.1.1 Clinical

Females are more affected than males. Age group affected is 20–40 years. Mandible and maxilla are affected equally. Peripheral type is seen usually in the anterior gingival region. In maxilla, they are seen anterior to the first molar, while in mandible posterior to the first molar. It can present with swelling and pain [39].

19.3.1.2 Radiologically

It presents as a unilocular or multilocular lesion with a well-defined sclerotic border. If calcification is present, it can appear as radiopaque flakes.

19.3.1.3 Pathology

The microscopy of central and peripheral type is similar. It is composed of scattered, small, inactive odontogenic epithelium in strands, cords or nests in a variably cellular fibrocollagenous stroma [40]. Calcification is variable, and when it is extensive, it is called ossifying variant of odontogenic fibroma. When granular cell appearance is noted within the odontogenic epithelium or stromal cells, it is called granular cell variant. Central odontogenic fibroma can be associated with central giant cell granuloma sometimes. Periepithelial amyloid deposition (cuffing) is noted rarely in central type.

19.3.1.4 Treatment and Prognosis

Enucleation and curettage are the usual line of treatment. Central lesions are treated by conservative laser excision, while simple excision is enough for peripheral lesions. The tumour may recur rarely, and it may be due to insufficient removal [41].

19.3.2 Odontogenic Myxoma

Myxomas of bone always occur in the jaws suggesting that they may be of odontogenic origin as they resemble mesenchymal portion of the tooth germ.

19.3.2.1 Clinical

They occur mostly in young adults, and there is a slight female predilection. About two-thirds of cases occur in mandible and one-third in maxilla, commonly in the molar regions. Occasionally, extraosseous cases occur in gingiva. Usually, it presents as a slowly growing swelling and rarely produces severe facial deformities. Unilateral sinonasal obliteration may mimic nasal polyposis.

19.3.2.2 Radiology

They present as a multilobular unilocular swelling resembling a cyst-like rarefying expansile

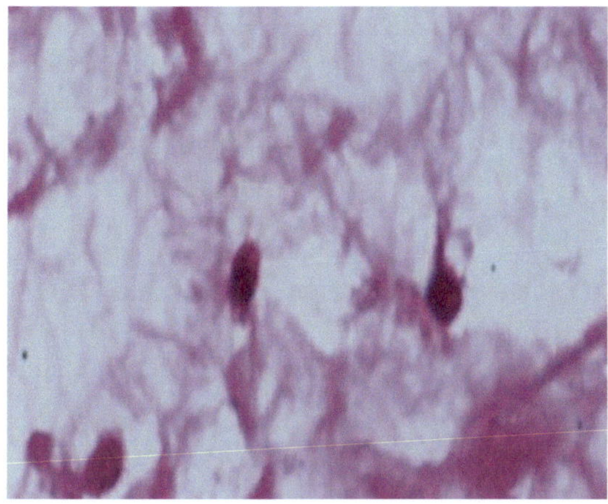

Fig. 19.5 Odontogenic myxoma: stellate cells in a myxoid stroma, H&E ×100

lesion of the jaws. Most of them present as multilocular translucencies with internal bony septa in a stepladder-like or tennis racket-like pattern, but this is rarely seen. They are usually fine and curved in appearance.

19.3.2.3 Pathology

Grossly, it is soft and semi-translucent with a glistening surface. Microscopically, loose stellate cells dominate with long anastomosing cytoplasmic processes (Fig. 19.5). The intercellular substance is somewhat granular and basophilic intensely staining with alcian blue [42]. Occasionally, they may contain binucleate cells and bizarre large nuclei mimicking atypia. Sometimes, zones within myxoma may show considerable fibromatous quality but have no clinical significance. The term odontogenic myxofibroma may be used when more of collagen is present [43]. The stromal elements of tooth bud may mimic myxoma, but tooth buds are sharply circumscribed, and periphery shows epithelial cells. Odontogenic myxomas permeate the medullary cavity of bone due to matrix secretion. This gives rise to a pseudomalignant growth pattern [44, 45].

19.3.2.4 DD

Myxoma resembles chondrosarcoma, osteosarcoma and even fibrosarcoma with myxoid features and should be differentiated from it. Tuberous sclerosis and naevoid basal cell carcinoma syndromes are seen to be associated with them.

19.3.2.5 Treatment and prognosis

Even though they can recur like ameloblastoma, they will not metastasize usually. Treatment is wide local excision. 25% can recur [46]. Hence, long-term follow-up is needed.

19.3.3 Cementoblastoma

Cementoblastoma is a benign odontogenic tumour. Calcified cementum-like tissue is deposited directly on a tooth root in this mesenchymal tumour. It is a rare tumour accounting for 1–6% of all odontogenic tumours.

19.3.3.1 Clinical

Majority of the tumours are seen in those aged less than 30 years. >75% of the cases are seen among mandibular molars and premolars. The second common sites are maxillary molars and premolars. Cementoblastomas cause buccal and lingual/palatal expansion of the affected bony cortical plates. It presents with sharp tooth pain similar to toothache [47]. The tumour is slow growing and becomes large if left untreated.

19.3.3.2 Radiologically

It appears as a large radiopaque mass continuous with the tooth from which it originates. They have a capsule, and it is seen as a thin film of uniform lucency around the periphery. Radiology is pathognomonic showing expansion of the cortical plate with deviation of the surrounding tooth roots as the tumour grows [47].

19.3.3.3 Pathology

Grossly, it appears as a calcified mass that is attached to the root or roots of tooth from which it originates. Microscopy shows thick trabeculae of calcified cementum-like material. It is deposited on an intact or partially resorbed root. It is strongly basophilic. There are many irregular lines resembling Paget disease of bone. The central part is more mature, while periphery is cellular consisting of trabeculae rimmed by active cementoblasts with fibrovascular stroma [48].

19.3.3.4 DD

The histology resembles osteoblastoma, but osteoblastomas in jaws are not attached to roots of tooth.

19.3.3.5 Treatment and Prognosis

Treatment is conservative. It can recur if incompletely removed.

19.3.4 Cemento-Ossifying Fibroma

Cemento-ossifying fibroma is a distinct type of ossifying fibroma occurring in tooth-bearing areas of the jaws. It is a benign fibro-osseous lesion, which is odontogenic in origin. Other types are trabecular, juvenile and psammomatous types. They are considered under chondro- and fibro-osseous lesions [49].

19.3.4.1 Clinical

Cemento-ossifying fibromas are slow-growing lesions presenting with painless bone expansion. The tumour is seen more in females and occurs in the second and third decades of life. They occur in mandibular molars and premolars.

19.3.4.2 Radiologically

It is seen as a well-defined lytic lesion with varying degrees of sclerosis. The amount of hard tissue present determines the degree of sclerosis.

19.3.4.3 Pathology

There will be single mass or large fragments grossly. Microscopically, they are encapsulated lesions. It contains calcified tissue in variable amounts and a hypercellular fibrovascular stroma. The calcified material may look like bone or cementum. No bony infiltration is seen.

19.4 Malignant Odontogenic Tumours

The malignant odontogenic tumours are rare. Even though they all share similar clinical and radiographic features, they differ primarily in their histologic features. The features pointing towards malignancy in odontogenic tumours are rapid growth, asymmetry, pain, paraesthesia, anaesthesia and an ill-defined destructive osteolytic process.

19.4.1 Ameloblastic Carcinoma

Ameloblastic carcinoma is a rare primary malignant odontogenic tumour of epithelial origin. It is the malignant counterpart of ameloblastoma. The tumour shows cellular atypia and can metastasize [50]. It consists of less than 1% of all odontogenic tumours. BRAF V600E mutation has been found as in other ameloblastic neoplasms.

Ameloblastic carcinoma is of two types—primary and secondary.

Ameloblastic carcinoma—primary type: These are ameloblastomas with cytological atypia.

Ameloblastic carcinoma—secondary type: Intraosseous—arises in a pre-existing benign ameloblastoma.

19.4.1.1 Clinical

Ameloblastic carcinoma presents with swelling, pain, rapid growth, trismus, toothache, facial asymmetry and dysphonia. It occurs in more than 45 years' age group. The common site of the tumour is the posterior mandible. Maxilla is rarely involved.

19.4.1.2 Radiology

It is seen as an ill-defined radiolucent lesion with cortical bone perforation and/or soft tissue invasion. Rarely, it can originate from a pre-existing ameloblastoma.

19.4.1.3 Pathology

Both primary and metastatic ameloblastic carcinomas have ameloblastoma-like appearance with cytological atypia. But they lack the classic features of ameloblastoma like reverse polarity and peripheral palisading. The important diagnostic features include pleomorphism, increased nuclear cytoplasmic ratio, abnormal mitoses and vascular or neural invasion. Sometimes, areas of necrosis are seen focally [51]. Even though they present with increased mitotic rate, the increase in mitosis alone is not helpful to diagnose malignancy.

19.4.1.4 DD

The differential diagnosis includes ameloblastoma, malignant ameloblastoma, primary intraosseous squamous cell carcinoma and clear cell odontogenic carcinoma.

19.4.1.5 Treatment and Prognosis

Radical resection is the choice of treatment. But the prognosis is poor. Lung metastasis occurs frequently than locoregional lymph node metastasis. Malignant lesions have 30% recurrence rate and 22% metastatic rate. Radiotherapy and chemotherapy seem to be less useful for the treatment of ameloblastic carcinomas [50, 52].

19.4.2 Primary Intraosseous Carcinoma

Primary intraosseous carcinomas are rare. In 1913, Loos described this tumour as a central epidermoid carcinoma of the jaws. They arise from the odontogenic epithelium seen as remnants of odontogenesis, or from the epithelial lining of an odontogenic cyst or other precursor epithelial lesions.

19.4.2.1 Clinical

The clinical manifestations of the cases are not specific. They may present with progressive swelling of the jaw, pain and loosening of the teeth. Large lesions may cause cortical bone destruction and perforation. Cervical lymph node metastasis is common. The tumour is observed in a wide age range with a mean age of 55–60 years. It frequently occurs in the corpus and posterior region of the mandible. Maxillary cases are mostly located in the anterior region.

19.4.2.2 Radiology

Radiographically, there is a radiolucent lesion with irregular cortical border.

19.4.2.3 Pathology

Microscopy shows malignant squamous cells but without features of ameloblastoma. Keratinization is rare. It is a diagnosis of exclusion usually.

19.4.2.4 DD

One has to exclude other malignant odontogenic carcinomas, metastatic carcinomas, intraosseous salivary gland carcinomas and carcinomas of the maxillary region. Immunohistochemistry helps to rule out these entities. Suei et al. proposed three criteria for diagnosing this tumour:

1. To differentiate it from surface mucosal squamous cell carcinoma, overlying mucosa should be intact without any ulcer.
2. To rule out any other odontogenic carcinoma, the biopsy specimen has to be sampled thoroughly. The sections should show squamous cell carcinoma without any cystic component or other odontogenic tumour cells.
3. To rule out metastasis from unknown primary, the chest radiograph must be clear or free from any tumour at the time of diagnosis and for a follow-up period of more than 6 months.

19.4.2.5 Treatment and Prognosis

Primary treatment is radical resection with neck dissection. Adjuvant radio- or chemotherapy may be beneficial. However, distant metastasis to lung is rare. Even though the cases arising from cysts may have a better prolonged survival, the prognosis is poor.

19.4.3 Clear Cell Odontogenic Carcinoma

Clear cell odontogenic carcinoma is a rare malignant, translocation-associated odontogenic epithelial neoplasm consisting of nests of clear cells and fibrous hyalinized stroma. Fluorescent in situ hybridization demonstrates EWSR1 rearrangements in vast majority (88%) of cases [1, 2]. Hansen described this entity in 1985.

19.4.3.1 Clinical

Majority of cases are asymptomatic. But non-specific symptoms like root resorption and soft tissue invasion can occur. The most common site is the mandible and usually seen in females. Most of the tumours are seen in 4–7 decades. Rarely they can present with cervical lymphnode metastasis [53].

19.4.3.2 Radiology

It presents as a destructive radiolucent lesion with poor margins. Soft tissue involvement is common as the lesion often perforates bone. They can also present as jaw swelling with loosening of the teeth.

19.4.3.3 Pathology

Microscopy shows vacuolated and clear cells in sheets or groups, separated by a hyalinized stroma. These cells show a material which is diastase-resistant periodic acid-Schiff (PAS) positive and mucicarmine negative. This is helpful to rule out salivary gland neoplasms. The cells show mild atypia and occasional mitosis.

19.4.3.4 DD

Other clear cell-rich neoplasms, especially metastatic renal cell carcinoma, should be excluded. Other tumours to be differentiated are clear cell salivary gland tumours, clear cell variant of calcifying odontogenic tumour, sclerosing odontogenic carcinoma, epithelial myoepithelial carcinoma and clear cell variant of mucoepidermoid carcinoma [54]. The differentials considered are ameloblastic fibroma, desmoplastic fibroma and squamous odontogenic tumour when it shows ameloblastic appearance.

19.4.3.5 Treatment

The treatment is complete surgical resection. Adjuvant radiotherapy is also given in some cases.

19.4.4 Ghost Cell Odontogenic Carcinoma

Ghost cell odontogenic carcinoma is an extremely rare malignant epithelial tumour. It has features of calcifying cystic odontogenic or dentinogenic ghost cell tumour. It arises de novo in most of the cases or arises from benign precursor ghost cell odontogenic lesions (40%). 50% of the reported cases are from Asia. Aberrations of Wnt signalling pathway with beta-catenin overexpression occur in these tumours similar to calcifying cystic odontogenic tumours.

19.4.4.1 Clinical

The tumour has no specific signs and symptoms. All are slow growing with ulceration, root resorption or soft tissue invasion. Maxilla is commonly affected than mandible.

19.4.4.2 Radiology

The tumour presents as a destructive radiolucent lesion with ill-defined borders. Evidence of benign precursor lesions can be seen in previous films if arising from benign lesions.

19.4.4.3 Pathology

Ghost cells with marked pleomorphism, necrosis and infiltrative growth pattern are essential for the diagnosis. Evidence of precursor benign tumours may be present. The ghost cells are large having pale-staining cytoplasm without nuclei and occur in varying numbers. Ameloblastomatous areas with peripheral palisading, reverse polarization and stellate reticulum are also seen. The malignant epithelial cells are seen in sheets, cords or islands in a fibrous stroma [55] (Fig. 19.6).

19.4.4.4 DD

Differential diagnoses include ameloblastic carcinoma, benign epithelial odontogenic neoplasm, calcifying cystic odontogenic tumour and calcifying epithelial odontogenic tumour.

19.4.4.5 Treatment

Wide local resection is the treatment like other oral carcinomas [56].

19.4.5 Sclerosing Odontogenic Carcinoma

Sclerosing odontogenic carcinoma is a rare malignant epithelial tumour. Even though it was first described in 2008, it has been added for the first time in WHO classification in 2017 only. Only 15 cases have been reported to date.

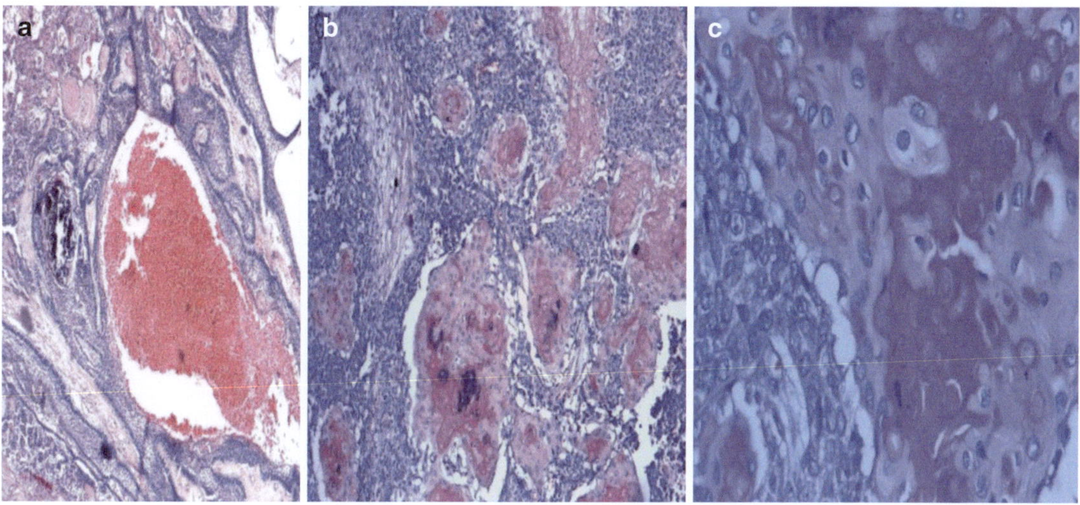

Fig. 19.6 Odontogenic ghost cell carcinoma: (**a**) Ameloblastoma like epithelial proliferation and haemorrhagic areas, H&E ×100. (**b**) Epithelial islands with ghost cells, H&E ×250. (**c**) Ghost cells, H&E ×400

19.4.5.1 Clinical

The most frequent sites are the premolar and molar areas of the mandible and rarely anterior and molar regions of the maxilla with no sex predilection. They are thought to arise from odontogenic epithelial rests and malignant transformation of odontogenic cyst epithelial lining. They sometimes cause expansion of the surrounding jawbone and increased mobility of involved teeth. If the lesion involves mental or inferior alveolar nerve, it may cause paraesthesia.

19.4.5.2 Radiology

Radiographically, there is an ill-defined radiolucency or mixed radiolucent-radiopaque character with frequent cortical bone destruction, and it can mimic a fibro-osseous lesion. Tumour has been reported to extend beyond radiographic margins.

19.4.5.3 Pathology

Grossly, it appears as a firm expansile mass with poorly defined pushing borders with erosion of surrounding bone and teeth. It may infiltrate adjacent muscle, fat and sinus membranes. The microscopy shows polyhedral epithelial cells in single file cords and strands within a dense sclerotic stroma. There is no keratinization. Mitosis or nuclear pleomorphism is rare. Diagnosis is extremely difficult on small biopsies as the histology mimics other head and neck neoplasms. Even though the cells look bland, the tumour shows aggressive infiltrative growth into muscle and nerve. Marked sclerosis in the surrounding stroma may lower down the rate of metastasis.

19.4.5.4 DD

Since it is a very rare tumour, other odontogenic tumours and metastasis should be excluded before the diagnosis.

19.4.5.5 Treatment

The primary treatment is surgical resection. They are low-grade malignant tumours.

19.4.6 Odontogenic Sarcoma

Odontogenic sarcoma is an extremely rare malignant odontogenic tumour. The epithelial component is benign, and the mesenchymal component is malignant. Commonest among them is ameloblastic fibrosarcoma. It is thought to originate from a precursor lesion like ameloblastic fibroma [57].

19.4.6.1 Clinical

The tumour occurs in young adults (mean age 30 years). The common site is mandible. They are seen as expansile mass. Pain and paraesthesia are the clinical symptoms.

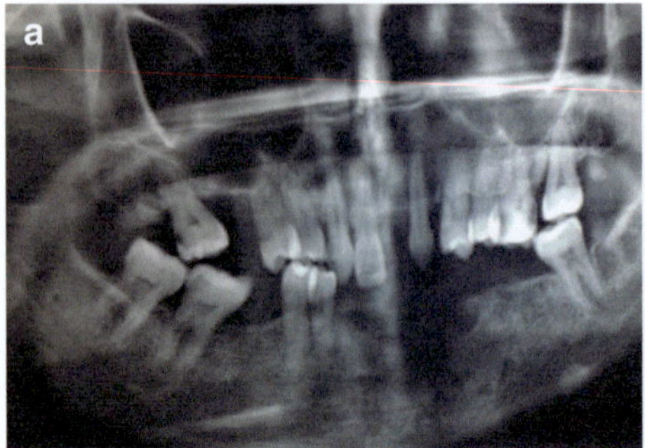

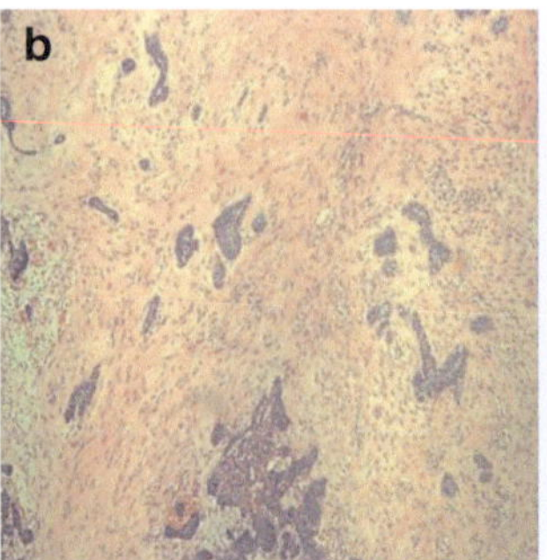

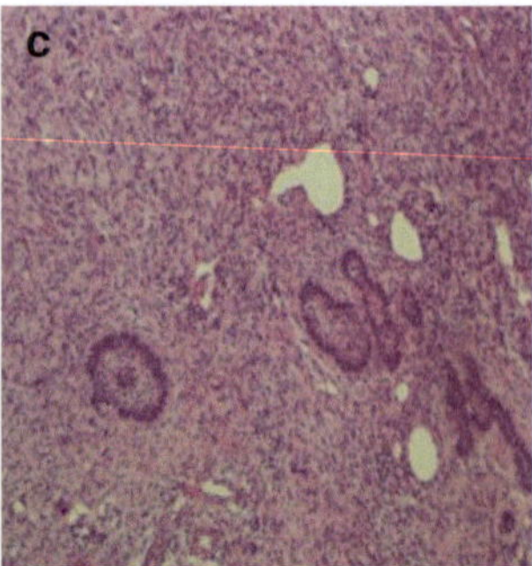

Fig. 19.7 Ameloblastic fibrosarcoma. (**a**) Destructive lesion mandible. (**b**) Benign odontogenic epithelium in a fibrous stroma, H&E ×40. (**c**) Overgrowth of mesenchymal component (fibrosarcoma), H&E ×100

19.4.6.2 Radiology

The radiograph shows an expansive, multilocular radiolucent lesion with cortical erosion or with irregular margins.

19.4.6.3 Pathology

The epithelial component is benign. The basaloid odontogenic epithelium similar to ameloblastoma with an overgrowth of malignant mesenchymal component is seen (Fig. 19.7). When dentin is present within the malignant stroma, it is called ameloblastic fibrodentinosarcoma, and when enamel is present within the malignant stroma, it is called fibro-odontosarcoma [58, 59]. The mesenchymal component shows increased mitosis, variable degrees of cellularity and cytological atypia. Stromal cells can be arranged in a herringbone or storiform pattern.

19.4.6.4 Treatment

The treatment is wide local excision with free surgical margins.

19.4.7 Odontogenic Carcinosarcoma

These tumours are very rare mixed malignant tumours [60].

19.4.7.1 Clinical

Odontogenic carcinosarcoma develops in the posterior mandible. Only two cases have been reported in the maxilla. It can occur at any age.

19.4.7.2 Radiology

Presents as a lytic lesion with ill-defined borders.

19.4.7.3 Pathology

Both the epithelial and mesenchymal components of the tumour are cytologically malignant with high proliferation index.

19.4.7.4 DD

Care should be taken not to misdiagnose a spindle cell odontogenic carcinoma as odontogenic carcinosarcoma.

19.4.7.5 Treatment

Surgical resection is the treatment.

19.5 Odontogenic Cysts

Developmental cysts occur along the lines of fusion and in relation to teeth. It accounts for 10% of odontogenic cysts. Dentigerous cysts and odontogenic keratocysts are the most common types, while calcifying odontogenic cysts and glandular odontogenic cysts are uncommon types.

19.5.1 Dentigerous Cyst

The name dentigerous cyst is derived from Latin word, meaning tooth bearing. It is also called follicular cyst. They can become very large and

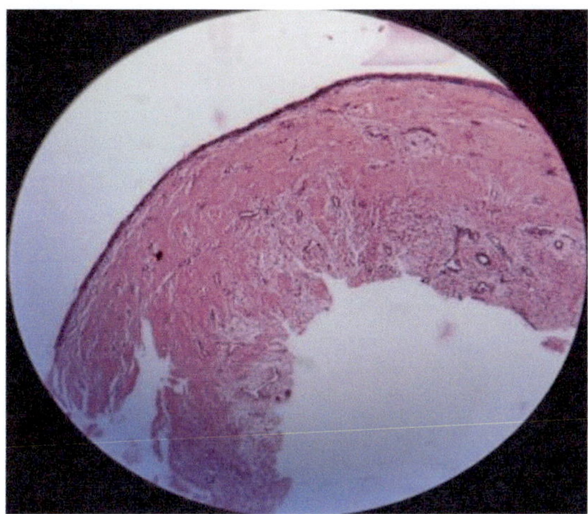

Fig. 19.8 Dentigerous cyst: Thin uniform odontogenic epithelial lining arising from reduced enamel epithelium of 2–3 cell layers with bland connective tissue capsule, H&E ×40. Picture courtesy: Dr. Heera, Professor of Oral Pathology

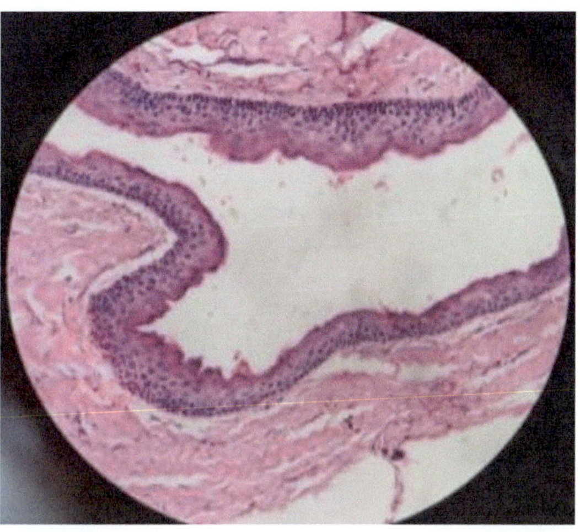

Fig. 19.9 Uniform ribbon-like epithelial lining with basal tall columnar cells with palisaded nuclei resembling tombstone or picket fence. The surface parakeratin shows corrugations, H&E ×100. Picture courtesy: Dr. Heera, Professor of Oral Pathology

displace the tooth causing expansion of bone. It is formed when fluid accumulates between the crown of an impacted tooth and the overlying epithelium [12].

19.5.1.1 Radiology

The crown of the molar tooth buried in the cyst is seen projecting into it.

19.5.1.2 Pathology

Dentigerous cysts are lined by nonkeratinized squamous epithelium and contain thin watery fluid (Fig. 19.8).

19.5.1.3 Treatment and Prognosis

The treatment is enucleation and curettage. Large cysts are decompressed initially. Rarely, malignant tumours like squamous cell carcinoma and ameloblastoma can arise from dentigerous cysts [12].

19.5.2 Odontogenic Keratocyst

These cysts are seen associated with the crown of an unerupted tooth or along the root of a tooth. If it is not associated with tooth formation, it is called primordial cyst. Those arising along the root of the tooth is called radicular cyst. These cysts can occur as part of Gorlin syndrome (basal cell nevus syndrome).

19.5.2.1 Clinical

These cysts can occur in all ages. But it is rare before 10 years. Males are commonly affected. Mandible is the preferred site. Third molar and ramus are commonly affected.

19.5.2.2 Radiology

50% of them are unilocular.

19.5.2.3 Pathology

The cyst is lined by basal cuboidal or columnar cells above which a 6–8-layered squamous epithelium is seen (Fig. 19.9). Cysts contain straw-coloured material or creamy keratinous material.

19.5.2.4 Treatment and Prognosis

Small cysts are enucleated with complete removal of cyst wall. Large cysts may need peripheral ostectomy. Recurrences are common if not completely removed.

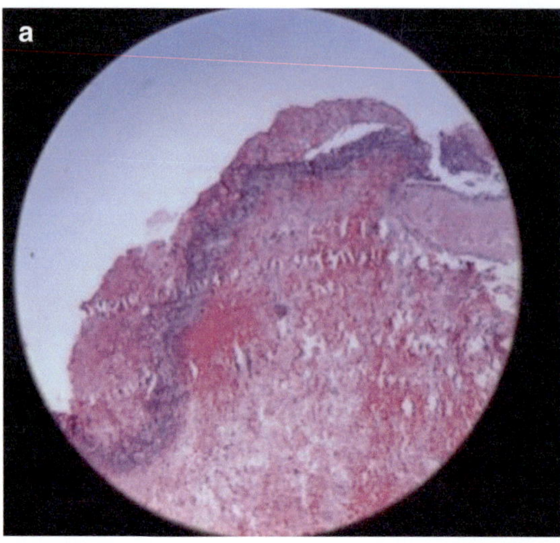

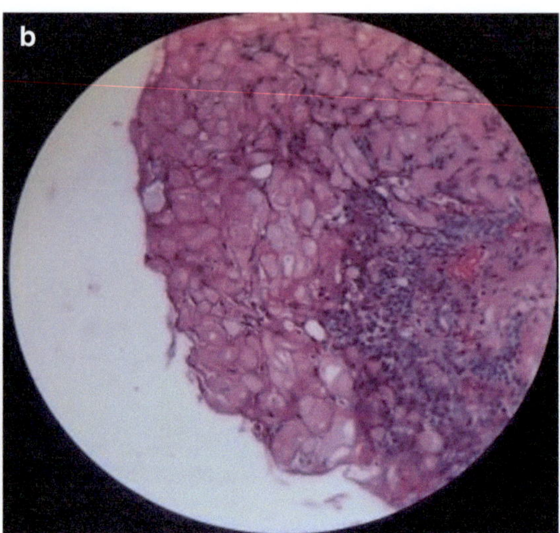

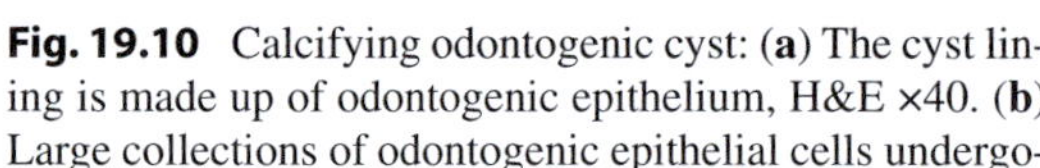

Fig. 19.10 Calcifying odontogenic cyst: (**a**) The cyst lining is made up of odontogenic epithelium, H&E ×40. (**b**) Large collections of odontogenic epithelial cells undergoing aberrant keratinization referred to as ghost cells, H&E ×100. Picture courtesy: Dr. Heera, Professor of Oral Pathology, Govt. Dental College, Thiruvananthapuram

19.5.3 Calcifying Odontogenic Cyst

Calcifying odontogenic cyst is a cystic or partially cystic tumour [1]. The lining is similar to ameloblastoma. Prominent keratinization, dentin-like material or melanin can be seen in the lesion (Fig. 19.10).

Points to Remember

- Ameloblastomas, adenomatoid odontogenic tumours, calcifying epithelial odontogenic tumours, odontogenic ghost cell tumours, squamous odontogenic tumours, ameloblastic fibromas, ameloblastic fibro-odontomas or odontomas are some of the common odontogenic tumours.
- Ameloblastoma is the commonest odontogenic tumour which we encounter during our practice.
- Immunohistochemistry is of limited value in the diagnosis of odontogenic tumour, while radiology plays a crucial role in its diagnosis.
- Malignant odontogenic tumours are very rare and aggressive.

References

1. El-Naggar AK, Chan JK, Grandis JR, Takata T, Slootweg PJ, editors. WHO classification of head and neck tumours. International Agency for Research on Cancer; 2017.
2. Wright JM, Vered M. Update from the 4th edition of the World Health Organization classification of head and neck Tumors: odontogenic and maxillofacial bone tumors. Head Neck Pathol. 2017;11:68–77.
3. Bassey GO, Osunde OD, Anyanechi CE. Maxillofacial tumors and tumor-like lesions in a Nigerian teaching hospital: an eleven year retrospective analysis. Afr Health Sci. 2014;14:56–63.
4. Sham E, Leong J, Maher R, et al. Mandibular ameloblastoma: Clinical experience and literature review. ANZ J Surg. 2009;79:739–7.
5. Filizzola AI, Bartholomeu-Dos-Santos TCR, Pires FR. Ameloblastomas: clinicopathological features from 70 cases diagnosed in a single Oral pathology service in an 8-year period. Med Oral Patol Oral Cir Bucal. 2009;19:e556–61.
6. Effiom O, Ogundana O, Akinshipo A, et al. Ameloblastoma: current etiopathological concepts and management. Oral Dis. 2018;24:307–16.
7. Hertog D, Bloemena E, Aartman IHA, et al. Histopathology of ameloblastoma of jaws; some critical observations based on a 40 years single instituition experience. Med Oral Patol Oral Cir Bucal. 2012;17:e76–82.
8. Cadavid AMH, Araujo JP, Coutinho-Camillo CM, et al. Ameloblastomas: current aspects of the new

WHO classification in an analysis of 136 cases. Surg Exp Pathol. 2019;2:17.

9. Speight PM, Takata T. New tumour entities in the 4th edition of the World Health Organization classification of head and neck tumours: odontogenic and maxillofacial bone tumours. Virchows Arch. 2018;472:331–9.
10. Milman T, Ying G-S, Pan W, et al. Ameloblastoma: 25 year experience at a single institution. Head Neck Pathol. 2016;10:513–20.
11. Philipsen HP, Reichart PA. Squamous Odontogenic tumor(SOT): a benign neoplasm of the periodontium. A review of 36 reported cases. J Clin Periodontol. 1996;23:922–9263.
12. Cawson AR, Binnie HW, Speight P, Barrett WA, Wright MJ, editors. Lucas's pathology of tumors of the oral cavity. 5th ed; 1998.
13. Haghighat K, Kalmar JR, Mariotti AJ. Squamous odontogenic tumor: diagnosis and management. J Periodontol. 2002;73:653–6. https://doi.org/10.1902/jop.2002.73.6.653.
14. Leider AS, Jonker LA, Cook HE. Multicentric familial squamous odontogenic tumor. Oral Surg Oral Med Oral Pathol. 1989;68:175–81. https://doi.org/10.1016/0030-4220(89)90189-8.
15. Wright JM Jr. Squamous odontogenic tumor like proliferations in odontogenic cysts. Oral Surg Oral Med Oral Pathol. 1979;47:354–8. https://doi.org/10.1016/0030-4220(79)90259.
16. Lin YL, White DK. Squamous odontogenic tumor. Oral Maxillofac Surg Clin North Am. 2004;16:355–7. https://doi.org/10.1016/j.coms.2004.03.003.
17. Pindborg JJ. A calcifying epithelial odontogenic tumor. Cancer. 1958;2:838–43.
18. Basu MK, Matthews JB, Sear AJ, Browne RM. Calcifying epithelial odontogenic tumour: a case showing features of malignancy. J Oral Pathol. 1984;13(3):310–9.
19. Singh N, Sahai S, Singh S, Singh S. Calcifying epithelial odontogenic tumor (Pindborg tumor). Natl J Maxillofac Surg. 2011;2:225–7.
20. Gotmare SS, Pereira T, Shetty S, Kesarkar KS. Pindborg tumor pathology with special stains. Indian J Pathol Microbiol. 2018;61:239–41.
21. Kaushal S, Mathur SR, Vijay M, Rustagi A. Calcifying epithelial odontogenic tumor (Pindborg tumor) without calcification: a rare entity. J Oral Maxillofac Pathol. 2012;16(1):110–2.
22. Germanier Y, Bornstein MM, Stauffer E, Buser D. Calcifying epithelial odontogenic (Pindborg) tumor of the mandible with clear cell component treated by conservative surgery: report of a case. J Oral Maxillofac Surg. 2005;63(9):1377–82. https://doi.org/10.1016/j.joms.2005.05.298.
23. Rick GM. Adenomatoid odontogenic tumor. Oral Maxillofac Surg Clin North Am. 2004;16:333–54.
24. Rajendran R. In: Rajendran R, Sivapathasundharam B, editors. Shafer's text book of oral pathology. 6th ed. Noida: Elsevier; 2009. p. 282–3.
25. Philipsen HP, Reichert PA, Zhang KJ, Nikai H, Yu KX. Adenomatoid odontogenic tumor: biologic profile based on 499 cases. J Oral Pathol Med. 1991;20:149–58.
26. Trodahl JN. Ameloblastic fibroma. A survey of cases from the Armed Forces Institute of Pathology. Oral Surg. 1972;33:547–58.
27. Gupta DRS, Tandon A, Mehrotra D, Gupta OP. Ameloblastic fibroma: report of 3 cases and literature review. Int J Oral Maxillofac Pathol. 2011;2:59–63.
28. Lalitha C, Goyal S, Perka L, Kodangal S. Ameloblatic fibroma. J Indian Acad Oral med Radiol. 2016;28:199–202.
29. Vij R, Vij H. Ameloblastic fibroma: An uncommon entity. BMJ Case Rep. 2013;2013:pii: bcr20130102799.
30. Ide F, Kikuchi K, Kusama K, Muramatsu T. Primordial odontogenic tumour: is it truly novel? Histopathology. 2015;66:603–4. https://doi.org/10.1111/his.12595.
31. Bologna-Molina R, Pereira-Prado V, Sánchez-Romero C, González-González R, Mosqueda-Taylor A. Primordial odontogenic tumor: a systematic review. Med O ral Patol Oral Cir Bucal. 2020;25(3):e388–94.
32. Poomsawat S, Ngamsom S, Nonpassopon N. Primordial odontogenic tumor with prominent calcifications: a rare case report. J Clin Exp Dent. 2019;11(10):e952–6.
33. Custódio M, Araujo JP, Gallo CB, Trierveiler M. Gingival complex odontoma: a rare case report with a review of the literature. Autops Case Rep. 2018;8(1):e2018009. https://doi.org/10.4322/acr.2018.009. PMID: 29515984; PMCID: PMC5828291
34. Koh KJ, Park HN, Kim KA. Gardner syndrome associated with multiple osteomas, intestinal polyposis, and epidermoid cysts. Imaging Sci Dent. 2016;46(4):267–72.
35. da Silva Rocha OKM, da Silva Barros CC, da Silva LAB, de Souza Júnior EF, de Morais HHA, da Costa Miguel MC. Peripheral compound odontoma: a rare case report and literature review. J Cutan Pathol. 2020;47(8):720–4. https://doi.org/10.1111/cup.13676.
36. Kämmerer PW, Schneider D, Schiegnitz E, Schneider S, Walter C, Frerich B, Kunkel M. Clinical parameter of odontoma with special emphasis on treatment of impacted teeth-a retrospective multicentre study and literature review. Clin Oral Investig. 2016;20(7):1827–35. https://doi.org/10.1007/s00784-015-1673-3. Epub 2015 Nov 27. PMID: 26612404.t. PMID: 32134132
37. de Arruda JAA, Monteiro JLGC, Abreu LG, de Oliveira Silva LV, Schuch LF, de Noronha MS, Callou G, Moreno A, Mesquita RA. Calcifying odontogenic cyst, dentinogenic ghost cell tumor, and ghost cell odontogenic carcinoma: a systematic review. J Oral Pathol Med. 2018;47(8):721–30.

38. Etemad-Moghadam S, Baghaee F, Dadafarid Z, Alaeddini M. A 44-year analysis of ghost cell odontogenic tumour subtypes in an Iranian population. J Craniomaxillofac Surg. 2014;42(7):1154–9.
39. Santoro A, Pannone G, Ramaglia L, Bufo P, Lo Muzio L, Saviano R. Central odontogenic fibroma of the mandible: a case report with diagnostic considerations. Ann Med Surg (Lond). 2015;1(5):14–8. https://doi.org/10.1016/j.amsu.2015.11.004. PMID: 26793312; PMCID: PMC4687461
40. Kabiraj A, Singh A, Khaitan T, Jaiswal A. Odontogenic fibroma of the maxilla—an atypical presentation. Iran J Pathol. 2016;11(5):435–8. Epub 2016 Dec 24. PMID: 28974961; PMCID: PMC5604105
41. Chrcanovic BR, Freire-Maia B, Gomez RS. Small central odontogenic fibroma mimicking hyperplastic dental follicle and dentigerous cyst. J Maxillofac Oral Surg. 2014;13(3):332–6. https://doi.org/10.1007/s12663-011-0221-1. Epub 2011 Apr 22. PMID: 25018609; PMCID: PMC4082542
42. Jun Li T, Sun SL, Luo HY. Odontogenic Myxoma: a clinicopathologic study of 25 cases. Arch Pathol Lab Med. 2006;130(12):1799–806.
43. Dietrich EM, Papaemmanouil S, Koloutsos G, Antoniades H, Antoniades K. Odontogenic fibromyxoma of the maxilla: a case report and review of the literature. Case Rep Med. 2011;2011:238712.
44. Gupta S, Grover N, Kadam A, Gupta S, Sah K, Sunitha JD. Odontogenic myxoma. Natl J Maxillofac Surg. 2013;4(1):81–3.
45. Banasser AM, Bawazir MM, Islam MN, Bhattacharyya I, Cohen DM, Fitzpatrick SG. Odontogenic myxoma: a 23-year retrospective series of 38 cases. Head Neck Pathol. 2020;14(4):1021–7.
46. Kourda-Boujemâa J, Farah-Klibi F, Rammeh S, Adouani A, Zermani R, Ben J-BS. Odontogenic myxoma: About four cases and review of the literature. Ann Pathol. 2010;30(3):168–75.
47. Brannon RB, Fowler CB, Carpenter WM, Corio RL. Cementoblastoma: an innocuous neoplasm? A clinicopathologic study of 44 cases and review of the literature with special emphasis on recurrence. Oral Surg Oral Med Oral Pathol Oral Radiol Endod. 2002;93(3):311–20. https://doi.org/10.1067/moe.2002.121993.
48. Jelic JS, Loftus MJ, Miller AS, Cleveland DB. Benign cementoblastoma: report of an unusual case and analysis of 14 additional cases. J Oral Maxillofac Surg. 1993;51(9):1033–6. https://doi.org/10.1016/S0278-2391(10)80051-5.
49. El-Mofty SK. Fibro-osseous lesions of the craniofacial skeleton: an update. Head Neck Pathol. 2014;8(4):432–44. https://doi.org/10.1007/s12105-014-0590-0.
50. Devenney-Cakir B, Dunfee B, Subramaniam R, Sundararajan D, Mehra P, Spiegel J, Sakai O. Ameloblastic carcinoma of the mandible with metastasis to the skull and lung: advanced imaging appearance including computed tomography, magnetic resonance imaging and positron emission tomography computed tomography. Dentomaxillofac Radiol. 2010;39(7):449–53.
51. Kishore M, Panat SR, Aggarwal A, Upadhyay N, Agarwal N. Ameloblastic carcinoma: a case report. J Clin Diagn Res. 2015;9(7):ZD27–8.
52. Roy Chowdhury SK, Ramen S, Chattopadhyay PK, Moorchung N, Rajkumar K. Ameloblastic Carcinoma of the mandible. J Maxillofac Oral Surg. 2010;9(2):198–201.
53. Krishnamurthy A, Ramshankar V, Majhi U. Clear cell odontogenic carcinoma of the mandible and temporomandibular joint with cervical lymph nodal metastasis. Natl J Maxillofac Surg. 2014;5(2):221–3.
54. Walia C, Chatterjee RP, Kundu S, Roy S. Clinical enigma: a rare case of clear cell odontogenic carcinoma. Contemp Clin Dent. 2015;6(4):559–63.
55. Sukumaran R, Somanathan T, Kattoor J. Odontogenic ghost cell carcinoma with pulmonary metastasis. J Oral Maxillofac Pathol. 2015;19(3):371–4.
56. Rappaport MJ, Showell DL, Edenfield WJ. Metastatic ghost cell odontogenic carcinoma: description of a case and search for actionable targets. Rare Tumors. 2015;7(3):5813.
57. Bertoni F, Del Corso G, Bacchini P, Marchetti C, Tarsitano A. Ameloblastic Fibrosarcoma of the mandible evolving from a prior Ameloblastic Fibroma after two years: an unusual finding. Int J Surg Pathol. 2016;24(7):656–9.
58. Muller S, Parker DC, Kapadia SB, Budnick SD, Barnes EL. Ameloblastic fibrosarcoma of the jaws. A clinicopathologic and DNA analysis of five cases and review of the literature with discussion of its relationship to ameloblastic fibroma. Oral Surg Oral Med Oral Pathol Oral Radiol Endod. 1995; 79(4):469–77.
59. Kunkel M, Ghalibafian M, Radner H, Reichert TE, Fischer B, Wagner W. Ameloblastic fibrosarcoma or odontogenic carcinosarcoma: a matter of classification? Oral Oncol. 2004;40(4):444–9.
60. Kim IK, Pae SP, Cho HY, Cho HW, Seo JH, Lee DH, et al. Odontogenic carcinosarcoma of the mandible: a case report and review. J Korean Assoc Oral Maxillofac Surg. 2015;41(3):139.

MIX
Papier aus verantwortungsvollen Quellen
Paper from responsible sources
FSC® C105338

If you have any concerns about our products,
you can contact us on
ProductSafety@springernature.com

In case Publisher is established outside the EU,
the EU authorized representative is:
Springer Nature Customer Service Center GmbH
Europaplatz 3, 69115 Heidelberg, Germany

Printed by Libri Plureos GmbH
in Hamburg, Germany